D1734010

Pathology of
Multiple Pregnancy

Virginia J. Baldwin

Pathology of Multiple Pregnancy

With 199 Illustrations in 316 Parts

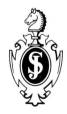

Springer-Verlag
New York Berlin Heidelberg London Paris
Tokyo Hong Kong Barcelona Budapest

Virginia J. Baldwin, M.D.
British Columbia's Children's Hospital
Department of Pathology
4480 Oak Street
Vancouver, B.C. V6H 3V4 Canada

Library of Congress Cataloging-in-Publication Data
Baldwin, Virginia J.
    Pathology of multiple pregnancy / Virginia J. Baldwin.
      p.   cm.
    Includes bibliographical references and index.
    ISBN 0-387-94011-1. — ISBN 3-540-94011-1
    1. Multiple pregnancy—Complications. I. Title.
    [DNLM: 1. Diseases in Twins. 2. Pregnancy Complications.
    3. Pregnancy, Multiple. 4. Twins, Monozygotic. WQ 235 B182p 1993]
    RG567.B35   1993
    618.2′5—dc20
    DNLM/DLC
    for Library of Congress   92-48343

Printed on acid-free paper.

© 1994 Springer-Verlag New York Inc.
All rights reserved. This work may not be translated or copied in whole or in part without the written permission of the publisher (Springer-Verlag New York, Inc., 175 Fifth Avenue, New York, NY 10010, USA), except for brief excerpts in connection with reviews or scholarly analysis. Use in connection with any form of information storage and retrieval, electronic adaptation, computer software, or by similar or dissimilar methodology now known or hereafter developed is forbidden.
The use of general descriptive names, trade names, trademarks, etc., in this publication, even if the former are not especially identified, is not to be taken as a sign that such names, as understood by the Trade Marks and Merchandise Marks Act, may accordingly be used freely by anyone.
While the advice and information in this book are believed to be true and accurate at the date of going to press, neither the authors nor the publisher can accept any legal responsibility for any errors or omissions that may be made. The publisher makes no warranty, express or implied, with respect to the material contained herein.

Production managed by Ellen Seham, manufacturing supervised by Jacqui Ashri.
Typeset by ATLIS Graphics & Design, Inc., Mechanicsburg, PA.
Printed and bound by Edwards Brothers, Inc., Ann Arbor, MI.
Printed in the United States of America.

9 8 7 6 5 4 3 2 1

ISBN 0-387-94011-1 Springer-Verlag New York Berlin Heidelberg
ISBN 3-540-94011-1 Springer-Verlag Berlin Heidelberg New York

This text is dedicated to the multiplets—the twins and supertwins. I hope that what we have learned from you will help those yet to come.

Foreword

It is almost exactly twenty years since Virginia J. Baldwin, M.D., first became part of my laboratory at the Chicago Lying-In Hospital as a special trainee in placentology. She demonstrated quickly the capacity for close attention to detail so evident in the pages that follow of this important compilation on twinning. She was able to spend this time with my late colleague, Prof. John R. Esterly and myself, and later, with Drs. William Blanc and Kurt Benirschke, because of the supportive environment created in Vancouver by the then chairman of pathology, Prof. David F. Hardwick. She was thus in an institution with a large obstetrical service and active interests in reproductive pathology with the intellectual climate so vital to thoughtful work. This wonderful book is the logical product of that skill given the opportunity to exercise it. Such circumstances are all too rare these days; my own career goes back to the time when it was the norm to give a scholar or researcher the time to work at length on a matter of importance, undistracted by grant deadlines or the necessity for competition for resources that is occasionally destructive of creative insight. This may be an unrecognized benefit of the Canadian health care system, which, while less dedicated to research in general, is large enough for universities with medical institutions to be able to provide the occasional niche for genuine scholarly endeavor. In my own more recent career, I have tried to find that in the American system; my current post in Memphis is perhaps the best that can be obtained on our side of the border.

It was through this environment that Dr. Baldwin became aware of the embryo collection so well managed by Dr. Betty Poland. That function made great use of photodocumentation. The benefit of an expert photographic unit is generously evidenced in this book, a treasure of mostly original photographs illustrating very broad experience.

You, the reader, have before you a carefully crafted work, one very well illustrated and drawing from the richness of twin literature. Twins do continue to fascinate and the reader benefits from Dr. Baldwin's evident fascination. She gives us a synopsis of the history of twinning, the early concepts, and then goes into an exposition on mechanisms. I was personally gratified to see her treatment of the less well known phenomenon of dispermic monovular twinning, and in particular the discussion of the seeming paradox of paternal factors.

Over thirty years ago I became the father of twins in a family with two other sets of twins close by entirely on my side of the family with their paternal grandmother as the link. To be more precise, I have twin daughters, twin grandnephews (via my sister and her elder daughter), and a pair of male–female twin great uncles and aunts (siblings of my maternal grandmother). This may be of interest because examination of the placenta of my twins, and later, at age 12, of their blood groups (ABO, Rh, MNS) and fingerprints, strongly indicated dispermic monovular twinning. Now, by the much more comprehensive techniques so well summarized by Dr. Baldwin in Chapter 2, similar cases would have a larger data matrix of proof, especially DNA studies. As she well emphasizes, the likelihood is that this "third" type of twinning is more common than is generally considered. Nevertheless, as she is at pains to emphasize, there is a lot that remains unknown about the mysteries of twinning.

Dr. Baldwin provides food for thought for the speculative mind as well in her discussion of the relationship of children derived from monofollicular in vitro polyfertilization and other marvels of the age. This is one of the compelling features of a work rich with detail. The pathologist can be left behind so quickly as interventionist medicine expands and becomes complexly interrelated. Even a researcher so well versed in these matters (witness her familiarity with the homeobox genes) may not have it all in hand, or more likely in these kinds of projects, on the desk or floor nearby. Invasive intrauterine diagnostic probes have been shown to contribute to the confusion of membrane interpretation.

In a study by Megory et al.,[1] a disruption of the common membrane between the twin sacs, found at 39 weeks, was attributed to funipuncture at 24 weeks but not to earlier amniocenteses at 17 and 21 weeks. The extent of entanglement illustrated by these authors is impressive. Their study indicated the placental membranes were dichorionic-diamniotic on fused dichorionic placental disks. Thus the title of the article is somewhat misleading; it should have been something like "Postcordocentesis Fenestration of Common Dichorionic Twin Membranes." A datum missing from the account is the location of the twins with respect to the sacs at the time of delivery. The possible role of earlier punctures is not explored. Nevertheless, such cases deserve wide publicity so that accumulative experience will be available by which to assess both the clinical impact of such procedures on the fetuses and newborns and the effect on the placental specimen. Certainly the entanglement of the umbilical cords from fused dichorionic placentas is something outside of the expected natural experience.

The method used by Dr. Baldwin in examining placentas is very well described. The suggestion that the interested pathologist keep an independent record of especially interesting cases is a good one, particularly when one has teaching duties. For continuing research, however, more detailed access to computerized data or summaries is required.

The value of this book to clinicians is contained in Chapter 4. The citation to Ahn and Phelan[2] as authority that 20% to 40% of twins may remain undiagnosed until onset of labor, or even until delivery, comports with the teaching of the 1940s and 1950s, but is no longer acceptable in the United States, even just 5 years later. In fact, modern obstetricians who fail to determine the number and relative location of multiple fetuses by ultrasound are close to *res ipsa loquitur* malpractice and would certainly receive a summons should anything go wrong! This chapter also contains useful information on the various other clinical factors that may have an impact on fetal development, with emphasis on possible discordancy between twins. This chapter is an artful weaving of the literature and the immediate Vancouver experience. The scope and richness of detail exists nowhere else, not in her other papers, nor in any of the contributions of Perrin, Benirschke, Blanc,

Naeye, or myself. This obstetrical snapshot of twins is matched by instant photography of the newborn and the effect of twinning on various postnatal disorders and subsequent development. Any such compilation must be viewed (a) as the limited field of the source material (we are all slaves to our data source), and (b) as a very firm foundation on which to build future observations.

Here Dr. Baldwin reaches the high plane of pathologist as natural historian, not only in the immediate descriptive sense, but in the older nineteenth century meaning as one whose field of study is all of nature and the interrelationship of the living world upon the evolving rocks of time. She prepared us to make use of this perspective by the background of basic human biology in Chapters 1 through 3. Chapter 5 carries this sense to its fruition, the mortality of twins. This is a meaty chapter, worthy of a major review article or brief monograph when combined with Chapter 6, on the morbidity of twins. I suppose this shows the bias of the pathologist, to put the chapter for mortality ahead of the chapter for morbidity; perhaps I merely expose my clinical side from years ago, to raise such a question! When Chapters 5, 6, and 7 (anomalous development) are taken together, one has the essence of the overall twin problem. It is most seemly, and very good, that Dr. Baldwin has eschewed the use of statistical methods. She occasionally gives us the relative frequency between two aspects or categories, but makes no effort to divine statistical significance. This is good because in the first place embryonic development and lesion formation is not a statistical field as presently understood, and in the second place these details might well require a file of all the twins born in North America over an equivalent period of time, *if* one could write the comparative matrix table for analysis. True to her calling as natural historian, she is content to show general relationships, many time- or stage-dependent, confident that future work is likely to show whether variations are significantly different in a causal way.

Beginning with Chapter 8 we find three exquisite sections on the very special problems of monozygous twinning, including much original work on the vascular anastomoses of such placentas and the twin transfusion syndrome. Chapter 10 considers the problem that physicians most often encounter in patient counseling, explanation of why some so-called identical twins are not in fact identical, and why they sometimes show discordant or very different anomalies or other diseases. While I endorse her conclusion that the age-old question of teratoma versus amorphous fetus remains open, it does no harm to wonder whether a rule of thumb actually might exist, theoretically. Clearly, the suggestion that DNA typing be done, or chromosome counts be determined, would be of assistance. So far, the consequences of in vitro fertilization have not shed light on this subject.

In Chapter 10, on anomalies of monozygous duplication, we have a compilation that appears nowhere else in the literature, comparing a set of specific references, by which to obtain a common vocabulary and more precise definitions. This section is a worthy advance in the field, and I hope that the system of analysis provided here will be adopted by others. The addition of her own material gives cohesion to a fragmented, sometimes occult, subject. This section has much to recommend it.

The final chapter, Chapter 11, which discusses triplets and higher combinations, also contains much new information. The section reminds me of that old aphorism, turned upside down, that prematures are not simply small children, they are not even just small newborns; this implies they are a different form of human existence. Likewise, triplet and quadruplet sets, while often containing twins, are not simply "larger" twinnings. They represent another order of human development. Perhaps in the future someone will have collected an experience in these higher orders of fetal life equivalent to Dr. Baldwin's collection of twins. The true sequel of this book can then be written. For the present, this most valuable book should spur additional efforts on the pathology of twinning, and in particular, the pathology of twin placentas.

In conclusion, there is treasure trove in this tome, much to recommend it to many kinds of physicians and biologists, and a solid rock on which to build newer edifices of scholarship.

Douglas R. Shanklin, M.D., F.R.S.M.
Professor of Pathology and of Obstetrics and Gynecology
University of Tennessee, Memphis;
Chief of Perinatal Pathology and of Developmental Neuropathology;
Formerly, Pathologist-in-Chief,
Chicago Lying-In Hospital,
University of Chicago

References

1. Megory E, Weiner E, Shalev E, Ohel G. Pseudomonoamniotic twins with cord entanglement following genetic puncture. *Obstet Gynecol* 1991;78:915–917.
2. Ahn MB, Phelan JP. Multiple pregnancy: antepartum management. *In:* Gall SA (ed). Twin Pregnancy. *Clinics in Perinatology* 1988;15:55–69.

Preface

The pathology of having more than one human conceptus at a time has been referred to as the history of sibling rivalry before birth.[1] In addition to the psychosocial, sociological, and ethical issues raised by human multiples, or twins and supertwins as they are also called,[2] the scientific aspects of human twinning and higher multiples are part of a number of disciplines. In addition to all the concepts of disease and developmental disorders encountered in singleton infants, the pathology of multiple pregnancy includes considerations of basic processes in reproduction and embryology, normal development and teratology, and genetic and environmental influences on development. Similarly, the placentology of multiple conceptions adds several dimensions to the interpretations required in singletons. It is no wonder that multiple reproduction has attracted medical attention over the years.

The quality and usefulness of much of the information that has been reported concerning multiple gestations is in direct proportion to the precision and completeness of the pathology—the descriptions and interpretations. Many pathologists have contributed to our knowledge of the scope of the pathology of multiple pregnancy, and the pediatric pathologist particularly has had a special interest and background on which to draw. In addition, a number of astute obstetricians, pediatricians, neonatologists, and perinatologists have provided valuable insights, and research scientists have deepened our understanding of the basic processes. My debt to these excellent contributions is acknowledged by references to their work on which I have been privileged to build.

The stimulus for this monograph came from the research for a chapter on the pathology of multiple pregnancy for Wigglesworth and Singer's[3] *Textbook of Fetal and Perinatal Pathology*. When the editors gently indicated that they could not possibly accept everything I wanted to include, valuable though it was, it occurred to me that it would be helpful to have a single volume that provided an expansion of the information available on the pathology of twins and higher multiples. Parents of multiples, their families, and the multiples themselves, are becoming more active in their search for information, as witness the proliferation of twin societies, associations of parents of multiples, and lay publications related to multiple births. As a result, in addition to the questions arising from the scientific curiosity of those who care for multiples, there is an increasing need for these caregivers to be able to answer their patient's questions, accurately and understandably. Also, as part of the enhanced concern regarding management liability in human reproduction in general, there has been an increasing focus on problems of outcome in multiple gestation in particular. Thus, it has been my plan in this volume to provide useful information across the spectrum of the pathology of multiple pregnancy, based on information from the literature and a review of a large number of related cases.

It is for all those interested in human multiple reproduction that this monograph is intended, including direct caregivers and indirect support staff, and particularly those in a position to interpret the pathologic findings when problems occur. It is my hope that they will find something interesting and useful in these pages.

References

1. Gonzales-Crussi F. *Notes of an Anatomist*. London: Pan Books; 1986:19.
2. Noble E. *Having Twins. A Parent's Guide to Pregnancy, Birth and Early Childhood*. Boston: Houghton Mifflin; 1991:3.
3. Baldwin VJ. Pathology of multiple pregnancy. In: Wigglesworth JS, Singer DB, eds. *Textbook of Fetal and Perinatal Pathology*. Oxford: Blackwell Scientific; 1991:221–262.

Acknowledgments

This volume would not have been possible without the general support and specific contributions of the following individuals, and my indebtedness to them is hereby acknowledged:

David Hardwick, who was responsible for introducing me to the specialty of pediatric pathology in the first place, and who helped me pursue possibilities that he saw before I did.

Douglas Shanklin, who was my guide as I began to learn about placental pathology, who read the first draft of this monograph, and who made many valuable suggestions, reminding me in particular of my debt to the work of such pioneers as Hertig, Gruenwald, and others.

Kurt Benirschke, who started providing challenging personal encouragement when I was a resident in training and who continues to be an enthusiastic and informative colleague and resource.

James Dimmick, for constant encouragement as I worked through this manuscript, including reading the entire text to find problem areas that I had overlooked.

Ann Hungerford, who gave me the tools that changed writing from a dreaded drudgery to a rewarding challenge.

John Kingsmill, who read my writing with great patience and reminded me of my duty to use understandable language and readable style.

Christine Kirkham, for remarkable transcription and formatting skills including being able to read my writing when I could not.

The staff at Springer-Verlag, who displayed remarkably diplomatic patience and encouragement through the inevitable delays.

Finally I would like to acknowledge the literature research provided by Pat Price, the line drawings provided by Kevin Dimmick, the technical and secretarial support of the staff in Anatomic Pathology at the British Columbia's Children's Hospital, and my professional colleagues in pathology for making allowances for my distracted periods.

Contents

1
Introduction and Twin Studies

"The position of woman in any civilization is an index of advancement of that civilization; the position of woman is gauged best by the care given to her at the birth of her child. Accordingly, the advances and regression of civilization are nowhere seen more clearly than in the story of childbirth."[1]

The mystery of childbirth has been associated with beliefs and practices arising from humankind's imagination and ingenuity, and these have been yielding only gradually to increasing knowledge of the physiology of reproduction as such information has been more widely understood. When pregnancy resulted in the birth of more than one child at a time, the mystery was compounded and the fascination with multiple births persists.[2–4] Fortunately for the infants and mother, this interest is now largely benevolent social and scientific curiosity, although for some people there is still the uneasy sense that twins, particularly "identical" twins, have an added dimension to life that ordinary singletons are denied and cannot understand. This "specialness" of twins is exemplified in the twin cult of the Yoruba in Africa, who have had the highest twinning rate in the world.[5]

The psychosocial and cultural consequences of multiple pregnancy have evolved with advancing scientific knowledge. Until fairly recently, the response to a multiple birth has spanned the gamut from destruction to deification of the infants and/or parents, usually the mother, by the other members of their community.[6,7] In Western societies, the community response has mellowed to active curiosity, with intermittent newspaper or television reports of "curiosities" or feature articles in periodicals,[8,9] fictional stories and films,[3] and nonfiction books including an occasional remarkably understandable presentation of scientific information for a lay audience.[10] At the same time, the parents and families of twins and supertwins have themselves sought more information about their special offspring. A number of national and regional societies

have been formed,[7] such as the Parents of Multiple Births Association of Canada, special interest publications ranging from single topic pamphlets to newsletters and periodicals directed to families with multiples are now available, and parents of multiple births meet regularly to exchange support and ideas. Even the special needs of families who are mourning the loss of one or more multiples are reflected in the establishment of specific grieving support groups, such as the Center for Loss in Multiple Births based in Alaska. And finally, the multiples themselves are seeking each other out in twin clubs and associations, to share the uniqueness of their special experience in life. This can sometimes lead to interesting situations. Double identical-twin marriages may come from groups of twins, and while legally the offspring would be double first cousins, they are in fact genetically brothers and sisters.[4] The quest for information represented by these social movements is the spur behind the development of community home–based businesses such as Twins and More in Langley, British Columbia, developed by a new mother of twins, and geared to filling the unmet needs of families with multiples for everything from birth announcements to strollers.

The social and cultural curiosity about human multiple births is reflected in the scientific community, and the scientific interest in aspects unique to multiple gestation has focused on two main fronts, the pathology of multiple pregnancy and epidemiologic twin studies. In studies of the pathology of multiple pregnancy, there has been particular interest in both the patterns and aberrations of monozygotic or single egg twinning, which include some of the most bizarre anomalies of human reproduction. The epidemiologic value of studying twins was first proposed by Galton[11] in 1876. He stated that twins could be studied to improve our understanding of the relative roles of genetic and environmental influences in human development and disease, and twin studies have dealt with a broad range of conditions indeed.

Role of the Pathologist

The pathologist is the one person in a position to provide the basic information that is critical to the validity of any study of twins and supertwins. This can be done in the day-to-day service pathology of normal and abnormal multiple gestation, and, as a consequence of that service role, in any research into the pathophysiology and epidemiology of human multiples.

The importance of the observations made by the service pathologist in his or her daily practice cannot be overestimated, because careful delineation of the placentation and documentation of the findings at postmortem examination is critical to an accurate interpretation of comparisons among infants of multiple gestation. The placentas of all multiple gestations are examined to define the pattern of placentation, as it may contribute to zygosity determination. Any gross or microscopic asymmetry detected in the placenta of a multiple gestation may provide information that is critical to the explanation of asymmetric growth or abnormal perinatal outcome of the infants, and this may have both medical and legal significance. Careful autopsies of infants of multiple gestation who die in utero or perinatally may provide important information as to the cause and/or mechanism of death, and in cases where only one fetus or infant died, the findings may have significance for the survivor. Again, there are potentially both medical and legal aspects to the findings and interpretation of some of these cases. Central to the clinicopathological correlations that are made in multiple pregnancy are the concepts that the mother and uterus represent an "environment" for the conceptus, influencing it/ them from fertilization onward, and that the human uterus is best suited for only one infant at a time. These concepts enlarge the scope of possible patho-

physiologic mechanisms that the pathologist examining the products of multiple pregnancy must consider.

The value of carefully documented accurate observations of pathology in multiple pregnancy to research studies of twins and supertwins is particularly evident in questions of discordant/concordant development, anomalies, and disease. Much is made in these studies of the zygosity of the individuals, as interpretations of hereditary or environmental influences are deduced based on the degree of supposed genetic identity. As can be imagined, if zygosity determination is not accurate, or if the lesion/disorder being studied is erroneously described, explained, or ascribed as to its genetic or environmental cause, any conclusions from such a study would be open to question. As this text is focusing on the pathology of multiple pregnancy, concerns regarding twin studies are discussed briefly below.

Because the pathologist has such an important role to play in both the service and research aspects of the pathology of multiple pregnancy, it is suggested that, if they are in a position to be dealing with the placentas and/or infants of multiple gestations, they make themselves aware of the additional considerations such cases require. It is to this end that this text has been prepared. The aim is to provide a discussion of the special (and truly fascinating) additional lesions possible in the products of multiple pregnancy, with particular attention to specific techniques of examination and suggested interpretation of findings.

Information Sources and Outline of Text

The literature on multiple gestations is extensive. Interest in twins and higher multiples predates written history and the mythology of many races, cultures, and societies, includes stories of twins.[3] The scientific description of multiples date back at least to Hippocrates[3] and the volume of literature has increased steadily since. The number of articles per year concerning various aspects of multiple gestation is now in the hundreds.

It has been necessary to be selective in the sources used for this text. The standard references and texts on twins, multiple pregnancy, and the placentation of multiple pregnancy provide valuable starting points for basic review.[6,12–22] There are also bibliographic collections available such as for the Scandinavian literature on twins,[23] and specific aspects of the study of twins.[24] Information has been selected from review articles that correlate a large number of cases of a particular disorder, and this is supplemented with instructional descriptions of small groups or single case reports. A broad survey has been undertaken with a view to providing a sense of scope rather than a catalogue of specifics beyond what is illustrative.

The choice has been made for this text to focus on aspects of multiple gestation that would be of particular interest to the pathologist concerned with details of lesions and descriptive analysis, as well as pathophysiology. Directions for future investigations are indicated where appropriate, so that others can build on what I have learned, as I have done from those before me. It is hoped that the discussions may be of interest and assistance to others in perinatal medicine as well: obstetricians, neonatologists, perinatologists, obstetric and special care nursery nurses, and individuals in related paramedical fields.

The text is divided into 11 chapters. This first, introductory chapter is completed with a brief discussion of twin studies, particularly the factors to be considered such as sources of variability when one is evaluating the reported results.

The mechanisms of twinning are described in Chapter 2. The pathophysiology and biological influences on multiple-egg conceptions and single egg origins of plural conceptions are described with some comments on the rates. General comments regarding zygosity determination with reference to specific methods are included.

Describing the placentations in multiple pregnancy may be a challenge and Chapter 3 is dedicated to the placenta. The possible patterns of disks and membranes are described with a discussion of the factors that may influence these patterns. The vascular patterns of the umbilical cord and chorionic vessels are emphasized. Suggested examination techniques are provided. The concept of molar disease (choriomas) and twins is discussed.

A multiple pregnancy is considered a high-risk pregnancy from the obstetric point of view and the potential risks are discussed in Chapter 4. Maternal disorders that predate pregnancy and gestational complications of multiple pregnancy are described briefly as well as the concept of a combined pregnancy. Difficulties with labor and delivery such as interval delivery and perinatal asphyxia are discussed. Premature delivery is virtually the rule when there is multiple pregnancy and the problems associated with this are also discussed in this chapter.

The mortality of twins is increased over that of singletons, and mortality rates and causes are discussed in Chapter 5. Associations of twin mortality with placentation patterns, fetal sex, birth order, and gestational age are discussed. Both natural and iatrogenic fetal death are described and the different patterns at the different gestational ages are described in detail.

There is an increased morbidity among twins compared to singletons and low birth weight is a particular concern. In Chapter 6, definitions and standards are provided with a discussion of causes, rates, and the concept of intrapair variation as it relates to birth weight. Also, the pattern of infections, neoplasia, system-related morbidity, and other disorders of twins are described.

Anomalous development of twins has long been a subject of study, and Chapter 7 describes the results of general reviews of twin anomalies as well as specific malformations. In addition, there is a discussion of chromosomal anomalies in twins and malformations related to the twinning process itself.

There are those who consider that monozygotic twinning is itself an anomaly, and that the monochorionic monozygotic twin is at greatest risk for maldevelopment. In Chapter 8, there is a discussion of monoamniotic twins. In Chapter 9, the consequences of intertwin vascular anastomoses are presented in detail. These include the placental vascular anatomy and possible hemodynamics as well as a description of the clinically significant patterns of anastomosis. The twin transfusion syndrome can occur acutely or chronically or as a combined phenomenon, and the chronic pattern may be unremitting or may fluctuate spontaneously. When fetal death occurs in relation to twin transfusion, it may be spontaneous or induced. The pathologic findings in all aspects of the twin transfusion syndrome are presented in some detail.

Some of the most bizarre anomalies of human reproduction are represented by anomalies of monozygotic duplication, and these are discussed in Chapter 10. Asymmetric duplication includes endoparasitic, ectoparasitic, and chorangiopagus parasitic twinning anomalies. Symmetric duplication includes the gamut of patterns of conjoined twins. A description is provided along with suggested mechanisms of pathology.

In the discussion that follows, reference is generally limited to twin gestations in order to make the concepts and data clearer. However, the concepts also apply to higher multiples, and abnormalities specific to triplets, quadruplets, and higher multiples are discussed in Chapter 11.

Where appropriate, the information available from the literature has been augmented by data identified as "Survey '91 Review." These data are derived from a review of over 1,100 placentas from multiple gestations where all infants survived, approximately 100 placentas with special features such as an undiagnosed twin, and close to 600 autopsies on one or more members of 355 sets of multiple gestation. The survivor group consists of placentations from two successive tertiary obstetric/neonatal units and these were examined from 1973 to 1991 inclusive, with incomplete ascertainment of all available twin placentas in the unit for the first 5 years and 95% to 100% ascertainment thereafter. The autopsy group consists of infants and placentas from twin autopsies from 1958 to 1991 inclusive, and there were in addition 26 cases where autopsy permission was refused but the placenta could be examined. The review also encompasses placentas from higher multiples, placentas with embryonic or early fetal death of one or both twins, and occasional special situations such as following intervention procedures, and these are described in relevant sections in later chapters. The population base is approximately 2.5 million people in the western province of British Columbia, Canada, and is largely Caucasian with a fairly stable European and native Indian population, and an increasing proportion of people from Asia and the Indian subcontinent. African and South American groups are infrequently represented. The majority of the twin deliveries in the province were referred to the tertiary obstetric/neonatal units mentioned above, either as undelivered mothers, or delivered infants requiring care. In addition, 1% to 2% of the placentas surveyed were submitted from other hospitals for pathology consultations to the pediatric pathol-

ogy staff serving these clinical units. In the discussions of mortality, the term "perinatal mortality" refers to death of a live-born infant any time between birth and 7 completed days of life; neonatal death is 8 to 28 days; infant death is 29 days to 1 year.

Twin Studies

One of the hazards of being a twin is being pursued through life by a growing number of twin researchers.[25-30] The extensive literature on twin studies has arisen from one basic premise—that by comparing a feature in so-called "identical" and "fraternal" twins (more precisely, monozygotic and dizygotic, respectively), the different degrees of genetic and environmental influences on that feature can be determined. This "nature versus nurture" concept has been applied to everything from attributes of personality to the incidence of cancer, and while some insights have been gained, there are aspects to these studies that impair the value of their interpretations.[14,31,32]

In their review of multiple pregnancy, Benirschke and Kim[33] note three considerations to keep in mind when reviewing the data from twin studies. First, an excess of perinatal mortality among members of multiple gestations, especially the monozygotic type, removes these cases from longitudinal study of disease and naturally biases other studies against more lethal conditions when deaths and autopsy data are excluded.[34] Second, the zygosity of twins is still often not ascertained accurately, so that discordant monozygotic twins may not be identified and concordant dizygotic twins may be mislabeled as monozygotic. Statistical determinations of zygosity that have been used in large numbers of individuals should not be used to derive incidence figures in the small numbers encountered in most disease/defect studies. Gruenwald[35] went so far as to suggest that because monochorionicity adds to the burden of pathology beyond the genetics of monozygosity, these cases should actually be omitted from twin studies. Third, it is still not appreciated just how much environmental influences may affect the developing conceptus, even exerting an effect prior to conception by virtue of influences on the maternal environment, so that some environmental effects are wrongly labeled as due to genetic influences. Even the simple crowding effect of several infants in the uterus can alter fetal growth, either directly or through maternal disease. For example, pregnancy-induced hypertension is increased in multiple gestation.[36] Also, the development of one twin can profoundly influence the development of the co-twin, to create some of the most remarkably phenotypically dissimilar infants, who, however, originated from one egg and are thus "identical". Therefore, studies that suggest that the twinning process itself is not a factor in malformations,[37] or that all twin pairs have a relatively similar intrauterine environment[38] should be evaluated critically. It can be argued that aberrations of twinning as described above may be missed in ordinary studies, but that it may be reasonable to suppose the number of such cases is small and not likely to influence the results of most twin research.[29]

There are other factors to be considered that affect ascertainment of cases for twin studies. Retrospective twin studies from different populations may not be comparable because of different reporting requirements or definitions of death. For example, reported fetal mortality in Norway begins at 16 weeks of gestation, whereas in Minnesota fetal death is reported only if it occurs at 20 weeks of gestation or beyond. Also, an infant who dies minutes after birth is classed as a neonatal death in Minnesota, but a fetal death in Norway.[39] Other biases of ascertainment are legion and include variations in the thoroughness of examination and styles of reporting the findings,[40] assumptions that lead to attribution of environmental versus genetic contributions to the observed variations,[24,41] and such simple things as the observation that female pairs are more likely to volunteer for twin studies than male pairs.[42]

It is also difficult to know how much value to place on the various twin studies in light of the apparent magnitude of early pregnancy loss of twins (see Chapter 5). Is this loss biased to anomalous, diseased, or otherwise abnormal twins, to monozygotic or to dizygotic twins? Would the answers materially affect rates or statistics? Is this pattern of fetal death in early pregnancy an irreducible load that perhaps has no bearing on the patterns of mortality and morbidity later in gestation, and therefore may not be of any significance in twin studies of survivors? More information about the nature of early pregnancy wastage of twins may help answer these questions.

Part of the difficulty in assessing twins is that the sources of variability are nearly infinite and some, while rare, can be quite striking. Some have already been referred to and others are detailed in discussions that follow in Chapters 2 and 7, but an outline now is instructive. At fertilization, the number of sperm/egg combinations is variable, leading to variations in chromosomal composition. Also, there may be an influence of characters in the cytoplasmic mass that may not be represented equally in some twin zygotes.[43] Postzygotic mitotic chromosomal behavior during early divisions of the conceptus may lead to mosaics, or chromosomally different individuals that may or may not be phenotypically similar. Implantation may be asymmetric or otherwise abnormal, and certainly the geography of implantation may determine whether dichorionic conceptuses will have distinct or fused gestational sacs. Intertwin vascular connections across a shared chorionic mass can lead to striking fetal asymmetries and blood chimeras. The basic genetic makeup of the zygote, namely the attributes derived from the parents that may determine the fetal response to unfavorable influences during gestation, is a well-recognized source of variability. The unfavorable influences during gestation may consist of aspects of maternal anatomy or physiology, intrauterine phenomena of interfetal or placental origin, and intrafetal processes. Even the consequences of labor and delivery may lead to markedly dissimilar fetal outcomes and characteristics that are completely unrelated to events up to that point. These potential sources of variability must always be considered when data from twin studies are being evaluated.

The pathologist can improve the value of twin studies by providing precise and thorough descriptions of placental pathology and autopsy findings, and making clinicopathological correlations based on knowledge and experience. In addition, clinical colleagues could be encouraged to be concerned about zygosity determination and pathologists may be in a position to facilitate the laboratory services required, either locally or regionally.

References

1. Haggard HW. *Devils, Drugs and Doctors*. London: William Heinemann, 1929:3.
2. Corney G. Mythology and customs associated with

twins. In: MacGillivray I, Nylander PPS, Corney G, eds. *Human Multiple Reproduction*. Philadelphia: WB Saunders, 1975:1–15.

3. Gedda L. *Twins in History and Science*. Springfield: Charles C Thomas; 1961:3–32.

4. Scheinfeld A. *Twins and Supertwins*. Philadelphia: JB Lippincott; 1967.

5. Oruene TO. Cultic powers of Yoruba twins: manifestation of traditional and religious beliefs of the Yoruba. *Acta Genet Med Gemellol*. 1983;32:221–228.

6. Bryan EM. *The Nature and Nurture of Twins*. London: Bailliere Tindall; 1983:1–9.

7. Noble E. *Having Twins. A Parent's Guide to Pregnancy, Birth and Early Childhood*. Boston: Houghton Mifflin, 1991:1–18.

8. Rogers J. Me, myself and us: twins. *Sci Dig*. 1980;Nov/Dec:92–97.

9. Rosen CM. The eerie world of reunited twins. *Discover*. 1987;6(9):36–46.

10. Ingram J. *Twins: An Amazing Investigation*. Toronto: Greey de Pencier; 1988.

11. Galton F. The history of twins as a criterion of the relative powers of nature and nurture. *J Anthropol Inst G Br Irel*. 1876;5:391–406.

12. Newman HH. *Multiple Human Births*. New York: Doubleday, Doran; 1940.

13. Strong SJ, Corney G. *The Placenta in Twin Pregnancy*. Norwich: Pergamon Press; 1967.

14. Bulmer MG. *The Biology of Twinning in Man*. Oxford: Clarendon Press; 1970.

15. MacGillivray I, Nylander PPS, Corney G. *Human Multiple Reproduction*. Philadelphia: WB Saunders; 1975.

16. Potter EL, Craig JM. *Pathology of the Fetus and the Infant*. 3rd ed. Chicago: Year Book Medical Publishers; 1975:207–237.

17. Fox H. *Pathology of the Placenta*. London: WB Saunders; 1978:73–94.

18. Gedda L, Parisi P, Nance WE, eds. Twin Research 3, Proceedings of the Third International Congress on Twin Studies. Twin biology and multiple pregnancy. *Prog Clin Biol Res*. 1981;69A.

19. Shanklin DR, Perrin EVDK. Multiple gestation. In: Perrin EVDK, ed. *Pathology of the Placenta*. Contemporary Issues in Surgical Pathology. Vol. 5 (Roth LM, series ed.). New York: Churchill Livingstone; 1984:165–182.

20. Gall SA, ed. Twin Pregnancy. *Clin Perinatol*. 1988;15(1):1–162.

21. Benirschke K, Kaufmann P. *Pathology of the Human Placenta*. 2nd ed. New York: Springer-Verlag; 1990:636–753.

22. Baldwin VJ. Pathology of multiple pregnancy. In: Wigglesworth JS, Singer DB, eds. *Textbook of Fetal and Perinatal Pathology*. Oxford: Blackwell Scientific; 1991:221–262.

23. Schwartz RM, Keith LG, Keith DM. The Nordic contribution to the English language twin literature. *Acta Obstet Gynecol Scand*. 1986;65(6):599–604.

24. Price B. Bibliography on prenatal and natal influences in twins. *Acta Genet Med Gemellol*. 1978;27:97–113.

25. Christian JC. The use of twin registers in the study of birth defects. *Birth Defects*. 1978;14(6A):167–178.

26. Twins at Jerusalem. Editorial. *Lancet*. 1980;2:244–245.

27. Gedda L, Parisi P, Nance WE, eds. Twin Research 3: Proceedings of the Third International Congress on Twin Studies. Intelligence, personality and development. Epidemiology and clinical studies. *Prog Clin Biol Res*. 1981;69B,C.

28. Gedda L, Brenci G, Tripodi F. Twin Research, past and present. In: Bonne-Tamir B, Cohen T, Goodman RM, eds. Proceedings of the 6th International Congress of Human Genetics. *Prog Clin Biol Res*. 1982;103A:345–350.

29. Hrubec Z, Robinette CD. The study of human twins in medical research. *N Engl J Med*. 1984;310:435–441.

30. Farber SL. *Identical Twins Reared Apart*. New York: Basic Books; 1981.

31. Allen G. Twin research: problems and prospects. In: Steinberg AG, Bearn AG, eds. *Prog Med Genet*. 1965;4:242–269.

32. Allen G. Errors of Weinberg's difference method. In: Gedda L, Parisi P, Nance WE, eds. Twin Research 3: Twin Biology and Multiple Pregnancy. *Prog Clin Biol Res*. 1981;69A:71–74.

33. Benirschke K, Kim CK. Multiple pregnancy. *N Engl J Med*. 1973;288:1276–1284,1329–1336.

34. Emanuel I, Huang S-W, Gutman LT, Yu F-C, Lin C-C. The incidence of congenital malformations in a Chinese population: the Taipei collaborative study. *Teratology*. 1972;5:159–169.

35. Gruenwald P. Environmental influences on twins apparent at birth. *Biol Neonate*. 1970;15:79–93.

36. Marivate M, Norman RJ. Twins. *Clin Obstet Gynecol*. 1982;9(3):723–743.

37. Lamm SH, Hoffman HJ. An etiologic interpretation of birth defect incidence and coincidence rates in twin pairs. In: Nance WE, ed. Twin Research: Biology and Epidemiology. *Prog Clin Biol Res*. 1978;24(B):143–148.

38. Layde PM, Erickson JD, Falek A, McCarthy BJ. Congenital malformations in twins. *Am J Hum Genet*. 1980;32:69–78.

39. Hoffman HJ, Bakketeig LS, Stark CR. Twins and

perinatal mortality: a comparison between single and twin births in Minnesota and Norway, 1967–1973. In: Nance WE, ed. Twin Research: Biology and Epidemiology. *Prog Clin Biol Res*. 1978;24(B): 133–142.

40. Hay S, Wehrung DA. Congenital malformations in twins. *Am J Hum Genet*. 1970;22:662–678.

41. Price B. Primary biases in twin studies. *Am J Hum Genet*. 1950;2:293–352.

42. James WH. Gestational age in twins. *Arch Dis Child*. 1980;55:281–284.

43. Myrianthopoulos NC. Congenital malformations in twins: epidemiologic survey. *Birth Defects*. 1975; 11(8):1–39.

2
Twinning Mechanisms and Zygosity Determination

Our concepts of the possible mechanisms of twinning, the rates of these different mechanisms, and the factors that influence those rates have developed considerably in recent years with the aid of technical advances in two disciplines—prenatal diagnosis and DNA analysis. The increasing use of ultrasound examination in early pregnancy has identified far more pregnancies that begin with a multiple gestation than pregnancies that actually end with multiple infants delivered (see Chapter 5). Studies to date suggest that much of this early loss is of one particular type of twins, so our concepts of the rates of the different mechanisms of twinning may need to be revised. Also, it used to be that twins either looked alike (identical) or not (fraternal) and that was all that could be said. Now, it is possible to determine which parent provided a specific portion of the genome in each twin, and subtle and unusual varieties of biologic mechanisms of twinning that were only theoretical constructs before can be refuted or confirmed (see below). Finally, the influences governing twinning are increasing as the modes of twinning multiply. These recognized influences now include endogenous hormones and genetic predispositions, a variety of exogenous influences on natural ovulation, exogenous hormonal induction of ovulation, and extracorporeal manipulation of embryos. Benirschke and Kaufmann[1] provide an extensive discussion of a number of forces underlying twinning, particularly endocrine influences, with comparative observations from other animals. In spite of this complexity, it is still useful to consider that the majority of multiple births arise from either a single egg or multiple eggs, and that these two broad groups can be considered separately, recognizing that in the higher multiples, combinations can occur. It may be helpful to refer to the diagrams indicated throughout the following discussion.

Multiple Egg Conceptions

In multiple egg or polyovular conceptions, two or more individual eggs are each fertilized by individual sperm to create separate and genetically distinct embryos (types 1, 2, 3, and 4 in Fig. 2.1). Polyovulation can occur naturally, or it can be induced by exogenous hormones. The eggs may come from a single follicle, from separate follicles maturing together in the same cycle, or possibly from sequential cycles (superfetation). The eggs may be fertilized by sperm from one source, either by coitus, or in the laboratory (artificial insemination, or in vitro fertilization), or from separate sources by coitus (superfecundation) with the same or different partners.

Natural Polyovulation

Natural polyovulation is subject to a number of influences, many of which may have a common denominator—an effect on the levels of pituitary gonadotropins and hence ovarian stimulation.[2–6] A genetic predisposition to polyovulation is reflected in a number of remarkable family trees with numerous sets of twins in several generations.[7–10] This is usually considered to be matrilineal,[11] acting on the hormonal axis of ovulation induction, but a paternal role would seem to exist as well,[8,10] although just

Type   Process   Terminology

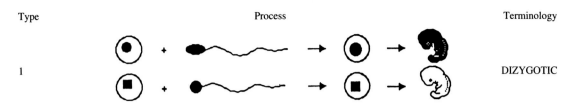

1   DIZYGOTIC

Two eggs from separate follicles in polyovular cycle with two sperm from one coitus; two genetically distinct zygotes and embryos; two corpora lutea; commonest pattern of polyovular twinning.

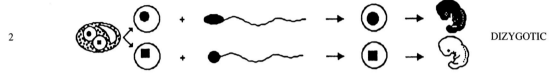

2   DIZYGOTIC

Two eggs from binovular follicle in one cycle with two sperm from one coitus; two genetically distinct zygotes and embryos; one corpus luteum; frequency unknown, likely uncommon.

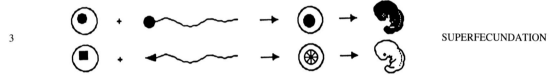

3   SUPERFECUNDATION

Two eggs from polyovular cycle and two sperm, each from separate source; two genetically distinct zygotes and embryos; DNA studies necessary to prove separate paternity if sperm from different coitus partners within lifespan of eggs from one cycle; frequency unknown.

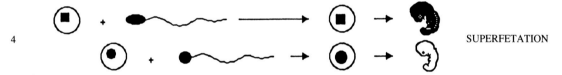

4   SUPERFETATION

Two eggs from sequential cycles and two sperm from same or separate source; two zygotes at different times; two embryos at different developmental stage; genetically distinct; other causes fetal asymmetry *must* be ruled out; existence still debated.

FIGURE 2.1. Patterns of combinations of eggs and sperm with polyovular twinning.

how this can be exerted at the cellular or biochemical level remains to be determined.[12] An increased rate of twinning in mothers of triplets has been reported, consisting of both polyovular and monovular twins at two to three times the rate in the general population.[13] Recurrent spontaneous twinning is at twice the background rate,[14,15] with some truly exceptional examples of individual fecundity reported, such as a woman who had a total of 15 sets of twins, triplets, and quadruplets, with no singleton births with any of her three husbands.[10] This recurrence may be related to the pituitary-ovary endocrine axis of the mother, but an association of twinning with decreased levels of α_1-antitrypsin

activity has been noted,[7] and a deficiency of this enzyme might allow enhanced sperm passage through cervical mucus and thus greater fertilization opportunities with natural polyovulation. The relationship of increased twinning rates in patients surgically treated for Stein-Leventhal syndrome[16] and in sibships of patients with ovarian dermoids or teratomas[17] to the maternal neuroendocrine axis is not clear, as the types of twins were not clarified. The remarkable variation in the incidence of polyovular twinning as it is identified in different racial groups is considered to be due to genetic differences, although the very high frequency in the Ibadan Nigerians has been attributed to dietary influences on hormone levels.[18] It has been thought that some as yet unidentified component of the "native" diets may be influencing hormonal levels and hence twinning, when compared to European diets. Seasonal variations in twinning rates have been attributed to the influence of levels of daylight on hormonal function.[2,19] Chronic malaria has been reported to increase twinning rates, possibly by altering hormonal levels in a manner similar to the effects of malnutrition.[20,21] Socioeconomic conditions alone do not appear to affect twinning when corrections are made for maternal age.[22] Socially disadvantaged narcotic addicts have been reported to have an unexpectedly high incidence of twins (10.5%) but the type of twins was not clear and the connection remains undefined.[23] There has been recent attention to the observation of increased twinning among human immunodeficiency virus (HIV)-infected mothers, possibly related to neuroendocrine effects of coincidental drug use, but the true extent of this trend is still being investigated.[24] Finally, there is a greater tendency for polyovular twinning with advanced maternal age, as well as, but independent of, increasing parity,[9,11,25] but the explanation is not known.

Multiovular follicles have been suggested as a potential source of polyovular twinning (type 2 in Figure 2.1). However, although multiovular follicles were seen throughout the reproductive age span in a large proportion of the adult women whose ovaries were examined, an association with polyovular twinning was discounted because the number seen bore no discernible relation to the woman's endocrine status or history of twin births, and the ability of such follicles to ovulate was considered to be impaired.[26] The fecundity of such ova is uncertain, so it may be difficult to verify this type of twinning process. Interestingly, a binovular follicle was seen in an aspirate for in vitro fertilization and both zygotes were viable to the eight cell stage in the laboratory.[27] The embryos from the binovular follicle were developing within a common septum pellucidum, raising the possibility that such closely apposed embryos might aggregate naturally in the blastocyst stage to create whole body chimeras from completely fused fraternal twins.[28] Therefore, while not a frequent event, this mode of polyovulation may not be as rare as originally thought.

Exogenous Stimulation of Polyovulation

The use of so-called fertility drugs has led to increasing numbers of plural births, due largely to superovulation with fertilization of multiple eggs.[29] Although the exact mechanisms are not known, the effect of these drugs does not appear to be directly dose related, and single egg twins have been reported as well.[30] The gonadotropins, human or synthetic, act on the ovary to stimulate ovulation. Rates of 17% to 40% multiple pregnancy have been reported,[29,31] with a large number of high multiple births of three to nine infants. Clomiphene citrate acts on the hypothalamus and pituitary, interferes with normal estrogen receptors, and results in release of increased levels of endogenous gonadotropins. Rates of 0% to 13% multiple pregnancy have been reported, mostly twins.[29,31] Superfetation has been suggested as a risk if a second induction cycle takes place on top of an undetected pregnancy from an immediately preceding induction cycle.[32] Another proposed mechanism that might permit superfetation in some individuals is a transient diminution of hypothalamic-pituitary inhibition at the time of the luteal-placental steroid shift.[33] It has been suggested that the difference in twinning rates between clomiphene (8–10%) and gonadotropin (25–30%) stimulation may be due to a greater incidence of resorptions. In 78 cases of exogenously stimulated ovulation, resorptions were observed in 64% of clomiphene multiples and 0% of gonadotropin multiples.[34] Bromocryptine reportedly lowers prolactin levels at the pituitary, allowing normal ovulation, and is not associated with any increased risk of multiple pregnancy, spontaneous abortion, or congenital malformations.[31] The assumption that the multiple gestations associated with exogenous hormones are polyovular in origin was supported by detailed zygosity determinations in a case of septuplets following gonadotropin stimulation,[35] although other studies suggest that monovular twinning rates are also increased by artificial induction of ovulation.[30]

In the Survey '91 Review there were 12 twin placentas from recorded Clomid pregnancies. All were dichorionic, two-thirds were a fused single disk, and one-third were known dizygotic because of unlike sex of the twins. Of the eight same-sex pairs, six were male pairs, a rather higher proportion than seen overall in twins (see Chapter 3).

Unfortunately, zygosity determination was not pursued in these cases. In one case, four embryos had been seen on the initial scan, but no sign of the two involuted embryos were identified on the delivered dichorionic fused placenta of the male twins at 32 weeks.

In Vitro Fertilization

In vitro fertilization of eggs with sperm and subsequent placement of the developing embryos back into the uterus at four- to eight-cell stages is now well documented. The incidence of multiple pregnancy after in vitro fertilization–embryo transfer (IVF-ET) depends on the number of embryos replaced, with reported rates up to 23% multiples at delivery.[36] The results of one study suggest that the actual rate is probably higher if the incidence of multiples is noted in early pregnancy—embryonic and fetal death removed 51% of the multiple conceptuses noted initially.[37] The tendency has been to reduce the number of embryos placed in the uterus, in order to reduce the risk of too many "takes," to try to avoid the subsequent intervention procedures that have been used (see Chapter 5). If the other embryos are frozen for implantation at a later date, we may need to broaden our definition of twins to include infants who are conceived at the same time although not born at the same time.[38] The risk of heterotopic/combined pregnancies is increased with IVF-ET, with survival of the intrauterine conceptus only.[39] (Combined pregnancies are discussed further in Chapter 4.) The majority of multiples from IVF-ET are thought to be dizygotic, although zygosity studies are not usually detailed.[40] A higher than expected incidence of single-egg twinning has been reported as well, although the source of the stimulus is not clear[30,41] (see the section on single-egg twins that follows). The patterns of placentation and fetal outcome are not usually specified in any detail in reports of outcome of IVF-ET pregnancies.

In 8 of the 15 cases of twins from IVF-ET in the Survey '91 Review, the number of embryos replaced was known and ranged from three to seven. There was spontaneous reduction in six cases with no residue of the 18 other conceptuses on the delivered placentas, and the two cases with elective reductions are described further in Chapter 5. In one case, gamete intrafallopian transfer (GIFT) had been used and a tubal ectopic implantation was removed laparoscopically at 6 weeks. The 13 deliv-

ered placentations were all dichorionic (see Chapter 3) and fused or separate in equal numbers. The placentas were appropriately grown by weight for the gestational dating (34 weeks to term) in all cases, with only two developmental abnormalities, one marginally inserted umbilical cord, and one very asymmetrically partitioned disk. There were no diagnostic microscopic abnormalities in 11 cases, and one case was described as having villi that were diffusely mature for dates without dysmaturity. The lack of significant pathology in the majority of the placentas agrees with a recent report except for a much higher frequency of anomalous cord insertions, 13.3% marginal and 10% velamentous out of 30 cords from 15 sets of twins in the series described.[42]

The infants from the 13 Survey '91 Review IVF-ET twin sets were assumed dizygotic (boy/girl) in five cases, but the zygosity of the five girl/girl and three boy/boy sets was not pursued. The major finding in the infants at birth was growth discordance by weight in seven sets, with the weight of the smaller twin ranging from 9% to 44.5% less than the weight of the larger twin. No gross or microscopic asymmetry in the placentation was discerned in six cases. In the seventh, the female twins had been asymmetric since early gestation and at birth at 34 weeks differed by 44.5% in weight, although both did well postnatally. The smaller twin was attached to only one-fourth of the placental volume with only three chorionic vascular pairs (Fig. 2.2) and the parenchyma was ischemic with increased fibrin. There is one case report of an IVF-ET dizygotic pair that differed by 50%, but no placental details were given other than the comment that the discordant growth was attributed to "placental insufficiency," a term that was not explained.[43] This degree of growth asymmetry is encountered in spontaneous multiples and has a number of potential causes (see Chapter 6), so the relationship to the process of IVF-ET remains undetermined. One wonders if there is a difference in cell numbers or growth potential in the returned embryos that successfully implant that might be a reflection of the in vitro manipulation.

Superfecundation, Superfetation

Superfecundation (type 3 in Fig. 2.1) is defined as the fertilization of separate eggs during a polyovular cycle by sperm from closely spaced coitus with

FIGURE 2.2. This asymmetric dichorionic diamniotic fused twin placenta came with twin girls (A and B) following in vitro fertilization–embryo transfer (IVF-ET). Zygosity studies were not pursued. Growth was discordant from early in pregnancy and at birth at 34 weeks the smaller twin was 44.5% lighter than her co-twin but both did well. The smaller twin (B) was attached to only one-quarter of the placental volume with only three major chorionic vessel pairs from a marginally inserted cord and the villus parenchyma was ischemic with increased fibrin. The association, if any, between the procedure and discordant growth is not determined.

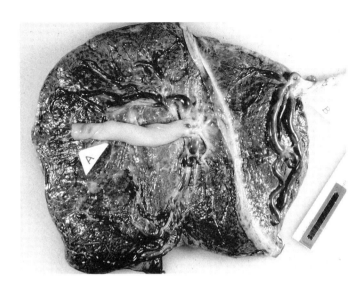

separate males, also known as heteropaternal superfecundation.[44] It has been suggested that in an ancient society the presence of a fetus papyraceous may have been taken as evidence of superfecundation, providing a rationale for contraception during pregnancy when birth control was otherwise generally proscribed.[45] Modern superfecundation has been reported, based on skin color and blood groups,[46] and has been documented using human leukocyte antigen (HLA) haplotypes.[47,48] It would seem that superfecundation could be a theoretical possibility if sperm used for artificial insemination came from pooled donor semen, although this is not the usual practice. Superfecundation as a result of closely spaced coitus with the same partner would not be separable from dizygotic twinning after one coitus.

Superfetation (type 4 in Fig. 2.1) is defined as the fertilization of ova from sequential cycles. Based on our knowledge of the hormonal events following conception, this mechanism of twinning is difficult to accept, except possibly with exogenous hormones.[32] It seems that much of the argument for superfetation comes from markedly discordant birth weights or Dubowitz scores of the twins in the cases that have been considered to represent superfetation.[49–51] Unfortunately, however, the discussions make no reference to other potential causes of weight or developmental discordance, such as asymmetric chorion development, or placental parenchymal pathology such as villitis, to name only two possible contributing mechanisms. It has also been pointed out that concordant neurological

scores can be seen in twins even with very discordant weights, against the concept of superfetation.[52] An intriguing observation that might have relevance to this theoretical construct was reported for experiments with triton eggs by Spemann in 1901 to 1903 (reported by Gedda[53]). When the egg was partially constricted by a hair soon after fertilization so that the nucleus was entirely in one side, segmentation of the cytoplasm followed nuclear division on that side only. With time, nuclear material spread through the constriction to the other cytoplasmic mass and segmentation began there, creating "twin" embryos of different size and developmental stage from one zygote. Proof of this mechanism of twinning in humans remains to be seen.

Single-Egg Origins of Plural Conceptions

Single-egg origins of plural conceptions are difficult to explain. Even describing the simplest possibility—combining one sperm with one egg to create a zygote that then undergoes a twinning process to create two monozygotic and theoretically genetically identical embryos (type 1 in Fig. 2.3)—does little to define the process, and a number of theories have been proposed to explain this twinning process. The concepts of the other possible mechanisms of single egg twinning, the polar body twinning shown as type 2(a) and 2(b) in Fig. 2.3, have

Type   Process   Terminology

1   MONOZYGOTIC

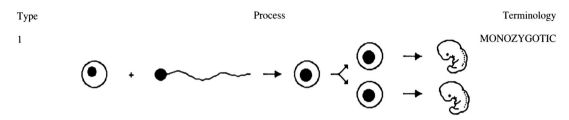

One egg and one sperm; twinning of one zygote or derivitive blastomeres or embryonic disk creating genetically identical embryos; majority of single-egg twinning; see Chapter 7 for possible sources of variation in this pattern.

2a   DISPERMIC
                                                                                           MONOVULAR

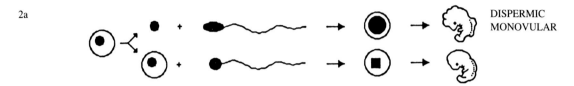

First polar body and secondary oocyte (from primary oocyte) both fertilized by one sperm each; creates abnormal triploid zygote and embryo, and diploid zygote and embryo; proven with chorangiopagus twin (Chapter 10).

2b

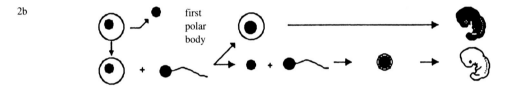

Interaction of sperm with secondary oocyte in fertilization releases second polar body (tertiary oocyte), which is fertilized by second sperm; genetically distinct but more similar than polyovular dizygotic; DNA studies needed to identify details of maternal genomic component.

FIGURE 2.3. Patterns of combinations of egg and sperm with monovular twinning.

been defined more clearly based on information available from the application of newer DNA technologies.[54–56] In these latter patterns, the process is termed dispermic monovular twinning because in both cases the zygotes are genetically distinct—the paternal contribution is obviously distinct, and even though the maternal contribution is from one egg, the individual chromatids in the polar body and mature oocyte are potentially dissimilar as a result of chromatid interchanges during meiosis (Fig. 2.4). Not only are the genetic/chromosomal possibilities more complex with single-egg twinning than with polyovular twinning, but also the spectrum of the physical appearance of the twins and the patterns of their respective gestational sacs is more varied. In most cases, the patterns of the components of the gestational sacs can be explained embryologically by the concept that the twinning event may take place at any time during the first 2

weeks after fertilization,[57,58] but other explanations are needed in some cases of polar body twinning that would seem to bypass the accepted patterns.

Monozygotic Twinning

Theories that try to explain how one zygote becomes two individuals focus on the "twinning event." It has been suggested that this process consists of "splitting" of the developing embryo, with the two halves developing as separate individuals.[59] Alternatively, multiple embryos may arise from one zygote if more than one inductive or organizing focus or axis develops.[60] In both theories, there is the concept of a delay in development as a factor in single-zygote twinning, and this suggests that monozygotic twinning is an anomalous embryonic process and thus itself a malformation. It may be that if the twinning process takes

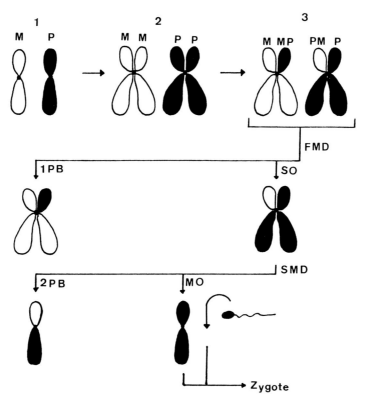

FIGURE 2.4. Meiosis related to polar body twinning. This is a simple representation of one source of variation in the genome of the oocyte and polar bodies to supplement the description of polar body twinning in Fig. 2.3, type 2a and 2b. At step 1, one chromosome pair in the primary oocyte is represented nonspecifically, with one chromatid maternally derived (M) and one paternally derived (P). In step 2, each chromatid splits longitudinally except at the centromere so there are now four chromatids in close association, two identical maternally derived (MM) and two identical paternally derived (PP). In step 3, there is the potential for exchange of genetic material across the chromatids in this tetrad so different combinations of genetic material can be created compared to the original maternally and paternally derived chromatids, repre-

sented as M and MP, and P and PM. In the first meiotic division (FMD) the dyads go to separate "cells," one becomes part of the first polar body (1PB) and the other part of the secondary oocyte (SO). How random this step is may vary with different chromosomes. As the sperm begins fertilization, the second meiotic division (SMD) takes place. The dyad splits—one chromatid enters the second polar body (2PB) and the other exists briefly in the mature oocyte (MO) until joining with the sperm to create the zygote. Again the basis for which chromatid goes where is not known. It can be seen that the chromosomal number in the first polar body is $2n$, like the primary and secondary oocytes, while in the second polar body and mature oocyte it is n. This has relevance to the ploidy of polar body twinning as noted in Fig. 2.3.

place after several cell divisions have occurred from the original zygote, then there has been the opportunity for some mis-segregation of cytogenetic or cytoplasmic material. There would then be two populations of cells with potentially different and repelling cell surface characteristics, tending to promote the evolution of two separate individuals (Hall JG, 1992, personal communication). The differences that could exist at this stage could be the

result of mitotic crossing over, postzygotic nondisjunction, influences of genomic imprinting and/or pattern of X chromosome inactivation, anomalous homeobox genes, and cytoplasmic segregation, especially mitochondria.[61–66] This mechanism of a primary abnormality prior to twinning can apply to either the splitting or codominant axis theories, can explain the discordant growth and development encountered in supposedly identical monozygotic twins (see Chapter 7), and may also be the source of some "vanished" twins (See Chapter 5).

In the *"splitting" theory* of monozygotic twinning, it is suggested that a minor arrest occurs in the very early development of the fertilized ovum, and that this can lead to a division in the blastocyst or embryonic area[59] (Fig. 2.5). This arrest or delay is attributed to environmental conditions disturbing the rate of growth after fertilization. Development of individual embryos from separated blastomeres that originated from one fertilized egg has been documented experimentally in subvertebrates and primitive vertebrates,[53] but what the stimulus for separation of the cells might be in vivo was difficult to extrapolate until the sources of cell differences as mentioned above were identified. Alternatively, an incomplete septum pellucidum could allow some of the blastomeres to separate through the defect, with the potential for two separate embryos to develop. It has been suggested that the timing of this split determines the appearance of the infants and their gestational sac components, the idea being that the longer the time from fertilization to separation, the less separate the embryos will be. This theory is useful as it can explain a number of twinning anomalies. For example, this theory might explain the varieties of incompletely separated twins if the split was late and incomplete (see Chapter 10). It may also account for some discordantly developed twins, if the split was complete but not symmetrical. Finally, it might help explain mirror image structural and functional variations in monozygotic twins, such as facial clefts and handedness,[67] and might also be considered in the pathogenesis of other problems of situs in twins, such as the polysplenia/asplenia syndromes.

The *codominant axis theory* was supported by observations on plants, fish, and humans that suggested that monozygotic twinning was the result of an unusual budding process produced by an early interruption of the development rate[68] (Fig. 2.6). The theory was that there are many potential points in the developing embryo at which an embryonic axis might arise, and when one has arisen, it normally suppresses the potential ability of the other points to form an axis, so that only one axis develops, although the factors that determine why one point dominates are not known. There may be a small cluster of cells acting as a field enforcer or gradient establisher, and if this cell cluster is abnor-

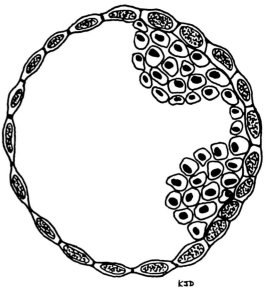

FIGURE 2.5. The splitting theory of monozygotic twinning with two separate inner cell masses becoming evident at the blastocyst stage. Depending on whether the separate cell masses are mixtures of embryonic and placental progenitor cells, or embryonic precursors only, i.e., depending on when the twinning process took place after fertilization, the accompanying placentation could be dichorionic or monochorionic, and diamniotic or monoamniotic.

mal, two organizing centers may evolve instead of one.[60] In some circumstances, instead of one point proliferating at a disproportionate rate to form the embryonic shield, two such points could be established with more or less equal rates of proliferation, both of which might be somewhat less active than the single point would be. The development of three or four codominant axes would be considerably less likely, because if one axis usually suppresses all others, two would probably be even more effective at suppressing any more. This formation of two points of rapid gastrulation, from which would grow the axes of the embryos, would be the initial step in double formations. Homeobox genes are known to influence morphogenetic field development along the established axis, may have a role to play in the creation of that axis, and so may be implicated in axis anomalies as well.[65]

The intrinsic potential for twinning (and hence aberrations of twinning) may exist in all eggs, and external conditions, such as unusual tubal or intrauterine factors that delay implantation, could be the

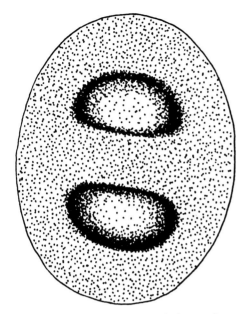

FIGURE 2.6. The codominant axis theory of monozygotic twinning. In this schematic portrayal of the surface of the embryonic plate or disk, two cell clusters have emerged creating two embryonic shields with parallel axes instead of a single embryonic mass. This twinning process would be more limited in time than the separate blastocyst stage embryonic cell masses, and monochorionic placentation with diamniotic or monoamniotic membranes would be most likely.

forces that allow more than one growing point to express itself. The eggs of some species are more prone, or more able, to develop several codominant axes,[60] possibly representing an aspect of genetic contribution to monozygotic twinning.[69]

The codominant axes theory can be used to explain developmental abnormalities of monozygotic twinning.[70] If these axes were sufficiently separate, then separate twins could develop. If they were incompletely separated, the resultant twins might be either symmetrically abnormal as with conjoined twins, or asymmetrically duplicated (see Chapter 10). As this theory is invoking a stimulus or defect in the embryonic cell mass, it suggests that this method of twinning would be limited to a monochorionic pattern of placentation.

The concept of a delay in development as a factor in monozygotic twinning could be invoked at several stages. A prolonged interval between ovulation and fertilization has been reported to lead to increased monozygotic twinning in the rabbit.[71] Al-ternatively, a delay in the development of a dominant axis could allow codominant axes to develop. It may be possible to blend the splitting and codominant axes theories by suggesting that the delay in appearance of the axes is the result of the time needed for separation of the developing cell mass and its reaggregation into two clusters, each with sufficient organizing material to initiate embryonic tissues.[72] Whatever takes place, this delay could be due to some environmental influence, such as suboptimal oxygen,[68,73] coupled with a possible hereditary susceptibility to codominant axes, perhaps on the basis of cytoplasmic or sex chromosomal components.[50] The influence of sex chromosomes is suggested by the excess of females in aberrations of single-egg twinning. Until inactivation of one of the X chromosomes, at about day 8 to 9, the extra gene mass slows cell division. If X inactivation is triggered by an intracellular time clock, then there will be fewer cells at the time of inactivation. This may in turn make the XX embryo more susceptible to abnormalities that result in twinning. There may also be a role for genomic imprinting as to which X chromosome is inactivated and when.[74] Also, hereditary and/or environmental factors could augment the process by delaying implantation into the uterine wall. Hypothetically, such a delay could lead to a brief period of less than ideal nutrition of the developing embryo, because beyond the normal implantation stage it should be nourished by the endometrium, rather than by uterine luminal fluids.

Monovular Dispermic (Polar Body) Twinning

The possibility of fertilization of a polar body as well as an oocyte from the same egg, leading to twin conceptuses, arose from observations in 1914 of the maturation and fertilization of ova in warm-blooded animals such as the mouse, although the hypothesis had been suggested as early as 1894 (reported by Gedda[75]). The polar body was theorized to be a mature germinal cell with a haploid chromosome set, capable of being fertilized. A number of other workers supported this possibility,[75] but proof of its occurrence had to await methods of DNA analysis, in order to document that this was indeed a mechanism for the creation of genetically distinct individuals from one egg.

Theoretically, polar body twinning could take

place at two points in the sequence of meiosis (see Fig. 2.4). If dispermic fertilization took place after the first meiotic division of the egg (type 2a of Fig. 2.3), fertilization of the secondary oocyte with one sperm would lead to discharge of the second polar body and creation of one diploid zygote. If a second sperm simultaneously fertilized the first polar body, a triploid zygote would result. This possibility was proven with the results of tests of histocompatibility antigen haplotypes in a malformed triploid acardiac twin—two maternally derived chromosome sets were detected and both maternal HLA haplotypes, the latter observation reflecting crossover during the prophase of meiosis I.[76] The dispermic component of the twins was confirmed by finding different paternal HLA haplotypes in each twin. An interesting additional observation in this twin pair was that, as with all acardiac/normal twin sets, both twins were enclosed in the same chorion. In monozygotic twinning, the pattern of the arrangement of the twins and the components of their respective gestational sacs depends on the embryologic development over time in relation to the timing of the twinning event, with more complete sets of membranes around each twin the sooner after fertilization that the twinning event occurs. In this case, however, the twinning event could hardly have been earlier, and yet they were both within the same outer layer of the gestational sac. The suggested explanation was that the proximity of the ovum and its first polar body in the perivitelline space within the zona pellucida could permit the implantation and subsequent development of the twins as distinct cell masses within a common trophoblast, leading to nonidentical twins within a single chorion but with separate amnions. This suggestion was entirely consistent with the early observations by Hertig[77] on the development of the extraembryonic structures. In other words, if one embryo is capable of providing the trophoblast, this in turn leads to the necessary extraembryonic structures of mesoblastic origin, as the degree of mesoblast formation is correlated with the degree of trophoblast development. However, amnion induction requires the presence of the embryo, and an "included" embryo could therefore provide its own amnion.

If dispermic fertilization took place at the second meiotic division (type 2b in Fig. 2.3), the implication would be that one sperm fertilized the secondary oocyte, creating a normal diploid zygote and the second polar body, which in turn was fertilized by a second sperm, creating a second diploid zygote. These monovular zygotes would be not quite as genetically distinct with respect to nuclear DNA as zygotes from two separately ovulated eggs. The initial volume of cytoplasmic material would seem to be very different, but there is also the concept of a tertiary oocyte—a second polar body that has more of the secondary oocyte's cytoplasm than usual, possibly on the basis of anomalies of cytoskeletal mechanisms necessary for the usual remarkably asymmetric second meiotic division.[78] It is not known what significance either of these concepts might have for the ultimate development of the zygotes, especially the extrafetal membranes.

Dispermic monovular twinning raises several interesting questions regarding the development of extraembryonic membranes in the gestational sacs, and the potential for confusion as to the exact type of twinning mechanism involved. It was suggested above that the proximity of the oocyte and polar body would permit the development of the two distinct zygotes within one trophoblastic shell. Another contributing factor might be that the gestational sac membranes originate from the zygote with the greater cytoplasm, and the polar body zygote is included only if it is close enough. It may be that polar body zygotes do not have enough cytoplasm to provide for a gestational sac, and that they only survive if they can be included within the sac of the oocyte zygote. If this is the case, then dispermic monovular twins would only occur within a common outer layer or chorion. If they were both girls or both boys, they would be assumed to be monozygotic unless detailed genetic studies were done, an unlikely investigation unless one twin was abnormal. A relevant pilot study of blood groups found discrepancies among minor blood groups in 3 of 12 sets of monochorionic twins.[79] These could be dispermic monovular twins or monozygotic twins with mitotic crossing over. If it was a boy/girl pair, it would be assumed to be dizygotic, unless the placenta was examined with a willingness to accept and attempt to explain the apparent incongruity of such a situation.

The existence of chimeras, individuals that appear to be a mixture of cells from two genetically distinct sources, has been known for some time and

FIGURE 2.7. This was a monochorionic diamniotic placenta with twin A an externally normal 1,965-g female with 100% 46,XX karyotype from skin fibroblasts, and twin B an externally normal 2,360-g male with 100% 46,XY karyotype from skin fibroblasts. Both twins had a 50:50 mixture of their karyotypes in cultures of blood lymphocytes. The placenta was formalin fixed and torn between the cord insertions, as shown, when received. No anastomoses were visible on the surface, but a full-thickness section from chorion to maternal surface parallel to the tear halfway between the tear and cord B on a line to cord A (dotted line) contained two true cross sections of large subchorionic vessels that might have reached the (torn) base of cord A, although this could not be confirmed. It was suspected that this was an example of monovular dispermic twinning, and studies are continuing to try to confirm this.

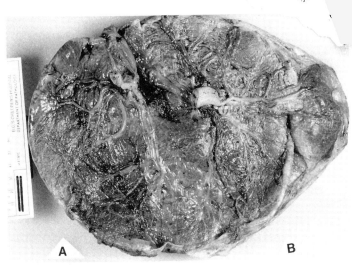

they can be whole body or blood chimeras.[80] The origin of whole-body chimerism is not understood, but in some cases may be related to zygote fusion after fertilization of eggs from a binovular follicle,[28] and it may not be detected unless there is a mixture of sex chromosomes with accompanying gonadal abnormality. Blood chimeras must arise through vascular anastomoses between the twins at some point of their development. Adequately documented anastomoses between twins who are each in their own chorionic sac is extremely rare, implying that blood chimeras must be monovular twins within a single chorion. A recent case from the Survey '91 Review illustrates the problems and appears to confirm this interpretation. A 1,965-g externally normal girl (twin A in Fig. 2.7) and a larger 2,360-g and also externally normal boy (twin B in Fig. 2.7) were delivered at 35 weeks' gestation, with only mild respiratory distress in the male complicating the immediate newborn period. The formalin-fixed placenta submitted weighed 775 g in the trimmed state, and 40% of the chorionic surface drained to twin A and 60% to twin B. Unfortunately the parenchyma was torn between the insertions of the cords and although one potential vascular anas-tomosis was identified, it could not be confirmed (Fig. 2.7). No separating membranes could be identified grossly but a bilaminar amniotic membrane was found microscopically. The apparent discrepancy between the pattern of the extraembryonic membranes and the boy/girl twin pair suggested the possibility of dispermic monovular twinning. The blood lymphocytes from each infant were a 1:1 mixture of normal 46,XY and 46,XX cell lines, and this has persisted 3 years later, suggesting blood chimerism. The skin fibroblasts from the boy grew only normal 46,XY cells, and from the girl, only normal 46,XX cells. Detailed DNA investigations are in process.

If, on the other hand, the polar body zygote is capable of forming a set of extraembryonic membranes and hence its own gestational sac, any pattern of membranes would be possible, analogous to monozygotic twinning, and genetically distinct twins from dispermic monovular twinning would be identified as dizygotic twins. The real frequency of this pattern of twinning is surely underestimated unless it is suspected, so that the special genetic studies to prove the monovular origin can be performed.

gle-Egg Twinning as an Anomaly

foregoing discussion on the possible mecha-
n   ms of single-egg twinning suggests that single-
egg twinning is an anomalous embryonic process,
and thus itself a malformation. This concept is
reinforced by the greater frequency of all malformations in single-egg twins (see Chapter 7) and a
particular increase in some malformations that may
have implications for both the mechanism of twinning and the malformation in question. Examples of
such malformations include chromosomal loss,[81,82]
anterior neural tube defects,[83] sirenomelia,[84] caudal duplication,[85] esophageal atresia,[86] and the
Duhamel anomalad (reduction/fusion anomalies of
pelvis and legs with associated visceral defects).[70]
It is not clear whether the twinning process predisposes to these anomalies, or whether the circumstance causing the anomaly has also led to the
twinning (see Chapter 7).

There have been a number of suggestions for the
forces or circumstances responsible if single egg
twinning is an anomaly. It has been generally stated
that there is no genetic predisposition to single egg
twinning in contrast to the recognized familial
aggregates of polyovular twinning. However, a
number of reports, with various studies to confirm
monozygosity, have suggested that in some families genetic factors contribute to the occurrence of
single-egg twins and that this influence could be
passed through the mother or father.[69,87–89] Another large study of the incidence of twinning in the
families of 950 zygosity-determined, unselected
twin pairs under complete ascertainment, confirmed a propensity to monozygotic twinning as
well as to dizygotic twinning, which could be
inherited through the maternal line. They also found
a paternal role in dizygotic twinning but did not
confirm a paternal role in monozygotic twinning.[8]
It has been suggested that recent use (within 9
months) of oral contraceptives may increase the
possibility of single egg twins, although no mechanism was proposed.[90] If this were true, it might
suggest that the familial forces in single egg twinning had a hormonal component.

The rather remarkable uniformity of ratios of
apparent monozygotic twinning worldwide suggests an underlying random spontaneous biologic
event, and this could consist of any of the changes
mentioned above, such as mitotic crossing over.[61]

Depending on the nature of the genetic change, cell
surface characteristics could be affected with profound influences on cell–cell interactions including
the induction of twinning. These changes could
theoretically result in such asymmetric twinning
that one twin was lost early (the vanishing twin),
and virtually any degree of discordance up to simply
minor variations in external features such as hair
color or dermatoglyphics (Hall JG, Kalousek DK,
1992, personal communications).

A review of the sex ratios of twins has shown an
excess of female sets among twin pairs at the least
separated end of the spectrum, and this seems to
hold to a lesser degree in all single egg conceptions.
One study reported the sex ratio of males to males
plus females to be 0.514 for singletons and two-egg
twins, 0.496 for all single-egg twins, 0.42 for
monochorionic single-egg twins, 0.23 for conjoined twins, and 0.25 for sacral teratomas.[91] This
confirmed a previous observation of a decreased
frequency of males in twins, a tendency that increased with higher multiples—males were 51.59%
of singletons, 50.85% of twins, 49.54% of triplets,
and 46.48% of quadruplets.[92] These data lead to a
number of questions. Is the female zygote or early
embryo more prone to division or development of
codominant axes, and if so, why? Alternatively, is
there a selective loss of male conceptions prior to
identification, and if so, why? Is the female chromosome carrying sperm better able to fertilize the
polar body? No satisfactory explanation for this
apparent trend is yet suggested, although a relationship to the greater mass of the X chromosome and
its effect on early cell division prior to inactivation,
and the influence of which X chromosome is inactivated with respect to the remaining genome, may
be important.[74]

The rate of single-egg/zygote/embryo twinning
has been reported to be higher after in vitro fertilization and embryo replacement than after physiologic conception,[93] but it has been stated that the
majority of plural births after in vitro fertilization
are polyembryonic.[40] It seems that this debate will
require careful zygosity studies of the fetuses and
infants of multiple gestations after in vitro
fertilization/embryo transfer before it is resolved.
Perhaps the extracorporeal manipulation that
IVF-ET entails could provide the stimulus and
delay in embryonic development that has been
suggested is important to single-egg twinning. This

possibility has been denied by those who consider that it is the artificial induction of ovulation that precedes the IVF-ET that predisposes to zygotic division or an enhanced survival of monozygotic twins, rather than the in vitro conditions.[30]

Rates of Multiple Conceptions

It is very difficult to determine the incidence of multiple reproduction because of differences in definitions used in reporting. In many reports, stillborns and spontaneous abortions are not included, so the rates given represent only successful multiple pregnancies and not the incidence of multiple conceptions. Also, statistics on overall twinning rates in any population are only as good as the birth reporting practices of the area. With these reservations, the reported rates for twins demonstrate geographic trends that seem to follow racial lines. The highest rates are encountered among black populations in Africa, 1 twin birth in 33 births among the Ibo of eastern Nigeria,[21] 1:30 in Ghana,[25] 1:28 in Mozambique,[94] and 1:22 among the Yoruba of western Nigeria.[21] The rate is reduced to 1:79 among blacks in the United States.[73] Average rates among caucasians are 1:80 to 1:100, based on 1:67 to 1:100 from collated data from Europe,[95] 1:59 to 1:100 in the former Czechoslovakia,[96,97] 1:51 in Norway,[98] and 1:78 in Germany,[99] and in the United States 1:53 in Minnesota,[98] 1:86 in Florida,[100] and 1:100 for the Collaborative Perinatal Project in the United States.[73] The lowest rates occur in Asian populations with 1:100 reported from Taipei,[101] and rates in Japan ranging from 1:108[19] to 1:178.[95] Other populations provide intermediate values, such as 1:71 to 1:118 in India[102,103] and 1:112 in Mexican Americans.[104]

We are now aware that there is a remarkably high rate of loss of multiple conceptions during the pregnancy and that the observed twinning rates at delivery seriously underestimate the actual rate of twin conceptions. Multiple pregnancies may constitute more than 12% of all natural conceptions, but only 2% of these may survive to term as twins.[105] In one study, 60% of the twins conceived in 30 twin pregnancies were lost at various times during pregnancy, and fewer than half of the gestations terminated with a living twin pair.[106] Statistics on the rates for the different types of twins, polyovular or monovular, are therefore subject to reservation related to the rate of fetal loss with multiple gestation, particularly for monozygotic twinning because monozygotic twins have been found to represent an unusually high proportion of fetal death (see Chapter 5).

Statistics on the rates for the different types of twins are also significantly hampered by inexact determinations of the type of twinning. While determination of the type of twinning is most probably accurate on the basis of the sex of the infants and the pattern of the gestational membranes in just over 50% of cases,[22] most studies of twinning rates are retrospective and details of placentation are not known. Thus, considerable effort has been spent on other ways of determining the zygosity of like-sex twins. As many of the studies are retrospective statistical analyses, a statistical approach has been developed known as Weinberg's rule.[107,108] This differential method of assigning monozygotic and dizygotic rates uses a formula based on the assumption that the number of like-sexed dizygotic twins is equal to the number of unlike-sex dizygotic twins, so that the number of monozygotic twin pairs can be calculated as the total number of twin pairs, less two times the number of unlike-sex twin pairs. This method has been used to gain an overall impression of the distribution of large numbers, but it is not helpful in dealing with assignation of zygosity in small groups or specific cases. More specific methods of zygosity determination are discussed in the following section, and one of the most comprehensive reports of zygosity assessment was by Cameron et al.[109] They used extensive studies to determine zygosity prospectively in 1,424 twin pairs (live-born and stillborn) from Belgium and England, and their data identified 31% as monozygotic and 69% as dizygotic in origin.

While reports of relative rates of monozygotic and dizygotic twinning must be assessed with consideration of the methods used to determine zygosity, the statistics that are available suggest that the rate of monozygotic twinning is relatively uniform worldwide and that the geographic/racial variations are in dizygotic twinning.[12,28,57,73,110–113] A decline in dizygotic twinning has been reported more recently,[67,114–116] but the reasons for this have not been clarified.

In summary, the overall rates of multiple gestation, as well as rates of specific types of plural

TABLE 2.1. Methods of zygosity determination.*

Method	Comment
Physical features	Discordant genital sex probably indicative of dizygosity, whether monovular or polyovular in origin. Other features suggestive, but not reliable.
Placenta	
Membrane patterns	Monochorionicity (histologically proven) indicates monovular origin, although dispermic monovular dizygosity cannot be detected unless the twins are of discordant sex.
Placental alkaline phosphatase	Phenotypic differences imply genotypic differences and hence probable dizygosity.
Cytogenetics	Amnion, chorionic fibroblasts, and cytotrophoblast can be cultured, although fetal blood is more appropriate.
Blood components	
Blood groups	Red cell antigens of ABO, Rh, MNSs, Kell, and Duffy systems most common. Probability of monozygosity increases with number of concordant systems and discordance in any system generally taken as indicating dizygosity.
Red cell isoenzymes	Acid phosphatase, phosphoglucomutase, peptidase A and B, adenylate kinase; a difference in any one is tentative evidence of dizygosity.
Histocompatibility antigens	Platelets or white cells; very specific.
Cytogenetics	
Chromosomal polymorphism	From cultures of lymphocytes/other tissues as needed; very specific.
Direct DNA analysis	Minisatellite DNA "fingerprints" used prenatally and postnatally; polymerase chain reaction (PCR) analysis of specific gene regions may become standard in cases where greatest detail required.
Miscellaneous	Used in unusual cases, such as characterization of chimeras.
Secretor status	
Tissue isoenzymes	
(e.g., hepatic)	

*Consult text and Chapter 7 regarding influences that might affect the interpretation of these zygosity tests in some cases.

births, need to be reassessed to include fetal death during pregnancy, accurate prospective determination of zygosity, and recognition of the racial influences on the different types of twinning.

Zygosity Determination

Much has been made in the preceding sections of the importance of accurate determination of zygosity, and a number of methods are available (Table 2.1). The significance of zygosity to the validity of twin studies has been emphasized, but genetic identity is also important to disease risks and occasionally even therapy of the twins in later life. With newer techniques, Cameron et al.[109] were able to expand the original methods outlined by Benirschke and Kim[2] to 13 variables in three categories. Currently, DNA technology is being used more often[47,76] and may eventually replace all other tests. Some studies of zygosity determination include detailed frequency tables and relative probabilities of zygosity.[12,117,118]

Zygosity studies are perhaps more easily initiated at the time of delivery of the twins, because cord blood is an ideal source of material for these studies and the twin placenta(s) are readily available for careful pathologic examination. However, blood tests and chromosomal studies can be performed long after birth, even by a reference laboratory at some distance from the patient. Determination of zygosity will be a problem with fetal death, especially in early pregnancy, unless tissue maceration has not progressed beyond possible chromosomal culture, either from the fetus or placenta. The degree of certainty of zygosity determination depends on the test system used, and in the paragraphs that follow, the methods are described in order of ascending certainty. It must be remembered, however, that newer knowledge of genetic diversity, even in monozygotic twins, makes the interpretation of small differences problematic.[61] Concordance after superficial testing is not equivalent to monozygosity and many tests may not be sensitive enough to detect small differences.

The pathologist contributes to zygosity determination by providing carefully documented placental findings, indicating those sets of twins for whom studies other than physical examination and placental membrane patterns are required—like-sex dichorionic twin pairs. In addition, the pathologist may be in a position to provide the laboratory facilities needed for the other test systems referred to below, but it is usually the perinatal or pediatric clinician who is responsible for initiating the additional studies needed.

Physical features

The physical appearance of twins has been used for centuries to define the different types of twinning, and the terms "identical" and "nonidentical/fraternal" have become enshrined in the language as equivalent to single-egg or monozygotic and polyovular or dizygotic twins, respectively. In general, anatomic intrapair differences in monozygotic twins are smaller than those in dizygotic twins, but it is well recognized that zygosity diagnosis cannot be based on physiomorphic or biometric data alone, in spite of sometimes apparent dramatic identity at first glance.[119] In fact, monozygotic twinning is associated with some of the most discordant and bizarre twin pairs seen in man (see Chapter 10). Of all the physical features that are accessible during a routine physical examination, the most certain is the genital sex. With the exception of unusual postzygotic mitotic errors (see Chapter 7), or discordant anomalies of sexual development, discordant sexuality of external genitalia indicates dizygosity, although not whether polyovular or monovular in origin.

Placenta

The placenta can be studied for the structure of the separating membranes and analyzed for placental enzymes, and it can provide cell cultures for chromosomal and DNA studies. Histologic evaluation of the separating membranes between the twins should be done routinely (see Chapter 3). Monochorionicity (diamniotic or no separating membrane) is almost certainly an indication of monovular origin, although dispermic monovular dizygosity cannot be detected. The degree of conjunction of the disks in dichorionic placentations is of no assistance in zygosity determination, because up to one-half of dizygotic twins will have a single disk placentation (see Chapter 3). If the pattern of the placental membranes and the fetal sexes are known, zygosity can be assigned in just

over 50% of twin deliveries.[109] There are three allelic autosomal genes for placental alkaline phosphatase, from which six phenotypes can be determined, and up to 60% of dizygotic twins can be identified with this assessment based on phenotypic differences.[109] Cytogenetic and DNA studies can be performed on placental cell cultures, although cord blood or venous blood from the infants would be more appropriate, particularly if there is any concern regarding placental mosaicism wherein fetus and placenta have different chromosomal attributes.[120]

Blood Components

The cells in cord blood or peripheral blood can be used in several test systems for zygosity studies: blood groups and isoenzymes can be determined from red cells, histocompatibility antigens can be identified on white cells and platelets, lymphocytes can provide cell cultures for cytogenetic/chromosomal analyses, and DNA can be extracted for amplification techniques. The blood group systems most frequently used are ABO, Rh, MNSs, Kell, and Duffy, and the probability of monozygosity increases with the number of concordant systems, while discordance in any system is taken as indicating dizygosity,[121] with the reservations already noted. A sequential test system based on relative gene frequencies of the different blood group antigens in the population in question may be more efficient than a random search.[122] At least four red cell enzymes can be differentiated with starch gel electrophoresis: acid phosphatase, phosphoglucomutase, and peptidase A and B with six phenotypes each, and adenylate kinase with three phenotypes, and a difference in any one of the isoenzymes is tentative evidence of dizygosity.[109] The HLA system is sufficiently specific that it can be used to detect different paternity in cases of superfecundation,[47] but it would appear that DNA technology will eventually be the most reliable test system.

Chromosomes and DNA Analysis

Chromosomal polymorphisms, using banding techniques, may detect dizygosity,[121] but direct analysis of chromosomal DNA is the definitive tool to determine the degree of genetic identity. Four advantages of current DNA technology are that only one sample of material is required, only a small sample is needed, the sample does not have to be fresh, and the specificity for each person far exceeds any other test system available. Minisatellite DNA probes can determine zygosity by providing DNA "fingerprints," and have been used prenatally[123] as well as postnatally.[124,125] The polymerase chain-reaction amplification of specific gene sequences from DNA seems to provide the ultimate tool for analysis of the genetic origin of twins,[54-56] and may eventually supersede all other tests.

Other Zygosity Assessments

Additional methods of zygosity assessment may be used in unusual situations. For example, characterization of dizygotic chimeras may include secretor status, hepatic or other tissue isoenzymes, karyotypes of several tissues, assays for specific markers, and mixed lymphocyte cultures.[126] Reciprocal skin grafts may not be completely reliable, as it has been suggested that for complete acceptance, there has to have been vascular sharing during gestation, not just monozygosity.[56]

Summary

Our concepts of the types of twinning possible are being revised by the application of highly sophisticated DNA technology, but it may be the pathologist who identifies the unusual cases, the ones that "don't fit" and warrant further investigation. The rates of twinning are being revised too, based on early pregnancy evaluations by ultrasound. Again, it is the pathologist who can confirm and define the pattern of fetal mortality of twins. Finally, zygosity assignment may be critical to the individual twin pair and to broader-based twin studies, and placental findings by the pathologist determine which twins need additional and more costly studies. This central role of the pathologist in twin studies and zygosity assignment is readily fulfilled in the most basic histopathology laboratory because all that is needed is informed curiosity and competent ability to make and read microscopic tissue sections. The next chapter provides the basic information for pathologic examination of the placenta.

References

1. Benirschke K, Kaufmann P. *Pathology of the Human Placenta*. 2nd Ed. New York: Springer-Verlag; 1990:643–652.
2. Benirschke K, Kim CK. Multiple pregnancy. *N Engl J Med*. 1973;288:1276–1284,1329–1336.
3. Nylander PPS. The causation of twinning. In: MacGillivray I, Nylander PPS, Corney G, eds. *Human Multiple Reproduction*. Philadelphia: WB Saunders; 1975:77–86.
4. Nylander PPS. Frequency of multiple births. In: MacGillivray I, Nylander PPS, Corney G, eds. *Human Multiple Reproduction*. Philadelphia: WB Saunders; 1975:87–97.
5. Nylander PPS. Factors which influence twinning rates. In: MacGillivray I, Nylander PPS, Corney G, eds. *Human Multiple Reproduction*. Philadelphia: WB Saunders; 1975:98–106.
6. MacGillivray I. Epidemiology of twin pregnancy. *Semin Perinatol*. 1986;10(1):4–8.
7. Lieberman J, Borhani NO, Feinleib M. Twinning as a heterozygote advantage for $\alpha_1$antitrypsin deficiency. In: Nance W, ed. *Twin Research: Biology and Epidemiology*. Prog Clin Biol Res. 1978; 24B:45–54.
8. Parisi P, Gatti M, Prinzi G, Caperna G. Familial incidence of twinning. *Nature* 1983;304:626–628.
9. Wenstrom KD, Gall SA. Incidence, morbidity and mortality, and diagnosis of twin gestations. *Clin Perinatol*. 1988;15(1):1–11.
10. Gedda L. *Twins in History and Science*. Springfield: Charles C Thomas; 1961:67–99.
11. Allen G. The parity effect and fertility in mothers of twins. In: Nance WE, ed. Twin Research: Biology and Epidemiology. *Prog Clin Biol Res*. 1978; 24B:89–97.
12. Bulmer MG. *The Biology of Twinning in Man*. Oxford: Clarendon Press; 1970:9.
13. Eriksson AW. Twinning in families of triplets. *Acta Genet Med Gemellol*. 1990;39:279–293.
14. Hendricks CH. Twinning in relation to birth weight, mortality and congenital anomalies. *Obstet Gynecol*. 1966;27:47–53.
15. Blickstein I, Borenstein R. Recurrent spontaneous twinning. *Acta Genet Med Gemellol*. 1989;38:279–283.
16. Stein IF. Multiple pregnancy following wedge resection in the Stein-Leventhal syndrome. *Int J Fertil*. 1964;9:343–350.
17. Edmonds AW, Hawkins JW. Relationship of twins, teratomas, and ovarian dermoids. *Cancer Res*. 1941;1:896–899.
18. Nylander PPS. Causes of high twinning frequen-

cies in Nigeria. In: Nance WE, ed. Twin Research: Biology and Epidemiology. *Prog Clin Biol Res.* 1978;24B:35–43.

19. Sekiya S, Hafez ESE. Physiomorphology of twin transfusion syndrome: a study of 86 twin gestations. *Obstet Gynecol.* 1977;50:288–292.

20. Cox ML. Incidence and etiology of multiple births in Nigeria. *J Obstet Gynecol Br Cwlth.* 1963;70:878–884.

21. Egwuatu VE. Triplet pregnancy: a review of 27 cases. *Int J Gynecol Obstet.* 1980;18:460–464.

22. Myrianthopoulos NC. An epidemiologic survey of twins in a large, prospectively studied population. *Am J Hum Genet.* 1970;22:611–629.

23. Thornton L, Clune M, Maguire R, Griffin E, O'Connor J. Narcotic addiction: the expectant mother and her baby. *Ir Med J.* 1990;83(4):139–142.

24. Lallemant-Le Coeur S, Lallemant M. Twinning among HIV-infected mothers. *Lancet.* 1992; 339(Jan 4):66–67.

25. Bonney GE, Walker M, Gbedemah K, Konotey-Ahulu FID. Multiple births and visible birth defects in 13,000 consecutive deliveries in one Ghanaian Hospital. In: Nance WE, ed. *Twin Research: Biology and Epidemiology.* Prog Clin Biol Res. 1978;24B:105–108.

26. Gougeon A. Frequent occurrence of multiovular follicles and multinuclear oocytes in the adult human ovary. *Fertil Steril.* 1981;35:417–422.

27. Zeilmaker GH, Alberda AT, van Gent I. Fertilization and cleavage of oocytes from a binovular human ovarian follicle: a possible cause of dizygotic twinning and chimerism. *Fertil Steril.* 1983;40:841–843.

28. Benirschke K. Origin and significance of twinning. *Clin Obstet Gynecol.* 1972;15:220–235.

29. Wyshak G. Statistical findings on the effects of fertility drugs on plural births. In: Nance WE, ed. Twin Research: Biology and Epidemiology. *Prog Clin Biol Res.* 1978;24B:17–33.

30. Derom C, Derom R, Vlietinck R, Van den Berghe H, Thiery M. Increased monozygotic twinning rate after ovulation induction. *Lancet.* 1987;8544(May 30):1236–1238.

31. Spirtos NJ, Hayes MF, Magyar DM, Cossler NJ. Spontaneous abortion following ovulation induction. In: Hafez ESE, ed. *Spontaneous Abortion.* Hingham: MTP Press; 1984:81–98.

32. Bsat FA, Seoud MA-F. Superfetation secondary to ovulation induction with clomiphene citrate: a case report. *Fertil Steril* 1987;47:516–517.

33. Monga M, Reid RL. Superfoetation in the human: a case report. *J Soc Obstet Gynecol Can.* 1992; 14(2):81–84.

34. Schneider L, Bessis R, Simonnet T. The frequency of ovular resorption during the first trimester of twin pregnancy. *Acta Genet Med Gemellol.* 1979;28:271–272.

35. Cameron AH, Robson EB, Wade-Evans T, Wingham J. Septuplet conception: placental and zygosity studies. *J Obstet Gynecol Br Cwlth.* 1969; 76:692–698.

36. Beral V, Doyle P. Births in Great Britain resulting from assisted conception, 1978–1987. *Br Med J.* 1990;300:1229–1233.

37. Andrews MC, Muasher SJ, Levy DL, Jones HW, Garcia JE, Rosenwaks Z, Jones GS, Acosta AA. An analysis of the obstetric outcome of 125 consecutive pregnancies conceived in vitro and resulting in 100 deliveries. *Am J Obstet Gynecol.* 1986; 154:848–854.

38. In vitro baby born 15 months after twin. *The Vancouver Sun.* 1990;Jan 9:A6.

39. Rizk B, Tan SL, Morcos S, Riddle A, Brinsden P, Mason BA, Edwards RG. Heterotopic pregnancies after in vitro fertilization and embryo transfer. *Am J Obstet Gynecol.* 1991;164:161–164.

40. Yovich JL, Stanger JD, Grauaug A, Barter RA, Lunay G, Dawkins RL, Mulcahy MT. Monozygotic twins from in vitro fertilization. *Fertil Steril.* 1984;41:833–837.

41. Edwards R, Mettler L, Walters D. Identical twins and in vitro fertilization. *J In Vitro Fertil Embryo Trans.* 1986;3:114–117.

42. Englert Y, Imbert MC, van Rosendael E, Belaisch J, Segal L, Feichtinger W, Wilkin P, Frydman R, Leroy F. Morphological anomalies in the placenta of IVF pregnancies: preliminary report of a multicentric study. *Hum Reprod.* 1987;2:155–157.

43. Sauer MV, Lobo RA, Paulson RJ. Successful twin pregnancy after embryo donation to a patient with XY gonadal dysgenesis. *Am J Obstet Gynecol.* 1989;161:380–381.

44. Wenk RE, Houtz T, Brooks M, Chiafari FA. How frequent is heteropaternal superfecundation? *Acta Genet Med Gemellol.* 1992;41(1):43–47.

45. Feldman P. Sexuality, birth control and childbirth in orthodox Jewish tradition. *Can Med Assoc J.* 1992;146:29–33.

46. Gedda L. *Twins in History and Science.* Springfield: Charles C Thomas; 1961:127.

47. Terasaki PI, Gjertson D, Bernoco D, Perdue S, Mickey MR, Bond J. Twins with two different fathers identified by HLA. *N Engl J Med.* 1978;299:590–592.

48. Májský A, Kout M. Another case of occurrence of two different fathers of twins by HLA typing. *Tissue Antigens.* 1982;20:305.

49. Nance WE, Winter PM, Segreti WO, Corey LA, Parisi-Prinzi G, Parisi P. A search for evidence of hereditary superfetation in man. In: Nance W, ed. Twin Research: Biology and Epidemiology. *Prog Clin Biol Res.* 1978;24B:65–70.

50. James WH. Gestational age in twins. *Arch Dis Child.* 1980;55:281–284.

51. Nance WE. Malformations unique to the twinning process. In: Gedda L, Parisi P, Nance WE, eds. Twin Research 3: Twin Biology and Multiple Pregnancy. *Prog Clin Biol Res.* 1981;69A:123–133.

52. Dubowitz V, Dubowitz LMS. Inaccuracy of Dubowitz gestational age in low birth weight infants (Letter). *Obstet Gynecol.* 1985;65:601–602.

53. Gedda L. *Twins in History and Science.* Springfield: Charles C Thomas; 1961:101–105.

54. Miller WL. Recombinant DNA and the pediatrician. *Pediatrics.* 1981;99:1–15.

55. Landegren U, Kaiser R, Caskey CT, Hood L. DNA diagnostics—molecular techniques and automation. *Science.* 1988;242:229–237.

56. Rudd NL, Dimnik LS, Greentree C, Mendes-Crabb K, Hoar DI. The use of DNA probes to establish parental origin in Down syndrome. *Hum Genet.* 1988;78:175–178.

57. Benirschke K, Driscoll SG. *The Pathology of the Human Placenta.* New York: Springer-Verlag; 1967:91–179.

58. Strong SJ, Corney G. *The Placenta in Twin Pregnancies.* Norwich: Pergamon Press; 1967:14–77.

59. Golan A, Amit A, Baram A, David MP. Unusual cord intertwining in monoamniotic twins. *Aust NZ J Obstet Gynecol.* 1981;22:165–167.

60. Boklage CE. On the timing of monozygotic twinning events. In: Gedda L, Parisi P, Nance WE, eds. Twin Research 3: Twin Biology and Multiple Pregnancy. *Prog Clin Biol Res.* 1981;69A:155–165.

61. Coté GB, Gyftodimou J. Twinning and mitotic crossing over: some possibilities and their implications. *Am J Hum Genet.* 1991;49:120–130.

62. Hall JG. Genomic imprinting: review and relevance to human diseases. *Am J Hum Genet.* 1990;46:857–873.

63. Solter D. Differential imprinting and expression of maternal and paternal genomes. *Annu Rev Genet.* 1988;22:127–164.

64. Storrs EE, Williams RJ. A study of monozygous quadruplet armadillos in relation to mammalian inheritance. *Proc Natl Acad Sci USA.* 1968;60:910–914.

65. De Robertis EM, Oliver G, Wright CVE. Homeobox genes and the vertebrate body plan. *Sci Am.* 1990;263(1):46–52.

66. Winchester B, Young E, Geddes S, Genet S, Hurst J, Middleton-Price H, Williams N, Webb M, Habel A, Malcolm S. Female twin with Hunter disease due to nonrandom inactivation of the x-chromosome: a consequence of twinning. *Am J Med Genet.* 1992;44(6):834–838.

67. Gedda L, Brenci G, Franceschetti A, Talone C, Zipparo R. A study of mirror imaging in twins. In: Gedda L, Parisi P, Nance WE, eds. Twin Research 3: Twin Biology and Multiple Pregnancy. *Prog Clin Biol Res.* 1981;69A:167–168.

68. Stockard CR. Developmental rate and structural expression: an experimental study of twins, "double monsters" and single deformities, and the interaction among embryonic organs during their origin and development. *Am J Anat.* 1921;28:115–277.

69. Segreti WO, Winter PM, Nance WE. Familial studies in monozygotic twinning. In: Nance WE, ed. Twin Research: Biology and Epidemiology. *Prog Clin Biol Res.* 1978;24B:55–60.

70. Smith DW, Bartlett C, Harrah LM. Monozygotic twinning and the Duhamel anomalad (imperforate anus to sirenomelia): a non-random association between two aberrations in morphogenesis. *Birth Defects.* 1976;12(5):53–63.

71. Bomsel-Helmreich O. Delayed ovulation and monozygotic twinning in the rabbit (abstract). *Acta Genet Med Gemellol.* 1974;23:19.

72. Zwilling E. Survival and non-sorting of nodal cells following dissociation and reaggregation of definitive streak chick embryos. *Dev Biol.* 1963;7:642–652.

73. Myrianthopoulos NC. Congenital malformations in twins: epidemiologic survey. *Birth Defects.* 1975;11(8):1–39.

74. Burn J, Corney G. Zygosity determination and the types of twinning. In: MacGillivray I, Campbell DM, Thompson B, eds. *Twinning and Twins.* Chichester: John Wiley; 1988;7–25.

75. Gedda L. *Twins in History and Science.* Springfield: Charles C Thomas; 1961:128–129.

76. Bieber FR, Nance WE, Morton CC, Brown JA, Redwine FO, Jordon RL, Mohanakumar T. Genetic studies of an acardiac monster: evidence of polar body twinning in man. *Science.* 1981; 213:775–777.

77. Hertig AT. On the development of the amnion and exocoelomic membrane in the pre-villus human embryo. *Yale J Biol Med.* 1945;18:107–115.

78. Boklage CE. Twinning, nonrighthandedness, and fusion malformations: evidence for heritable causal elements held in common. *Am J Med Genet.* 1987;28:67–84.

79. Mortimer G. Zygosity and placental structure in monochorionic twins. *Acta Genet Med Gemellol.* 1987;36:417–420.

80. Benirschke K, Kaufmann P. *Pathology of the Human Placenta*. 2nd ed. New York: Springer-Verlag; 1990:718–720.

81. Uchida IA, Freeman VCP, Gedeon M, Goldmaker J. Twinning rate in spontaneous abortions. *J Hum Genet*. 1983;35:987–993.

82. Flannery DB, Brown JA, Redwine FO, Winter P, Nance WE. Antenatally detected Kleinfelter's syndrome in twins. *Acta Genet Med Gemellol*. 1984;33:51–56.

83. Windham GC, Sever LE. Neural tube defects among twin births. *Am J Hum Genet*. 1982;34:988–998.

84. Wright JCY, Christopher CR. Sirenomelia, Potter's syndrome and their relationship to monozygotic twinning (a case report and discussion). *J Reprod Med*. 1982;27:291–294.

85. Rowe MI, Ravitch MM, Ranniger K. Operative correction of caudal duplication (dipygus). *Surgery*. 1968;63:840–848.

86. German JC, Mahour GH, Wooley MM. The twin with esophageal atresia. *J Pediatr Surg*. 1979; 14:432–435.

87. Harvey MAS, Huntley RMC, Smith DW. Familial monozygotic twinning. *J Pediatr*. 1977;90:246–248.

88. Shapiro LR, Zemek L, Shulman MJ. Genetic etiology for monozygotic twinning. *Birth Defects*. 1978;14(6A):219–222.

89. Schinzel AAGL, Smith DW, Miller JR. Monozygotic twinning and structural defects. *J Pediatr*. 1979;95:921–930.

90. Macourt DC, Stewart P, Zaki M. Multiple pregnancy and fetal abnormalities in association with oral contraceptive use. *Aust NZ J Obstet Gynecol*. 1982;22:25–28.

91. James WH. Sex ratio and placentation in twins. *Ann Hum Biol*. 1980;7:273–276.

92. Potter EL, Craig JM. *Pathology of the Fetus and the Infant*. 3rd ed. Chicago: Year Book Medical Publishers; 1975:207–237.

93. Mettler L, Riedel H-H, Grillo M, Michelmann HW, Baukloh V, Weisner D, Semm K, Bastert G, Hack HJ. Schwangerschaft und geburt monozygoter weiblicher zwillinge nach In-vitro-fertilization und Embryotransfer (IVF-ET). *Geburtshilfe Frauenheilkd*. 1984;44:670–676.

94. Bugalho A, Strolego F, Carlomagno G. Outcomes of twin pregnancies at the Hospital Central of Maputo: retrospective study of 315 consecutive twin deliveries, January 1–September 30, 1987. *Int J Gynecol Obstet*. 1989;29:297–300.

95. Marivate M, Norman RJ. Twins. *Clin Obstet Gynecol*. 1982;9(3):723–743.

96. Onyskowova Z, Dolezal A, Jedlicka V. The frequency and character of malformations in multiple births (a preliminary report). *Teratology*. 1971; 4:496–497.

97. Zahálková M. Perinatal and infant mortality in twins. In: Nance WE, ed. Twin Research: Biology and Epidemiology. *Prog Clin Biol Res*. 1978; 24B:115–120.

98. Hoffman HJ, Bakketeig LS, Stark CR. Twins and perinatal mortality: a comparison between single and twin births in Minnesota and in Norway, 1967–1973. In: Nance WE, ed. Twin Research: Biology and Epidemiology. *Prog Clin Biol Res*. 1978;24B:133–142.

99. Grothe W, Rüttgers H. Twin pregnancies: an 11 year review. *Acta Genet Med Gemellol*. 1985;34:49–58.

100. Robertson EG, Neer KJ. Placental injection studies in twin gestation. *Am J Obstet Gynecol*. 1983;147:170–174.

101. Emanuel I, Huang S-W, Gutman LT, Yu F-C, Lin C-C. The incidence of congenital malformations in a Chinese population: the Taipei collaborative study. *Teratology*. 1972;5:159–169.

102. Chandra P, Harilal KT. Plural births—mortality and morbidity. In: Nance WE, ed. Twin Research: Biology and Epidemiology. *Prog Clin Biol Res*. 1978;24B:109–114.

103. Shah SB, Patel DN. Twinning and structural defects. *Indian Pediatr*. 1984;21:475–478.

104. Ho SK, Wu PYK. Perinatal factors and neonatal morbidity in twin pregnancy. *Am J Obstet Gynecol*. 1975;122:979–987.

105. Boklage CE. Survival probability of human conceptus from fertilization to term. *Int J Fertil*. 1990;35:75–94.

106. Robinson HP, Caines JS. Sonar evidence of early pregnancy failure in patients with twin conceptions. *Br J Obstet Gynecol*. 1977;84:22–25.

107. Åkesson HO, Smith GF, Thrybom Br. Twinning and associated stillbirths in Sweden, 1871-1960. *Hereditas*. 1970;64:193–198.

108. James WH. Excess of like-sexed pairs of dizygotic twins. *Nature*. 1971;232:277–278.

109. Cameron AH, Edwards JH, Derom R, Thiery M, Boelaert R. The value of twin surveys in the study of malformations. *Eur J Obstet Gynecol Reprod Biol*. 1983;14:347–356.

110. Corney G. Twin placentation and some effects on twins of known zygosity. In: Nance WE, ed. Twin Research: Biology and Epidemiology. *Prog Clin Biol Res*. 1978;24B:9–16.

111. Layde PM, Erickson JD, Falek A, McCarthy BJ. Congenital malformations in twins. *Am J Hum Genet*. 1980;32:69–78.

112. Hrubec Z, Robinette CD. The study of human twins in medical research. *N Engl J Med*. 1984;310:435–441.

113. Shanklin DR, Perrin EVDK. Multiple gestation. In: Perrin EVDK, ed. *Pathology of the Placenta*. New York: Churchill Livingstone; 1984:165–182.

114. James W. A hypothesis on the declining dizygotic twinning rates in developed countries. In: Nance WE, ed. Twin Research: Biology and Epidemiology. *Prog Clin Biol Res*. 1978;24B:81–88.

115. Lazar P, Hemon D, Berger C. Twinning rate and reproductive failure. In: Nance WE, ed. Twin Research: Biology and Epidemiology. *Prog Clin Biol Res*. 1978;24B:125–132.

116. Twins at Jerusalem (Editorial). *Lancet*. 1980;2:244–245.

117. Smith SM, Penrose LS. Monozygotic and dizygotic twin diagnosis. *Ann Hum Genet*. 1955;19:273–289.

118. Corney G, Robson EB. Types of twinning and determination of zygosity. In: MacGillivray I, Nylander PPS, Corney G, eds. *Human Multiple Reproduction*. Philadelphia: WB Saunders; 1975:16–39.

119. Gedda L. *Twins in History and Science*. Springfield: Charles C Thomas; 1961:155–214.

120. Kalousek DK, Dill FJ. Chromosomal mosaicism confined to the placenta in human conceptions. *Science*. 1983;221:665–667.

121. Fisher RA, Sheppard DM, Lawler SD. Twin pregnancy with complete hydatidiform mole (46,XX) and fetus (46,XY): genetic origin proved by analysis of chromosome polymorphism. *Br Med J*. 1982;284:1218–1220.

122. Das Chaddhuri AB. Effecient sequential search of genetic systems for diagnosis of twin zygosity. *Acta Genet Med Gemellol*. 1991;40:159–164.

123. Kovacs B, Shahbahrami B, Platt LD, Comings DE. Molecular genetic prenatal determination of twin zygosity. *Obstet Gynecol*. 1988;72:954–956.

124. Hill AVS, Jeffreys AJ. Use of mini-satellite DNA probes for determination of twin zygosity at birth. *Lancet*. 1985;2:1394–1395.

125. Azuma C, Kamiura S, Nobunaga T, Negoro T, Saji F, Tanizawa O. Zygosity determination of multiple pregnancy by deoxyribonucleic acid fingerprints. *Am J Obstet Gynecol*. 1989;160:734–736.

126. Gilgenkrantz S, Marchal C, Wendremaire Ph, Seger M. Cytogenetic and antigenic studies in a pair of twins: a normal boy and a trisomic girl with chimera. In: Gedda L, Parisi P, Nance WE, eds. Twin Research 3: Twin Biology and Multiple Pregnancy. *Prog Clin Biol Res*. 1981;69A:141–153.

3
The Placenta in Multiple Pregnancy

The pathologist's contribution to the analysis of multiple pregnancy is twofold—surgical pathology of the placentation, and autopsy pathology of any deceased fetus(es) or infant(s). The easiest and most obvious examination is documentation of placental morphology, but unfortunately this is still often quite incomplete.

Some aspects of the pathology of the placenta in multiple pregnancy have received attention for years, and particularly outstanding is the late 19th century contribution of Schatz to the study of vascular communications.[1,2] Systematic approaches to all aspects of the pathology of the placenta in multiple gestation have been contributed by Strong and Corney,[2] Boyd and Hamilton,[3] Benirschke and Driscoll,[4] Potter and Craig,[5] Fox,[6] Shanklin and Perrin,[7] and Benirschke and Kaufmann,[8] and these excellent references can be consulted for additional details and other examples of the topics discussed in this chapter.

The first of two aspects of placenta examination in multiple gestation is the examination for those lesions that are also encountered in singleton gestations. The gross and microscopic appearances of single artery umbilical cords, meconium staining of membranes, premature separation or abruption of the maternal surface, villitis, and villus ischemia and villus infarcts, to mention only a few examples, are the same in multiples' placentas as in those of singletons. These lesions are discussed in detail in the other chapters dealing with placental pathology in general, in many of the volumes cited above.[4–8] Some of these lesions are particularly important in the placentas of multiple pregnancy, and they are discussed in the relevant sections that follow. For example, much of the perinatal mortality and morbidity in multiple gestation is attributable to preterm delivery, and some of the potential factors initiating labor may be identified on the placenta. In fact, it was their studies of placentas from twin pregnancies that led Benirschke and Driscoll[4] to the conclusion that ascending infection was the major pathogenetic mechanism of chorioamnionitis. They found that the membranes of the leading twin were the only ones that were inflamed or were the more severely inflamed of the two in all those cases where placental anatomy could be correlated with birth order (Fig. 3.1.) In another example, asphyxia of the second fetus is a particular concern in twin pregnancies and evidence for a possible cause, such as a cord problem or abruption, and its duration and severity, such as meconium staining, may be assessed in the placenta.

The second aspect of placental morphology with twins or greater multiples includes those features unique to, and due to, the multiple nature of the gestation. Specifically, these are the pattern of the disk and membrane relationships, and the pattern and degree of anastomoses of the chorionic vasculature. While the disk and membrane relationships do not always identify the zygosity of the infants, the patterns of placentation may have other significance for fetal development, particularly overall growth.[9,10] The consequences of the various patterns of intertwin anastomotic vascularization can be bizarre (see Chapter 9) and can influence twin development from early gestation to the neonatal period. If the placental examination is inadequate in these cases of suboptimal outcome, an erroneous attribution of causation may be made with inaccu-

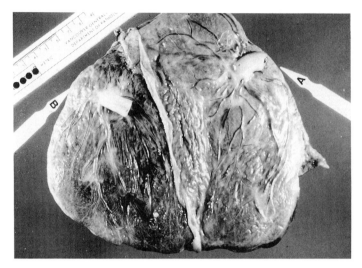

FIGURE 3.1. In this dichorionic diamniotic fused twin placenta at 25 weeks' gestation, the cloudiness of twin A's portion of the chorionic surface is due to marked fetal and maternal acute inflammation. The surface in side B is clear grossly, although there was early mild acute inflammation on that side as well microscopically. This differential picture supports the concept of acute chorioamnionitis as an ascending infection, with greater infection and inflammation in the sac over the cervix.

rate conclusions drawn and inappropriate counseling given. Therefore, before the discussion of the findings in multiple gestation placentas, it is important to review the process of examination of the twin placenta.

Examination of Twin Placentas—Procedures and Techniques

Careful examination of the placentation (placenta or placentas) from a multiple gestation is important, and need not be viewed as an intimidating prospect. A great deal of information can be gained from efficient examination, even on a busy surgical pathology service, and special cases can be identified and set aside to be processed with more painstaking techniques at a more convenient time. Those in the fortunate position of having research space, time, and funding can employ the specialized injection procedures and dissection studies described in the references given.

Placentas from multiple gestations are sufficiently infrequent in most hospitals that all should be examined, whether in the local laboratory or at a larger reference center. Fresh tissues are easier to examine and more valuable information can be obtained from them than from fixed specimens, but examination of a fixed placenta is better than no examination at all.

The most important procedure, prior to the examination of a multiple pregnancy placentation, is accurate identification of the umbilical cords. Speculations as to birth order can sometimes be made on the basis of patterns of membrane rupture, thickness of umbilical cords correlated with stated fetal weights, evidence of ascending infection in one sac, or maceration changes associated with a dead twin, but there is no guaranteed method of reconstruction of the gestation without proper labeling of the cords. This becomes particularly critical when the placental findings based on birth order must be correlated with ultrasound appearances, birth complications, fetal/infant death, or perinatal problems. The potential medicolegal implications are self-evident. One approach might be to suggest to clinical colleagues that they mark the cord of the first-born twin by transfixing it with a safety pin—an item that can be sterilized and placed on every delivery tray.[11] Once the cords have been distinguished in the case room, it is also helpful for this information to be indicated appropriately on the requisition accompanying the specimen, e.g., "cord A marked with pin," or some such phrase, because not everyone will mark the cords the same way, no matter what the guidelines might be. How the cords have been assigned must be part of the report. If there was no indication, the pathologist must make some differentiation and dictate that information into the report.

In their approach to twin placentas, Shanklin and Perrin[7] emphasize the value of clinical information

FIGURE 3.2. Most placentas from multiple pregnancy can be examined adequately with the equipment illustrated—forceps, scissors, scalpel, knife, ruler, weight scale and syringe.

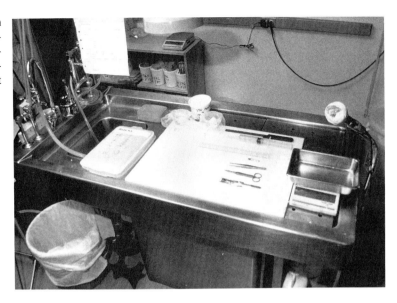

that includes general and obstetric maternal history, family history, details of the current pregnancy, labor and delivery, and details of the infants' sex, weight, condition, and course. Such information certainly enhances interpretation of the placental findings. Knowledge of ultrasonic findings during pregnancy is also useful, particularly with regard to relative fetal growth, fluid volumes, and embryonic or fetal death during pregnancy.

The actual physical setup for the placental examination, the procedure for recording the results and submitting tissues for processing, and the storage of tissues, reports, and pictures will vary in different laboratories. Blood precautions are required, and having a sink adjacent is convenient. The specific equipment required is minimal and likely already available in most anatomic pathology services (Fig. 3.2):

sharp medium-length scissors
medium-sized nontoothed forceps
scalpel with #22 blade; long bladed sharp knife
    may be preferred by some
long metal ruler
direct weight scale with a dish large enough for a
    placenta; metal pie plate is perfect
50 cc syringe and #20, #18, and #25 needles.

In addition, an overhead light with a magnifying lens is often helpful, and a nearby photography setup is invaluable. On a busy service with restricted assistance, dictation of findings during the examination and processing of sections taken from fresh tissue is efficient and adequate for most specimens. Representative portions of tissue can be saved in a small container when storage areas are at a premium, and blocks, slides, and reports can be stored, along with other surgical cases, in accessioned numerical sequence. If a checklist form is used to record findings, it must be designed with enough flexibility to accommodate the variations encountered in multiple placentations. Some may prefer a narrative approach, and with computerized reporting, the several phases of gross and microscopic dictations, with conclusions and diagnoses, have to be transcribed only once, a considerable saving of secretarial time and of paper, if only one printed copy is produced. The reports are distributed as usual for the individual service, but a pathologist specifically interested in placental pathology may find it valuable to keep his or her own record of all or selected cases for purposes of reference and follow-up.

Initial Orientation

Twin placentations may consist of two separate disks and gestational sacs, two distinct disks with shared/overlapping sac membranes, or one disk with various membrane patterns. If the twin placentation consists of two separate disks, each with its own cord and membranes (Fig. 3.3), each can be processed in turn, usually in order of birth. Obser-

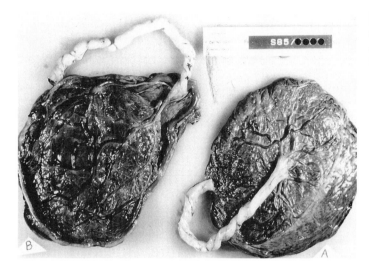

FIGURE 3.3. Twin placentation—dichorionic diamniotic; separate pattern—separate and distinct placentas; each with attached cord and membranes.

vations are made analogous to those made of a singleton placenta. Particular note is made of anomalies of the cord and cord insertion, and it is important to record the relative sizes/weights of the disks in order to collate this information with the fetal weights. The usual sections are taken for histologic examination (Fig. 3.4). When the disks are separate but have partially fused or overlapping membranes (Fig. 3.5), note is made of the appearances—the percentage of overlap—and a section

taken of the septum as outlined below. The single-disk or fused placenta can be oriented on a flat surface with the first delivered twin's portion to the right (Fig. 3.6). It may take some manipulation of the specimen to orient the disk, membranes, and cords to as near as possible the intrauterine position, but this is helpful in appreciating the overall arrangement of the specimen.

The subsequent examination of the fused/single disk, as described in the following sections, is done in a specific order so as to make the most efficient use of the examiner's time. It is wise to develop an habitual approach to the basics of the examination, so that inevitable interruptions do not lead to forgotten data.

Cords and Membranes

When processing a single-disk twin placenta, it is helpful to examine the components from both twins in each segment of the examination in turn, rather than try to do all the observations for one twin and then the other. The cord of the first twin is measured and examined as usual for the number of vessels, insertion site/manner, and any abnormalities, before being removed 1 cm from the placental surface and serially sectioned along its length. If the insertion is velamentous, the distance from the margin of the placenta should be recorded and the path of the intramembranous vessels described with comments as to their type, intactness, and final insertion onto the placenta. If there are no abnormalities, two portions are submitted for histological examination,

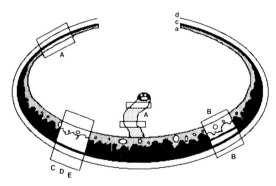

FIGURE 3.4. The amnion (a), chorion (c), and decidual (d) layers of the placenta. In block A are the membrane roll and two cross sections of the umbilical cord, one each at the fetal and placental ends. In block B, there is one random section of fetal surface, making sure that chorionic vessels and amnion are included, plus a random section of maternal surface. In blocks C, D, and E are random full-thickness sections of mid- to lateral (but not peripheral) parenchyma from fetal to maternal surfaces. Additional sections are taken as the findings indicate.

FIGURE 3.5. Twin placentation—dichorionic diamniotic—separate disks with shared overlapping membranes pattern. The disks are distinct, but the adjacent reflected membranes have fused, and can overlap one (a) or both (b) placentas. In (a), the white line indicates the margin of the disk that is hidden by the membrane overlap.

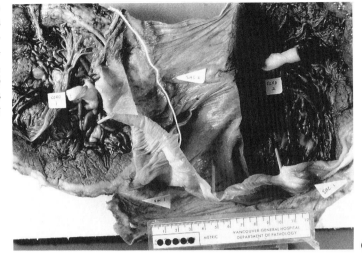

(a)

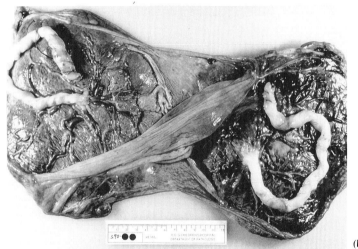

(b)

one each from the placental and fetal ends of the cord. Any lesions are sectioned as well. The outer free membranes, the chorion laeve, of this twin's side of the placenta are examined next as usual, determining the rupture site, if possible, and recording the same features as with a singleton placenta. A membrane roll is submitted for histology in the usual manner, but do not remove all the remaining membranes yet (Fig. 3.7). Then the cord and membranes of the other twin are examined and described similarly, noting in addition the distance between the insertions of the two cords.

Septum

The nature of the membrane wall between twins who share a single placental disk is critical informa-tion. This wall may still be intact, or may have been the site of rupture as the second twin was born. This may be a tentative clue to birth order if the cords were not marked in the case room (Fig. 3.8). The line of attachment of the septum on the disk surface is described with an indication of the proportions of the chorionic plate on either side, and the relation of its attachment to the apparent vascular equator of the two chorionic circulations (Fig. 3.9). An initial assessment as to the membranes it contains can be made. If it contains chorion, it will be firmly fixed to the placental surface with a ridge along its base of attachment because it is continuous with the underlying parenchyma. (This ridge can be seen in Fig. 3.1.) It will be variably opaque, depending on the thickness of the chorion layers, and the amnion layers can be dissected off either

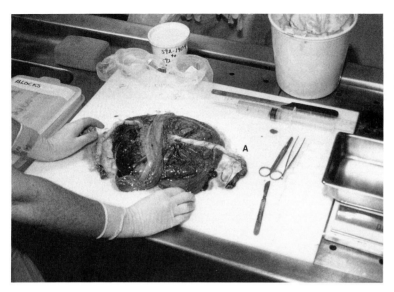

FIGURE 3.6. The single-disk twin placenta can be oriented so that the first delivered twin's portion (A) (indicated by one suture tie) is on the right. This orientation can be maintained so as to be clear which twin's portion is being examined throughout the process.

side. If it consists of amnion only, two layers will be definable, it generally will be quite filmy, and it is easily removed from the chorionic surface because it is not attached. A membrane roll sample of the separating membranes is submitted for histology, and may be accompanied by a section of the site of attachment at the chorionic plate, the "T" section. All the remaining membranes can be trimmed off at the placental margin, but be sure to continue to keep track of which cord is which (Fig. 3.10).

The amnion lining of the gestational sac tends to separate from the underlying chorionic surface more readily as gestation proceeds, and it is often nearly completely separated in the delivered term placenta. Thus, if no septum or separating membrane is identified, great care must be taken to make sure that there is a continuous and complete covering of amnion over the chorionic surface between the cord insertions, and/or that there is no remnant of diamniotic separating membrane attached to remnants of the chorion laeve. An apparent single sac that is actually due to complete separation of the amnion is more common than a truly single monoamniotic sac.

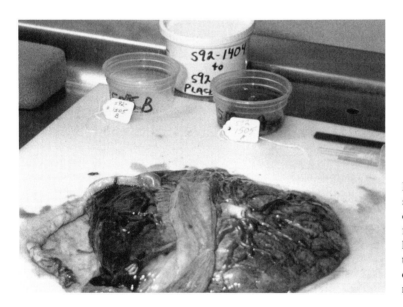

FIGURE 3.7. At this stage of the stepwise examination of a single-disk twin placenta, the cord and free membranes of the first twin have been described and sections taken. The cord and membranes of the second twin are examined next, followed by the septum.

FIGURE 3.8. In this dichorionic diamniotic fused twin placenta, the outer membranes of sac A (cord with suture tie) are torn. Through the gap can be seen the rupture site in the separating membranes or septum, through which twin B was born. All other membranes of sac B were intact. This pattern of membrane rupture may be a clue to birth order if the cords are not labeled.

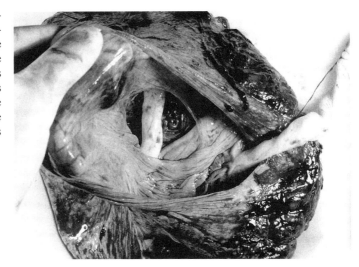

FIGURE 3.9. The line of attachment of the septum between the twins in a single-disk placenta is worth noting. In the dichorionic diamniotic placenta (a), the thick membrane is usually located at the chorionic vascular equator between the twins, so that its attachment (arrowheads) serves as a way of describing the partitioning of the chorionic surface to each twin. In this case, the division is nearly symmetrical. In the monochorionic diamniotic placenta (b), the septum contains amnion only, so the attachment can be quite independent of the chorionic vascular equator between the twins, and in this case is at 90° to the zone between the circulations (a slightly curved line between the arrowheads and through the diamond). However, the respective proportions of chorionic surface vascularized from each twin still need to be recorded. This diamniotic layer is quite filmy compared to a septum with chorion in it. In this picture it has been rolled in order to make it more visible.

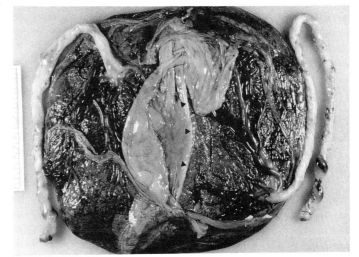

(a)

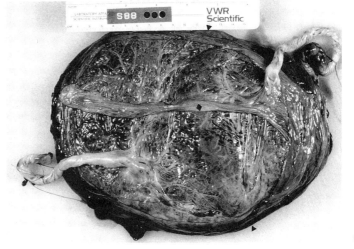

(b)

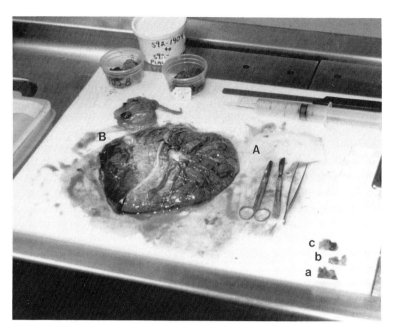

FIGURE 3.10. At this stage of the stepwise examination of a single-disk twin placenta, the cords and free membranes of both twins have been described and sampled, as has the septum. Cord and membranes of twin A are in block a, and of twin B in block b, and the septum in c. Alternatively, specimens from twin A's side can be sequential in blocks a–e, then the septum in f, and then blocks from twin B's side. The specific routine is less important than the routine use of a complete process.

Chorionic Vessels and Injection Studies

Both the overall pattern of chorionic vascularization, and the specific pattern of intertwin vascular connections, are critical observations to make of twin placentas. Particularly important is the relative proportion of the chorionic surface occupied by vessels from each twin. Asymmetries of this pattern can be significant regarding overall fetal development in any pattern of twin placenta, but particularly with the fused or single disk, regardless of the type of septum (Fig. 3.11). Intertwin vascular anastomoses are frequent in those fused placentas with a septum of amnion only, or with no septum at all, and often very significant to fetal development, so every effort should be made to demonstrate and provide detailed descriptions of any anastomoses in these cases. Contrary to some reports,[12] it cannot be assumed that vascular anastomoses are always present in a monochorionic placenta. Also, contrary to these same reports, anastomoses in fused placentas with septa that contain chorion are rare and require precise documentation.

Vascular anastomoses between the twins can be of two main types—surface artery to artery (arterial) or vein to vein (venous) connections, or arteriovenous connections through the parenchyma (parenchymal). In compound anastomoses, bidirectional or surface and parenchymal connections are present from the same vessels. In order to see the vessels better, it is helpful to strip the amnion from the surface of the placenta, along the vascular equator, the zone where the circulations approach each other. Visual identification of the direct surface anastomoses (Fig. 3.12), arterial or venous, can often be confirmed by simply shunting blood back and forth by compressing the vessels. Generally, the arteries are the superficial vessels and the veins the deeper vessels on the chorionic surface,[4,7] although the peripheral branches may occasionally reverse this pattern.[13] When in doubt, trace the vessel back toward the umbilical cord insertion. Confirmation of these surface anastomoses can be made by injection. "Third circulation" anastomoses, arterial-capillary-venous parenchymal anastomoses, can be suspected grossly by identifying unaccompanied vessels from each twin that terminate close to each other on the chorionic surface (Fig. 3.12). Ordinarily, each artery has an accompanying vein and they penetrate the chorionic plate within millimeters of each other. An artery from one twin that penetrates the chorionic surface adjacent to a vein from the other twin is a potential site of a shared cotyledon. This requires confirmation by injection and sectioning of the subjacent lobes, an obvious drawback of the examination of the fixed placenta.

Each examiner has his or her own preferred

FIGURE 3.11. Asymmetric vascularization of the chorionic surface in a single-disk twin placenta can be seen whether the septum contains chorion (a) or not (b). In the dichorionic diamniotic placenta (a), vessels from twin A occupy about one-third of the surface, and vessels from twin B about two-thirds. These were girl/boy twins and the girl (A) was 35% smaller than her co-twin boy (B), even though twin B also had a single artery cord. In the monochorionic diamniotic placenta (b), the vascular equator is closer to cord B than cord A (along a curved line joining arrows) in spite of the placement of the septum, so that the vascularization is asymmetric, about one-third to B and two-thirds to A. The smaller twin B was only 10% less than her co-twin in weight, but there were intertwin anastomoses that likely modified the effect of the chorionic asymmetry; an arterial and a parenchymal shunt from A to B were demonstrated.

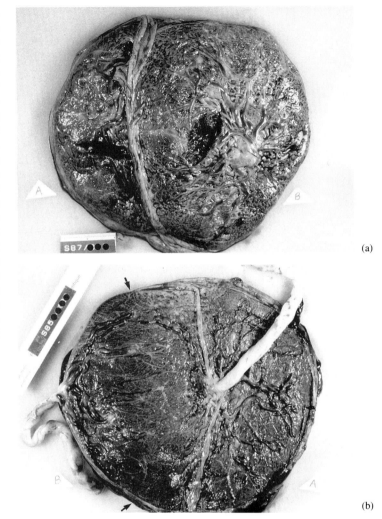

(a)

(b)

method of injection of chorionic vessels of placentas, and each method has advantages and drawbacks. If permanent records are desired, injected radiopaque materials can be x-rayed, or colored material, such as milk, trypan blue suspension, or India ink, that will not diffuse out of the vessels, can be photographed. Care is required with these methods to prevent extravasation of the injected material, which would interfere with interpretation and documentation. An advantage of ink particles is that they can be seen in the vessels injected even after histologic processing. A variety of complex perfusion techniques have been described[14,15] and they may provide more accurate and complete assessment of vascular connections, particularly of parenchymal anastomoses, than less time consuming

methods. Depending on the circumstances, however, satisfactory compromises are possible. Forceps and a 50-cc syringe with a 21 or 25 gauge needle are adequate for most specimens, using air as the injected material. There are reported disadvantages with air—for example, that a meniscus may prevent adequate perfusion of small vessels.[2] However, injected vessels can be photographed (Fig. 3.13a), and shared cotyledons may be identifiable as an area of pale or bloodless villi in the placenta slices, so an estimate of the volume of the shared area can be made (Fig. 3.13b). Injection is made close to the areas of suspected anastomosis to avoid artifactual filling of nearby branches (Fig. 3.14), and the injection pressure is slow and steady to avoid disrupting the parenchyma. The size of vessel

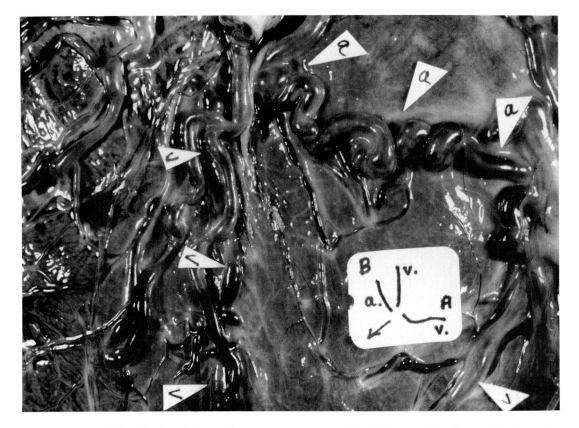

FIGURE 3.12. In this close-up view of the vascular equator between two cords in a monochorionic diamniotic placenta from which the septal membranes have been removed, three intertwin vascular anastomoses are shown. There is a convoluted arterial (aaa) anastomosis between the bases of the cords and a more wavy venous (vvvv) anastomosis that is longer and partly out of the picture. In the center is an arteriovenous or parenchymal anastomosis that is actually a compound anastomosis, where one artery from cord B connects through the parenchymal villus tissue circulation to both a vein of its own plus a vein from cord A. This is drawn on the label for clarity.

that can be injected is limited only by the skill of the examiner.

Details of any anastomosis identified should be recorded, including the size and type of vessels involved, an indication as to which twin the vessels came from in arterial or venous connections of different sized vessels, and the twin of origin of the arteries and veins of parenchymal and compound shunts. The written description can be supplemented by drawings and photographs and, in complex cases, a line drawing may be particularly helpful (Fig. 3.15). For those who are interested in visual shorthand, a scheme such as in Fig. 3.16 may be useful as well.

Disks

Finally, the mass of the placental parenchyma can be analyzed. The overall shape and outline of the disk is described, and it is measured and weighed. The maximum diameter of the disk and its width at 90° are measured. Thickness can be assessed in the intact placenta, or after serially slicing the parenchyma. In the intact placenta, a scalpel blade is inserted from the maternal surface to the chorionic surface perpendicularly to the examining table. The level of the surface of the decidual plate is noted on the blade with the thumb, or forceps, and then measured against a ruler. Such measurements can

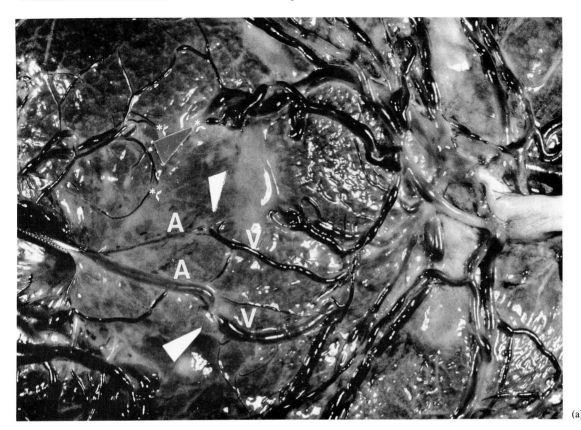

(a)

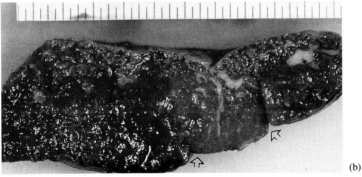

(b)

FIGURE 3.13. While there may be some drawbacks to the use of air as an injection medium for demonstration of intertwin vascular anastomoses, injected vessels such as the parenchymal anastomosis in (a) can be photographed for documentation, and the volume of the shared cotyledon can be assessed by the volume of pale villi (between arrows) in the placental cross section (b), created by the injected air displacing fetal blood in villus capillaries. Note that in (a), air can be seen in both the artery (A) and vein (V) of the two parenchymal anastomoses (white card pointers), involving vessels of 2-mm diameter in the larger one and 0.5- to 1-mm diameter in the smaller one. Note also how the artery and vein of these two anastomoses insert near each other and without accompanying respective vein or artery. This is in contrast to the three pairs of vessels at each of the three points of the dark card pointer (small white stars) where vessels of the artery-vein pair are both from the same umbilical cord, two from one side and one from the other. (Forceps are seen blocking the backflow of air in the largest anastomosis.)

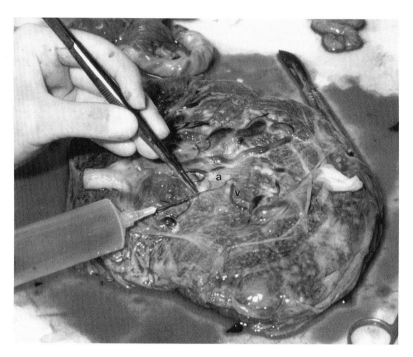

FIGURE 3.14. Injection to demonstrate parenchymal (arteriovenous) or compound anastomoses is done by locating an artery (a) from one twin that enters the placenta near a vein (v) from the other twin. Air is injected into the artery near this spot with slow, steady pressure, preventing backflow with forceps and noting if air comes up into the vein.

be made at several points in the intact placenta to gain an estimate of variation in thickness. This method of measurement should not be done until after any injection studies are completed. It may be useful to determine placental volume by displacement, but certainly placental weight must be recorded as usual, to the nearest 5 g. The chorionic and maternal surfaces are examined as usual, with comments made as to differences between the two sides, particularly of color and texture of the maternal surface. Finally, the placenta is serially sliced at 1-cm intervals, from the maternal surface, parallel to the axis between the cords if possible. Comparisons are made between the chorionic tissues of each side, the volume of shared cotyledons is determined if possible, and any other features noted as usual. Routine histologic sections consist of chorionic surface from each side, including vessels and amnion, maternal surface from each side, and full thickness blocks from each side, as in Fig. 3.4. Further sections are dictated by the findings.

Histology

The histologic review of the tissues from twin placentas is the same as of singleton placentas with the addition of documentation of the components of the separating membranes and a comparison of the findings in the villous tissues from each twin. Even monochorionic twin placentas can have considerably discordant microscopic findings in the villus tissue, and this discrepancy may be clinically significant (see low birth weight discussion in Chapter 6).

Triplets or More

The approach to placentations from higher multiples of gestation is simply a methodical expansion of the above techniques with careful attention to precise documentation of membrane relationships and vascular patterns.

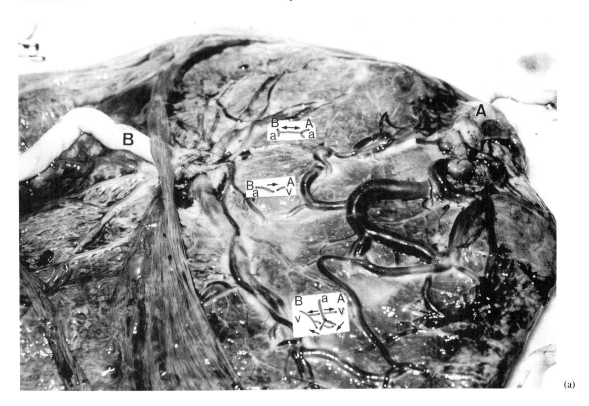

(a)

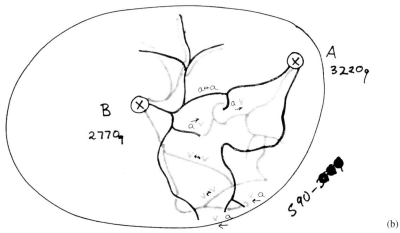

(b)

FIGURE 3.15. Although a written text description of demonstrated anastomosis is essential, some cases benefit with the use of drawings as well. In this case, a close-up of the region of anastomosis has been photographed (a) with superimposed labels identifying the twin of origin (A and B), vessel type [artery (a), vein (v)], and direction of flow (arrows). A supplemental drawing (b) to clarify the pattern of anastomosis is also helpful and can become part of the record and referred to in discussion. (Reprinted with permission from Baldwin VJ, *Developmental Pathology of the Embryo and Fetus*, JB Lippincott, 1992).

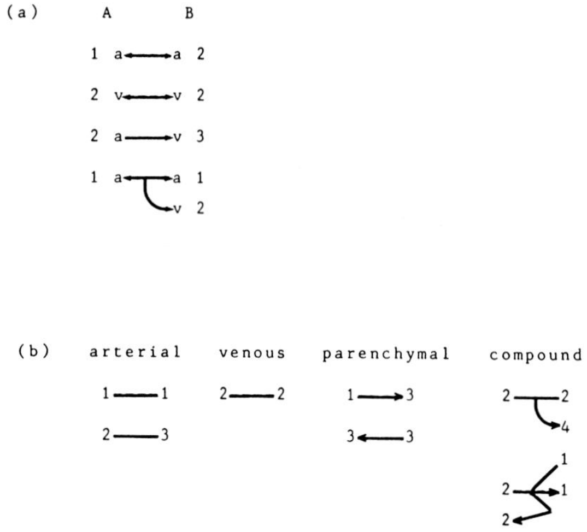

(a)   A   B

     1 a ← a 2

     2 v ← v 2

     2 a → v 3

     1 a ⊤ a 1
            └ v 2

(b)   arterial   venous   parenchymal   compound

       1 —— 1   2 —— 2   1 —→ 3   2 ⌐ 2
                                                      └ 4
       2 —— 3   3 ←— 3
                                                        1
                                                  2 ⧼ 1
                                                  2

FIGURE 3.16. Using shorthand schemes like these, inter-twin vascular anastomoses can be recorded for quick assessment and comparative evaluations. In (a), the origin and type of vessels are indicated—twin A, twin B, artery (a), vein (v), and the size of the respective vessels in millimeters. The direction of flow can be indicated by arrows. In this way, arterial, venous, parenchymal, and compound anastomoses can be represented. In (b), the type of anastomosis is listed at the top and the assumption is made that twin A is on the left and twin B on the right. The size of the vessels is shown in millimeters and the arrows are used to indicate probable unidirectional flow. Where no arrows are present, the implication is that flow could be in either direction. This method is helpful if there are numerous anastomoses in one case, particularly complex compound patterns. With either method, additional information could be added to suit the individual case and examiner's preference.

Patterns of Disks and Membranes

The patterns of placentation in multiple pregnancy depend on the type of twinning (polyovular or dizygotic, monovular or monozygotic), the timing of the twinning process in monozygotic twins, and the relative location of implantation in the uterus for all polyovular and some monovular twins. Variations in the reported rates of the different patterns depend on the rates of polyovular twinning, and the population of origin must be considered when reviewing such data.[16,17] For example, in Africa, with a high dizygotic rate, 95% of the placentas are dichorionic placentas and only 5% are monochorionic placentas, but the Caucasian rate, from the United States and England is 80% and 20%, respec-

tively. The following discussion of patterns of placentation may be augmented by reference to Figs. 2.1, 2.3, 3.17, and 3.18.

Patterns of Placentation and Zygosity

When the conceptuses arise from separate ova, *polyovular or dizygotic,* they may be of opposite or same sex, and each embryo has the full complement of membranes, both amnion and chorion. The proximity of implantation in the uterine wall determines whether the gestational sacs are completely separate, share membranes, or actually fuse into an apparent single mass with a dividing septum. These are called, respectively, dichorionic diamniotic separate (DCDA-S), dichorionic diamniotic with shared membranes (DCDA-SM), and dichorionic diamniotic fused (DCDA-F). When dichorionic disks are distinct masses, the reflected membranes may be fused at some point over their convexity, depending on their positional relationship in the uterus, and these often become pulled apart during delivery and the disks may be submitted as separate specimens. Frequently, however, the placentas have obviously grown close to each other, not close enough for the disks to fuse, but close enough for the membranes to overlap the adjacent disk, as in Fig. 3.5. This pattern of irregular chorionic fusion may be unilateral or bilateral, and is attributed to intra-amniotic fluid pressures affecting the direction of expansion of the sac.[8] Although chorionic surface vessels are less well developed under the overlap, there is no other apparent effect on placental development or fetal well being.

When there is a dichorionic septum dividing the surface of a single-disk placenta, it is firmly attached to the chorionic surface, its line of attachment parallels the vascular equator or watershed of the chorionic plate vessels between the circulations from each twin, and it roughly demarcates the border between the chorionic tissues of each twin.[2,17] Because the developing embryos are each invested with a layer of chorion, any conjunction of membranes between them will always contain chorionic tissue. This zone of apposed chorions may or may not be visually separable into two layers, either grossly or microscopically. An unfortunate and erroneous interpretation occasionally encountered in placenta reports is that the finding of a single band or layer of chorion between the two

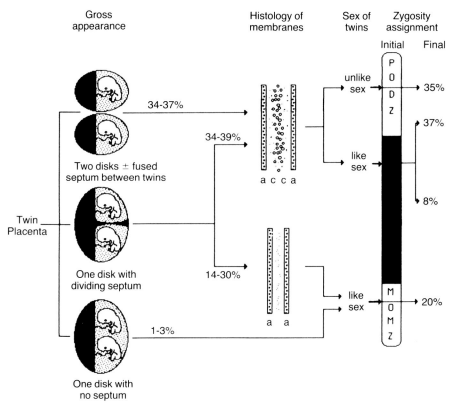

Gross appearance · Histology of membranes · Sex of twins · Zygosity assignment

FIGURE 3.17. This diagrammatic flow chart of the possible patterns of twin placentation can be consulted with photographic examples of these specimens in Fig. 3.18. The possible patterns flow through the gross appearance of the whole specimen and the microscopic layers of the separating membranes with the range of reported percentages of each (see Table 3.1). The black zone in the bar of initial zygosity assignment represents that group of twin sets for whom zygosity determination by other tests is required. The percentages on the left side of the flow chart represent the range of relative percentages from the literature and Survey '91 Review, while the percentages on the right side represent Cameron's[11] data. a, amnion, c, chorion, PODZ, polyovular dizygotic, MOMZ, monovular monozygotic.

amnions in the septum is interpreted as constituting a "monochorionic" pattern. The finding of any chorionic tissue between the layers of amnion, whether as wisps of chorionic tissue, or two distinct layers, constitutes a dichorionic placentation.

The placentation of *monovular monozygotic* and thus usually like-sex twins has been described as occurring in three possible patterns: separate complete gestational sacs (dichorionic diamniotic) with separate or fused disks, as with polyovular dizygotic twins; a single disk and chorionic sac with separate amniotic sacs inside [monochorionic diamniotic (MCDA)]; or a single cavity and placental disk [monochorionic monoamniotic (MCMA)]. The pattern has been considered to be determined by the timing of the twinning process, which is thought to be randomly distributed over the first 14 days of development, leading to decreasing barriers between the twins as the separation occurs later in development, and culminating in conjoined twins with a single cord and a single sac.[4,18] Thus, the finding of only one common outer shell of chorion would indicate a monovular monozygotic twin pair, as this pattern is not known to occur with polyovular dizygotic twin pairs. If there is a bilaminar septum of amnion, the location of the apparent attachment to the chorionic surface can be quite arbitrary, as the membranes are not truly adherent to the underlying chorion, and may be even at 90° to the vascular equator (see Fig. 3.9b).

The problem of interpretation of zygosity from the pattern of placentation arises in those situations

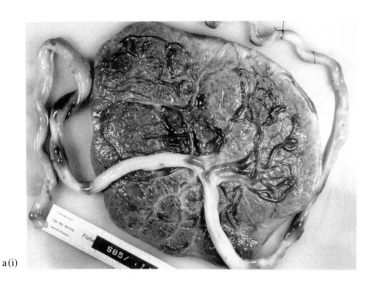

a(i)

FIGURE 3.18. Possible patterns of placentation of twins: (a) Gross examples: (i) monochorionic monoamniotic, cords very closely inserted; (ii) monochorionic monoamniotic, cords further apart; (iii) monochorionic diamniotic—note very delicate membrane layer across middle of disk (one cord inserts at separating membranes);

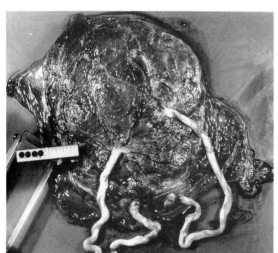

a(ii)

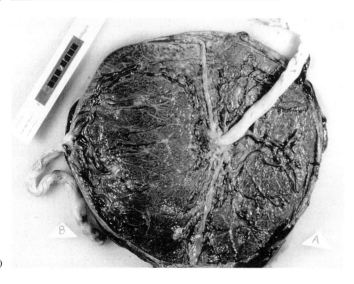

a(iii)

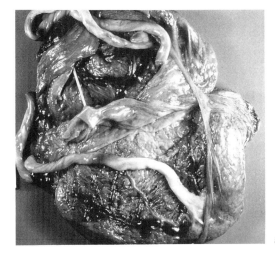

a(iv)

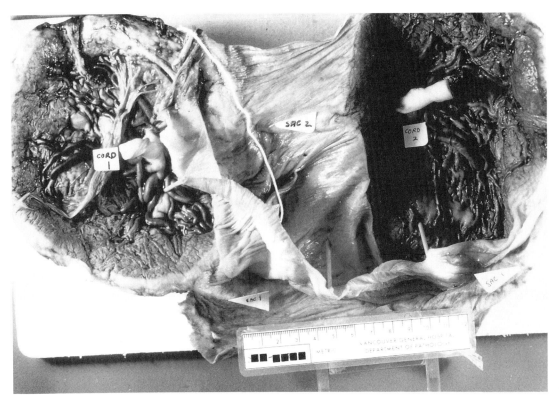

a(v)

FIGURE 3.18. *Continued.* (iv) dichorionic diamniotic, fused disk with thick separating membrane across middle; (v) dichorionic diamniotic, separate disks but shared overlapping membranes—white cord outlines edge of one disk;

of dichorionic diamniotic placentations with like-sex twins, because this pattern can be seen with either polyovular dizygotic twinning or monovular monozygotic twinning. Cameron[11] stated in 1968 that the degree of fusion of the chorionic disks is not an indication of zygosity, and although this com-ment had been made before and has been reempha-sized since, this misinterpretation is still made. While dichorionic monozygotic twin placentas have been reported to be fused six times more frequently than they were separate,[19] others have found that dichorionic monozygotic placentas were

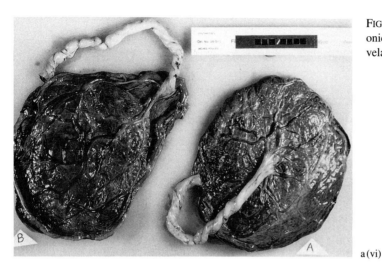

a(vi)

fused or separate with equal frequency.[4,20,21] Thus, it is unreliable to assume that twins of the same sex with a single placenta are monozygotic, and it is also inaccurate to conclude that separate placentas are a good indication of dizygosity. It is these sets of twins who require the additional zygosity testing described in Chapter 2, if their genetic identity is to be determined.

Because the degree of fusion of the chorionic disks is not a reliable indication of zygosity, it might be questioned whether this distinction is of any value. It has been suggested that differentiation as to whether dichorionic placentas were separate or fused was of doubtful biological significance and that such distinctions were not important.[22] However, more recent studies suggest that whether the disks are fused or separate is in fact an appropriate distinction to be recorded because it has implications for fetal growth.[9,10] These studies are described further in the discussion of low birth weight in Chapter 6.

The patterns of placentation that might be expected with *monovular dispermic* twinning remain to be determined. These twins are genetically distinct, strictly speaking are dizygotic, and yet seem to be associated with a monochorionic pattern of placentation, whether it is the first or second polar body that is fertilized. It was suggested in the discussion of this type of twinning in Chapter 2 that the explanation may be that only the large fertilized oocyte has the capacity to produce the placenta, and if the fertilized polar body is near enough, it will be included. An unusual case reported by Nylander and Osunkoya[23] may be an example of this category. They carefully documented a case of normal heterosexual twins with a monochorionic placenta in western Nigeria, which has a very high twinning rate and where 95% of the placentas are dichorionic. The case they described was unique in 2,000 twin placentas they saw over a period of 3 years. There was a zone of chorion in part of the septum, just above the line of attachment to the chorionic surface, but there was none present in the remainder. In addition, there was a superficial vascular anastomosis across the chorionic surface in the zone where the membranes consisted of amnion only. "Chorion fusion," with breakdown of the chorionic layer, has been described in animals,[20] and although Nylander and Osunkoya's case was initially thought to represent the same process, it seems more likely that it represents an example of dispermic monovular twinning, because dispermic monovular twinning has been confirmed in humans while chorion fusion has not.

Although most twin placentations can be assigned to the patterns described above and represented in Figs. 3.17 and 3.18, there will be occasional specimens, such as the examples from the Survey '91 Review shown in Fig. 3.19, that tax our powers of observation and interpretation, and serve to remind us that no matter how many cases we have seen, there is always something new to explain (see Chapter 1 for the source of the Survey '91 Review cases). For example, dichorionic diamniotic fused placentas have been portrayed as quite neatly conjoined side by side with distinct chorionic surfaces

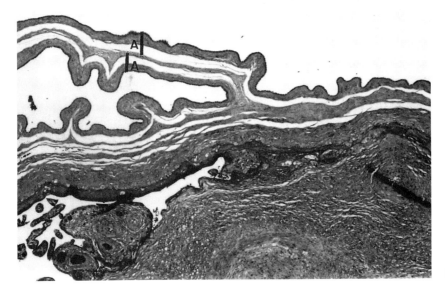

b(i)

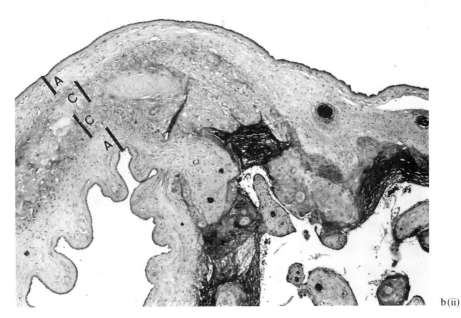

b(ii)

FIGURE 3.18. *Continued.* (b) Microscopic appearance of septum or separating membranes: (i) amnion only, from monochorionic placentation—only two layers of amnion (A) (tissue in middle is part of amnion connective tissue); (ii) amnion and chorion from dichorionic placentation—two layers of amnion (A) and two layers of chorion (C), which may be fused variably to look like one (note atrophic villi in chorion layer). (Reprinted with permission from Wiggelsworth and Singer, *Textbook of Fetal and Perinatal Pathology*, Chapter 8, Blackwell Scientific, 1991.)

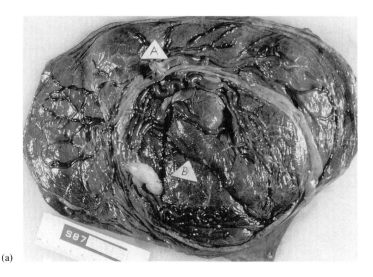

(a)

FIGURE 3.19. Twin placentas are occasionally puzzling in their gross form, and such cases can serve as a basis for rethinking the embryology. In the 31 week dichorionic diamniotic placenta in (a), instead of being side to side, one twin's sac (B) is "embedded" within the other twin's sac (A). These twin girls were weight discordant by 38%, with the smaller twin from the "enclosed" sac. The zygosity was not assessed and there were no reported perinatal problems. Careful histology of the various membranes indicated that the "internal" crescentic septum was the usual dichorionic diamniotic membrane, and that the short arc of the outer wall of the "contained" sac was the usual amnion and chorion, so that twin B was simply remarkably surrounded but not totally enclosed by twin A's gestational sac. The twin placenta with twin boys in (b) looks superficially like separate disks with shared membranes. However, the horizontal fold of membranes (arrowheads) was a diamniotic septum, so this was a monochorionic placentation. Two groups of vessels can be seen crossing between the disks. These originated from cord A, and one artery anastomosed with an artery from cord B in the outside group (at diamond). Thus, this would seem to be a monochorionic placenta with separate disks but with an anastomosis, a somewhat confusing situation based on most accepted descriptions of the types of twin placenta. The membranous zone between the disks contains a thin layer of involuted villus tissue microscopically, suggesting that the zones of villus tissue for each twin had been part of a single mass at some stage. This might have represented the result of an attachment to a uterine anomaly, although none had been commented on at the time of section delivery. Symmetrically grown 33 week twin boys had the unusual placenta in (c). In one-third of the septum between the twins, there were only two layers of amnion (above arrow, layers of amnion reflected apart), while in the remaining two-thirds there was an increasing amount of chorion between the layers of amnion, reaching 1.5 cm height in the septum at the margin. The fetal vessels were 3 cm apart in the dichorionic zone and although they came closer to-

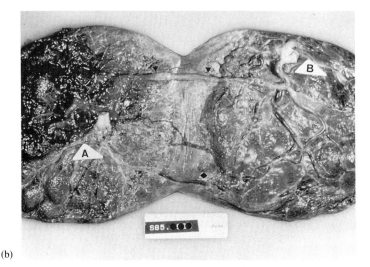

(b)

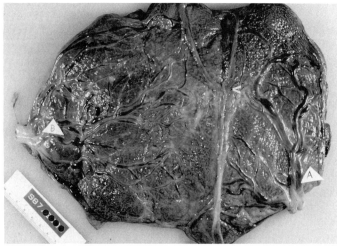

(c)

gether in the diamniotic zone, no anastomoses were demonstrated with injection. The twins were within 7% by weight, in spite of the marked asymmetry of the respective chorionic regions. Both were blood group A Rh negative, but no further zygosity studies were done.

TABLE 3.1. Statistical reports of patterns of placentation with twins.

| Author or source | Dichorionic diamniotic | | Monochorionic | | Dichorionic diamniotic | | |
	Separate	Fused	Diamniotic	Monoamniotic	Unlike-sex Dizygotic	Like-sex DZ	MZ
Benirschke and Driscoll (United States)[4]	35.2%	34.0%	29.6%	1.2%			
Cameron (Birmingham)[11]			----------------20%----------------		35%	37%	8%
Pauls (World Review)[26]				.83%			
Nylander (Nigeria)[27]	41.5%	50.3%	4.8%	0.2%			
Soma et al. (Japan)[28]	20.3%	18.5%	56.6%	4.6%	14.8%		
Cameron et al. (Birmingham and Ghent)[14]			19.5%	2.5%	34%	35%	9%
Robertson and Neer (United States)[15]	37.5%	37%	---------------25.5%---------------		40.4%	-----59.6%-----	
Shanklin and Perrin (Chicago and Florida)[7]	34.4%	36.6%	26.4%	3.2%			
Survey '91 survivor data (British Columbia, Canada)	36.8%	30.8%	31.8%	.6%	35.1%	-----64.9%-----	
Survey '91 mortality data (British Columbia, Canada)*	23.3%	17.2%	43.4%	5.7%	40%	-----47.5%-----	

*Survey '91 mortality data—the sex of the other twin was not known in 12.5% of the cases of dichorionic placentas with unilateral twin mortality.
DZ, dizygotic; MZ, monozygotic.

and sacs, and a tidy straight septum between. However, in Fig. 3.19a is a dichorionic diamniotic placentation with one twin's sac apparently completely enclosed within the other. These twins must have implanted remarkably close together, but why the gestational sacs grew in this fashion instead of in opposite directions is not known. Also, monochorionic placentas have been represented as being single-disk placentations, with or without a septum, but in Fig. 3.19b is a monochorionic placenta with two apparently quite distinct disks, a horizontally oriented bilaminar amniotic septum, and one artery to artery anastomosis proven by injection. Whether the microscopically detected involuted zone of villus tissue between the "disks" was due to an unusual implantation as perhaps on an undetected partial uterine septum or represented another possible placental pattern with dispermic monovular twinning was not determined. A related example of two apparently distinct disks and monochorionic membranes and intertwin anastomosis has been reported, but there was no suggestion of villus tissue between the disks.[24] Possible pathogenesis of this unusual pattern was not suggested. Finally, the septum in fused placentas has been represented as either amnion–amnion, or amnion–chorion–chorion–amnion. In Fig. 3.19c is a single-disk twin placenta, with a septum that is partly amnion only and partly contains chorion. The interposed layer of chorion was not extensive, but is reminiscent of Nylander and Osunkoya's[23] case, although their twins were a boy and a girl. Zygosity studies were strongly suggested in this example, but unfortunately were not pursued.

It is generally assumed that the membrane patterns are established early and persist throughout pregnancy. This is likely true in the majority, but prenatal disruption of the diamniotic septum has been reported with the suggestion that some apparently monoamniotic placentas at delivery may have been diamniotic earlier.[25] This has implications for fetal survival and is discussed further in Chapter 8. Careful pathologic examination of all apparently monoamniotic placentas is indicated.

Distribution Frequencies of Patterns of Twin Placentas

A number of researchers interested in multiple pregnancy have recorded the distribution frequencies of the various patterns of disks and membranes from twin pregnancies in their regions of practice. A limited selection of these are summarized in

Table 3.1, along with the data from the Survey '91 Review, for comparison. The comment made at the beginning of this discussion of placenta patterns concerning the importance of knowing the population from which the data are derived is exemplified by the very different distributions reported from Nigeria and Japan, reflecting the notable differences in rates of polyovular dizygotic twinning in

Fig. 20.

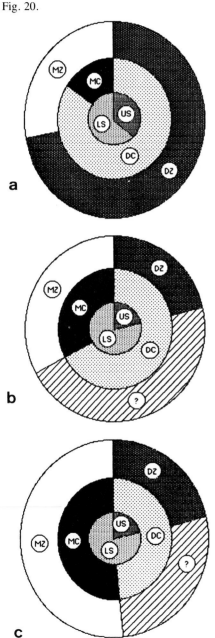

those countries compared to the others. Sometimes, clusters of numbers have more meaning if represented in a different manner, such as in Fig. 3.20a. The data chosen for this figure are those of Cameron[11] because of the thoroughness of his study, and the fact that his values approximate many of the other studies of North American and European populations.

The question might be asked why one might be interested in noting the relative distributions of patterns of placentation in a twin population. There are at least three useful observations that can be made, based on data from Survey '91 as an example. First, if the data from 909 of the survivor-group placentas are represented in a fashion analogous to that of Cameron (Fig. 3.20b), it is evident that, barring the situation of dispermic monovular twinning, preliminary zygosity assignment is possible in 56% of the twin sets, based on knowledge of the sex of the infants and pattern of placentation. Without knowledge of the placental pattern, zygosity testing would be needed in over three quarters of the twin sets, an unwieldy task. Second, if the data from 251 cases from the autopsy group are illustrated as in Fig. 3.20c, and the relative distributions are compared to those in Fig. 3.20b, it is evident that monochorionic monozygotic twinning accounts for a disproportionate load of twin mortality when compared to the incidence in survivors. The causes for this disproportion are discussed in Chapters 8, 9, and 10. Third, the distribution of fetal sex in relation to separate or fused dichorionic placentations was assessed in the survivor group, and the results confirmed the previous observation that the degree of separation is no indication of zygos-

◄
─────────────────────────────────

FIGURE 3.20. The relative proportions of like-sex (LS) and unlike-sex (US) twins are compared to the patterns of monochorionic (MC) and dichorionic (DC) placentation, and monozygotic (MZ) and dizygotic (DZ) origins. The (?) zone represents zygosity undetermined. In (a) the distributions are of the data from Cameron[11] with complete zygosity determination. In (b) and (c), monochorionicity was equated with monozygosity and unlike sex with dizygosity, recognizing the limitations of those conclusions. The distribution patterns in (b) represent data from the Survey '91 Review survivor group, and in (c) the data from the Survey '91 Review autopsy group. The disproportionate load of monozygotic monochorionic twins in the autopsy group is evident.

ity—of 216 unlike-sex and presumably dizygotic twin pairs, 47.2% had a single placental disk.

It has been suggested that monozygotic twinning is more frequent in female zygotes, accounting for the increased proportion of female sets with increasing proximity of the twins[29] (see Chapter 2). The distribution of like-sex pairs in relation to patterns of placentation was examined in 692 survivor-group pairs and 189 autopsy-group pairs from the Survey '91 data. There was no significant difference in the rate of male pairs to female pairs in the dichorionic placentas, whether separate or fused, or in the monochorionic diamniotic placentas, and in all cases they were nearly equally represented. In contrast, female pairs accounted for 70% of the monochorionic monoamniotic placentas, and were in excess in both the survivor and autopsy groups. (See Chapter 8 for a further discussion of monoamniotic twinning.)

Because many commentaries on twinning refer to the problem of space in the uterus when there is a multiple conception, the Survey '91 survivor group placental weights were assessed and related to fetal weights and membrane patterns. Total placenta weight gradually increased in a manner analogous to singleton placentas from 26 weeks to 41 weeks, but with such a broad scatter at each gestational age that no useful trends could be developed for specific patterns of placentation. Similarly, when fetoplacental ratios [total weight of twins divided by total placenta weight(s)] were calculated in cases with concordant twin growth, there was a rising trend in the ratios from 30 to 42 weeks, but again, such a broad scatter at each gestational age that no differentiation could be discerned among monochorionic, dichorionic fused, or dichorionic separate placentations. The hypothesis had been that separate placentas might attain a greater total weight than single-disk placentas, so that fetoplacental ratios would be lower with concordant, appropriately grown twins, but this was not supported by data available. In reported studies of growth of normal dichorionic separate twin placentas, the mean gross placental weights of the separate placentas at each gestational age from 33 weeks onward were at or slightly below the lowest weight in the range for singleton placentas at the same gestational age, perhaps a reflection of constrained space.[30,31] The relationship of placental patterns to fetal weight is discussed further in Chapter 6.

An interesting and clinically useful side issue is related to the pattern of placentation, particularly the nature of the septum in single-disk twins. If one twin fetus is discordantly affected with a condition that leads to elevated amniotic alpha-fetoprotein and acetylcholinesterase levels, the amniotic fluid of the normal twin may contain falsely high levels of these compounds as well, if the septum consists of amnion only.[32] Knowledge of this possibility is obviously critically important to the counseling process with prenatal diagnostic procedures.

Vascular Patterns

The pattern of vascular development of the twin placenta can have a tremendous impact on fetal growth and therefore warrants careful attention. Included in this concept are the vessels of the umbilical cord, the chorionic surface vessels, and intertwin vascular anastomoses.

Umbilical Cord

Anomalies of the umbilical cord are more frequent in placentas of multiple gestations, and include aberrant insertions and absence of one umbilical artery. Marginal and velamentous insertions, including insertions into the separating membranes, may occur as a function of intrauterine crowding, with secondarily distorted placental growth.[33] In other cases, they are associated with other abnormalities of placental vascularization and may represent a more complex developmental error. Similarly, the absence of one umbilical artery may be an isolated finding, or may be part of a malformation complex in the affected twin. In some cases, the anomalous cord has a combination of lesions, such as only one umbilical artery and a velamentous insertion, and in other cases both twins have anomalous cords, with either concordant or discordant lesions. It is interesting to note that in one study the incidence of marginally inserted umbilical cords in singleton placentas after in vitro fertilization–embryo transfer was 15.9%, compared to 5.6% in spontaneous singletons, and 10.6% for dichorionic, and 22.1% for monochorionic twins.[34] The significance of this observation as it relates to placenta development remains to be determined.

TABLE 3.2. Patterns of anomalous cord insertion in twins—percent of infants with anomalous insertions.

Anomaly	Comparative singleton frequency*	Pattern of placentation				Reference
		Dichorionic— separate	Dichorionic— fused	Monochorionic diamniotic	Monochorionic monoamniotic	
Velamentous	1.1	3.4	7.0	11.4	–†	(33)
		2.7	12.6	23.3	0.0	(11)
		0.0	10.0	10.0	–	(7)
Marginal	6.89	6.2	10.0	19.5	16.6	(33)
		1.0	6.0	27.0	–	(7)
Velamentous and marginal		9.6	17.0	31.0	16.6	(33)

*Singleton frequencies derived from averaged reported frequency in 194,365 infants for velamentous cords and 94,822 infants for marginal cords (35).
†–, not stated.

In addition to the overall increased incidence of anomalous insertions in multiple gestations compared to singletons, the frequency increases with increasing proximity of the twins, as demonstrated by the reported patterns from three studies as summarized in Table 3.2. The differential rates in the dichorionic placentas, comparing separate and fused, may be associated with irregular expansion of the fused placenta.[11]

The pattern of cord insertions has significance beyond descriptive completeness. In dichorionic diamniotic fused placentas, the umbilical cords may insert into the separating membranes at varying distances above the placental surface. Shanklin and Perrin[7] found that half the cords inserted in this fashion in their cases and both cords did so in two cases. The importance of this pattern is the potential for vasa praevia in reference to the second twin, with the risk of rupture and fetal bleeding after rupture of the second sac.[8] Also, there is an increased association of fetal malformations with anomalously inserted umbilical cords, although it is not clear whether the anomalous cord provides a threshold for manifestation of the fetal anomaly, or whether both are the effect of a common teratogenic influence. Up to 5.3% of infants with marginal cords, and 8.5% of infants with velamentous cords, have been reported to have structural defects consisting of malformations, deformations, and disruptions.[36] In addition to fetal anomalies, an extensive review of velamentous cord insertions reported an association with increased abortion, prematurity, polyhydramnios, abnormal presentation, premature rupture of membranes, postpartum hemorrhage, and decreased fetal weight.[37] Finally, Potter and

Craig[5] suggested that if one cord was attached peripherally, and was supplied by only a small portion of the placenta, the inadequate size of the capillary bed might be responsible for problems with fetal development.

The absence of one umbilical artery is more frequent in multiple gestations, ranging from 3.6%[33] to 35%[38] of the twins studied, and is also associated with detrimental development and perinatal outcome, as it is when it occurs in singletons.[39] The frequency of the anomaly is greater in autopsied twins than survivors, reflecting the associated malformations, particularly in monochorionic twins. An interesting observation is that most twins are discordant for this anomaly, although concordance occurs more often with monozygotic than dizygotic twins. This raises the question of the relative roles of genetic programming or predisposition, environmental stimuli, and abnormalities of the twinning process itself in the genesis of structural defects, particularly in single-egg twins. This question has not been answered for single artery umbilical cords, but will be raised in other contexts in subsequent chapters. Whatever the genesis of single umbilical artery cords, there is an effect on fetal growth—in twins discordant for single artery cords the smaller twin had the anomalous cord in 82.4%.[39] Just why single artery cords are associated with impaired growth is not clear, particularly when it has been reported from one study that 77% of fetuses with single umbilical arteries had normal Doppler systolic-to-diastolic ratios.[40]

Observations based on a review of 1,177 survivor group and 345 autopsy group twin placentas from the Survey '91 Review cases generally reinforce the

TABLE 3.3. Frequency of umbilical cord anomalies in Survey '91 twins—percent of infants affected.

	Number	Marginal insertion	Velamentous insertion	Single artery cord
Surviving infants	2,354	6.6%	5.3%	1.3%
Total infants from sets with one or both deceased	470	14.5%	8.3%	4.9%
Deceased infants only*	345	17.7%	11.0%	5.8%

*The deceased group includes twins who died and autopsy was refused, but the placenta was examined.

above comments. In Table 3.3, the increased frequency of velamentous cords is noted, as well as the increased frequency of all cord anomalies associated with perinatal mortality. The majority of the anomalies occurred in like-sex pairs, reflecting the greater frequency in monochorionic placentas, and all anomalies were increased in monochorionic twins who died, as shown in Table 3.4. It is not known why single artery and marginal cords seem to have a male–male predominance in the deceased group. All anomalies occurred with equal frequency in first- and second-born twins. Concordance of anomalous insertions accounted for 11.6% of marginal cords and 10.2% of velamentous cords in the survivors, but this tripled in the deceased twins to 38.7% and 31.6%, respectively. Concordance of single artery cords was 13.3% in survivors, but no concordance was noted in the deceased twins. Two-thirds to four-fifths of the concordant cord anomalies were in monochorionic placentas in all groups. Combinations of lesions were described in a few cases—absence of one umbilical artery occurred twice as often in velamentous as in marginal cords.

The above data incorporate several interpretations that are relevant. Single-artery cords include a few with lengthy segmental absence of one artery, probably representing an aberrantly long anastomosis above the placenta insertion, because that segment likely creates similar blood flow patterns as a full length absence. Velamentous cords include those inserted into the separating membranes of dichorionic fused placentas, as the basic pattern is analogous to insertion into the free membranes. The velamentous distance ranged from a centimeter above the placental surface to 18 cm at the apex of the gestational sac, and the vessel pattern ranged from a few short distance intramembranous vessels to a cascade of tortuous vessels through the septum and/or reflected membranes (Fig. 3.21). Cord insertions into the diamniotic septum were described in 11 monochorionic placentas of survivors, but this was not considered pathogenetically analogous to free membrane velamentous cords, although the risk of vasa praevia would be greater than in dichorionic septa because of the thinner nature of the membrane.

It was suggested above that anomalous develop-

TABLE 3.4. Distribution of umbilical cord anomalies in Survey '91 twins—percent of total numbers of the anomaly related to pattern of membranes and sex of twins.

	Velamentous insertion		Marginal insertion		Single artery	
	Surv	Dec*	Surv	Dec	Surv	Dec
Pattern of membranes						
Dichorionic—separate	15.6	27.1	18.2	11.7	16.1	15.8
Dichorionic—fused	38.5	13.5	23.4	13.3	29.0	5.3
Monochorionic	41.8	51.3	56.5	71.7	45.2	63.1
Dichorionic—not stated	4.1	8.1	1.9	3.3	9.7	15.8
Sex of twins						
Male-female	10.2	10.5	9.0	8.1	13.4	5.3
Male-male	35.1	36.8	37.4	61.3	33.3	73.7
Female-female	39.1	39.5	42.0	29.0	33.3	21.0
Sex not known	15.4	13.2	11.6	1.6	20.0	0.0

*The deceased group includes twins who died and autopsy was refused, but the placenta was examined.
Surv, survivors; Dec, deceased.

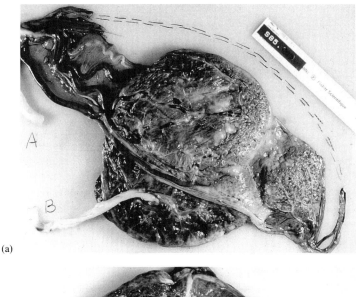

(a)

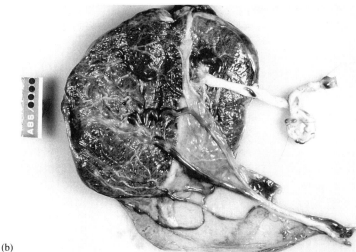

(b)

FIGURE 3.21. Anomalous insertions of the umbilical cord are more common with single-disk twin placentas and these are two remarkable examples. In (a), cord A has a velamentous insertion into the apex of the sac, with vessels in the free membranes and a few in the septum. (The dotted line indicates the cut ends of membranous vessels that were severed in order to flatten the placenta for the photograph.) In (b), there are prominent septal branches from the cord inserted into the separating membranes. Both examples are dichorionic diamniotic placentas. The problem of assessing the importance of discordant chorionic volume compared to anomalous cord insertions is exemplified by both these cases. In case (a), the male twins were 44% discordant by weight at 33 weeks, with the smaller twin from the smaller chorionic volume (B), raising the question of how important the abnormal cord insertion of twin A really was. In case (b), the smaller twin (by 33%) was from the larger chorionic volume, but with the velamentous cord insertion, suggesting that the anomalous insertion was important in this case.

ment of "body stalk" or umbilical vasculature might have an influence on fetal growth and development, so additional associations were studied in the Survey '91 Review. In 23 placentas, the chorionic surface served by the anomalous cord (9 marginal, 10 velamentous, 4 single umbilical artery) had fewer than normal surface chorionic vessels, with as few as three vascular pairs. In 18 of these cases, the placenta was monochorionic, suggesting a more generalized disturbance in vascular development than just crowding in the uterus. The relationship of discordant fetal growth to anomalous cord insertions was also examined. In 33 surviving twin sets, with marginal insertion of the cord of one of the twins, the birth weights were discordant, with the smaller twin more than 15% lighter than the larger,

and in two-thirds of these the smaller twin had the anomalous cord. Similarly, there were 22 sets with an assignable velamentous cord in one twin and a weight discordance of greater than 15%, and in close to 91% the smaller twin had the anomalous cord. In seven cases of velamentous/marginal pairs, the smaller twin was on the velamentous side in five. Dichorionic and monochorionic placentas were equally represented in both groups. There was no correlation with single-artery cords. The subject of discordant weight in twins is discussed further in Chapter 6.

The length of the umbilical cords of term twins has been measured and found to be an average of 7.9 cm shorter than term singletons.[41] There was no differentiation based on placental pattern provided.

One study of weight concordant twin pairs found greater concordance of cord lengths in monochorionic pairs than like-sex and unlike-sex dichorionic pairs, suggesting a genetic influence on cord length.[42] None of the survivor placentas in the Survey '91 Review had the entire cord for assessment, because of cord gas sampling in the case room and varying lengths initially left on the infant, so the reported measurements were not helpful. It was noted, however, that at least 21 twin placentas in the last 18 months of the survey had one or both cords still attached or submitted with the placenta that measured at or longer than the singleton mean for the gestational age,[43] and more than half were same-sex male pairs. This observation is obviously incomplete, but is presented as a suggestion for further study. The length of the cord seems to be influenced by the amount of fetal activity, and the shorter length in twins may reflect this on the basis of the cramped twin-filled uterus. There seems to be a relationship also between fetal activity and the development of the twist or helix of the cord—an increased incidence of cords without spiraling has been described in twins.[44] As straight cords were also increased among intrauterine fetal deaths, the suggestion was that shorter straight cords may be associated with an adverse prognosis, although whether due to the unusual cord or as part of a process that affected the cord as well is not determined.

The only other relatively prominent finding in the umbilical cords consisted of 12 survivor cases with true knots, one of which had a triple knot. However, it could not be determined from the reports available for review if these had been placed as a means to differentiate the twins, or were in fact congenital, so the value of the observation is undetermined. This difficulty reinforces the need for a standard procedure to identify the umbilical cords in the case room.

Chorionic Vessels and Intertwin Anastomoses

The normal development of vessels in the chorionic fetal surface of the placenta leads to a variety of vessel branching patterns from the site of cord insertion to the periphery of the disk.[45] The chorionic arteries generally pass over the chorionic veins, although in occasional cases a more peripheral vein may be superficial to the corresponding artery.[13] The umbilical cord arteries each branch dichotomously, producing eight or more terminal chorionic plate arteries, and are accompanied by parallel branching of the umbilical vein with 12 to 20 pairs of adjacent artery and vein branches that penetrate the chorion within a few millimeters of each other.[13,45] Additional penetrating vessels branch from these surface vessels to supply the fetal villus units, variously referred to as cotyledons or lobules, and the arteries are connected to the veins through short and broad villus capillaries. There are no vascular anastomoses between capillaries of adjacent villi and no arterial, venous, or arteriovenous anastomoses within or between cotyledons, an observation of some importance when considering intertwin anastomoses.[13]

The pattern of chorionic vessels in twin placentas is influenced by the type of twinning and pattern of placentation. In dichorionic separate placentas, the chorionic circulations are distinct and the pattern in each disk will vary in relation to the insertion site of the cord. When the disks are separate but the membranes overlap, the chorionic vessels in the area of the overlap are buried in the surface chorionic connective tissues and are not as visible from the surface as usual, but appear otherwise normal. In dichorionic fused placentas, the respective chorionic vascular territories of each twin are demarcated by the attachment line of the septum, which constitutes the periphery of the respective placental masses. The vessel patterns follow the cord insertion pattern and there is a higher incidence of anomalous cord insertions and consequent variant chorionic vessel patterns in this group, perhaps because of the positional effects of the growth and fusion of the disks.[46] Intertwin vascular anastomoses in dichorionic placentas are virtually unknown, even between what appear to be adjacent vessels in the septum, and any claim to the contrary must be documented unequivocally. These comments on vascular patterns apply to any dichorionic placentas, whether polyovular or monovular in origin.

When the twins share a disk with only a bilaminar septum of amnion, or no septum at all, the potential exists for vascular connections to occur between the two adjacent developing chorionic circulations. As indicated in the discussion of the examination of the placenta, there can be three types of anastomoses—

artery to artery and vein to vein on the chorionic surface, and an arteriovenous connection through villus capillaries. Further consideration of the anatomy and the possible physiology of intertwin vascular anastomoses is presented in Chapter 9, with the potential clinical and pathological consequences.

The observation of asymmetry of the chorionic mass and pattern of chorionic surface vessels has been made above and related to impaired fetal growth. Not all discordantly grown twins have asymmetric placentas, and not all asymmetric placentas are associated with discordant growth, but the observation of relative placental mass and twin growth is a useful one to make. In 200 consecutive survivor-group twin pairs who were discordantly grown by weight, with adequate identification of placental mass for each twin, 80% of the smaller twins were lighter than the larger twin by 15% or more, and 20% differed by 10% to 15%. Discordant size dichorionic placentations were the only placental variation identified in 33.5% of the over 15% group and 46% of the 10% to 15% group. Slightly more than half were dichorionic separate patterns, and like-sex pairs were twice as common as unlikesex pairs in both separate and fused patterns. The smaller sized separate disk, or the smaller part of the fused disk, belonged to the smaller twin in 93% of the over 15% group and 89% of the 10% to 15% group. It is not known whether the smaller placenta impaired the growth of the fetus, or both were small secondary to some other influence. The smaller placental mass was almost always associated with decreased numbers of chorionic vessel branches, suggesting an early problem with placental growth. It is not known how many of the like-sex discordantly grown dichorionic pairs might represent asymmetric single-egg twinning, monozygotic or dispermic monovular. The possible influence of implantation site is not discernible in this material. Asymmetry of placental mass/area was a common feature of discordant survivor monochorionic twins, but the relative roles of reduced placental mass, reduced numbers of chorionic vessels, abnormal cord insertions, and intertwin vascular anastomoses are difficult to discern and they often occur together. The problem of discordant twin growth is discussed more fully in Chapter 6, as other causes, such as discordant villus disease and discordant ischemic pathology, are also important.

Other Findings

The placentas from the survivor group of the Survey '91 Review were assessed for any additional reported abnormalities. When chorioamnionitis was present and where birth order was defined, the inflammation was present in the first sac, or was more severe in the first sac when both were affected, as noted by Benirschke and Driscoll.[4] There was no increase in accessory lobes, extrachorial membrane attachments, placenta fenestrata, or other shape abnormalities compared with singletons. Embryonic remnants in the cord, trophoblastic cysts, discrete chorangiomas, and chorangiomatosis were reported with less frequency than in singletons, although incomplete reporting of small lesions is always a possibility. There was no unusual clustering of infarcts, thrombi, intervillous fibrin, focal villus edema, avascular villi, villous immaturity, decidual necrosis with or without premature separation, calcium, intravillus hemorrhage, edema of the cord, or hemorrhagic endovasculopathy. When a history of maternal hypertension, diabetes, or blood group incompatibility was present, any histologic abnormality was the same as seen in singleton placentas. In cases where the histologic appearance of the villi was not compatible with the dates, the villi looked more mature in the majority, suggesting a problem with maternal blood flow to the placental mass. It is not surprising that there was little microscopic pathology in these survivor-group placentas from the survey. In those cases where there was significant villus pathology, it was usually correlated with impaired fetal growth and the affected cases are considered in Chapter 6.

Twinning and Trophoblast Disease

An interesting aspect of placental pathology in multiple gestation is the occurrence of gestational trophoblastic disease, and there are three relationships to be considered—twins with trophoblastic disease, molar and other twin pregnancies in the same woman, and molar twins.

Twins may develop gestational trophoblastic disease. "Homozygous" twin sisters (basis for identity was not stated) have been described, who developed molar pregnancies within 8 months of each other.[47] The first occurred in the primigravid twin who had postmolar choriocarcinoma at the time of hysterectomy, and the second was in the multigravid twin who had had a normal pregnancy 6 years earlier.

Molar pregnancies (choriomas) may occur in other pregnancies of mothers who have had twins, and an excess of choriomas among other pregnancies of mothers with twins has been reported at 6.7 times the expected incidence.[48] The choriomas were seen before and after the twin gestation, and the majority of the twins were dizygotic. In none of the molar pregnancies was there evidence of twinning. The significance of this observation remains to be determined.

One of the earliest "associations" of molar pregnancy in multiple gestation might be the case of a fantastic "multiple" gestation reported to have occurred in the year 1276 and described by Mayer[49] in which 365 "infants" likely represented carefully counted molar vesicles, appropriately segregated as to "sex," and duly baptized. However, there is also more scientific evidence for the suggestion that coexistent chorioma and normal fetus may represent dizygotic twinning.

Molar Twins

The biologic significance of the various patterns of gross and microscopic morphology of choriomas is being refined with detailed genetic studies. Particularly interesting have been the findings when a fetus and molar placental tissues coincide. Choriomas have been divided by their histologic appearance and cytogenetic origins into the diffusely abnormal androgenetic chorioma or "complete mole" and the more irregularly abnormal triploid variant chorioma or "partial mole" in which the histologic appearance depends on which parent provided the extra haploid set.[50,51] The triploid variant choriomas are occasionally associated with a recognizable but abnormal fetus. When the extra haploid set is paternal in origin, the fetus may die early, the placenta is more vesicular grossly, and in some cases may resemble a "complete mole". When the extra haploid set is maternal in origin, the placenta is less cystic and the fetus may survive longer. The differentiation is more than academic

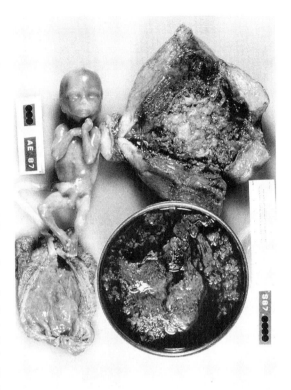

FIGURE 3.22. In this case of twin chorioma, the normal male fetus and his placenta are seen together with a mass of molar tissue that was androgenetic 46,XX. The uterus is also present in this picture. (Courtesy Dr. Dagmar Kalousek, Embryopathology Service, British Columbia's Children's Hospital, Vancouver, Canada.)

because there is a risk of persistent disease with androgenetic choriomas.

Before sophisticated genetic analysis was possible, five patterns of concurrent fetus and molar placental tissue were described.[52] The least amount of molar tissue consisted of very focal vesicular degeneration in a single placenta, such as a single cotyledon, of uncertain cause and significance. A pattern of multifocal vesicular degeneration throughout a single placenta, or a pattern of completely molar single placenta, is now known to represent the triploid variant chorioma. In the fourth pattern, there was extensive but quite distinct molar change in a portion of a single placenta and it was suggested that this might represent an origin in multiple gestation. The most convincing "molar twin" was the fifth pattern, two separate placentas, one normal and one molar.

The occurrence of an apparently normal fetus and

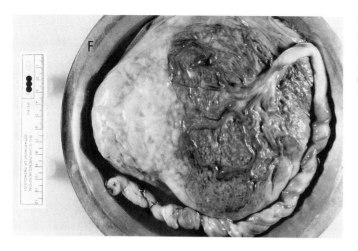

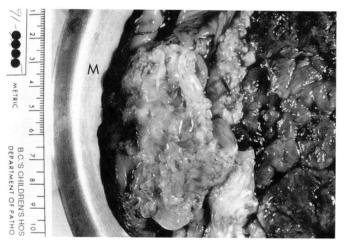

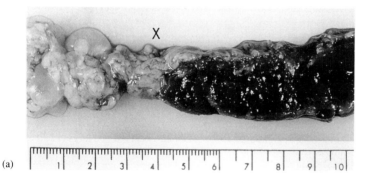

(a)

FIGURE 3.23. In this case of possible dizygotic twin chorioma, the views of the fetal (F), maternal (M), and cross section (X) of the 35 week placenta display the sharply demarcated zone of molar tissue in (a).

placenta with a separate molar placental mass, sometimes quite separately attached to the uterus,[53] appears to represent a dizygotic conception with one zygote developing into an androgenetic diploid chorioma.[54] A number of examples have been reported, and in 47 twin and 2 triplet conceptions, the associated twin or triplet consisted of 17 males and 10 females. Not all these cases were studied for cytogenetic origin, so triploidy with minimal manifestations was not ruled out.[54,55] These apparently twin fetus/chorioma pregnancies usually terminated in the second trimester with fetal death.[52,56–58] The data are incomplete, but there appear to be no greater risks for the normal twin compared to other

FIGURE 3.23. *Continued.* Microscopically (b) the distinctness of the junction zone (i) and the focal trophoblast hyperplasia (ii) in the largely infarcted molar tissue is shown. (Hematoxylin & eosin. Original magnification ×12.5 [b(i)], ×625 [b(ii)].

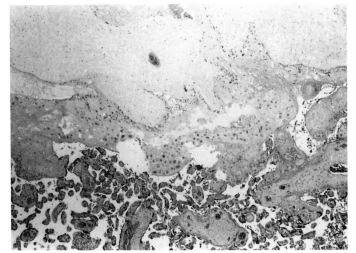

b(i)

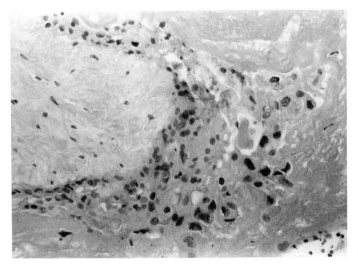

b(ii)

twins, other than those of prematurity, in those pregnancies that terminate beyond 31 weeks. This may be a reflection of the fact that over half of these cases had distinct molar and normal placentas. In contrast, in a larger more recent review, survival rate with a single placenta and localized molar change was 64%, higher than the 43.9% observed with distinct molar and normal placental masses. Only 5% of infants survived who had vesicles dispersed throughout a single placenta.[59]

More recently, a second pattern of normal fetus and molar placenta has been identified, in which the molar component is diploid, but morphologically resembles the variant chorioma pattern, either as a distinct zone of the otherwise normal single disk,[60] or intermingled with nonmolar villi throughout the placental tissue.[61] Without detailed marker analysis, the possibility of twinning in these and similar cases is not ruled out. It has been suggested on the basis of examination of restriction fragment length polymorphisms that there might be an entity of "diploid biparental conception with partial molar placental change."[62] The possibility that these cases may be examples of abnormally developing dispermic monovular twins, with the molar component perhaps arising from the fertilized polar body, or a uniparental disomy for an unknown chromosome, remains to be investigated.

Five examples of fetus with molar tissue were encountered in the Survey '91 Review. The first was electively terminated at 15 weeks of gestation, because of ultrasonic identification of an apparently diffusely abnormal molar pattern placenta, with an otherwise normal-appearing fetus. The termination led to fragmentation of the specimen, but no abnormalities were identified in the discernible fetal parts. The placental tissue grossly seemed to be uniformly vesicular, with cysts ranging from 5 to 8 mm and attaining a maximum of 1 cm. Microscopically, the placental tissues contained a mixture of apparently normal-appearing villus tissue, with a second population of tissue suggesting a "complete mole". Cultures of fetal skin and lung and placental chorion all grew a normal female karyotype. As this case occurred prior to the availability of more sophisticated studies, the exact nature of the molar tissue was not determined. The second example was terminated electively at 18 weeks, because of the identification of molar tissue. The chromosomally normal male fetus was appropriately grown, developmentally normal, and attached to a grossly and microscopically normal placenta (Fig. 3.22). The chorioma was separate and microscopically had features of both variant and "complete" chorioma. Cytogenetically, the chorioma was androgenetic 46,XX, suggesting dizygotic twinning.

The third example of fetus with molar placenta was one of partial molar transformation of an otherwise apparently normal placenta attached to a normal fetus, identified at 22 weeks of the gestation. Conservative management was elected and at 35 weeks a normal female infant was delivered with the affected placenta (Fig. 3.23a). Three-quarters of the placenta was grossly normal and the demarcation from the molar zone was abrupt. The molar zone was covered by normal amnion, but was completely abnormal with cysts of 2 to 3 mm in the majority and some up to 1 cm diameter. No definite maternal surface existed over the molar zone, but gray- tan tissue suggestive of necrotic decidua with old hemorrhage was mingled with the vesicles. The villus tissue in the normal portion looked more like 38 weeks with focal nonspecific villitis, occasional thrombus fragments in some stem vessels, and small segments of villus sclerosis. There was mild acute nonspecific fetal and maternal inflammation of cord, membranes, and placental surface. There were iron staining macrophages in the decidua of the membranes, and zones of decidual necrosis with hemorrhage were confirmed. The microscopic demarcation of normal and molar placenta was as abrupt microscopically as grossly, with no evidence

of molar change in any of the villi on one side, and total molar change on the other. Most of the molar tissue was infarcted with only those molar villi near the junction with the normal placenta remaining viable. Because of the infarction, it was hard to assess trophoblast proliferation, although a few zones were identified on viable villi near the junction zone (Fig. 3.23b). Lymphocytes from the infant, amnion, and chorion, and villi from the normal part of the placenta all provided normal 46,XX cells. The molar tissue did not grow, so it could not be completely characterized. The distinctness of the molar zone and the identifiable histology suggested that this might be another example of dizygotic twinning, with one twin a chorioma, but dispermic monovular twinning cannot be ruled out.

The other two cases were somewhat more fragmented, so the exact relationship of the molar tissue to normal placenta was not clear. In one, both the molar tissue and the normal placenta from the normal fetus were 46,XX, but not apparently further defined. The most recent case was unusual in that the placenta from the chromosomally normal male fetus was partially admixed with molar villi that also had a 46,XY karyotype, but made up of two paternal haploid contributions.

It is clear that the spectrum of molar twins requires further definition using the newer DNA technology. It is recommended that cases of fetus with molar placenta be investigated cytogenetically as well as morphologically. Fresh amnion, chorion, and villi from both the normal and cystic placental portions can be submitted for cytogenetic and DNA analysis (Kalousek DK, 1992, personal communication).

Conclusion

A relatively small expenditure of time and care taken for examination and documentation of placental findings in multiple pregnancy can have far-reaching implications. Careful pathologic examination of the placentation of twins can provide clinically important information, as well as stimulating observations that relate to the biology of twinning and intrauterine development of twins—a fair return for the effort expended. No less important is the fact that when adequate placental examinations are available for expert review and assessment, disputes regarding gestational care and outcome are more likely to be settled in favor of the defense.[63]

References

1. Kloosterman GJ. The "Third Circulation" in identical twins. *Ned Tijdschr Verlosk Gynaecol.* 1963; 63:395–412.

2. Strong SJ, Corney G. *The Placenta in Twin Pregnancy.* Norwich: Pergamon Press; 1967.

3. Boyd JD, Hamilton WJ. *The Human Placenta.* Cambridge: W Heffer; 1970:313–334.

4. Benirschke K, Driscoll SG. *The Pathology of the Human Placenta.* New York: Springer-Verlag; 1967:91–179.

5. Potter EL, Craig JM. *Pathology of the Fetus and the Infant.* 3rd ed. Chicago: Year Book; 1975:207–237.

6. Fox H. Pathology of the placenta. In: Bennington JL, ed. *Major Problems in Pathology.* Vol 7. London: WB Saunders; 1978:73–94.

7. Shanklin DR, Perrin EVDK. Multiple gestation. In: Perrin EVDK, ed. *Pathology of the Placenta. Contemporary Issues in Surgical Pathology.* Vol 5. Roth LM, series ed. New York: Churchill-Livingstone; 1984:165–182.

8. Benirschke K, Kaufmann P. *Pathology of the Human Placenta.* 2nd ed. New York: Springer-Verlag; 1990:636–753.

9. Corey LA, Nance WE, Kang KW, Christian JC. Effects of type of placentation on birthweight and its variability in monozygotic and dizygotic twins. *Acta Genet Med Gemellol.* 1979;28:41–50.

10. Buzzard IM, Uchida IA, Norton JA, Christian JC. Birth weight and placental proximity in like-sex twins. *Am J Hum Genet.* 1983;35:318–323.

11. Cameron AH. The Birmingham twin survey. *Roy Soc Med Proc.* 1968;61:229–234.

12. Bhargava I, Chakravarty A. Vascular anastomoses in twin placentas, and their recognition. *Acta Anat.* 1975;93:471–480.

13. Arts NFTh. Investigations on the vascular system of the placenta. Part I. General introduction and the fetal vascular system. *Am J Obstet Gynecol.* 1961;82:147–158.

14. Cameron AH, Edwards JH, Derom R, Thiery M, Boelaert R. The value of twin surveys in the study of malformations. *Eur J Obstet Gynec Reprod Biol.* 1983;14:347–356.

15. Robertson EG, Neer KJ. Placental injection studies in twin gestation. *Am J Obstet Gynecol.* 1983; 147:170–174.

16. Benirschke K, Kim CK. Multiple pregnancy. *N Engl J Med.* 1973;288:1276–1284,1329–1336.

17. Corney G, Robson EB. Types of twinning and determination of zygosity. In: MacGillivray I, Nylander PPS, Corney G, eds. *Human Multiple Reproduction.* Philadelphia: WB Saunders; 1975:16–39.

18. Corner GW. The observed embryology of human single ovum twins and other multiple births. *Am J Obstet Gynecol.* 1955;70:933–951.

19. Fujikura T, Froehlich LA. Twin placentation and zygosity. *Obstet Gynecol.* 1971;37:34–43.

20. Bulmer MG. *The Biology of Twinning in Man.* Oxford: Clarendon Press; 1970.

21. Ramos-Arroyo MA, Ulbright TM, Yu P-L, Christian JC. Twin study: relationship between birth weight, zygosity, placentation, and pathologic placental changes. *Acta Genet Med Gemellol.* 1988; 37:229–238.

22. Corney G. Placentation. In: MacGillivray I, Nylander PPS, Corney G, eds. *Human Multiple Reproduction.* Philadelphia: WB Saunders; 1975:40–76.

23. Nylander PPS, Osunkoya BO. Unusual monochorionic placentation with heterosexual twins. *Obstet Gynecol.* 1970;36:621–625.

24. Kim K, Lage JM. Bipartite diamnionic monochorionic twin placenta with superficial vascular anastomoses: report of a case. *Hum Pathol.* 1991;22:501–503.

25. Gilbert WM, Davis SE, Kaplan C, Pretorius D, Merritt TA, Benirschke K. Morbidity associated with prenatal disruption of the dividing membrane in twin gestations. *Obstet Gynecol.* 1991;78:623–630.

26. Pauls F. Monoamniotic twin pregnancy. A review of the world literature and a report of two new cases. *Can Med Assoc J.* 1969;100:254–256.

27. Nylander PPS. The value of the placenta in the determination of zygosity—a study of 1,052 Nigerian twin maternities. *J Obstet Gynecol Br Cwlth.* 1969;76:699–704.

28. Soma H, Yoshida K, Tada M, Mukaida T, Kikuchi T. Fetal abnormalities associated with twin placentation (abstract). *Teratology.* 1975;12:211.

29. James WH. Sex ratio and placentation in twins. *Ann Hum Biol.* 1980;7:273–276.

30. Ward BS. Cellular growth of the placenta in twin pregnancy late in gestation. *Placenta.* 1985;6:107–116.

31. Naeye RL. Do placental weights have clinical significance? *Hum Pathol.* 1987;18:387–391.

32. Stiller RJ, Lockwood CJ, Belanger K, Baumgarten A, Hobbins JC, Mahoney MJ. Amniotic fluid α-fetoprotein concentrations in twin gestations: dependence on placenta membrane anatomy. *Obstet Gynecol.* 1988;158:1088–1092.

33. Benirschke K. Placental morphogenesis. In: Wynn RM, ed. *Fetal Hemostasis. Vol 1: Proceedings of the*

First Conference. New York: New York Academy of Sciences; 1965;217–265.

34. Jauniaux E, Elkazen N, Leroy F, Wilkin P, Rodesh F, Hustin J. Clinical and morphologic aspects of the vanishing twin phenomenon. *Obstet Gynecol*. 1988;72:577–581.

35. Benirschke K, Kaufmann P. *Pathology of the Human Placenta*. 2nd ed. New York: Springer-Verlag; 1990:199–204.

36. Robinson LK, Jones KL, Benirschke K. The nature of structural defects associated with velamentous and marginal insertion of the umbilical cord. *Am J Obstet Gynecol*. 1983;146:191–193.

37. Ottolenghi-Preti GF. Sopra un rarissimo caso di gravidanza gemellare con un feto papiraceo e con inserzione velamentosa del funiculo del feto vivo. *An Ostet Ginecol Med Perinat*. 1972;93:173–199.

38. Sekiya S, Hafez ESE. Physiomorphology of twin transfusion syndrome: a study of 86 twin gestations. *Obstet Gynecol*. 1977;50:288–292.

39. Heifetz SA. Single umbilical artery. A statistical analysis of 237 autopsy cases and review of the literature. *Perspect Pediatr Pathol*. 1984;8:345–378.

40. Duerbeck NB, Pietrantoni M, Reed KL, Anderson CF, Shenker L. Doppler flow velocities in single umbilical arteries. *Am J Obstet Gynecol*. 1991; 165:1120–1122.

41. Soernes T, Bakke T. The length of the human umbilical cord in twin pregnancies. *Am J Obstet Gynecol*. 1987;157:1229–1230.

42. De Silva N. Zygosity and umbilical cord length. *J Reprod Med* 1992;37(10):850–852.

43. Naeye RL. Umbilical cord length: clinical significance. *J Pediatr*. 1985;107:278–281.

44. Lacro RV, Jones KL, Benirschke K. The umbilical cord twist: origin, direction and relevance. *Am J Obstet Gynecol*. 1987;157:833–838.

45. Boyd JD, Hamilton WJ. *The Human Placenta*. Cambridge: W Heffer; 1970:222–227.

46. Benirschke K. The placenta in twin gestation. *Clin Obstet Gynecol*. 1990;33:18–31.

47. LaVecchia C, Franceschi S, Fasdli M, Magioni C. Gestational trophoblastic neoplasms in homozygous twins. *Obstet Gynecol*. 1982;60:250–252.

48. De George FV. Hydatidiform moles in other pregnancies of mothers of twins. *Am J Obstet Gynecol*. 1970;108:369–371.

49. Mayer CF. Sextuplets and higher multiparous births: a critical review of history and legend from Aristote-

les to the 20th Century. *Acta Genet Med Gemellol*. 1952;1:118–135,242–275.

50. Szulman AE, Surti U. The syndromes of partial and complete molar gestation. *Clin Obstet Gynecol*. 1984;27:172–180.

51. Shanklin DR. *Tumors of the Placenta and Umbilical Cord*. Philadelphia: BC Decker; 1990:24–29.

52. Beischer NA. Hydatidiform mole with coexistent foetus. *Aust NZ J Obstet Gynecol*. 1966;6:127–141.

53. Yee B, Tu B, Platt LD. Coexisting hydatidiform mole with a live fetus presenting as a placenta previa on ultrasound. *Am J Obstet Gynecol*. 1982;144:726–728.

54. Fisher RA, Sheppard DM, Lawler SD. Twin pregnancy with complete hydatidiform mole (46,XX) and fetus (46,XY): genetic origin proved by analysis of chromosome polymorphisms. *Br Med J*. 1982;284:1218–1220.

55. Sauerbrei EE, Salem S, Fayle B. Coexistent hydatidiform mole and live fetus in the second trimester. *Radiology*. 1980;135:415–417.

56. Hohe PT, Cochrane CR, Gemlich JT, Austin JA. Coexistent trophoblastic tumor and viable pregnancy. *Obstet Gynecol*. 1971;38:899–904.

57. Ladehoff P, Maruszczak A. A pregnancy with a hydatidiform mole, thyrotoxicosis and live born infant. *Acta Obstet Gynecol Scand*. 1978;57:477–478.

58. Suzuki M, Matsunoba A, Wakita K, Nishijima M, Osanai K. Hydatidiform mole with a surviving coexistent fetus. *Obstet Gynecol*. 1980;56:384–388.

59. Vejerslev LO. Clinical management and diagnostic possibility in hydatidiform mole with coexistent fetus. *Obstet Gynecol Survey*. 1991;46:577–588.

60. Deaton JL, Hoffman JS, Saal H, Allred C, Koulos JP. Molar pregnancy coexisting with a normal fetus: a case report. *Gynecol Oncol*. 1989;32:394–397.

61. Feinberg RF, Lockwood CJ, Salafia C, Hobbins JC. Sonographic diagnosis of a pregnancy with a diffuse hydatidiform mole and coexistent 46,XX fetus: a case report. *Obstet Gynecol*. 1988;72:485–488.

62. Vejerslev LO, Sunde L, Hansen BF, Larsen JK, Christensen IJ, Larsen G. Hydatidiform mole and fetus with normal karyotype: support of a separate entity. *Obstet Gynecol*. 1991;77:868–874.

63. Schindler NR. Importance of the placenta and cord in the defense of neurologically impaired infant claims. *Arch Pathol Lab Med*. 1991;115:685–687.

4
Obstetric Aspects of Multiple Pregnancy

Pregnancy is a dynamic process of an evolving interaction of three complex biologic entities— mother, fetus, and placenta—that includes autonomous characteristics of each entity as well as systems of interactions in three dyads and one triad, as well as external and unknown sources of influence[1] (Fig. 4.1a). This way of considering the events during pregnancy can be used not only for the normal structural changes and functional processes, but also for abnormalities of structure and function, and for the consequences of these abnormalities on the other components of the triad. It may also help clarify just what is being assessed during antenatal, intrapartum, and postnatal testing. The presence of more than one fetus at a time adds another dimension to these interactions. As the types of twins become less and less separate, the potential for distortion of first the placental component, and then the fetal component, can be represented by the altered shapes needed to represent the interactions as in Fig. 4.1b,c and Fig. 4.1d,e respectively. These representations serve to remind us not only of the potential for feto-fetal interaction, particularly in monoamniotic twinning, but also of the maternal-fetal interaction system. Aspects of fetoplacental and maternoplacental interactions were described in Chapter 3, and the implications of monochorionicity are presented in Chapters 8, 9, and 10. This chapter highlights maternal-fetal and maternal-fetal-placental associations as they relate to the pathology of multiple pregnancy.

One of the major hurdles faced by a twin conception is diagnosis—diagnosis of the presence of twins, the possible pattern of twinning, and detection of abnormalities. Without an index of suspicion and the use of appropriate ultrasound examination techniques, 20% to 40% of twin conceptions may not be identified as such before labor and delivery.[2] Because this information assists the planning of optimal care, the absence of the diagnosis occasionally assumes medicolegal significance as well. Next, the potential complications of twinning differ according to the patterns of twinning and placentation, and in many cases it becomes important to determine the chorionicity of the twins in utero. In skilled hands, clinicopathological correlation of ultrasound findings of membrane thickness and the histology of the septum has provided a predictive accuracy of 83% to 100%.[3,4] Also, prenatal diagnosis and continuing monitoring of the twins may be required, and while a number of observations and tests are available, they are often technically more difficult than with singletons. Ultrasound examinations provide a valuable assessment of the twins on an ongoing basis, although the procedure is necessarily more time-consuming and painstaking.[5] It has been recommended that serial sonographic monitoring at 3- to 4-week intervals be used in uncomplicated twin gestations during the third trimester, with enhanced monitoring as indicated.[6] Genetic amniocentesis may be required, and, in skilled hands, bilateral karyotypes have been possible in 93% of twin pregnancies with few complications.[7] Caution is required in interpreting amniotic fluid alpha-fetoprotein concentrations, because there may be diffusion across a diamnion septum, creating falsely elevated values in a sac with a normal twin.[8] Elevated levels of maternal serum alpha-fetoprotein (MSAFP) have been used to detect twin conceptions and predict those that are at

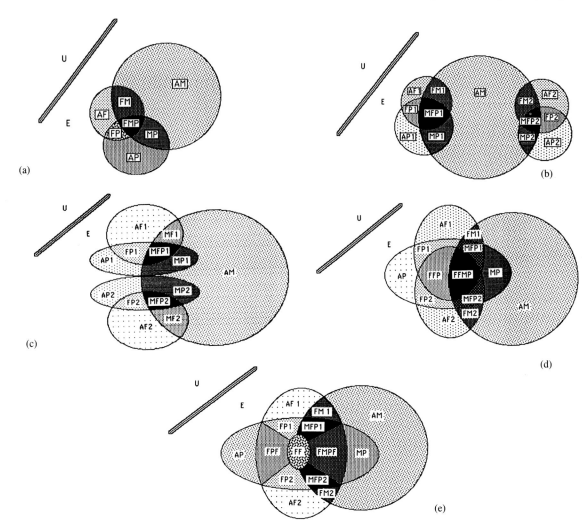

FIGURE 4.1. Fetal-maternal-placental interrelationships. These schematics represent the fetal, maternal, and placental interactions in singleton and twin pregnancies. A, autonomous; M, maternal; F, fetal; P, placenta; E, exogenous; U, unknown. (a) The overlapping circles represent the three biologic systems that interact during pregnancy with autonomous, dyad, and triad fields of activity, as well as external influences that are known and unknown. The autonomous categories are those parts of the fetus, mother, and placenta that are not directly connected with either of the other two components. The three dyads indicated are meant to represent both functional and anatomic interactions. The triad corresponds to the terminal villus. (b) This scheme represents dichorionic twins with separate gestational sacs. The appended numbers serve to distinguish the entities of each twin. (c) This scheme is of dichorionic twins with a single disk/fused

placenta. The appended numbers apply as in (b). The distortion of the placenta circles represents the observation that the growth of each can be affected by the proximity of the other, but there is no interconnection. (d) This represents monochorionic diamniotic twins. The placenta is represented by a single disk with distinct portions allocated to each twin. There are two new zones of interaction indicated. FFP represents intertwin vascular anastomoses on the placenta, and FFMP represents the shared placental cotyledons. (e) In this representation of monochorionic monoamniotic twins the placenta is a single structure. The distinctions between the twins are portrayed as less clear-cut because of the degree of vascular sharing encountered in these cases. There is a zone of feto-fetal interaction (FF) to represent the fact that the twins are in the same amniotic sac and can interact directly.

higher risk of a number of complications, including preterm birth, low birth weight, discordant growth, and perinatal death.[9] Twin-specific tables are not necessary, as race specific singleton ratios for MSAFP can be extrapolated to twins, using the same proportionate cutoff levels.[10] Fetal blood sampling from the umbilical cords is used in twin pregnancies at risk for acquired or inherited disorders that require blood for diagnosis.[11] The results of these investigations may lead to termination procedures, so the time and care required for accuracy of cord identification is essential. Fetal umbilical artery blood flow is now being assessed in multiple pregnancy, although it takes persistence to make sure that each cord is being assessed, and abnormal patterns are being correlated with increased fetal morbidity and mortality.[12]

The diagnosis of a twin conception has significant ramifications for all aspects of the course and management of the pregnancy, as can be determined from any one of a number of obstetric references,[13–16] and this chapter makes no attempt to reiterate those presentations. While it is theoretically true that all aspects of the maternal organism could influence the perinatal outcome of twins, the following discussion is limited to those maternal/gestational problems that have a reasonably direct association with fetal and placental pathology. In this context, then, there are three groups of obstetric concerns to consider: maternal disorders that affect twins; pregnancy complications that are increased with twins, including heterotopic pregnancy; and problems with labor and delivery of twins, including prematurity, fetal distress or trauma, and interval deliveries.

Maternal Disorders Affecting Twins

Maternal disorders would appear to affect twins the same as they do singletons, but the situations are complicated by the technical difficulties of assessing and monitoring two fetuses, and the possibility of discordant fetal effects and responses. Bilateral monitoring of twin fetuses has been reported in cases of rhesus isoimmunization and maternal immune (idiopathic) thrombocytopenic purpura, and discordant fetal responses have been described in these conditions as well as with maternal diabetes mellitus.

Discordant fetal response to an apparently homogeneous maternal state has been recognized for some time in *erythroblastosis fetalis due to rhesus isoimmunization* in twins.[17–19] In addition to problems of discordant severity, there are technical challenges in the diagnosis, monitoring, and management of two infants in the same uterus, although a successful outcome is possible in skilled hands.[19] The pattern seems to be that monovular twins will be equally affected, while asymmetry of response is expected when twins are dizygotic and thus discordant for blood group, but variations have been described. Twins that have the same Rh and ABO status have been reported to be equally affected[20] and variably affected,[17] but the variability in the latter group was not explained. In twins who have Rh identity, if they are different in their ABO groups and one is incompatible with the mother's ABO group, the ABO incompatible twin may have less damage from the Rh antibodies in primary Rh isoimmunization as they may not cross that twin's placenta as readily and may be blocked from the red cells.[20] Not all reviews of the relationship of ABO and Rh fetomaternal incompatibility agree that ABO incompatibility protects against subsequent Rh incompatible pregnancies.[21] In unlike-sex twins, it has been suggested that the female infants were better able to provide an effective erythropoietic response without producing the severe hepatocellular problems that cause hydrops, although there was no explanation as to the origin of this apparent sex difference.[19] The cases of perinatal death due to Rh isoimmunization have become much less frequent with the advent of preventive programs, and only older cases were present in the Survey '91 Review autopsy group: a set of female twins at 27 weeks' gestation of unknown placentation pattern equally affected, a presumably dizygotic pair with a severely affected stillborn macerated male with marked splenomegaly, and a liveborn female who was mildly hydropic but did well after two neonatal exchange transfusions (Fig. 4.2). In a more recent set of dichorionic separate-disk unlike-sex twins with maternal anti-Kell antibodies present, the male twin was well when delivered at 31 weeks, while the female was stillborn with evidence of hemolysis and hydrops.

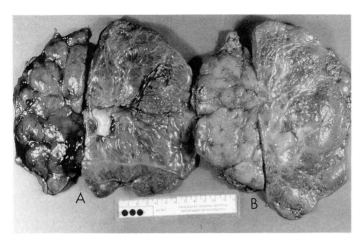

FIGURE 4.2. These two placentas are from an Rh isoimmunized dichorionic diamniotic twin pregnancy with a severely affected stillborn macerated male (pale placenta on right) and a less severely affected female who survived (placenta on left). Note the differential color of the villus tissue, due to different degrees of villus hydrops, although the size was not noticeably different.

Discordant fetal responses with *maternal immune (idiopathic) thrombocytopenic purpura* (ITP) have been reported in an unlike-sex twin pair with separate placentas.[22] Both twins were assessed by cordocentesis prenatally and while the female twin was more severely affected, she did not require special treatment after birth. The difference in severity of the thrombocytopenia was attributed to possible genetic differences in platelet antigens, although no details were provided, and/or a difference in permeability of the respective placentas to the maternal antibodies. Fetomaternal platelet incompatibility leading to fetal isoimmune thrombocytopenia could be discordant in a manner analogous to Rh isoimmunization, but does not appear to have been reported. In the Survey '91 Review, there was a set of monochorionic male twins at 37 weeks in which twin A had very low platelets, a massive intracerebral hemorrhage, and cutaneous and visceral petechiae, and he died at 43 hours of age, while the co-twin was less seriously affected and survived. The mother had immune thrombocytopenia. The apparent fetal asymmetry may be due in part to a greater antibody load in the larger twin A on the basis of intertwin vascular anastomoses with the smaller twin B. Also, the twins were delivered vaginally and this may have contributed to the manifestations in twin A.

Diabetes mellitus is also reported to be associated with asymmetric fetal responses. A pair of dichorionic male infants delivered to a diabetic woman were 1,000 g different in weight and although both did well, one was the classical macrosomic infant with hypoglycemia.[23] Although this discordant manifestation of the fetal effects of maternal diabetes was attributed to heterozygosity, and hence genetic variation in fetal responsiveness to the maternal disease, there was no indication as to how dizygosity was established. In the Survey '91 Review autopsy group, there were only two sets of twins with diabetic mothers, although twins may be more frequent than expected in insulin dependent diabetics,[24] and both sets were earlier cases with inadequate placental reporting. In one set of male monochorionic twins with a 1,500-g placenta, one twin was stillborn, but other causes of fetal death in monochorionic twins, such as vascular sharing and intertwin transfusions, were not ruled out. In the second set, the deceased male twin of unknown zygosity to the surviving male twin died at 15 days with aortic thrombosis and islet cell hyperplasia of the pancreas, massive intracerebral hemorrhage with multifocal anoxic neuronal necrosis, bronchopulmonary dysplasia, and renal failure. The source of these complications of the neonatal course after apparently spontaneous delivery at 34 weeks was not described.

Other maternal disorders and twin pregnancies are rarely reported specifically and tend to be limited to those situations where there is a risk associated with a hereditary disorder, and prenatal diagnosis of the twins is undertaken with a view to further management of the case.[11] Selective termination of discordantly affected fetuses is discussed further in Chapter 5. In one of the Survey '91 Review autopsy cases, monochorionic female twins born to a mother with myotonic dystrophy at 29 weeks appeared to be discordantly affected, with twin B dying at 3 weeks of age with diffuse skeletal muscle atrophy, growth retardation, severe brain damage, and bronchopulmonary dysplasia. Twin A was reportedly unaffected. The discordancy remains unexplained unless one of the mechanisms discussed in Chapter 7 can be invoked, such as genomic imprinting relating to which X chromosome was inactivated.

Acquired problems during pregnancy with twins are also rarely reported specifically. The potential teratogenic effect of exogenous agents is always a concern in pregnancy, so a successful pregnancy with well-grown and apparently normal unlike-sex twins in a mother receiving cyclosporin A immunosuppression after renal transplantation is of note.[25] In the Survey '91 Review, there were three interesting cases in this category of acquired maternal problems. A set of unlike-sex dichorionic-fused placenta twins was delivered prematurely at 22 weeks because of abruptio placenta, and they succumbed in 2 hours because of immaturity. The gestational dating was based on ultrasound measurements at 7 to 8 weeks of pregnancy when the twins were diagnosed. The interesting feature was that they were at the 90th percentile for growth, even using singleton data, even though the mother had had intestinal bypass surgery and had gained only 3 lbs to that point in pregnancy. A mother with malaria and a hemoglobin of 50 g/l delivered normally grown twins at 24 weeks who died within 24 hours of respiratory insufficiency. The placenta was small with poorly vascularized villi, but no parasites were seen. A woman with lipoid nephrosis was also hypertensive and delivered a macerated male twin at 28 weeks, while the undiagnosed second dichorionic female twin survived. The contribution of the maternal disease in this case was uncertain as there was also prolapse of the umbilical cord with the foot of twin A.

Among *maternal malformations* that might influence the outcome of a multiple gestation are malformations of the uterus. They are cited as a potential contributing factor to preterm labor and delivery with singletons,[26] so it might be suspected that the same problems would arise with twins. Exceptions are reported, however, and they serve to remind us to question why the general principle does not always seem to apply. Twins, one in each horn of a bicornuate uterus, have been retained until 31 weeks[27] and 35 weeks[28] of gestation. There were two relevant cases in the Survey '91 Review. A set of monochorionic twins, both in the same side of a bicornuate uterus, were stillborn at 26 weeks, attributed initially to "crowding" because of the uterine anomaly, but pathologically determined to be due to the twin-to-twin transfusion syndrome across vascular anastomoses. In another case, a set of female dichorionic twins was delivered by section at 31 weeks. One twin did well, but the other was growth retarded by 2 to 3 weeks and had died in utero 6 weeks previously. There was evidence of multifocal old and recent premature separation of the placenta, which was an unusual V-shape, with diffusely ischemic villus tissues with multiple infarcts on the side of the deceased twin. The placental form suggested a uterine anomaly and in fact a partial septum was present, with both twins apparently on the same side of the septum. Unfortunately, no note was made of the actual attachment of the placenta at the time of section delivery. It may be that septal attachments are not as well perfused, accounting for the pathology in the placenta and perhaps the fetal growth retardation and death. The adaptability of the uterus is demonstrated by the report of a woman with gonadal dysgenesis mosaicism and an initially hypoplastic uterus, who was able to carry normal triplets to 33 weeks' gestation, following in vitro fertilization and embryo transfer after medical hormonal therapy.[29]

The pathologist's role in situations of maternal disorders and a multiple pregnancy is to correlate observations of placentation and fetal/infant pathology with the maternal disorder, so as to identify relevant associations for future reference. Pathologic confirmation (or not) of prenatal diagnoses has quality assurance and medicolegal functions as well.

Gestational Complications of Multiple Pregnancy

Some of the problems that twins face in utero are the obstetric complications of having two or more fetuses growing in a space meant ideally for one.[30–39] The greater endocrine and circulatory loads of a multiple conception place increased burdens of adaptation on the mother, and the increased intrauterine volume potentially adds to her morbidity. The "exaggerated" physiologic adaptations to a multiple pregnancy means that different standards of "abnormality" need to be established as the singleton parameters may not apply for many test systems.[40] Twin gestations have been reported to have up to nearly three times the incidence of antenatal complications with singletons, but this discussion will focus on those complications with implications for fetal survival.

Hypertensive syndromes of pregnancy are a particularly important complication of any gestation and there seems to be a consensus that the incidence is increased with twins, although the degree reported varies from 3 to 15 times the occurrence with singletons. There are conflicting reports as to whether hypertension is more likely with dizygotic or monozygotic twins, and the definitive answer to this question might have relevance to the pathophysiology of maternal hypertension with twins.[41] Fetal growth retardation seems more important than fetal death for hypertensive mothers of twins, with a decrease in total fetal weights and greater interfetal growth discordance. Maternal death with twin gestations is reported rarely, but has been associated with pregnancy-induced hypertension.[42]

In the Survey '91 Review, survivor group, hypertension associated with fetal growth problems was more prevalent with dichorionic than monochorionic placentations, and the details are presented in Chapter 6. In the autopsy group, there were three cases of emergency section delivery for complicated maternal hypertension with death of one twin. One case is described above associated with a septate uterus. In the second, the concordant and appropriately grown monochorionic male twin who died was anemic and twin transfusion syndrome was considered responsible, until a major fetomaternal hemorrhage was diagnosed. The mother's hypertension had become clinically progressive at the same time, as asymmetric placental thickening due to hydrops was identified with ultrasound examination 2 weeks prior to the delivery at 34 weeks. The placenta did not have ischemic features. In the third, the autopsied growth retarded monochorionic 28-week female twin died at 42 hours of complications of prematurity, while the better-grown twin survived, but the placental attributes were incompletely recorded. In other words, while maternal hypertension was clinically severe enough to lead to operative delivery, the perinatal deaths are potentially attributable to unrelated events. It is noteworthy that all these cases were monochorionic twins.

Antepartum hemorrhage has been reported to be increased with twins, both due to placenta previa and premature separation/abruption, with rates of two to three times that of singletons, although not every survey reports an increase. Abruptio placenta has been listed as a cause of up to 4.5% of perinatal mortality in twins.[43] When there is more than one conceptus at a time, there is a theoretical risk of low implantations or unstable implantations, with vasa praevia a particular risk on the basis of the increased frequency of velamentous cord insertions in twins as noted in Chapter 3. However, only four twin pairs in the Survey '91 autopsy group were associated with complications of asphyxia or prematurity following spontaneous preterm delivery at 27 weeks and 29 weeks with abruptio placenta, and 26 weeks and 27 weeks with placenta praevia. The association of embryonic or fetal death with first trimester bleeding is discussed in Chapter 5.

There are conflicting reports of the incidence of *maternal anemia* with twins, from no increase to two to three times the rate seen with singleton pregnancies. Because of the greater maternal plasma volume expansion in twin gestations, the lower hemoglobin levels reported of around 100 g/l may simply represent an exaggeration of "normal" pregnancy anemia. Increased viscosity of maternal blood seems to be one of the critical factors determining placental perfusion in women with pregnancy-induced hypertension, and is associated with less than normal plasma volume expansion, particularly when fetal growth retardation occurs.[44] Perhaps the greater "normal" volume expansion with twin gestations serves to ensure perfusion of the larger mass of placental tissues, because no apparent fetal detriment has been reported attributed to maternal anemia.

Twin conceptions are at greater risk for *fetal developmental anomalies* and fetal death, and these represent diagnostic and management problems. The investigative techniques referred to in the introduction to this chapter may be used to identify and characterize fetal maldevelopment during pregnancy, with a view to more reasoned approaches to decision making, particularly regarding labor and delivery. The pathologist's role in those cases where there has been an antenatal diagnosis of a particular abnormality is to confirm (or not) the diagnosis at the time of postmortem examination, should that opportunity arise.

Antepartum fetal death is a potentially serious complication of multiple gestation for both the mother and surviving twin. Intrauterine fetal death in singleton conceptions with retention of the dead fetus may be complicated by a maternal defibrination syndrome.[45] Defibrination is also a risk when one fetus of a twin conception dies, due to either natural causes or iatrogenic intervention, and the pregnancy continues. This complication can be managed clinically so that the surviving infant can be delivered without threat to the mother.[46,47] In the case of a retained singleton death, this complication is attributed to thromboplastin entering the maternal circulation from the dead conceptus. However, maternal coagulopathy seems to occur so rarely in situations of retained intrauterine fetal death of one of a multiple gestation, that diffusing fetal thromboplastin must be an incomplete explanation. Fetal death of one monochorionic twin has been reported to be associated with a significant risk of intrauterine morbidity in the survivor on the basis of induced coagulopathy across vascular anastomoses. The evidence for this proposed pathogenetic mechanism is not altogether convincing and the topic is reviewed in detail in Chapter 9. Maternal coagulopathy (in the absence of pregnancy-induced hypertension) was not reported in any of the Survey '91 Review cases with intrauterine death of one fetus.

Diabetes mellitus in pregnancy is potentially serious for mother and infant, but the reported relationship of diabetes to twin pregnancy varies. Gestational diabetes mellitus is reported in twin pregnancies with the same frequency as singletons,[38] while another review suggests that both chemical and overt diabetes are higher in multiple gestations.[48]

Excessive amounts of amniotic fluid, hydramnios or *polyhydramnios,* can be a subjective finding, but have been noted to be more common in twin pregnancies.[14] Fetal mortality in these cases is high, 23% to 87%,[18] related to the underlying cause of the hydramnios, such as fetal malformation with chronic accumulations or twin transfusion with acute hydramnios, or to the possibility that the uterine distention leads to premature delivery,[49] although the latter association is disputed.[50] Acute hydramnios, developing within a few days, has been reported in 2% of twin pregnancies and occurs in the second trimester.[51] It is associated with normally developing monochorionic twins, but the precipitate course usually terminates the pregnancy in a few days.[52,53] In the Survey '91 Review autopsy group, hydramnios was recorded as the cause of preterm labor and delivery at 21 to 29 weeks in 12 cases, associated with twin transfusion in nine, and with monochorionic twins without documented anastomoses in three. The association of hydramnios and twin transfusion is discussed further in Chapter 9.

With potentially double the volume of intrauterine contents in twin gestations, it might be expected that *premature cervical effacement and dilatation* would be a problem, and an incidence two to three times higher than in singleton gestations has been observed (Farquharson D, Lindahl S, 1985, personal communication). The consequences of premature cervical ripening are ascending infection, premature rupture of membranes and premature labor, often in combination with prolapse of fetal parts, such as the umbilical cord. Because premature delivery is one of the main sources of perinatal morbidity and mortality with twins, cervical cerclage has been tried as a prophylactic measure, but with equivocal results.[54] In fact, in one study of cervical ripening and subsequent labor, a group of women were identified who had cervical dilatation and effacement for several weeks before the onset of labor, although what else characterized these patients, such as smaller twins, was not specified.[55] The importance of cervical dilatation to prematurity with multifetal pregnancies is attested to by continuing attempts to define better ways of monitoring the cervix, clinically[56] and ultrasonographically.[57] Cervical incompetence was listed as the cause of preterm delivery at 20 weeks in one set of the Survey '91 Review autopsy-group twins, and a cervical suture placed at 25 weeks in a second set was associated with preterm delivery the next day, with necrotizing chorioamnionitis of sac A and perinatal death of twin A with pulmonary and cerebral hemorrhage.

An obstetric complication unique to multiple conceptions is the occurrence of *heterotopic pregnancy* (combined uterine and extrauterine), or ectopic multiple implantations. The pattern of combined uterine and tubal (occasionally ovarian) concurrent pregnancies is to be differentiated from a compound multiple in which a current intrauterine pregnancy coexists with a remote residual tubal implantation.[58] The incidence of heterotopic multiple implantations seems to be increasing and may be related to techniques of assisted fertility coupled with the tubal pathology necessitating those techniques.[59] Bilateral simultaneous tubal pregnancies,[60] unilateral twin ectopic tubal gestations,[61] and ovarian twin pregnancies[62] have been reported. Although it has been suggested that unilateral tubal twins are more likely monozygotic, the evidence is questionable in many cases,[61] so the zygotic origin of these aberrantly implanted twin patterns remains to be determined. A heterotopic twin pregnancy with molar placental tissue with the intrauterine twin has been reported, but unfortunately without cytogenetic studies.[63]

Problems of Labor and Delivery

The obstetric complications in twin gestations continue into the process of labor and delivery, as evidenced by the volume of available literature on the proper conduct of parturition with twins. There is a consensus that the delivery of twins can be fraught with problems, but there seems to be little agreement on the details of how to anticipate, prevent, or manage the problems. From the perspective of the pathologist investigating suboptimal outcomes, complications of labor and delivery that contribute to prematurity, perinatal asphyxia, and fetal injury are of particular concern. Interval delivery of twins is rare, but of interest as well.

Perinatal Trauma

It is difficult to separate the potential complications of malpositioned or undiagnosed twins from those of birth order and discordant growth with respect to perinatal asphyxia and birth trauma, but the second twin seems to be at greater risk on all counts. Up to 58% of twins may be presenting as other than vertex,[64] more frequently the second twin.[65] After 165 days of pregnancy in a series of 100 twin sets, the fetal presentation was observed to stay the same in two-thirds of A twins and one-half of B twins; 44% were not vertex at delivery, 28% of A twins and 50% of B twins (Wittmann BK, 1987, personal communication). Breech presentation of the second twin has been reported to be associated with lower

birth weight and concomitant increased risks for perinatal asphyxia and birth trauma.[66] Fortunately, interlocking of twins seems to be rare, 0.1%, but the perinatal mortality is high, 31%.[18] The clinical decision as to the best route of delivery in any one case is always predicated on minimizing fetal compromise, and various combinations of vaginal and operative deliveries are recommended.[35,67] A somewhat contrasting review of 362 pairs of twins suggested that neither position nor presentation were significant factors in perinatal mortality or morbidity, and that there was no urgency to deliver twin B if electronic fetal heart rate monitoring was normal, thus avoiding potential trauma associated with urgent mechanically assisted delivery.[68] It was noted in this review as well that cesarian delivery did not preclude injury. It has been suggested that the reported increased risks for twin B represent the load of undiagnosed twins, as one cannot plan optimum management for that which is not known to exist.[67]

Reports of perinatal morbidity and mortality of twins specified as due to trauma are infrequent. Traumatic perinatal deaths of twins have been observed with the same frequency as of singletons,[69] but have also been reported as the cause of 11.5% of all perinatal twin deaths, 14.3% of twin A, and 4.1% of twin B deaths.[70] In a review of 362 twin pairs, 2% of the infants were described to have birth related injuries consisting of 10 small cephalohematomas and one large one that led to anemia and elevated bilirubin, a fractured clavicle and humerus during breech delivery of a 3,420-g twin B, two infants with transient facial nerve palsy, and one Erb's paralysis with paralysis of the left diaphragm after vertex delivery of a 2,100-g twin A. This review contained only one perinatal death due to asphyxia because the cervix clamped down on the aftercoming head of a 1,000-g second twin. In the Survey '91 Review autopsy group, there were three sets of twins with obstructed labor due to malposition: in a monochorionic set at 33 weeks, twin A's head was interlocked with the head of twin B who had died in utero with growth retardation and hydrops, but twin A survived after cesarian delivery; in a dichorionic-fused set, the heads of the male twins were interlocked at delivery at 28 weeks and twin A survived, but twin B died at 5½ months of age of complications of prematurity, primarily lung disease; in a dichorionic-separate set at 24 weeks, twin B was a transverse lie and eventually stillborn. In two sets, cord prolapse from twin B led to emergency deliveries, a traumatic breech extraction at 30 weeks, and an operative abdominal delivery at 39 weeks, but both B twins died with asphyxial lesions. In one case, the uterus clamped down after delivery of twin A at 24 weeks and twin B was stillborn. In one case of undiagnosed twins at 27 weeks, twin A died of complications of prematurity, while twin B survived; and in another case of undiagnosed twins at 25 weeks, the second twin was stillborn when delivered with the manually removed placenta after twin A who died neonatally with lesions of asphyxia and prematurity.

Perinatal Asphyxia

Transition of the fetus from the uterine to the external environment requires a switch from maternal blood flow around a somewhat distant structure (the placenta) as a source of oxygen, to an internal autonomously functioning lung/pulmonary blood flow system. This incredibly dramatic physiologic change is accomplished remarkably smoothly in the majority of cases, but the consequences of delayed or partially successful transitions are only too well known to pathologists, neurologists, and the courts. The causes, manifestations, and consequences of what is called perinatal asphyxia are subjects of intense interest with multiple gestations just as with singletons, and the undiagnosed second twin represents a particular problem.

The importance of perinatal asphyxia as a pathophysiologic process is that it probably accounts for the majority of fetal deaths. Chronic and/or acute disturbances of fetal oxygenation/perfusion would appear to be the final mechanism of intrauterine death at almost any gestational age. There are virtually no developmental anomalies that can be said to cause fetal death directly, although the abnormal development may contribute to fetal heart failure, may affect placental development and function, or impair fetal responses to asphyxia-causing stresses. Infectious agents can lead to fetal death directly, but do so rarely when compared to the numbers of fetuses who are live-born infected or survive the infection but are growth retarded or malformed. Perinatal asphyxia has been reported as the main cause of death for 15% of A twins and 25% of B twins without specifying the time of death.[40] In another survey, asphyxia was given as the main cause of 27% of singleton deaths, 34% of twin A deaths, and 42% of twin B deaths.[69]

It is obviously critical to be able to assess the status of a fetus prior to delivery, either before or during labor, in a sufficiently reliable and meaningful fashion so that appropriate measures can be undertaken to minimize the consequences of any disruptive events.[71] Cardiorespiratory compromise of fetal/neonatal well-being that may have neurologic/visceral sequelae consists of disruptive events and subsequent fetal responses that may or may not compensate for the stress. The pattern of fetal/neonatal response and its effectiveness may vary with the nature of the stress (acute or chronic, steady or intermittent, mild or severe), and the status of the fetus/infant (gestational age or maturity and size, preexisting compromise such as growth retardation), but the severity of the consequences may be unpredictable in the individual case. The ability to assess the situation will vary with the tools available and the stage of labor and delivery being assessed. Difficulties arise when detectable abnormalities in the fetus/newborn do not appear to correlate with clinical events, for example, heart rate tracing abnormalities during labor but good Apgar scores at birth, and yet clinical or pathological evidence of brain damage. The methods of assessing perinatal well-being in the fetus/newborn and the terminology used to describe the situations are being reassessed because it would seem that unhelpful generalizations have crept into usage.[71]

For the purposes of this discussion, the term "perinatal asphyxia" is used to encompass those antepartum, intrapartum, and immediate neonatal events that appear to affect fetal/neonatal oxygenation and/or circulation, with consequences for fetal/neonatal survival. These situations may have specifically definable pathologic causes, may be accompanied by pathologically recognizable manifestations of fetal/neonatal responses, and may have pathologically evident consequences in fetal/neonatal organ systems.[72–76]

The potential causes of perinatal asphyxia are the same for twins as for singletons, with additional risks for the second twin, particularly if undiagnosed, for monochorionic twins with vascular anastomoses, and for monoamniotic twins. Potential sources of the intrauterine asphyxia include problems of the maternal supply line, lesions at the fetomaternal junction, immunologically generated placental dysfunction, problems of maternal perfusion of the placenta, fetal vascular developmental anomalies, disorders, or dysfunction, or problems at the fetomaternal exchange site. The gross and microscopic appearances of these lesions in twins are the same as when they are seen with singletons. For example, in one survey of the 30% of twin deaths attributed to perinatal asphyxia, one-third were associated with antepartum hemorrhage (due to intrapartum premature separation in the majority), cord accidents (prolapsed cords or entangled monoamniotic cords) occurred in 16.6%, maternal toxemia and fetal growth retardation were important in 11% each, and dystocia and an undiagnosed second twin in 5.5% each. No cause for the asphyxia was identified in 16.6%.[77] The umbilical cord is of particular concern with twins. While anomalous insertions of the umbilical cord occur with singletons, it was noted in Chapter 3 that not only are they more common when there are multiple fetuses, but they are even more frequent with perinatal twin deaths (Table 3.3), and are recognized as a contributing factor to perinatal asphyxia.[78] Therefore, careful observation and documentation of the details of cord insertions may be critical information for the interpretation of perinatal asphyxia of twins. The effects of perinatal asphyxia also contribute to neonatal death, so potential intrauterine causes and manifestations must be sought in these cases as well. However, it is true that in many cases the underlying problem is not determined, and only the effect is evident, i.e., fetal death with or without lesions of fetal response or asphyxial damage.

The degree of increased risk for twin B, if in fact there is any, is not settled. Suggestions of an increased susceptibility of twin B have come from observations that lower Apgar scores were assigned to twin B twice as often as to twin A in both monochorionic and dichorionic twins.[79] However, other observations suggested that the differences in Apgar scores were associated more with low birth weight than birth order.[80] In one study, a biochemical disadvantage to the second-born twin was demonstrated regardless of route of delivery, zygosity, birth interval, or presentation,[81] while another found no significant differences as long as each twin weighed at least 1,500 g each.[82] The additional potential risks for the second twin consist of three main contributing factors—the higher incidence of growth retardation, the higher incidence of nonvertex presentation, and the effect of the contraction of the uterus after delivery of the first twin. The pathologist has an important role in clarifying these situations. Growth retardation adds an additional burden to the fetus' ability to cope with events causing asphyxia,[83] so that documentation of the pattern and degree of growth retardation and identification of contributing factors, such as placental disorders or fetal anomalies, is important.[84] Factors contributing to growth retardation in twins are discussed in Chapter 6. Malpresentation of the second twin can predispose to cord prolapse or may lead to delayed delivery, as referred to above, but when the relative risk of growth retardation is compared to malpresentation, most surveys report that fetal size is the more critical factor.[35] Uterine contraction after delivery of the first twin may actually prevent delivery of the second twin, or may be associated with premature separation of the placenta[26,35] and, at least theoretically, increasing compression of uterine placental vessels with compromise of the maternal supply line. Failure to anticipate a second twin may lead to Ergotrate being administered after the first delivery with potential complications for the second twin.[77]

Monochorionic twinning has additional risk factors for perinatal asphyxia. Twins who share circulations may be at risk for acute alterations in blood flow across the anastomoses following changes in amniotic fluid volume after rupture of membranes, or as a consequence of discordant hypotension in the fetuses, with consequences for oxygenation and perfusion. These situations are discussed more fully in Chapter 9. Monoamniotic twins are at risk for complications of feto-fetal interaction, and in fact most of the high mortality in this group is due to cord/fetal entanglements (see Chapter 8).

Accurate identification as to which twin is being assessed for all measures of fetal/neonatal well-being should go without saying, but it is so important that it is emphasized again with two additional comments. It was mentioned in the discussion of the placenta in Chapter 3 that the only time irrefutable identification of the umbilical cords can be made is in the delivery room, and that the explanation of the identification must be made known to the pathologist unless it is self-evident, such as one and two ligatures on the respective cords, for example. The pathologist who is investigating a perinatal twin death or a placenta in connection with a complicated neonatal course, may have the opportunity to review ultrasound reports, Doppler studies, fetal monitoring strips, or fetal blood sampling studies. Great care must be taken to be certain that the antenatal observations are correctly associated with the postnatal infants and designated placentation, particularly if the twins were delivered abdominally. Twin A in utero by ultrasound may not be twin A at section, and unless this is clarified, meaningful clinicopathologic correlation will be impossible.

The pathological findings that are attributed to fetal responses to perinatal asphyxial stresses, such as aspiration of amniotic debris, with or without meconium, and meconium staining of the placenta, are well described in texts of fetal and perinatal pathology and are the same in twins as in singletons.[72–76] An important additional observation that the pathologist can make is a comparison of these findings between the twins on the placenta(s), and in the twins themselves, should they come to autopsy.

Similarly, the pathologically evident consequences of perinatal asphyxia reflect tissue hypoxia/ischemia and are the same in twins as in

singletons.[72–76] Again, it is useful to compare the distribution and severity of these findings between the twins if both come to autopsy. The most extensively analyzed consequences of perinatal asphyxia are the lesions in the brain.[85,86] In a review of patterns and mechanisms of brain damage in twins, Norman[86] identified anoxic lesions due to perinatal asphyxia in 16.6% of her cases. She attributed differences in brain size, identified in three of five pairs of twins autopsied, to unequal blood supply during intrauterine growth. The third group of lesions consisted of cavitated and destructive lesions with or without abnormal neuronal migration. These were associated with cerebral ischemia and resulted from inequalities in perfusion that could have been due to a variety of vascular insults, such as abruptio placenta, placenta praevia, or other cord or placental catastrophes, as well as inequalities of monochorionic shunting.

In the Survey '91 Review of 324 sets of twins where one or both twins came to autopsy, there were 462 twin autopsies, and of these 4% of the twin sets had concordant asphyxial pathology, and asphyxial lesions were the only findings in 8.9% of the total number of autopsies (Table 4.1). Cases were classed in this category only if they were reported to have the accepted lesions,[72–76] includ-

TABLE 4.1. Comparative characteristics of twin deaths with lesions of asphyxia and/or prematurity: Survey '91 Review—autopsy group.

	Asphyxia alone	Asphyxia/prematurity	Prematurity alone	
Percent of twin autopsies	8.9	6.5	30.0	
Percent of twin sets concordantly affected	4.0	2.5	15.4	
Ratio male:female	1.4:1	1.5:1	1.5:1	
Ratio B:A	1.6:1	1.5:1	1.2:1	
Gestational age	21–40 weeks range	21–36 weeks range	21–24 wks = 26%	
	25–28 wks = 29%	25–32 wks = 90%	25–28 wks = 49.6%	
	37+ wks = 26.8%		29–32 wks = 17.2%	
Time of death	SB = 70%	<24 hrs = 40%	<24 hrs = 52%	
	<24 hrs = 19%	1–7 days = 33%	1–7 days = 21.5%	
	2–28 days = 11%	8–28 days = 7%	8–28 days = 18.7%	
		>28 days = 20%	1–9 mos = 7.8%	
Male/male:female/female twin sets	3:1	1:1	2:1	
Monochorionic:dichorionic placentation	1:1	1:1.7	1:2	
Causes				
Unknown	34%	73%	53%	
Other	Umbilical cord	29%	Cord prolapse 13%	Ascending inf.	18.7%
	Antepartum hem.	10%	Miscellaneous 14%	Antepartum hem.	9.3%
	IUGR	10%		Acute hydramnios	13%
	Twin transfusion	15%		Miscellaneous	6%
	Miscellaneous	2%			

SB, stillborn; IUGR, intrauterine growth retardation.

ing excessive amounts of aspirated amniotic debris with or without meconium, stress changes in the thymus and/or adrenals, and visceral hemorrhages, without other findings. The majority of twins with the diagnosis of perinatal asphyxia were male and twin B. The gestational dating spanned 21 to 40 weeks, with two peaks at 25 to 28 weeks and 37+ weeks. The majority were stillborn, or died within the first 24 hours. Of twin sets affected, male pairs were seen three times more often than female pairs. In one-quarter of the cases, mostly from the earlier years of the survey, the pattern of placentation was not recorded, and of the remainder 39% were monochorionic and 36% dichorionic with twice as many fused as separate disks. The cause of the asphyxial pathology in these Survey '91 cases was not defined/described in 34%. In 27% there were umbilical cord abnormalities that were considered contributory, including an abnormally long cord (104 cm), velamentous or marginally inserted cords, single artery cords, cord around the fetal neck, monoamniotic cord entanglement, and prolapsed cords. In 10% there was a diagnosis of placenta praevia, abruption, or fetomaternal hemorrhage, and in another 10% the asphyxiated twins were growth retarded (no predominance of A or B), associated with cord anomalies or asymmetric placental growth in all cases. In 15% asphyxial lesions were present in one or both of monochorionic twins with intertwin anastomoses and probable acute twin transfusion syndrome, with donor and recipient equally represented.

In this same group of twin autopsies surveyed, there was another group of infants who were reported to have asphyxial lesions plus lesions classically attributed to prematurity, particularly hyaline membrane disease. The comparative features of this group are also presented in Table 4.1. The excess load of male B twins is still present, although the male load in the twin sets is reduced. The peak of occurrence reflects the prematurity component, as does the more prolonged survival. This combined category was less evident in the later years of the survey, probably because of the increased numbers of longer survivals of prematurely delivered twins with complicated pathology masking any perinatal asphyxial lesions. The cause of the preterm delivery with asphyxia was not reported in the majority of the cases, twin B cord prolapse was identified in half the remainder, and antepartum hemorrhage,

resuscitation accidents, and delayed delivery for unstated reasons were also reported.

Prematurity and Sequelae

Although there have been marked improvements in obstetric management and perinatal care of twins, prematurity and its sequelae are still a major source of morbidity and mortality in multiple gestations,[68] although the reported magnitude of the problem varies. Part of the variation may be because problems can be encountered in defining prematurity as it relates to multiple pregnancy[34]—twins tend to be underweight for dates, although their length may be equivalent to a singleton of the same age.[87] Prematurity has been listed as the cause of up to 90% of neonatal twin deaths and 54% of fetal twin deaths, although it is not clear how intrauterine (fetal) death can be attributed to prematurity.[88] Premature delivery before 37 weeks occurred in 39% of twins, compared to 12% of singletons in one study,[69] while another reported that only 57% of twins were delivered at 40 weeks compared to 93% of singletons.[89] Death rates have been related to gestational age with 100% perinatal mortality reported at 21 to 24 weeks, 67% at 25 to 28 weeks, 27.7% at 29 to 32 weeks, 9% at 33 to 36 weeks, and 3.5% over 37 weeks.[90] The experience in 1984 to 1986 in the special care nursery from which some of the Survey '91 Review cases came showed a marked change in survival between 25 and 26 weeks (Ling E, 1987, presentation to grand rounds). At 25 weeks' gestation, 80% of twins and triplets died, at 26 weeks this had fallen to 57%, and mortality fell progressively to only 10% at 29 weeks. Both twins died in all sets up to 25 weeks, both died in 60% of sets at 26 weeks, and there were no sets where both died at 29 weeks. The clinical impression was that twins were functioning physiologically at a level equivalent to a singleton of 2 weeks earlier gestational age.

The causes of preterm delivery of twins are often the same as of singletons, such as ascending infection or antepartum hemorrhage, but there seem to be additional factors due to the presence of two fetuses instead of one, leading to excessive uterine distention as a labor stimulus.[89] A total weight of 5,450 g has been stated as the limit a uterus could accommodate,[79] although other data would not support this; combinations totaling over 8,000 g were carried easily to term in the Survey '91 Review.

Reports of twins in bicornuate uteri have been described in the preceding section on maternal uterine malformation. A factor contributing to premature delivery of twins may be the greater frequency of premature dilatation of the cervix, as discussed in the preceding section on gestational complications of multiple pregnancy. Although coitus with associated ascending infection has been reported as a contributing factor to preterm delivery of singletons,[91] no such association was reported in a similar study of twin pregnancies.[92] Excessive amounts of amniotic fluid may complicate twin pregnancies and stimulate preterm labor, suggested by the observation that measures aimed at reducing the volume of fluid have some success in prolonging pregnancy with twins.[93] However, although indomethacin can be an effective tocolytic agent and reduce amniotic fluid volume, it has been reported to have significant fetal toxicity, affecting cardiac function as well as renal output.[94] It has been suggested that one of the ways that uterine distention leads to preterm labor is by predisposing to preterm rupture of membranes, but premature rupture of membranes with twins has been reported to occur no earlier than with singletons, although the latency period with twins was significantly shorter.[95]

Gestational age at delivery has been correlated with patterns of placentation and fetal sex, with greater prematurity identified with monochorionic gestations and male twin pairs. One study reported that 14% of monochorionic twins were born at fewer than 28 weeks of gestation, compared to 4% of dichorionic same-sex twins and 2% of dichorionic opposite-sex twins,[96] while another observed that monochorionic twins delivered 10 days earlier than dichorionic twins and pregnancies of male/male twins were shorter than female/female twin or mixed-sex twin pairs.[97] Analysis of data from the Northwest University multihospital twin study also suggested that male twin pairs had shorter gestations than female twin pairs, or mixed sex twin pairs, although no apparent reasons distinguished that group.[98] Shanklin and Perrin[99] noted that 48% of twins with dichorionic fused placentas had been delivered by 38 weeks and 52% of twins with dichorionic separate placentas by 37 weeks, but 67% of monochorionic twins by 37 weeks. These observations may be related to problems of monochorionic twins as discussed further in Chapter 8.

The problem that twins face after premature delivery is the increased risk of complications, particularly hyaline membrane disease (HMD) and its sequelae, and intracranial hemorrhage. The lesions of prematurity identified pathologically in twins are the same as those described in singletons,[100–103] but they need to be supplemented with observations as to concordance or discordance of the presence and patterns of the lesions in any particular twin set.

Hyaline membrane disease occurs in twins for the same reasons of pulmonary immaturity as it occurs in singletons. In one report, HMD was diagnosed in 8% of A twins and 12% of B twins; HMD was the stated cause of perinatal death in 34% of all twins, and it was complicated by intracranial hemorrhage in 11.9% of the cases.[43] In another review of hyaline membrane disease in 294 twin pairs, it was noted that infants in the group with hyaline membrane disease were more premature, had lower birth weights, lower Apgar scores, were more often monozygotic, had been delivered by section more frequently, and had a higher mortality than the non-HMD group.[104] In 63% of the twin pairs, both twins were affected, and these infants had a lower gestational age and birth weight and were more often monozygotic. In 32% of the pairs, only twin B was affected and usually had lower Apgar scores and higher birth weight than the corresponding twin A. In only one pair was twin A affected alone. In the pairs where both twins were affected, they were equally affected in just over half, and twin B was more severely affected in the remainder. These authors suggested that monozygotic twins are particularly predisposed to HMD because they are more likely to be premature, and that twin B has a greater risk of the disease because of birth asphyxia. The increased risk of twin B may be related more to the altered labor and delivery events compared to twin A, because no increased risk for HMD was seen in second twins delivered abdominally, and malpresentation seemed more important than birth order in vaginally delivered twins.[105]

In addition to birth order, the incidence of HMD has been correlated with birth weight, sex of the twins, and whether or not there has been premature rupture of membranes. In one study, all the twins with HMD weighed less than 2,000 g, were less than 37 weeks' gestation, were equally at risk whether A or B, and nearly half died,[65] while another group reported that 1,500 g was the weight threshold.[106] While singleton male infants are at greater risk for HMD, no increased risk for male twins was noted in male/male or mixed-sex pairs over female pairs.[106] Premature rupture of the membranes appeared to reduce the risk of HMD for both twin A and B, although there was no mention of chorioamnionitis as a possible factor.[107]

The incidence of HMD in twins does not appear to have changed materially, except in reports of the use of steroids during labor, although mortality rates have declined.[64] In this context, it is of note that a study of lecithin/sphingomyelin (L/S) ratios in amniotic fluid of twins suggested that twin fetal lung maturation was usually synchronous and independent of sex, zygosity, and birth weight discordance, and that lung maturation occurred up to 4 weeks earlier in twins compared to singletons.[108] This contrasts with the local special care nursery experience as noted above—that twins appeared to be functioning at a level 2 weeks more immature than their gestational dating—and an explanation for this difference is not yet apparent.

The developmental immaturity of the paraventricular germinal matrix in the brain presents the other major risk of preterm delivery—subependymal matrix hemorrhage with intraventricular extension—occurring in as many as half of the infants of less than 1,500 g birth weight.[103] As with HMD, it appears that low birth weight is a more important predisposing factor than birth order or mode of delivery,[109,110] although one study reported that the only significant association with intraventricular hemorrhage in twins was respiratory distress.[111] In Norman's[86] series of brain damaged twins, periventricular infarction, also a lesion of prematurity, was found in 22% of her cases. Subependymal cell plate hemorrhage was present in 61% and it had ruptured into the ventricles in nearly half of the affected cases.

Persistent patency of the ductus arteriosus is a complication of the respiratory distress syndrome in the newborn, and the incidence and need for specific therapy is increased in twins.[112]

Necrotizing enterocolitis is another complication of prematurity and has been reported to be variably increased in first-born twins,[113] or equally represented in first- and second-born twins.[114] In the first instance, early feeding of the less-distressed first twin was considered important, while prematurity alone was considered the risk factor in the second report.

"Prematurity" as a cause of death in the Survey '91 Review was the diagnosis for those infants delivered preterm whose main clinical problems were related to HMD and its complications, and who had temporally associated lesions in other organ systems, such as necrotizing enterocolitis and subependymal cell plate hemorrhage. Excluded were those infants for whom the lesions of prematurity were simply complicating a more serious problem, such as a major malformation or one of the lesions of monochorionic monozygosity. Also excluded were those infants who died of "immaturity," that is, who were 20 to 23 weeks gestational age and who died shortly after birth with minimal findings pathologically. Some of the infants dying of "prematurity" also had a significant asphyxial component, but not all asphyxiated infants developed HMD. In some cases, when both twins died, twin A died with HMD, while twin B had only asphyxial lesions.

In the Survey '91 Review, complications of preterm delivery accounted for 30% of all autopsied twin deaths, and 44% of all live born twins autopsied; 15.4% of twin sets where both died were concordantly affected. The twin most likely to die of "prematurity" was a male, twin B, of less than 32 weeks of gestation, who would die at less than 7 days of age (see Table 4.1). He would have been a dichorionic twin twice as often as a monochorionic twin. In sets where both twins died of "prematurity," concordant male sets were twice as common as concordant female sets and 14% were male/female pairs.

A cause for the preterm labor and delivery was not identified in 53% of the Survey '91 cases. In 18.7%, there was pathologic evidence of ascending infection, associated in nearly half the cases with premature rupture of membranes (PROM) of up to 22 days, although not all cases of preterm labor with PROM, as long as 44 days in one case, had placental membrane inflammation. Antepartum hemorrhage had occurred in 15% of the cases with chorioamnionitis, while one third of all cases of antepartum hemorrhage and preterm labor (9.3%) were inflamed. In 13%, preterm labor appeared to be precipitated by acute hydramnios, both idiopathic and with twin transfusion. In 6%, preterm delivery was associated with a variety of situations, including bicornuate uterus, PROM without infection and with no apparent cause, cesarian delivery because of worsening maternal hypertension, and evident fetal distress.

All the infants who died of complications of prematurity before 7 days of age had pulmonary hyaline membranes and related lesions, including pulmonary interstitial emphysema in 34.3%, pneumothoraces in 14.7%, and notable pulmonary hemorrhage in 6.8%. In 49% of these infants, there was intracerebral hemorrhage ranging from small unruptured hemorrhages in the germinal matrix to large lesions with extensive intraventricular and subarachnoid extension. Periventricular leukomalacia was diagnosed in 2% and there were hypoxic/ischemic lesions of the liver and kidneys in 4%. Bronchopneumonia was recorded in 5%, due to *Pseudomonas* species, gram negative organisms (histologic diagnosis), or hemolytic streptococci, although no organism could be identified in some cases. Group B streptococci or *Candida* sepsis were present in 2% of very young infants dying within 24 hours, probably representing congenital infections. In half of the cases with histologic chorioamnionitis, there was no apparent evidence of fetal contamination, in 38% there was just aspiration of polymorphonuclear leukocytes in the lungs, in 9.5% a diagnosis of congenital pneumonia was made, and in 4% there was related fetal sepsis. (These cases were exclusive of those where fetal sepsis was the cause of death with minimal lesions of prematurity.) Changes of bronchopulmonary dysplasia[115] were already evident in 2% of these infants, with peribronchiolar fibrosis the main finding.

In the group of preterm twins who survived to 8 to 28 days, pulmonary pathology was the main contributing factor to neonatal death. In 73% of these infants, bronchopulmonary dysplasia (BPD), with or without pulmonary interstitial emphysema and chronic or terminal pneumothorax, was the major pathology. Late changes of germinal matrix hemorrhage, such as hydrocephalus, and periventricular infarctions, were reported in 58%. Hepatic lesions associated with intravenous alimentation were present in 7.6%, necrotizing enteropathy in 15% (acute and healed), aortic thromboses in 7.6%, and visceral infarcts in 7.6%. The BPD was complicated by staphylococcal bronchopneumonia in 10%, bronchopneumonia of uncertain agent in 10%, and systemic candidiasis in 5%. Signs of cor pulmonale were already present in 5%.

The preterm infants who survived the neonatal period had been born between 24 and 32 weeks, and lived up to 9 months. The majority of this group, 86%, had well developed BPD, usually with signs of cor pulmonale, and occasional additional complications, such as pulmonary hemorrhage, bronchopneumonia, or acute pneumothorax. The terminal event was often not well defined—the infant seemed to be getting progressively more difficult to ventilate, and it was concluded after considerable discussion and consultation with specialists, ethicists, and the parents, that therapy was only prolonging the dying process and was then withdrawn. These cases are important because they are very demanding ones, not only psychologically for the parents and staff, but financially for the institution. The pathologist has a very particular role in these cases—to make careful clinical-pathological correlations as a quality assurance and educational function for current and future decision making regarding care in similar cases. In addition to the lung lesions, there was evidence of prior germinal matrix hemorrhage or periventricular leukomalacia reported in 36% of these infants. Postnatal failure to thrive was a recurrent finding, although hepatic changes of intravenous alimentation were marked in only one case. In these infants, there were occasional additional findings, such as intratracheal granulation tissue, nephrocalcinosis, patent ductus arteriosus, and rather striking hypertrophy of the diaphragm in the longest survivor. The infants who died without major lung pathology succumbed to complications of hydrocephalus following intraventricular hemorrhage, and to acute necrotizing enteropathy.

Interval Delivery

On occasion, the fetuses of a twin or triplet pregnancy are delivered at intervals of days to months apart.[116] This is distinct from those multiple conceptions where one or two of twins or triplets die as an embryo or early fetus and degenerate but are retained, which is discussed further in Chapter 5. The initial delivery has occurred at 16 to 32 weeks of gestation, with the only survivors born at 31 and 32 weeks. The interval to the next delivery has ranged from 14 to 143 days with twins, 72 to 131 days with triplets when the second and third were delivered together, and intervals of 5 days and 16 days in one triplet set with all three delivered separately. Placental chorionicity was described in 14 of the 21 reported cases and the majority, 85.7%, were dichorionic or trichorionic. Zygosity assessment was not stressed, but four twin sets were unlike-sex, three triplet sets were at least dizygotic, and there were two monochorionic twin sets. The second delivered twin survived in 14 of 16 cases, the second triplet in 2 of 5 cases, and the third triplet in all cases. Of the 42 fetuses, 19 were male, 23 were female, and the sex of five of the first delivered fetuses was not recorded.

The pathophysiology of interval delivery is not understood, nor is the observation that when the retained fetus was female, the mean interval to delivery of the second fetus was 47 days longer than when the retained fetus was male—73.3 days (range 23–143) versus 26.5 days (range 5–56). Few fetal findings have been reported beyond the sex, gestational age, and death or survival. A variety of obstetric complications accompanied the second delivery, but any evidence of what might have caused the initial delivery had receded by the time the entire placentation was delivered following the last fetus.

Because of the intervals involved in these cases, most pathologists will not have the opportunity of seeing the entire process. Although reports are scanty, fetal pathology seems nonspecific. The placentations are usually described as having involuted or sclerotic but otherwise unremarkable portions or disks corresponding to the earlier delivered fetus, and a normal portion that may have evidence of premature separation or ascending infection.

In the Survey '91 Review, there were nine examples of interval delivery in the last 10 years, eight twins and one triplet, including the four cases reported separately.[116] Fetal pathology was available in only a few of the 14 fetal or perinatal deaths of the 19 infants. Mild to moderate growth retardation was described in two of the first born twins, and one first born twin had a velamentously inserted umbilical cord. The placentas were all multichorionic, and like-sex and unlike-sex pairs occurred with equal frequency. The cause of the first delivery was not determined, while the second occurred in a variety of clinical settings, including spontaneous premature rupture of the membranes, vaginal bleeding, or operative delivery after the detection of fetal distress in the survivor. The placental portion of the first twin was uniformly involuted and without distinguishing features, and the placental portion of the surviving twin was remarkable only for uncommon mild maternal inflammation of the membranes and placental surface (Fig. 4.3).

There were interesting observations in two placentas with a short delivery interval. In one case with an interval of 2 days at 26 weeks, the macerated male A twin was growth retarded by almost 4 weeks and had vascularized only one-third of the dichorionic- fused placenta. When the placenta was examined after delivery of the less growth retarded but also small male twin, portion A contained hemorrhagic endovasculopathy with avascular villi, while none was described in portion B. In a second case of interval delivery in triplets at 21 weeks, the first triplet was followed 42 hours later by the second and third triplets and the entire placentation. The placenta was trichorionic triamniotic with separate but abutting oval placenta portions, and histologically there were no distinguishing features in portions B and C. In portion A, which had been without fetal circulation for the interval of 42 hours, there were early lesions of hemorrhagic endovasculopathy (Fig. 4.4). It is suggested that these two observations have relevance to considerations of the pathogenesis of this interesting lesion.[117] Hemorrhagic endovasculopathy (HEV) is a histologically identified lesion of the fetal vessels in the subchorionic villous tissue of the placenta, of uncertain etiology and pathogenesis, and it has been associated with poor perinatal outcome, although it is also occasionally encountered in otherwise normal placentas. These observations in the two interval delivery cases would tend to support the concept that HEV is a reaction to reduced fetal blood flow, rather than a result of an infectious etiology. The fact that this lesion is associated with stillbirth and with perinatal distress would be compatible with this interpretation. In a case of stillbirth with advanced maceration, it may be difficult to determine whether the lesion occurred following fetal death or may have contributed to fetal demise, but in the living but distressed infant with a placenta containing large amounts of this lesion, one might suspect that the lesion was reflecting significantly impaired fetal perfusion, thus suggesting a search for causes of impaired fetal circulation.

Conclusion

To provide the most relevant clinical-pathological interpretation in cases of suboptimal outcome of twin gestation, the pathologist must consider the

FIGURE 4.3. These are two examples of the placenta from interval deliveries. In (a), the interval was 42 days, and the second twin and dichorionic diamniotic adjacent placentation was delivered at 32 weeks. The sex of the first twin was not known, the second twin was male. The vessels on the chorionic surface of A have collapsed completely and the villus tissue was sclerotic. The membranes of B were edematous and inflamed, but the villus tissue was immature and otherwise normal. Both cords contained three vessels. In (b), the interval was 143 days, with a male twin A delivered through an incompetent cervix at 19 weeks, followed by placement of a Shirodkar suture and twin B with the placenta at 40 weeks. The live-born female twin's portion of the dichorionic placenta was normal, while the portion from twin A was completely involuted, as seen from both the maternal (M) and fetal (F) surfaces.

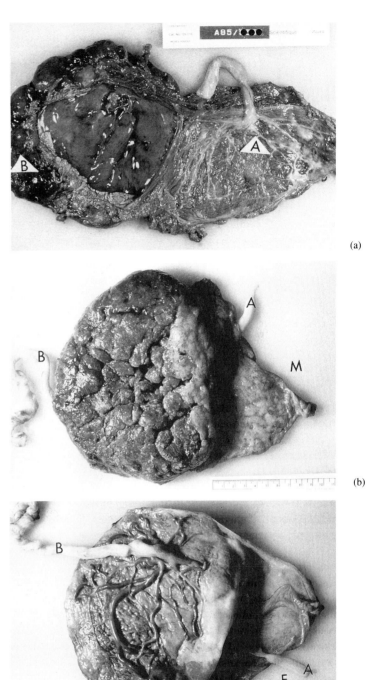

(a)

(b)

(b)

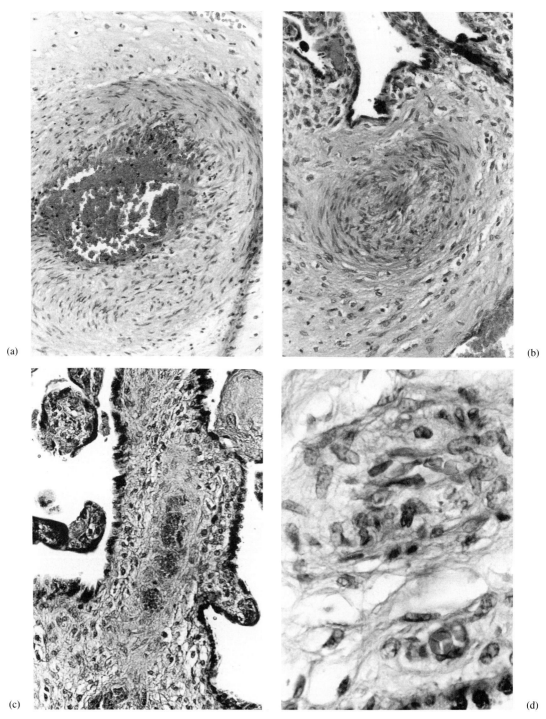

FIGURE 4.4. Vessel changes after interval delivery. In this case, the interval between delivery of triplet A, and triplets B and C with the trichorionic triamniotic placenta was 42 hours. Other than the presence of hemorrhagic endovasculopathy in triplet A's placenta, the placental portions were indistinguishable. Vascular lesions in triplet A's placenta included breakdown of the inner layers of a chorionic vessel wall with extravasation of red blood cells (a), sclerosis of a larger subchorionic vessel (b), and breakdown of capillary walls in the villi (c) and (d). These are in contrast to the normal villus tissue of triplet B (e) and C (f). [Hematoxylin and eosin; original magnifications ×62.5 (a–c,e,f), X320 (d)].

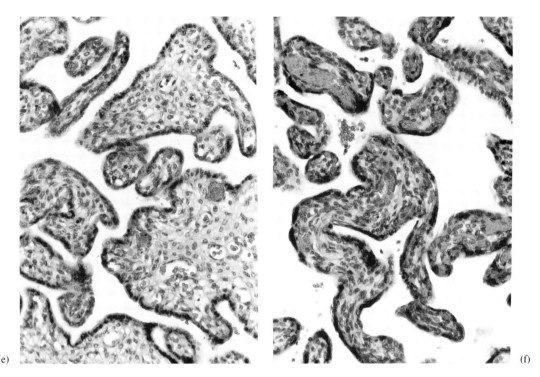

(e)   (f)

FIGURE 4.4. *Continued.*

possible maternal-fetal and maternal-fetal-placental interactions as diagrammed in Fig. 4.1. This is most easily achieved by regular consultation with clinical colleagues, both in a regular forum such as a mortality review committee, and with individuals on a case by case basis. Regular consultations not only enhance the pathologist's understanding of clinical events, but they also make clinicians more aware of and receptive to the pathologist's requirements for more clinical background and appropriate specimen handling and identification.

References

1. Baldwin VJ. The Placenta. In: Dimmick JE, Kalousek D, eds. *Developmental Pathology of the Embryo and Fetus.* Philadelphia: JB Lippincott; 1992:271–319.
2. Ahn MB, Phelan JP. Multiple pregnancy: antepartum management. In: Gall SA, ed. Twin Pregnancy. *Clin Perinatol.* 1988;15:55–69.
3. Townsend RR, Simpson GF, Filly RA. Membrane thickness in ultrasound prediction of chorionicity of twin gestations. *J Ultrasound Med.* 1988;7:327–332.
4. D'Alton ME, Dudley DK. The ultrasonographic prediction of chorionicity in twin gestation. *Am J Obstet Gynecol.* 1989;160:557–561.
5. D'Alton ME, Dudley DK. Ultrasound in the antenatal management of twin gestation. *Semin Perinatal.* 1986;10:30–38.
6. Coleman BG, Grumbach K, Arger PH, Mintz MC, Arenson RL, Mennuti M, Gabbe SG. Twin gestations: monitoring of complications and anomalies with US. *Radiology.* 1987;165:449–453.
7. Pijpers L, Jahoda MGJ, Vosters RPL, Niermeijer MF, Sachs ES. Genetic amniocentesis in twin pregnancies. *Br J Obstet Gynecol.* 1988;95:323–326.
8. Stiller RJ, Lockwood CJ, Belanger K, Baumgarten A, Hobbins JC, Mahoney MJ. Amniotic fluid α-feto-protein concentrations in twin gestations: dependence on placental membrane anatomy. *Am J Obstet Gynecol.* 1988;158:1088–1092.
9. Johnson JM, Harman CR, Evans JA, MacDonald K, Manning FA. Maternal serum α-feto-protein in twin pregnancy. *Am J Obstet Gynecol.* 1990; 162:1020–1025.
10. Drugan A, O'Brien JE, Gambino R, Johnson MP, Evans ML. Similarity of twin to singleton MSAFP ratio by race: no need to establish specific multifetal tables (Abstract). *Am J Obstet Gynecol.* 1992; 166:346.

11. Cox WL, Forestier F, Capella-Pavlovsky M, Daffos F. Fetal blood sampling in twin pregnancies. *Fetal Ther*. 1987;2:101–108.

12. Gaziano EP, Knox GE, Bendel RP, Calvin S, Brandt D. Is pulsed Doppler velocimetry useful in the management of multiple-gestation pregnancies? *Am J Obstet Gynecol*. 1991;164:1426–1433.

13. Ganesh V, Apuzzio J, Iffy L. Clinical aspects of multiple gestation. In: Iffy L, Kaminetzky HA, eds. *Principles and Practice of Obstetrics and Perinatology*. New York: John Wiley; 1981:1183–1192.

14. MacLennan AH. Clinical characteristics and management (multiple gestation). In: Creasy RK, Resnik R, eds. *Maternal-Fetal Medicine, Principles and Practice*. Philadelphia: WB Saunders; 1984:527–559.

15. Gall SA, ed. Twin pregnancy. *Clin Perinatol*. 1988;15(1):1–11,41–122.

16. Cunningham FG, MacDonald PC, Gant NF. *Williams Obstetrics*. 18th ed. Norwalk, CT: Appleton & Lange; 1989:629–652.

17. Beischer NA, Pepperell RJ, Barrie JU. Twin pregnancy and erythroblastosis fetalis. *Obstet Gynecol*. 1969;34:22–29.

18. Benirschke K, Kim CK. Multiple pregnancy. *N Engl J Med*. 1973;288:1276–1284,1329–1336.

19. Manning FA, Bowman JM, Lange IR, Chamberlain PF. Intrauterine transfusions in an Rh-immunized twin pregnancy: a case report of successful outcome and a review of the literature. *Obstet Gynecol*. 1985;65:2S-5S.

20. Knuppel RA, Shah DM, Rattan PK, O'Brien WF, Lerner A. Rhesus isoimmunization in twin gestation. *Am J Obstet Gynecol*. 1984;150:136–141.

21. Bowman JM. Fetomaternal ABO incompatibility and erythroblastosis fetalis. *Vox Sang*. 1986; 50:104–106.

22. Moise KJ, Cotton DB. Discordant fetal platelet counts in a twin gestation complicated by idiopathic thrombocytopenia purpura. *Am J Obstet Gynecol*. 1987;156:1141–1142.

23. Burke BJ, Sherriff RJ, Savage PE, Dixon HG. Diabetic twin pregnancy: an unequal result. *Lancet*. 1979;1:1372–1373.

24. Tchobroutsky C, Vray M, Papoz L. Fetal malformations in twin pregnancies of type 1 diabetic women. *Lancet*. 1991;337:1358.

25. Burrows DA, O'Neil TJ, Sorrells TL. Successful twin pregnancy after renal transplant maintained on cyclosporine A immunosuppression. *Obstet Gynecol*. 1988;72:459–461.

26. Cunningham FG, MacDonald PC, Gant NF. *William's Obstetrics*. 18th ed. Norwalk, CT: Appleton & Lange; 1989:731–736.

27. Booth JH. Twins in a double uterus. *BC Med J*. 1973;15:306–307.

28. Ahram JA, Toaff ME, Chandra P, Laffey P, Chawla HS. Successful outcome of a twin gestation in both horns of a bicornuate uterus. *Am J Obstet Gynecol*. 1984;150:323–324.

29. Bardequez AD, Ziegler DD, Weiss G. Multifetal pregnancy in a gonadal dysgenesis mosaic. *Obstet Gynecol*. 1990;76:502–504.

30. Nylander PPS, MacGillivray I. Complications of twin pregnancy. In: MacGillivray I, Nylander PPS, Corney G, eds. *Human Multiple Reproduction*. Philadelphia: WB Saunders; 1975:137–146.

31. Medearis AL, Jonas HS, Stockbauer JW, Domke HR. Perinatal deaths in twin pregnancy (a five year analysis of statistical studies in Missouri). *Am J Obstet Gynecol*. 1979;134:413–421.

32. Cetrulo CL, Ingardia CJ, Sbarra AJ. Management of multiple gestation. *Clin Obstet Gynecol*. 1980; 23:533–548.

33. MacGillivray I. Twins and other multiple deliveries. *Clin Obstet Gynecol*. 1980;7:581–600.

34. Marivate M, Norman RJ. Twins. *Clin Obstet Gynecol*. 1982;9:723–743.

35. Hays PM, Smeltzer JS. Multiple gestation. *Clin Obstet Gynecol*. 1986;29:264–285.

36. Polin JI, Frangipane WL. Current concepts in management of obstetric problems for pediatricians. II Modern concepts in the management of multiple gestation. *Pediatr Clin North Am*. 1986;33:649–661.

37. Wenstrom KD, Gall SA. Incidence, morbidity and mortality, and diagnosis of twin gestations. *Clin Perinatol*. 1988;15:1–11.

38. Kovacs BW, Kirschbaum TH, Paul RH. Twin gestations: I. Antenatal care and complications. *Obstet Gynecol*. 1989;74:313–317.

39. Spellacy WN, Handler A, Ferre CD. A case-control study of 1253 twin pregnancies from a 1982–1987 perinatal data base. *Obstet Gynecol*. 1990;75:168–171.

40. Campbell DM. Maternal adaptation in twin pregnancy. *Semin Perinatol*. 1986;10:14–18.

41. McMullan PF, Norman RJ, Marivate M. Pregnancy-induced hypertension in twin pregnancy. *Br J Obstet Gynecol*. 1984;91:240–243.

42. Neuman M, Ron-El R, Langer R, Bukovsky I, Caspi E. Maternal death caused by HELLP syndrome (with hypoglycemia) complicating mild pregnancy-induced hypertension in a twin gestation. *Am J Obstet Gynecol*. 1990;162:372–373.

43. Koivisto M, Jouppila P, Kauppila A, Moilanen I, Ylikorkala O. Twin pregnancy neonatal morbidity and mortality. *Acta Obstet Gynecol Scand Suppl*. 1975;44:21–29.

44. Sibai BM, Anderson GD, Spinnato JA, Shaver DC. Plasma volume findings in patients with mild pregnancy-induced hypertension. *Am J Obstet Gynecol.* 1983;147:16–19.

45. Pritchard JA. Hematological problems associated with delivery, placental abruption, retained dead fetus and amniotic fluid embolism. *Clin Hematol.* 1973;2:563–586.

46. Skelly H, Marivate M, Norman R, Kenoyer G, Martin R. Consumptive coagulopathy following fetal death in triplet pregnancy. *Am J Obstet Gynecol.* 1982;142:595–596.

47. Romero R, Duffy TP, Berkowitz RL, Chang E, Hobbins JC. Prolongation of a preterm pregnancy complicated by death of a single twin in utero and disseminated intravascular coagulation. *N Engl J Med.* 1984;310:772–774.

48. Dwyer PL, Oats JN, Walstab JE, Beischer NA. Glucose tolerance in twin pregnancy. *Aust NZ J Obstet Gynecol.* 1982;22:131–134.

49. Bender S. Twin pregnancy (a review of 472 cases). *J Obstet Gynecol Br Cwlth.* 1952;59:510–517

50. Hashimoto B, Callen PW, Filly RA, Laros RK. Ultrasound evaluation of polyhydramnios in twin pregnancy. *Am J Obstet Gynecol.* 1986;154:1069–1072.

51. Weir PE, Ratten GL, Beischer NA. Acute polyhydramnios—a complication of monozygous twin pregnancy. *Br J Obstet Gynecol.* 1979;86:849–853.

52. Steinberg LH, Hurley VA, Desmedt E, Beischer NA. Acute hydramnios in twin pregnancies. *Aust NZ J Obstet Gynecol.* 1990;30:196–200.

53. Radestad A, Thomassen PA. Acute polyhydramnios in twin pregnancy. *Acta Obstet Gynecol Scand.* 1990;69:297–300.

54. Newton ER. Antepartum care in multiple gestation. *Semin Perinatol.* 1986;10:19–29.

55. Neilson JP, Verkayl DAA, Crowther CA, Bannerman C. Preterm labor in twin pregnancies: prediction by cervical assessment. *Obstet Gynecol.* 1988;72:719–723.

56. Newman RB, Godsey RK, Ellings JM, Campbell BA, Eller DP, Miller MC III. Quantification of cervical change: relationship to preterm delivery in the multifetal gestation. *Am J Obstet Gynecol.* 1991;165:264–271.

57. Michaels WH, Schreiber FR, Padgett RJ, Ager J, Pieper D. Ultrasound surveillance of the cervix in twin gestations: management of cervical incompetency. *Obstet Gynecol.* 1991;78:739–744.

58. Novak E. Combined intra-uterine and extra-uterine pregnancy. *Surg Gynecol Obstet.* 1926;43:26–37.

59. Rizk B, Tan SL, Morcos S, Riddle A, Brinsden P, Mason BA, Edwards RG. Heterotopic pregnancies after in utero fertilization and embryo transfer. *Am J Obstet Gynecol.* 1991;164:161–164.

60. Edelstein MC, Morgan MA. Bilateral simultaneous tubal pregnancies: case report and review of the literature. *Obstet Gynecol Surv.* 1989;44:250–252.

61. Neuman WL, Ponto K, Farber RA, Shangold GA. DNA analysis of unilateral twin ectopic gestation. *Obstet Gynecol.* 1990;75:479–483.

62. Kalfayan B, Gundersen JH. Ovarian twin pregnancy. *Obstet Gynecol.* 1980;55(suppl 3):25S–27S.

63. Sze EHM, Adelson MD, Baggish MS, Contente N. Combined tubal and molar pregnancy: case report. *Am J Obstet Gynecol.* 1988;159:1217–1219.

64. Desgranges M-F, De Muylder X, Moutquin J-M, Lazaro-Lopez F, Leduc B. Perinatal profile of twin pregnancies: a retrospective review of 11 years (1969–1979) at Hopital Notre-Dame, Montreal, Canada. *Acta Genet Med Gemellol.* 1982;31:157–163.

65. Ho SK, Wu PYK. Perinatal factors and neonatal morbidity in twin pregnancy. *Am J Obstet Gynecol.* 1975;122:979–987.

66. McCarthy BJ, Sachs BP, Layde PM, Barton A, Terry JS, Rochat R. The epidemiology of neonatal death in twins. *Am J Obstet Gynecol.* 1981;141:252–256.

67. Warenski JC, Kochenour NK. Intrapartum management of twin gestation. *Clin Perinatol.* 1989;16:889–897.

68. Chervenak FA, Johnson RE, Youcha S, Hobbins JC, Berkowitz RL. Intrapartum management of twin gestation. *Obstet Gynecol.* 1985;65:119–124.

69. Zahalkova M. Perinatal and infant mortality in twins. In: Nance WE, ed. Twin Research: Biology and Epidemiology. *Prog Clin Biol Res.* 1978;24B:115–120.

70. Pettersson F, Smedby B, Lindmark G. Outcome of twin birth. Review of 1636 children born in twin birth. *Acta Pediatr Scand.* 1976;65:473–479.

71. Parer JT, Livingston EG. What is fetal distress? *Am J Obstet Gynecol.* 1990;162:1421–1427.

72. Gruenwald P. The pathology of perinatal distress. *Arch Pathol.* 1955;60:150–172.

73. Potter EL, Craig JM. *Pathology of the Fetus and Infant.* 3rd ed. Chicago: Year Book Medical Publishers; 1975:93–102.

74. Keeling JW. Intrapartum asphyxia and birth trauma. In: Keeling JE, ed. *Fetal and Neonatal Pathology.* London: Springer-Verlag; 1987:199–210.

75. Wigglesworth JS. Pathology of intrapartum and early neonatal death in the normally formed infant. In: Wigglesworth JS, Singer DB, eds. *Textbook of Fetal and Perinatal Pathology.* Oxford: Blackwell Scientific; 1991:285–306.

76. Ferguson WF. Perinatal mortality in multiple gestations (a review of perinatal deaths from 1609 multiple gestations). *Obstet Gynecol.* 1963; 23:861–870.

77. Benirschke K, Gille J. Placental pathology and asphyxia. In: Gluck L, ed. *Intrauterine Asphyxia and the Developing Fetal Brain.* Chicago: Year Book Medical Publishers; 1977:117–136.

78. Sekiya S, Hafez ESE. Physiomorphology of twin transfusion syndrome: a study of 86 twin gestations. *Obstet Gynecol.* 1977;50:288–292.

79. Grothe W, Ruttgers H. Twin pregnancies: an 11 year review. *Acta Genet Med Gemellol.* 1985; 34:49–58.

80. Young BK, Suidan J, Antoine C, Silverman F, Lustig I, Wasserman J. Differences in twins: the importance of birth order. *Am J Obstet Gynecol.* 1985;151:915–921.

81. Brown HL, Miller JM, Neumann DE, Sarpong DF, Gabert HA. Umbilical and blood gas assessment of twins. *Obstet Gynecol.* 1990;75:826–829.

82. Teberg AJ, Walther FJ, Pena IC. Mortality, morbidity and outcome of the small-for-gestational age infant. *Semin Perinatol.* 1988;12:84–94.

83. Brar HS, Rutherford SE. Classification of intrauterine growth retardation. *Semin Perinatol.* 1988;12:2–10.

84. Towbin A. Obstetric malpractice litigation: the pathologists' view. *Am J Obstet Gynecol.* 1986; 155:927–935.

85. Bejar R, Vigliocco G, Gramajo H, Solana C, Benirschke K, Berry C, Coen R, Reznik R. Antenatal origin of neurologic damage in newborn infants. II. Multiple gestations. *Am J Obstet Gynecol.* 1990;162:1230–1236.

86. Norman MG. Mechanisms of brain damage in twins. *Can J Neurol Sci.* 1982;9:339–344.

87. Crane JP, Tomich RG, Kopta M. Ultrasonic growth patterns in normal and discordant twins. *Obstet Gynecol.* 1980;55:678–683

88. Sehgal NN. Perinatal mortality in twin pregnancies (implications for clinical management). *Postgrad Med.* 1980;68:231–234.

89. Gedda L. Why can the study of twins be called Gemellology? In: Nance WE, ed. Twin Studies: Biology and Epidemiology. *Prog Clin Biol Res.* 1978;24B:1–8.

90. Keith L, Ellis R, Berger GS, Depp R. The Northwestern University multihospital twin study. I. A description of 588 twin pregnancies and associated pregnancy loss, 1971–1975. *Am J Obstet Gynecol.* 1980;138:781–789.

91. Naeye RL, Ross S. Coitus and chorioamnionitis: a prospective study. *Early Hum Devel.* 1982;6:91–97.

92. Neilson JP, Mutambira M. Coitus, twin pregnancy, and preterm labor. *Am J Obstet Gynecol.* 1989;160:416–418.

93. Lange IR, Harman CR, Ash KM, Manning FA, Menticoglou S. Twin with hydramnios : treating premature labor at source. *Am J Obstet Gynecol.* 1989;160:552–557.

94. Hallak M, Reiter AA, Ayres NA, Moise KJ. Indomethacin for preterm labor: fetal toxicity in a dizygotic twin gestation. *Obstet Gynecol.* 1991; 78:911–913.

95. Kurzel RB. Preterm PROM in twin gestations (abstract). *Am J Obstet Gynecol.* 1991;163:372.

96. Gruenwald P. Environmental influences on twins apparent at birth (a preliminary study). *Biol Neonate.* 1970;15:79–93.

97. Bleker OP, Hemrika DJ. Gestational age according to fetal sex in twins. *Am J Obstet Gynecol.* 1985;151:830–831.

98. Newton W, Keith L, Keith D. The Northwestern University multihospital twin study. IV. Duration of gestation according to fetal sex. *Am J Obstet Gynecol.* 1984;149:655–658.

99. Shanklin DR, Perrin EVDK. Multiple gestation. In: Perrin EVDK, ed. *Pathology of the Placenta. Contemporary Issues in Surgical Pathology.* Vol 5. Roth LM, series ed. New York: Churchill Livingstone; 1984:165–182.

100. Batcup G. Prematurity. In: Keeling JW, ed. *Fetal and Neonatal Pathology.* London: Springer-Verlag; 1987:179–198.

101. Potter EL, Craig JM. *Pathology of the Fetus and the Infant.* 3rd ed. Chicago: Year Book Medical Publishers; 1975:274–301,501–503.

102. Askin F. Respiratory tract disorders in the fetus and neonate. In: Wigglesworth JS, Singer DB, eds. *Textbook of Fetal and Perinatal Pathology.* Oxford: Blackwell Scientific Publications; 1991:661–674.

103. Larroche J-C. Fetal and perinatal brain damage. In: Wigglesworth JS, Singer DB, eds. *Textbook of Fetal and Perinatal Pathology.* Oxford: Blackwell Scientific Publications; 1991:807–838.

104. Verdusco R de la T, Rosario R, Rigatto H. Hyaline membrane disease in twins—a 7 year review with a study on zygosity. *Am J Obstet Gynecol.* 1976; 125:668–671.

105. Arnold C, McLean FH, Kramer MS, Usher RH. Respiratory distress syndrome in second-born versus first-born twins. *N Engl J Med.* 1987;317:1121–1125.

106. Ghai V, Vidyasagar D. Mortality and morbidity factors in twins. An epidemiologic approach. *Clin Perinatol.* 1988;15:123–140.

107. Yeung CY. Effects of prolonged rupture of mem-

branes on the development of respiratory distress syndrome in twin pregnancy. *Aust Pediatr J.* 1982;18:197–199.

108. Loveno KJ, Quirk JG, Whalley PJ, Herbert WNP, Trubey R. Fetal lung maturation in twin gestation. *Am J Obstet Gynecol.* 1984;148:405–411.

109. Pearlman SA, Batton DG. Effect of birth order on intraventricular hemorrhage in very low birth weight twins. *Obstet Gynecol.* 1988;71:358–360.

110. Morales WJ, O'Brien WF, Knuppel RA, Gaylord S, Hayes P. The effect of mode of delivery on the risk of intraventricular hemorrhage in nondiscordant twin gestations under 1,500 g. *Obstet Gynecol.* 1989;73:107–110.

111. Viscardi RM, Donn SM, Rayburn WF, Schork MA. Intraventricular hemorrhage in preterm twin gestation infants. *J Perinatol.* 1988;8:114–117.

112. Zanardo V, Foti P, Trevisanuto D, Zambon P, Stellin G, Milanesi O. Does the respiratory distress syndrome in twins and singletons run different risks of persistent ductus arteriosus? *Acta Genet Med Gemellol.* 1989;38:315–318.

113. Samm M, Curtis-Cohen M, Keller M, Chawla H. Necrotizing enterocolitis in infants of multiple gestation. *Am J Dis Child.* 1986;140:937–939.

114. Wiswell TE, Hankins CT. Twins and triplets with necrotizing enterocolitis. *Am J Dis Child.* 1988; 142:1004–1006.

115. Stocker JT. Pathology of hyaline membrane disease and acute reparative and long-standing "healed" bronchopulmonary dysplasia. In: Stocker JT, ed. *Pediatric Pulmonary Disease.* New York: Hemisphere; 1989:101–164.

116. Wittmann BK, Farquharson D, Wong GP, Baldwin VJ, Wadsworth LD, Elit L. Delayed delivery of second twin: report of four cases and review of the literature. *Obstet Gynecol.* 1992;79:260–263.

117. Sander CH, Kinnane L, Stevens NG, Echt R. Hemorrhagic endovasculitis of the placenta: a review with clinical correlation. *Placenta.* 1986; 7:551–574.

5
Mortality of Twins

It is tough to be a twin! The risks of disorder, disease, and death are greater for all members of a plural set from the moment of conception to the end of their life span, and encompass physical, psychological, and social threats.[1,2] There seems to be universal agreement on this concept although the reported statistical magnitude and details vary widely. It has been suggested that the frequency of twinning at conception may actually be as high as one in eight, and that for every live-born twin pair, there would appear to be at least six singletons who are actually sole survivors of twin conceptions, and in the remainder, the entire conception is lost, in the majority prior to clinical recognition.[3] Mortality of twins is thus a numerically important problem, and is the focus of this chapter. Morbidity of twins is discussed in Chapter 6, and Chapter 7 deals with anomalous development of twins.

Analysis of the patterns, rates, and causes of mortality in twins is a daunting project for three main reasons. The first hurdle in the reported studies is the problem of terminology and definitions, in three areas particularly: (a) not all reports agree on what constitutes fetal death, so that the lower limit for inclusion ranges from 16 to 28 weeks; (b) the methods of assigning zygosity are often only statistical inferences; and (c) categories of "cause" of death are rarely comparable between studies, definitions of the causes quoted may not be provided, and critical information such as patterns of placentation may not be provided.

The second obstacle in assessing twin mortality is the changing effect of technological advances in prenatal and perinatal diagnosis and management, in four areas especially: (a) the greater routine use of ultrasound examination in early pregnancy has revealed that twin conception is considerably more frequent than twin delivery, creating a new class of twin mortality to assess; (b) the technology of assisted reproduction is providing a new problem with more higher multiple conceptions, which is being "solved" with an ethically uncertain procedure of induced embryonic death; (c) the ability to diagnose fetal pathology antenatally has increased dramatically and selective terminations are being performed; and (d) the prenatal and perinatal care of multiple pregnancy has improved the survival of twins, so that data derived from earlier, even well done studies, have less predictive validity today.

The third source of complications in the assessment of twin mortality is the very complex nature of twins themselves, all the variable influences presented in the first four chapters of this volume. Twin mortality is related not only to the pattern of twinning, the sex of the twins, and the pattern of placentation, but also to the genetic and acquired biologic characteristics of the twins and the superimposed intertwin and maternal influences.

This catalogue of complications and considerations relevant to the study of mortality in twins leads to a reasonable question—Why bother? If it is generally accepted that twins die more often than singletons, of what value is analysis of the details? The answer is that there are good social/psychological, scientific, and medicolegal reasons for trying to define the patterns of twin mortality, and the interested pathologist has a key role in providing the best information possible for such analysis.

It could be questioned what the pathologist has to

contribute to the social/psychological benefit of analysis of twin deaths, but it may be that the pathologist is the only one who can provide the needed information. For example, when a twin conception is identified in early or midpregnancy but only one living infant is delivered, it is reasonable to expect a psychological impact on the mother, and maybe even the survivor sibling.[4–6] Substantive confirmation of the existence of the deceased twin, with further details where possible, such as fetal sex or type of twin, may help normalize the grieving process, which is likely underestimated and repressed in the face of a living infant to care for.[6] These considerations are even more relevant when unilateral twin death occurs late in pregnancy or in the perinatal period, with the additional concern of the significance of that death for the survivor. Careful documentation of the pattern of placentation and thoughtful assessment of the possible cause of death provides valuable information for counseling of the family. In the broader context of society in general, the pathologist provides continuous correlation of the anatomic/metabolic effects of perinatal care and confirmation (or not) of antenatal and perinatal diagnostic procedures. This is a critical component of the quality assurance process so necessary for the most efficient and effective use of our medical resources, human and financial. Trends detected in mortality (and morbidity) may point to necessary alterations in practice related to obstetric management and perinatal care.[7,8]

The scientific value of studies of twin mortality is perhaps self-evident but warrants a brief review of a couple of examples in this context. It has been noted in the discussion of placentation of twins that patterns of placentation are different in the group of live-born twins, compared to twins with single or concordant mortality, and the increased proportion of monochorionic twins in the mortality group is also seen in studies of embryonic and early fetal mortality.[9] This observation has contributed to the concept of monozygotic twinning as an anomaly; it also alters our concept of the rates of the different types of twins and leads to a reevaluation of the factors that might influence the occurrence of twins. In fact, the pathology of monochorionic monozygosity is so varied, three separate chapters are used in this monograph to discuss the patterns encountered. Also, since Galton[10] considered the influences of nature and nurture, the relative effect of genetic constitution and environmental forces on twin development has relied on the comparisons of a variety of findings in monozygotic ("identical") versus dizygotic ("nonidentical" or "fraternal") twins. Clarification of the contributions of environment and heredity is only possible when there is accurate assessment of the type of twinning, and knowledgeable evaluation of causes and mechanisms of death, disease, or malformations—provided by the pathologist. Chapter 1 should be consulted for a further discussion of problems of twin studies.

The pathologist has become an important part of the resolution of medicolegal disputes that revolve around unfortunate outcomes in multiple pregnancy, either as a witness of factual evidence from an examination of a placenta or one or more twin autopsies, or as an expert witness for an opinion concerning the findings.[11] In the first instance, the value of accurate and complete assessment and description of the placenta of a multiple gestation cannot be overstated,[12] and the same is true of the autopsy of any infants. In the second instance, knowledge of patterns of mortality related to the considerations discussed above provide the context for assessment and opinion in a specific case.

It is evident from the above comments that the pathologist has an opportunity and responsibility to provide the best information possible in cases of twin mortality. The examination and correlation of placental findings have been discussed in Chapter 3, and it must be emphasized that placental examination is an essential part of any perinatal autopsy of one or more fetuses/infants of a multiple conception. It is preferable to examine the placenta at the time of the autopsy, but as a minimum, the placental details must be part of the autopsy report. The autopsy techniques are the same as for singletons, whether embryo/fetus[13] or perinatal infant,[14–19] with additional special procedures in cases of anomalies of monozygotic duplication (see Chapter 10). When both twins are autopsied, the correlation of the findings in each with the other is often the most valuable aspect of the examination and warrants special attention.

Death of twins occurs during gestation, in the perinatal period, neonatally, and in infancy. Because the patterns of mortality and the apparent causes are different at these various times, the following descriptions will separate the discussions

FIGURE 5.1. Patterns of fetal death of twins.

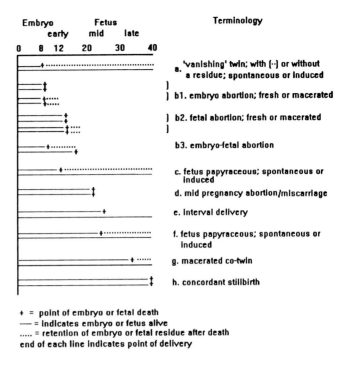

Embryo   Fetus
early   mid   late

a. 'vanishing' twin; with [··] or without a residue; spontaneous or induced

b1. embryo abortion; fresh or macerated

b2. fetal abortion; fresh or macerated

b3. embryo-fetal abortion

c. fetus papyraceous; spontaneous or induced

d. mid pregnancy abortion/miscarriage

e. interval delivery

f. fetus papyraceous; spontaneous or induced

g. macerated co-twin

h. concordant stillbirth

+ = point of embryo or fetal death
— = indicates embryo or fetus alive
..... = retention of embryo or fetal residue after death
end of each line indicates point of delivery

into fetal death and death after live birth, recognizing that often there is no absolute boundary between the nature of fresh stillbirth and early perinatal death.

Fetal Death

A pregnancy that starts as a multiple gestation may not continue as such because one or more of the fetuses dies in utero (Fig. 5.1). Fetal death has different causes and takes different forms at different times of the pregnancy, although the distinctions become less clear cut as the dead fetus is retained for a prolonged period of time. This section presents an overview of fetal death in the three trimesters of pregnancy and then discusses each in detail.

The extent of reproductive loss in the first trimester has been identified only relatively recently.[20] Ultrasound studies of early pregnancy have revealed that a surprising number of pregnancies start as multiples, but early embryonic or fetal death reduces the gestation to a singleton (Fig. 5.1a). This pattern of early death has been difficult to confirm because there is often little or no pathologic evidence of the dead twin's previous existence seen on the placenta of the surviving twin, who is delivered later in pregnancy. Other patterns of spontaneous twin death in the first trimester include embryo/fetal abortions, and retained dead fetus (Fig. 5.1b,c). More recently, in some cases of high multiple gestations, usually after ovulation induction procedures, selective embryocide is being undertaken to reduce the gestational maternal morbidity and fetal mortality.[21]

Second trimester loss is more easily recognized and takes several forms (Fig. 5.1c–f). If both fetuses die, they are usually spontaneously "aborted" or "stillborn." The terminology used depends on the timing of delivery and the legal definition of point of viability in the community where delivery takes place. If only one fetus dies, it may be delivered and the pregnancy continue (see Interval Delivery in Chapter 4), or it may be retained to become a fetus papyraceous within the membranes of the surviving fetus. Selective feticide may also be undertaken in the second trimester in rare cases where the life of a normal fetus is threatened by the effects of an abnormal fetus. The pregnancy is then able to continue so the normal infant can be delivered at maturity.[22]

Third trimester loss is the most familiar pattern of fetal mortality (Fig. 5.1e–h). If both fetuses die, the pregnancy will usually terminate spontaneously with delivery of stillborn infants who are more or less macerated, depending on the interval between death and delivery. If only one fetus dies, it may be delivered and the pregnancy may continue for a variable period of time until delivery of the remaining fetus. Alternatively, the dead fetus may be retained and be delivered as a macerated co-twin at the time of delivery of the surviving fetus.

The following discussion considers details of embryo/fetal twin death in early, middle, and late pregnancy, reviews rates and causes, and provides descriptions of the patterns of pathology seen.

Discordant Embryonic and Fetal Death in Early Pregnancy

Ultrasound studies of early pregnancy have identified a remarkable rate of loss of embryos and fetuses of multiple gestation in the first and early second trimester.[19,23–32] Although it might seem that knowledge of fetal death in early pregnancy is quite recent, one of the earliest described cases of a twin pregnancy in which one twin was a blighted ovum was by Guilleneau in 1594 (cited by Abrams[33]). In spite of this early interest, embryonic and fetal death in the first and early second trimester is the least understood pattern of fetal mortality in multiple pregnancy. It is possible that information that can be gained from study of these pregnancies will alter our concepts of the mechanisms and ratios of twinning, causes of fetal mortality, and methods of managing multiple pregnancy. The pathologist with an interest in multiple pregnancy is challenged to clarify the disorders and patterns of this early pregnancy fetal loss.

Patterns and Causes

Rates of early pregnancy loss of multiple gestation have been derived from pathology and ultrasound studies. Pathologically identifiable sets of twins have represented up to 3% of reported series of aborted embryos or fetuses,[9,34] and this is triple the rate for the occurrence of twins among late stillbirths or live-born infants.[34] Ultrasound studies have suggested that overall rates of early multiple pregnancy loss may be as high as 78% depending on the patient population, the timing of ultrasonography, and the number of scans performed.[30] Losses

from spontaneous multiple gestations have ranged from 63% to 100%.[20] Losses from induced multiple gestations have averaged 29%,[20,25] of which the highest rate of loss, 64%, was associated with clomiphene induction.[25] Comparisons of rates of fetal loss with the time during pregnancy that the twins were diagnosed has indicated that the loss occurs in the first and early second trimester.[23] Twin gestations identified by ultrasound at less than 10 weeks gestational age ended with delivery of singletons in 71% of cases. If twins were still present and viable at 10 to 15 weeks of gestation, then in 62% of cases the gestation was reduced to a singleton at delivery. If both twins were still viable after 15 weeks of gestation, they both survived to delivery.

The *pattern* of early gestational loss depends on the time in pregnancy when it occurs and may be subdivided into embryonic and fetal death, using 10 weeks' gestation as the dividing point. The twins may both die as embryos or as fetuses, or one may die as an embryo and one as a fetus. The pregnancy then terminates, and this pattern represents approximately one-third of the loss of twins[24,26] (Fig. 5.1b). Alternatively, one twin may die as an embryo or early fetus and the pregnancy continue with delivery of the survivor near term, a pattern seen in approximately two-thirds of cases, and termed the "vanishing twin" (Fig. 5.1a). The only apparent clinical sign of fetal death in this group may be an episode of slight vaginal bleeding, reported in up to 40% of cases,[27] and the process of embryonic or fetal death of one twin does not appear to affect the development of the survivor in most cases.[30] Death of one twin as a later fetus with survival of the co-twin to birth becomes an example of fetus papyraceous and is considered as a midpregnancy loss in the discussion that follows.

The *causes* of embryonic and fetal death in this period remain to be determined in the majority of cases. Part of the problem is that the presence of the multiple gestation may have been an early ultrasound diagnosis, and if death occurs at the embryonic stage and involves only one of the pair, there may be little or no residual tissue to assess at the time of delivery of the survivor. The explanation for a "vanishing twin," once the possibility of false positive or artifactual observations are ruled out, has focused on resorption, possibly of a blighted or lethally incomplete embryo, although the actual pathophysiologic process of such resorption is not clear. Even if the dead twin died as a fetus, what tissue remains may provide few clues as to a potential cause of death. Aborted twins at the embryo stage are more likely to be primarily abnormal, represented by one of the growth disorganizations, often with associated chromosomal errors.[9] Aborted twin fetuses tend to have the same variety of malformations as seen in aborted singletons, and the abortion is more likely to be associated with obstetric complications such as ascending infection or abruptio placenta.[9,13] The pathology of aborted twin embryos and fetuses is described in more detail in the next section.

Some of the observations made in studies of aborted twin embryos and fetuses may help define contributing factors to fetal death in the first trimester. For example, there is a high proportion of monochorionic conceptions among aborted twin embryos and fetuses, up to 85%, and this suggests that there may be some basic abnormalities of the monozygotic twinning process, such as asymmetric twinning, that contribute to embryonic/fetal death.[9] Alternatively, with multiple gestations, there may be implantation asymmetries that fail to provide adequate support for one or both embryos, leading to embryonic or fetal death. Lesser degrees of asymmetry of fetuses and placentas of twin gestations are well recognized later in pregnancy, suggesting that more severe forms may lead to earlier fetal death.

Elective first trimester embryo/fetal death has been termed selective abortion, selective termination, selective embryocide, selective continuation, multifetal pregnancy reduction, and selective embryo reduction, and has led to considerable discussion of the ethical as well as the clinical issues involved.[21,35–47] The indications, timing, and procedures used vary, and although elective reduction is almost always limited to multiple sets of three or more, it is included in this discussion of mortality of twins to allow a comparison of the pathology with that of natural or spontaneous reductions. The majority of cases are induced multiples, either by hormonal stimulation of polyovulation alone, or combined with extracorporeal fertilization and embryo replacement. Embryonic or fetal death has been obtained by aspiration techniques,[40,48] by injection of air,[49] sodium chloride,[21] or potassium chloride,[42–44,46] into the "selected" embryo/fetus

chest, pericardial sac, or heart, or by mechanical disruption with a needle.[41]

The pathologist's role in cases of early pregnancy twin death is twofold. First, the pathologist needs to provide clinicopathological correlation by identification of any embryonic or fetal residues on the placenta of surviving twins in pregnancies where fetal death has been documented by ultrasound during the pregnancy. Second, he or she must undertake careful examination and documentation of aborted embryos and fetuses in order to determine zygosity and possible causes for the gestational loss. It may be surprising to some pathologists who are not used to examining aborted embryos and fetuses just how much can be learned about and from them.

"Vanishing" Twins

Clinicopathological correlation of the "vanishing twin" phenomenon has been scanty, possibly because of the small volume of tissue in question, but in some cases superficially banal features of the delivered placenta may contain the evidence. Sulak and Dodson[50] provided clear documentation of a collapsed dichorionic second sac that presented grossly as a nondescript irregular plaque of thickened tissue in the reflected membranes of the placenta of the surviving twin. Jauniaux et al.[51] reported on three patterns of embryonic/fetal remnants. In five cases, they described a distinct marginal region of perivillus fibrin, although they make no comment as to the presence or absence of remnants of a gestational sac except in one case of later fetal death with a fetus papyraceous. One of these plaques did contain an embryonic remnant suggestive of vertebral segments, confirming the "vanished" twin. An unusual pattern was seen in one case of aborted fetuses where one had died several weeks earlier—an intermixture of normal and degenerate villi—but no explanation was suggested. Benirschke (in a personal communication[29]) reported finding a small separate dichorionic placenta with a 2 cm macerated fetus. Yoshida and Soma[52] reported nine cases of first trimester twin death with the involuted embryo represented by a chorionic cyst-like sac up to 7 cm diameter containing a stunted embryo or blighted umbilical cord, on the fetal surface of the surviving twin's placenta delivered at term.

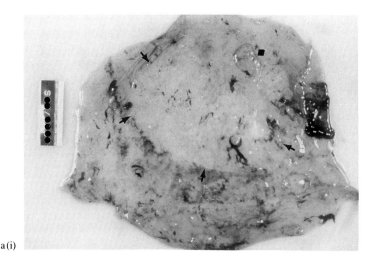

FIGURE 5.2. "Vanished" twins—clinical history of embryonic loss with pathologic confirmation of second conceptus. (a) The first twin died at about 11 weeks' gestation based on ultrasound findings. In the delivered placenta at term, there was a 12 × 0.2 cm plaque in the free membranes (arrows) 3 cm from the edge of the main placental mass (i). This plaque contained a smaller sac with a 3 × 2 × 1 mm embryo (diamond pointer) with limb buds and small ribs (ii). The male survivor was normal. The septum was dichorionic diamniotic. No cause for embryonic death defined.

a(i)

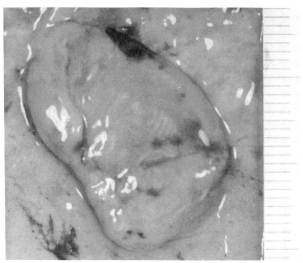

a(ii)

The Survey '91 cases of "vanishing" twin presented in three patterns—a history of embryo/fetal death with no discernible residue, a history of embryo/fetal death with a discernible residue, and an unexpected residue on the delivered placenta identified by the pathologist.

There were 23 placentas submitted with a history of vanishing twin, one with a vanishing triplet and one with two vanishing quadruplets, in which no evidence of the missing multiples could be found. When recorded, the missing multiple was identified as receding at 6 to 12 weeks of pregnancy, and coincidental antepartum hemorrhage was reported in five cases. In 13 cases, the sex of the surviving multiple was reported and 73% were male, including the two surviving male quadruplets and the male

dizygotic twin of the triplet survivor pair. This seems an unusual male preponderance but without an idea of the nature of the lost multiples, no further comment is possible. There were no reported problems in the well grown survivors and no significant placental abnormalities.

In eight cases accessioned in the last 8 years of Survey '91, there was a history of twins diagnosed by early ultrasound and there was a readily identified residue of the vanished twin in the delivered placenta of the surviving twin (Fig. 5.2). The first twin died at anywhere from 8 to 16 weeks' gestation and the survivor was delivered at 38 to 40 weeks. Only one set was known to be associated with drug-induced polyovulation (with clomiphene). The residue of the vanished twin was similar in all

FIGURE 5.2. *Continued*. (b) The first twin in this case was said to have died at about 15 weeks' gestation. The residual plaque in the free membranes of the delivered placenta (arrows) at 41 weeks was 12 × 8 × 0.1–0.2 cm and adjacent to the margin of the main placental mass (i). Even close up it is remarkably nondescript (ii). However, careful dissection identified a 7 × 5 cm zone within the plaque that contained embryo/fetal skeletal remnants (iii). This was a dichorionic diamniotic placentation and the male co-twin was normal. No cause of embryonic death was defined. [Hematoxylin and eosin, original magnification ×12.5 (iii).] (Reprinted with permission from Wigglesworth and Singer, *Textbook of Fetal and Perinatal Pathology,* Chapter 8, Blackwell Scientific Publications, 1991.)

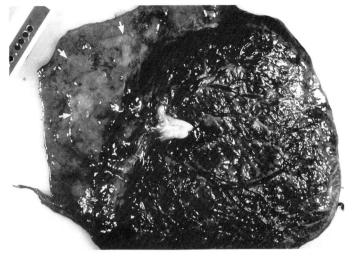

b(i)

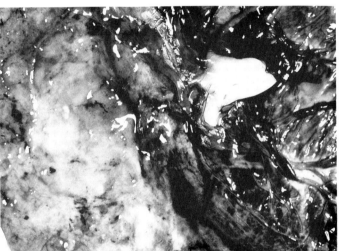

b(ii)

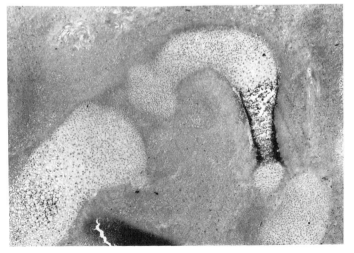

b(iii)

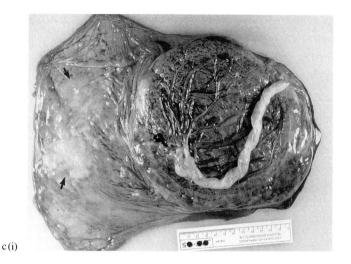

c(i)

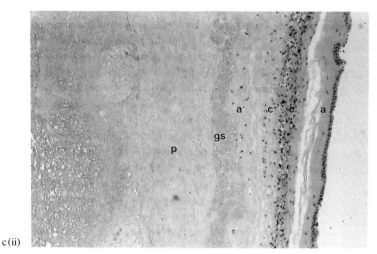

c(ii)

FIGURE 5.2. *Continued.* (c) Twins were diagnosed with ultrasound at 10 weeks and one had died by the next examination 2 weeks later. There was a 7 × 6 cm marginal plaque in the free membranes (i), which had a dichorionic diamniotic septum microscopically (ii), but no definite fetal remnant was seen. The male co-twin was slightly large for age with a longish cord (71 cm/57 cm) and a heavy placenta (665 g/450 g) with circumferential extrachorial membrane attachment. Mother was gestational diabetic and had been so in many of her 11 pregnancies. No cause of embryonic death was defined. (a, amnion, c, chorion layers from sac of surviving twin; a', amnion, c', chorion layers from "vanished" twin; gs, collapsed gestational sac from "vanished" twin; p, regressed placenta from "vanished" twin. [Hematoxylin and eosin, original magnification ×25 (ii).]

cases, and consisted of varying-sized plaques in the reflected membranes, adjacent to or at different distances from the disk of the surviving twin. The plaque ranged from 5 × 7 to 12 cm in diameter and was usually 1 to 5 mm in thickness. Occasionally, a portion of the plaque was a bit thicker and when such a region was dissected carefully, a collapsed gestational sac was entered. Histologic sections of these plaques identified them all as dichorionic placentations, and an occasional embryonic residue was noted, but no clue as to the cause of the twin death was identified. All surviving twins did well. Five were male and three female; only one was noted to have any problem and he was mildly large for gestational age. In seven cases, the placental pattern of the surviving twin was normal. In one case (Fig. 5.2c), the placenta was heavy, 665 g, had

a circumferential extrachorial (marginal) membrane attachment, and the umbilical cord was 71 cm long; the surviving twin was of normal growth but the mother was obese with recurrent insulin-dependent gestational diabetes mellitus in this pregnancy and in many of her 11 previous pregnancies.

In six placentas accessioned in the last 15 years of Survey '91, it was the pathologist who identified that the conception had originally been a twin gestation (Fig. 5.3). In five of the cases, the residue was similar to that described above—a plaque in the membranes of the placenta of the survivor. The plaques varied in size and macerated embryos were seen in three of them. All were dichorionic placentations. The sixth case was a particularly instructive example of the importance of careful examination of the placenta in cases of developmental anomalies

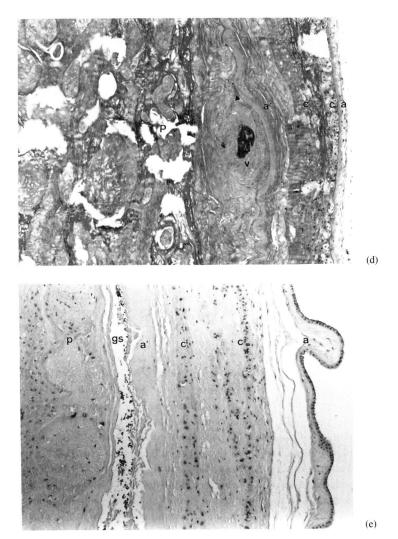

(d)

(e)

FIGURE 5.2. *Continued.* (d) This dichorionic diamniotic pattern of the separating membranes was documented overlying a 7 cm diameter circular plaque in the free membranes 3 cm from the margin of the main placenta in a term Clomid-induced twin pregnancy, where the first twin "disappeared" in the first trimester. No other embryonic remnant was found and the female survivor was normal. No cause of embryonic death was defined. (a, amnion, c, chorion layers of sac of surviving twin; a′, amnion, c′, chorion layers of sac of "vanished" twin; triangle is in collapsed gestational sac of "vanished" twin; v, residual chorionic surface vessel; p, involuted placental tissue. (Masson stain original magnification ×25).

(e) There appears to have been a rather remarkable degree of resorption in this case. One twin was reported to have loss of cardiac activity as seen by ultrasound examination at 15 to 16 weeks by dates, although it was said to be 9 to 10 weeks by size. At 41 to 42 weeks, a 3,200-g normal male infant was delivered spontaneously. In the marginal membranes near the cord insertion was an 8 × 6 cm rubbery grayish plaque that was 2 to 3 mm thick. The dichorionic nature of the septum was confirmed microscopically, but no definitive fetal remnant was detected. (a, amnion, c, chorion layers of sac of surviving twin; a′, amnion, c′, chorion layers of sac of "vanished" twin; gs, collapsed gestational sac of "vanished" twin; p, involuted placenta.

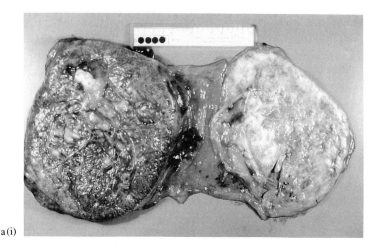

a(i)

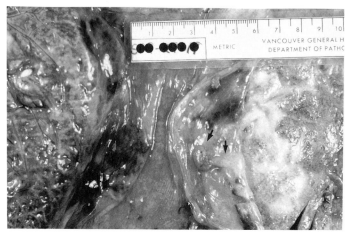

a(ii)

FIGURE 5.3. "Vanished" twins—no clinical history of detected twinning, but residual twin identified in placenta of live-born apparent singleton. (a) Dichorionic diamniotic twins with embryonic death at 6 weeks based on size of residue. The residue was a 16 × 12 × 0.5 cm plaque in the free membranes, 15 cm from the margin of the main disk (i). Careful dissection revealed a 10 × 6 cm cavity in this mass with a 15 mm crown–rump length macerated but definable embryo on a 2 cm body stalk (arrows) (ii). The main placental mass was normal. The sex of the survivor was not stated; no problems were reported. No cause of embryonic death was defined. [(ii Reprinted with permission from Wigglesworth and Singer, *Textbook of Fetal and Perinatal Pathology,* Chapter 8, Blackwell Scientific Publications, 1991:242.]

of a singleton (Fig. 5.3f). A female infant delivered spontaneously at 33 weeks had amyoplasia of the arms with contractures, and intestinal atresia from midjejunum to transverse colon. A number of causes were considered initially until the placental findings were available. In this case of unsuspected involuted twin, the second sac was on the surface of the survivor's placenta, contained a macerated embryo assessed to be 41 days of development by crown–rump length, and the placentation was confirmed histologically as monochorionic diamniotic. It was postulated that there had been intertwin vascular connections (as the majority of monochorionic twins do have them), and that there had been a hemodynamic or vascular insult that led to the death of one embryo with a lesser but still damaging effect on the other embryo who survived. There was no clue as to what that insult might have been. The size of the macerated embryo suggested that the damage

had occurred at about 8 weeks' gestation, the time at which the intestine is physiologically herniated into the body stalk, perhaps accounting for the intestinal lesions in the survivor, although the upper limb findings were not as readily explained. The finding of an involuted twin, with a potential explanation for the survivor's anomalies as due to a complication arising out of the monochorionic-monozygotic twinning circumstance, resulted in very different counseling regarding recurrence risks in the family. It might be argued that such cases are unusual, and perhaps the numbers do not justify the cost of time and effort to examine all placentas in cases of fetal anomalies. However, it is suggested that it would be very difficult to place a value on the importance of that finding to the family and to the process of genetic counseling in that situation.

It has been suggested above that severe asymmetry of the twinning process may be one mechanism

FIGURE 5.3. *Continued*. (b) Dichorionic diamniotic twin with embryonic death at 9 weeks based on size of residue. The residue was an irregular plaque in the free membranes of the normal immature (26 weeks) placenta. This plaque was 13 × 9 × 0.2–0.3 cm with one edge adjacent to the main mass. There was a visible fetoform mass with umbilical cord residue (i). Although readily seen without removal of the covering membranes, the septum was dichorionic microscopically. The embryo was 3.5 cm in crown–rump length with an optic vesicle and cardiac prominence, but no limb buds (ii). No information was provided about the survivor. No cause of embryonic death was defined. (Reprinted with permission from Wigglesworth and Singer, *Textbook of Fetal and Perinatal Pathology*, Chapter 8, Blackwell Scientific Publications, 1991:242.) (c) The dichorionic diamniotic septum collapsed over an undiagnosed twin was as easily defined in this case as in the other examples in this figure, but here the embryonic residue was particularly clear microscopically. The total residue was a 12 × 2 cm plaque in the membranes with a layer of adherent decidua. Microscopically, there were fetal remnants such as these vertebral and limb remnants, as well as evidence of the fetal sac, but no cause for the early death was determined. The survivor was said to be growth retarded at 34 weeks when delivered, but no other information was available.

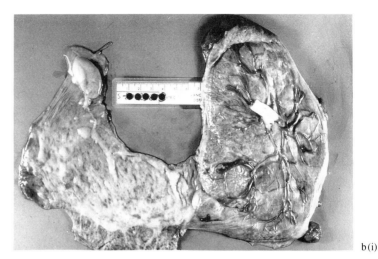

b(i)

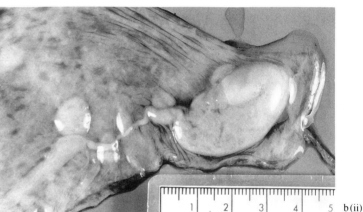

b(ii)

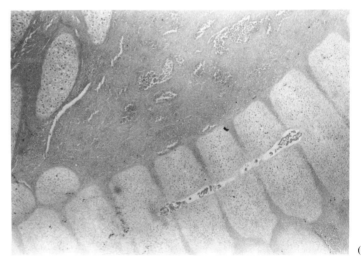

(c)

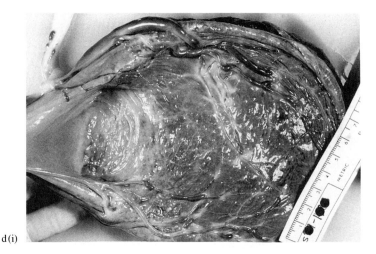

d(i)

FIGURE 5.3. *Continued.* (d) The location of the undiagnosed involuted twin was unusual in this case. The placenta was from an apparently normal preterm (30–31 weeks) male infant. The velamentous cord insertion was 6 cm from the placental margin, but the intramembranous vessels were wide ranging and inserted around half the circumference of the disk (i). In the zone within the innermost arcade of vessels was the second sac (ii). This sac was 10 cm diameter but no embryonic residue was found. There was little identifiable involuted villus tissue but the septum was dichorionic diamniotic histologically. This may be the residue of an originally empty sac twin but without early ultrasound findings no further comment is possible.

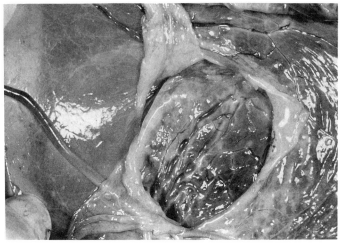

d(ii)

of discordant early embryonic or fetal death of twins. One such asymmetry could be discordant embryonic and/or placental chromosomal complements, in monozygotic or dizygotic twinning. Thus, it may be worthwhile to undertake cytogenetic evaluation of both portions of the placentation when a "vanished" twin or twin residue is detected, to attempt to identify such cases (Kalousek DK, 1992, personal communication).

Elective Embryo/Fetal Reduction

The pathology of elective embryo/fetal reduction procedures in the first trimester as identified at the time of delivery of the surviving multiples has been described rarely in the reported cases.[21,48,53] This is unfortunate because clinicopathological correlation serves a quality assurance function in these cases

particularly. The three cases of embryo reduction in the Survey '91 group are detailed here for comparison with the appearances of spontaneous reductions as described above. In the first case, a quintuplet pregnancy resulting from in vitro fertilization, and embryo transfer was reduced to twins in a staged procedure at 9 to 10 weeks of gestation.[21] In the reflected membranes of twin B in the dichorionic diamniotic fused placenta delivered with well grown normal male and female twins at 37 weeks, was a distinct 10 cm plaque and a marginal crescentic plaque, 10 × 4 cm. The distinct plaque contained a collapsed dichorionic sac and involuted villus tissue but no embryonic residue. The marginal plaque contained less detailed structures but was compatible with an involuted gestational sac. No evidence was found for a distinct third sac. It is possible that the first two terminations were repre-

FIGURE 5.3. *Continued*. (e) In this placenta from a normal female delivered spontaneously at 35 weeks to a well secundigravida with no reported gestational complications there was a gray-tan firm plaque 6 cm × 0.5 cm thick in the free membranes 10 cm from the nearest margin (arrows) (i). This contained a dissectable sac that had no microscopically detected embryonic residue in serial blocks of the entire mass, but a clear dichorionic septum was seen (ii). Cytogenetic analysis of cultured fibrous tissue from the plaque revealed 46,XX/46,XY, suggesting that it was the remains of a resorbed male conceptus. a, amnion, c, chorion layer of gestational sac of surviving twin; a′, amnion, c′, chorion layer of collapsed gestational sac (gs) of "vanished" twin. (Hematoxylin and eosin, original magnification ×25.)

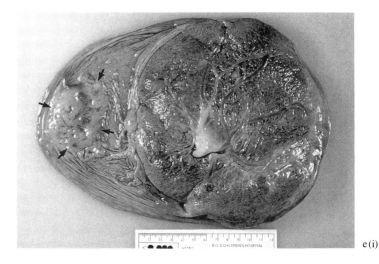

e(i)

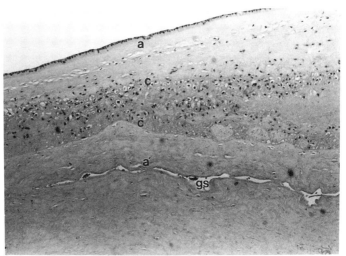

e(ii)

sented by the marginal plaque and the third, later termination by the residue further out in the membranes.

The second case of elective reduction provided several important lessons for the pathologist. Seven embryos were replaced into the uterus after in vitro fertilization and three sacs and three embryos were seen at 6 weeks. Three sacs again but now four embryos were seen a week later, with an appearance suggesting a monochorionic twin pair anteriorly, two embryos in a larger sac. A reduction to triplets at 11 weeks by means of intrathoracic potassium chloride into one of the anterior twin fetuses was effective immediately, but followed 6 hours later by death of the other anterior fetus. Appropriately grown and normal male and female twins were delivered by section at 33 weeks after the onset of pain at the previous cesarian site during spontaneous premature labor. The placentation was quite interesting (Fig. 5.4). The clarity of the Faxitron radiographs in this case prompted the use of x-ray examination thereafter of all placental masses that might represent involuted multiples. Unfortunately, the details of the sequence of fetal death was not known until after the gross prosection of the specimen, and the apparent distance between the residues led to them being treated as distinct gestational sacs. Histologic examination demonstrated that the membranes between A and B, A and "C," and B and "D" were unequivocally dichorionic, but the strong possibility that "C" and "D" were monochorionic could not be confirmed. The clinical events suggested that the anterior fetuses were monochorionic, because there were two in a larger

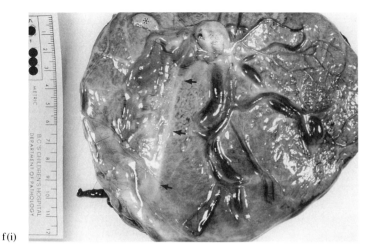

f(i)

FIGURE 5.3. *Continued.* (f) This was an unsuspected monochorionic diamniotic twin. On the delivered placenta can be seen a faint thickening of the surface membranes (arrows) and a small nodule of tissue (star) (i). When the membranes are reflected, an edematous cord (C) and associated embryo (E) are readily identified (ii). The gestational age of embryonic death was estimated at 8 weeks. The septum was confirmed diamniotic only (iii). The surviving twin had a number of anomalies that were potentially related to complications of monochorionic twinning and embryonic death as noted in the text. a, amnion of surviving twin; a′, amnion of embryo; gs, gestational sac space of embryo, v, chorionic vessel; p, placental villi). (Hematoxylin and eosin, original magnification ×12.5).

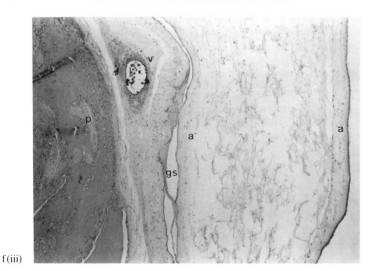

f(ii)

f(iii)

common sac than either of the other two fetuses had, and because the spontaneous death of the second fetus followed so soon after termination of the first. In fact, the differences in crispness of the appearances of the skeletons might suggest that "D" was the terminated fetus, while "C" was the one who died later, possibly as a result of some of the injected potassium chloride reaching the second twin across anastomoses, or as a response to hemodynamic shifts occurring across anastomoses after the death of quadruplet "D." This case points out the value to the pathologist of being very clear on the clinical events associated with an intervention procedure prior to any prosection of the specimen, in order to make the most of the placenta examination. The placental tissues of the surviving twins were well grown and normal aside from the relationship with each other and the involuted twins.

The third case involved the reduction of triplets to twins, in a 29-year-old primigravida. Triplets were conceived after seven cycles of hormonal therapy, because of panhypopituitarism following radiation for a craniopharyngoma. The mother had a cerebrovascular "accident" at 6 to 8 weeks with residual neuromuscular and neuropsychological deficit. At 11 weeks, one fetus was terminated with intrafetal injection of potassium chloride with immediate arrest of cardiac function. No adverse reactions were noted in the remaining fetuses and the mother was monitored carefully with no problems noted. Normal female twins were delivered by section at 34 weeks because of early labor and the mother's short stature and medical problems. The placenta was a dichorionic fused twin placenta with a 7-cm diameter and 5-mm-thick plaque in the membranes of triplet B, 5 cm from the margin (Fig. 5.5). Microscopically, the membrane mass was a dichorionic gestational sac with fetal remnants visible.

Documentation of Twin Residues

It can be concluded from the preceding discussion of the pathology of the "vanishing twin" that the closer we look, the more we can find. It is recommended that in all cases with a history of embryo or fetal loss in the first trimester, whether spontaneous or iatrogenic, with continuance of the pregnancy, that the placentation delivered with the survivor(s) be subject to careful pathologic examination, in-

cluding radiographs, photography, histology, and cytogenetics in spontaneous cases, undertaken with full knowledge of the clinical events. Should the pathologist be the first to suspect an originally twin or multiple gestation, the same techniques provide valuable documentation. It is helpful to try to determine the developmental size of the embryo/fetal residue, usually on the basis of crown–rump length or external developmental features,[13] and to determine the chorionicity of the membranes around the deceased multiple. Although the death of a multiple in early (first trimester) gestation seems to be accepted as having no adverse consequences for the mother or remaining fetuses in most cases, confirmation of the multiple nature of the conception, with as many details as possible, is a valuable contribution to the record of that gestation, with additional quality assurance benefits in cases of prenatal diagnosis of fetal death or in cases of elective interventions.

Spontaneous Concordant Embryo/Fetal Death

A separate category of first trimester embryo/fetal death in multiple pregnancy consists of spontaneously aborted embryo and/or fetus twins. In a detailed review of the material obtained from 1,939 pregnancies that terminated with spontaneous abortion of complete embryos or fetuses, 53 sets of twins were encountered, a rate of 2.7%.[9] There were 25 sets of embryos (defined as less than 8 weeks postovulatory age or 30 mm crown–rump length), 26 sets of fetuses (defined as 8 to 18 weeks postovulatory age and 30 to 165 mm crown–rump length), and two sets of embryo and fetus. Eighty-eight percent of the embryos were abnormal, mostly growth disorganized. Nine embryo pairs were discordant for the degree of growth disorganization and three of the pairs had a chromosomal anomaly. Twenty one of the 25 embryo pairs were identified as monozygotic because they had only one chorion, but zygosity could not be determined in the remainder. Twenty one percent of the fetuses were abnormal with a variety of malformations similar to those identified among singleton abortuses. Zygosity could be determined in 15 of the 26 fetal sets, and in 13 they were monozygotic. In 5 of these 13 sets there were discordant anomalies.

There were several additional interesting find-

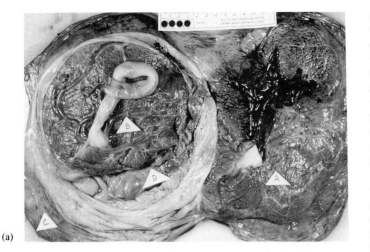

(a)

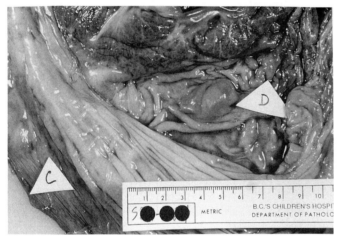

(b)

FIGURE 5.4. Elective reduction of in vitro fertilization–embryo transfer quadruplets to triplets at 11 weeks' gestation with spontaneous death of a second anterior fetus 6 hours later. Normal male and female twins were delivered at 33 weeks. The gestational sac of twin B had the appearance of being contained within the gestational sac of twin A, although the disks were distinct and separated by a zone of membranes 3.5 to 10 cm in width containing attenuated villus tissue (a). An ill-defined area of membrane thickening in the membranes of twin A and extending into the separating membranes between A and B contained an oval mass $4 \times 2.5 \times 0.7$ cm with visible extremities, ribs, and retinal pigment (quadruplet C) (b,c). A second less-defined oval mass $3 \times 2 \times 1$ cm (quadruplet D) was present in the combined membranes of A and B 7 cm from the margin of disk B (b,d). A thin membranous sac appeared to surround this remnant with a thick plaque in the membranes nearby. Because "D" seemed less distinctly fetal than "C," the remnants were x-rayed, and this confirmed the fetal nature of "D," although the appearance of the skeleton was not as crisp as of "C" (e). (a,c,d: Reprinted with permission from Baldwin VJ, *Developmental Pathology of the Embryo and Fetus*, JB Lippincott, 1992:325.)

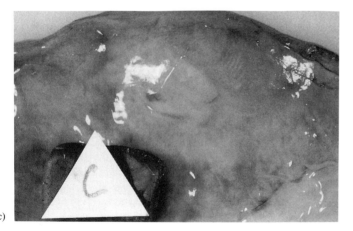

(c)

FIGURE 4. *Continued.*

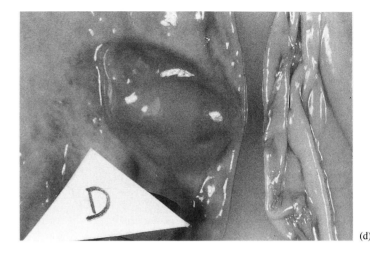

(d)

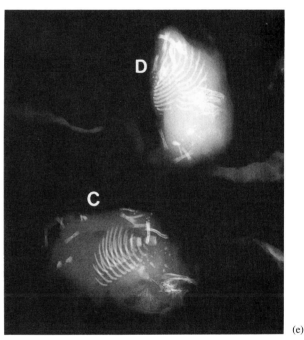

(e)

ings in this reported review of aborted embryos and fetuses. The ratio of females to males was 3 : 1, although the authors did not speculate further on the significance of this. Eighty-five percent of these dead twins were monozygotic, based on the fact that they were monochorionic, a proportion that is considerably higher than the usual 20% of monochorionic gestations in late pregnancy. Also, these monochorionic twins were lost as embryos in 60% of the cases, tending to support those who consider that monozygotic twinning is itself an abnormality, and therefore more prone to complications. It was also noted that separate placentas favored equal growth of the embryos or fetuses, an observation that supports the previous discussion (Chapter 3) of the importance of recording whether placentas are fused or separate.

In the Survey '91 group of concordant embryo/fetal twin deaths and abortions, there was an overlap of early (first trimester) and mid- (second trimester) pregnancy losses. In the legal jurisdiction of the survey cases, fetuses that are delivered after 20 completed weeks of pregnancy, whether they are live-born or stillborn, must be registered with the

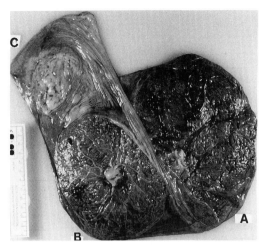

(a)

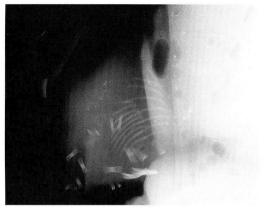

(b)

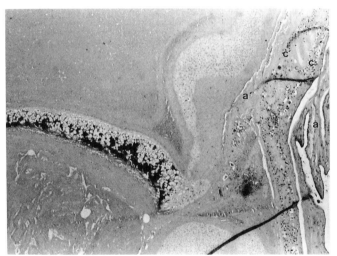

(c)

FIGURE 5.5. Elective reduction of hormonally induced triplets at 11 weeks' gestation. Normal dichorionic female twins (zygosity not further defined), delivered at 34 weeks. The triplet residue was a third dichorionic sac, 7×0.5 cm, located 5 cm from the margin of a dichorionic diamniotic fused twin placenta of the survivors (a). The delicate fetal skeleton can be seen with x-ray (b). The dichorionic pattern of membranes was identifiable, as were skeletal residues (c). a, amnion, c, chorion layers of surviving twin's sac; a', amnion, c', chorion layers of terminated twin's sac.

Provincial government department of Vital Statistics, District Registrar of Births, Deaths and Marriages, regardless of their degree of development or state of preservation. Thus, the Embryopathology Service examines embryos of fewer than 10 weeks' gestation and fetuses of 10 to 20 weeks' gestation. The rare fetus who is born with signs of life prior to 20 weeks is treated as a live-born fetus of greater than 20 weeks. A useful protocol for examination of embryos and fetuses has been described in detail by Kalousek et al.[13] and their atlas is recommended. Because the cases from the Survey '91 group were all examined by the same protocol, it was felt that the results could be presented as a group, rather than making a somewhat artifactual cutoff at 13 weeks' gestation. Also, there is the problem of how to classify those macerated fetuses that may have a developmental age of 13 weeks or less at death, but that were not delivered until the second trimester. Maceration at this gestational age makes it very difficult to decide if the fetal size by measurement was the gestational age at death, or if there was growth retardation before death, with death later than the size alone indicates. Correlation of pathologic findings with ultrasound measurements of growth may be helpful, but too few measurements are available as yet at this gestational age in cases such as these. At the earlier end of this period, there is a problem of how to classify a specimen that is morphologically embryonic, but the gestational age is said to be greater than the embryonic period. The choice has been made therefore to use the reported gestational age as the classifying criterion, with the thought that discrepancies of developmental age may be instructive.

FIGURE 5.6. These slightly discordant-sized empty sacs represent a spontaneous dichorionic diamniotic embryonic twin abortion of uncertain menstrual dating. Both provided normal 46,XX karyotypes but maternal contamination was not ruled out. (Courtesy of Dr. Dagmar Kalousek, Head, Embryo Pathology Service, British Columbia's Children's Hospital, with permission.)

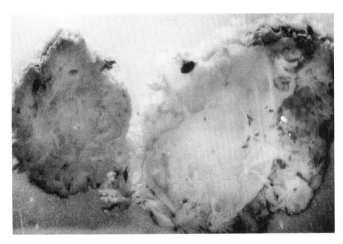

Embryonic Loss

In the Survey '91 Review, there were 16 sets of twin embryos examined. Half were monochorionic, one-quarter dichorionic, and one-quarter of undetermined chorionicity. The embryonic sex was detected in eight pairs and all were female; five were monochorionic and chorionicity was undetermined in three. The stated gestational age at termination was 12 weeks in the majority and all were spontaneous. The cause of the abortion, other than the anomalous conception itself, was not evident except in one case with severe inflammation that followed placement of an intrauterine contraceptive device 2 weeks previously at 10 weeks of gestation. Correlation of stated gestational age and developmental age was not possible in many cases because of an inability to stage the specimen even though the gestational age was known in some, and the absence of accurate dating when the developmental age could be assigned in others. Seventy-five percent of the embryos were demonstrably abnormal, and the remainder were too damaged to assess or the sac had ruptured and there was no embryonic tissue remaining. Twelve embryos, 37.5% of the total, were present as empty sacs (growth disorganized embryos, type 1), including four sets with concordant empty sacs, all dichorionic (Fig. 5.6). Ten embryos, 31%, were concordantly chromosomally abnormal and all female: two sets of monosomy X, one set with trisomy 21, one set with double trisomy of 7 and 16, and one set with mosaic triploidy (68,XX/69,XXX). In one pair, the chromosomally normal monochorionic female embryos had midfa-

cial dysplasia and slightly discordant delayed limb-bud development.

These findings reinforce the trend of observable abnormality in this group of twin losses as reported by Livingston and Poland[9] that reproductive loss of twins in the embryonic period is of lethal chromosomally abnormal conceptions in the majority, with an excess of monochorionic and female sets.

Embryo/Fetal Loss

There were four cases of double mortality, where death of the twins did not appear to have occurred at the same time, but they were delivered together. A female fetus delivered electively at 19½ weeks' gestation, because of elevated amniotic fluid alpha-fetoprotein and positive acetylcholinesterase test that suggested a neural tube defect, was found to be developmentally normal but accompanied by a macerated female co-twin of 9 weeks' developmental size.[54] This case has been reported previously in order to draw attention to the possibility of falsely elevated amniotic fluid markers of neural tube defects in cases of a surviving twin following embryo/fetal death of a co-twin. The placenta was too fragmented to determine the membrane pattern, but diffusion of alpha-fetoprotein across diamniotic intertwin membranes has been reported.[55] There were three sets of twins delivered at 19 to 19½ weeks with one twin macerated and one twin well preserved with intervals of 0.5, 1.0, and 3.5 weeks between the fetal deaths in each pair. The cause of death of the macerated fetus was not determined. Delivery was elective in one case following the diagnosis of fetal death, and spontaneous in the other two associated with bleeding and ascending infection. Two cases were dichorionic, one undetermined, and there was one each of female/female, male/male, and male/female pairs. There were so few cases in this category of discordant timing of fetal death that no pattern of pathology was detected.

Fetal Loss

There were 56 sets of twin fetuses delivered before 20 weeks of gestation in the Survey '91 group and these were segregated into two distinct patterns— *well-preserved acutely aborted fetuses* (61%) and *macerated fetuses* that had been retained for a period of time after fetal death before being aborted (39%) (Fig. 5.1b2). There are some interesting differences in the characteristics of the two groups and these are recorded in Table 5.1. The prominence of female pairs noted in the embryonic group is seen in the well-preserved fetus group, but not in the macerated group, and remains unexplained. The prominence of monochorionic twins in fetal loss data persists, although it is not quite as high in the well-preserved fetal abortion group, perhaps because of the different pattern of pathology between the well-preserved and macerated group. There were two peaks of fetal death in the well-preserved group at 14 to 15 weeks and 18 to 19 weeks, while fetal death in the macerated group was assessed to have occurred in the 12- to 15-week range in the majority. The probable age of the fetus at the time of

fetal death in the macerated group was estimated from bone lengths (hand, foot, or femur lengths), although it was recognized that if there had been a period of intrauterine growth retardation prior to death, the estimate of date of death would be an error toward an earlier date. For purposes of discussion, the measurements were taken at face value. The apparent periods of retention ranged from 1 week in two cases to 7 to 8 weeks in six cases, but could not be determined in seven cases due to insufficient data regarding the actual gestational age of the pregnancy at delivery.

The patterns of pathology identified in these fetal twin deaths differed between the two groups as well. The obstetric complications that contributed to the abortion of well preserved fetuses consisted of significant ascending infection in 44% of the cases (Fig. 5.7), occasionally with a history of vaginal bleeding, abruptio placenta alone in 12%, and in one case abortion was due to an infection following amniocentesis. Delivery of 23% of the well-preserved twins was induced because of ultrasonographically detected fetal anomaly, including conjoined twins, concordant multiple recurrent anomalies, discordant anencephaly, concordant hemoglobinopathy, discordant neural tube defect, and a chorangiopagus parasiticus twin pair. Four otherwise normal twins had anomalous cord insertions, a concordant pair with marginal cords and one each with marginal and velamentous insertions in separate twin sets. There were three sets with possible twin-to-twin transfusion syndrome, based on discordant fetal development and monochorionic placentations, but anastomoses were not confirmed.

TABLE 5.1. Comparisons of well-preserved and macerated aborted twin fetuses.

Characteristics	Well-preserved	Macerated
Sex distribution		
Female pair	68.6%	45.5%
Male pair	17.1%	50.0%
Female/male	14.3%	0
Unidentified	0	4.5%
Chorionicity/zygosity		
Monochorionic/monozygotic	40.0%	63.7%
Dichorionic/dizygotic	17.1%	4.5%
Dichorionic/zygosity unknown	20.0%	9.0%
Undetermined	22.9%	22.8%
Timing of fetal death	14/15 wks—31.4%	12–15 wks—59.0%
	18/19 wks—34.3%	16–19 wks—22.7%
	scattered—34.3%	scattered—18.3%
Major pathology identified	Obstetric complications 55.8%	Fetal malformations 50%

FIGURE 5.7. This monochorionic diamniotic twin pregnancy terminated spontaneously at 14 weeks with evidence of ascending infection in the sac of twin A; note the opacity of the chorionic surface on side A. The twins were otherwise normal and well preserved.

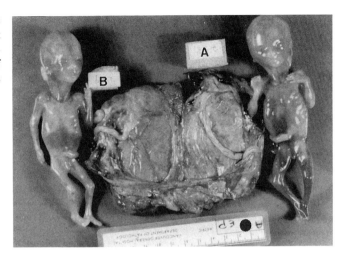

There was one pair with evidence of severe fetomaternal hemorrhage. The cause of the twin abortion was not determined in five cases. In contrast, there were considerably more malformations identified in the macerated twins. There were three chorangiopagus parasiticus pairs, and the other anomalies encountered are noted in Table 5.2, with examples in Fig. 5.8. There were two monoamniotic pairs with cord entanglement, and two monochorionic sets with possible twin-to-twin transfusion syndrome. In eight pairs the cause of intrauterine fetal death was not detected.

Midpregnancy Loss

We have seen in the discussion of first trimester loss that the death of one embryo or fetus does not necessarily lead to termination of the pregnancy,

TABLE 5.2. Anomalies identified in macerated twin fetal abortions.

Twin type	Twin A	Twin B
Monochorionic/male pair	Malrotation large bowel	Microcephaly
	Hypospadius III	Phocomelia upper limbs
	Bilobed right lung	Abnormal ossification of thoracic and cervical vertebral bodies
		Absence of toes bilaterally
		Absence of scrotum
		Absent left hemidiaphragm
		Absent anterior thoracic and abdominal wall with marked distortion visceral positions
		Abnormal development facial structures
?Chorionicity/female pair	Single umbilical artery	Transposition of the great vessels and ventricular septal defect
Monochorionic/male pair	Hypoplasia body stalk with eventration of abdominal viscera	Normal
	Anorectal agenesis	
	Agenesis external genitalia	
	Agenesis right kidney	
Dichorionic/male pair (Fig. 5.8a)	Growth retardation	Anencephaly
	Single umbilical artery on left	Midline cleft soft palate
	Abnormal ossification of humeral heads	
	Possible dwarfing process	
Monochorionic/male pair	Single umbilical artery	Normal
Monochorionic/female pair (Fig. 5.8b)	Normal	Amniotic band left arm
Monoamniotic/male pair	Single umbilical artery	Single umbilical artery

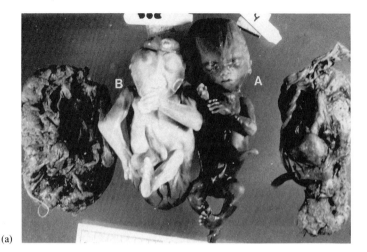

(a)

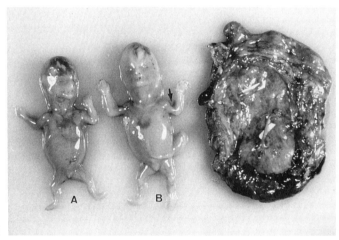

(b)

FIGURE 5.8. Examples of anomalies found in macerated concordant twin fetal abortions. (a) This dichorionic male twin pair was delivered spontaneously at 19 weeks. Twin A was growth retarded with a bone age of 14 to 16 weeks and abnormal ossification of the humeral heads. A specific osteochondrodystrophy was not identified. The anencephalic co-twin also had a midline cleft of the soft palate. Cytogenetic analysis was not possible as the specimen was formalin fixed when received. (b) These macerated female monochorionic twins were delivered spontaneously at 16 weeks. They were both 10 weeks developmental age and twin B had a constricting amniotic band on the left arm (removed to show indentation at arrow) and most of the amnion had separated from the inner surface of the placenta (small pieces of white card are placed under the umbilical cords to display them to better advantage). The cause of the fetal death was not determined.

and the same is true in some cases of fetal death in the second trimester. Because the fetus in such cases is much larger, it is sometimes easier to determine the type of twinning and possible contributing factors to fetal death. Midpregnancy losses of twins may be spontaneous or induced, and these are discussed in turn.

Spontaneous Fetal Death

Spontaneous fetal death in the second trimester presents in one of three ways (Fig. 5.1c–f). In one pattern, death of one or both fetuses may result in delivery of the entire contents of the uterus at once. The incidence and patterns of concordant twin mortality in midpregnancy are difficult to extract from the literature, primarily because the apparent limit of biological viability ex utero is in the middle of this trimester. The patterns of twin mortality in

the previable portion of the second trimester have been described in the previous section. Mortality of twins in the latter half of the second trimester is usually represented in reports of overall perinatal mortality of twins, particularly if the lower weight categories are assessed. Further discussion of these cases is therefore presented in the sections on late pregnancy loss and perinatal mortality that follow. Alternatively, one twin may be delivered and the pregnancy continues with the survivor. The features of interval delivery have been described in Chapter 4. The third alternative is that the dead fetus may be retained, becoming compressed to a fetus papyraceous or fetus compressus by the growing sac of the surviving twin as the fluid in its own sac is resorbed. The majority of the literature on midpregnancy twin death focuses on this situation of discordant fetal death with retention of the dead fetus, and that is the focus of the remaining discussion in this section.

The spontaneous death of one twin in the second trimester with retention of the dead fetus as a *fetus papyraceous* until its delivery with the survivor is not common and may be marked by few clinical signs. The overall rate of fetus papyraceous has been reported up to 0.54% of twin pregnancies and is reportedly higher in triplets,[56] sometimes with two papyraceous fetuses and a normal survivor.[57–59] There may have been a history of a period of rapid uterine growth followed by slowed or normal growth, sudden onset or improvement of toxemia, limited vaginal bleeding, sudden lower abdominal pain, or brief escape of small amounts of amniotic fluid, although the mother does not seem to be otherwise affected at the time or later. Such a history should alert the pathologist to check the placental tissues for residues of the dead twin.

The *cause of death* of these fetuses that will become papyraceous is not known in the majority of cases. Anomalous insertions of the cord, particularly velamentous insertions, have been implicated,[56,60,61] although just how anomalous cord insertions affect the fetus at these early stages is not known. Monochorionic twins may succumb due to a severe twin transfusion syndrome,[62–64] and cord entanglements of monoamniotic twins can lead to fetal death.[65] As many as 50% of papyraceous fetuses are said to have been growth retarded at the time of intrauterine fetal death,[66] but the criteria of impairment of fetal growth are unclear.

The largest reported review of fetus papyraceous was of 150 cases where intrauterine fetal death had occurred at less than 28 weeks of gestation, following which the dead fetus was retained until delivery of the viable twin at or near term.[60] The study data suggested that there was no increased risk of intrauterine fetal death for twins of monochorionic as compared to dichorionic placentation. Although there was a high percentage of cases in which the sex was not stated, males seemed more likely to die in the second trimester than females, since the surviving twin of monochorionic placentations was male in 39.6% of the cases and female in 20.8%. In most cases the pregnancies were uncomplicated, the surviving twin approached singleton standards of birth weight, and while no definite cause for the intrauterine fetal death was identified, abnormalities of the umbilical cord were common. In monochorionic twins, 47% of the cases in which the cord was mentioned had some abnormality that might have contributed to the fetal death. These consisted of amniotic bands, velamentous insertions, true knots or a single umbilical artery. Unexpectedly, in three monoamniotic cases, no cord problems were reported. Of the dichorionic twins, 27% of cases with descriptions of the cord mentioned significant lesions such as fetal entanglement, very short cords, velamentous insertions, and single umbilical artery. In this early report, vascular anastomoses were not mentioned in the monochorionic cases.

The *fetal remnant* is usually attached to a part of the placenta of the survivor and presents as a compressed mass that varies in the extent of identifiable features. The fetus may be sufficiently well preserved that autopsy examination is possible to look for major anomalies and to identify the sex. Measurements can also be made to assess growth, but it may be difficult for the pathologist to determine the time of death of the papyraceous fetus. The size may suggest death at a certain date but the clinical data may suggest a different date.[67] In some of these cases it is possible that growth was initially impaired or arrested by the process that eventually led to fetal death. Unless there are extensive intertwin vascular communications, cessation of the fetal circulation in that portion of the placentation associated with the dead twin leads to gradual reduction of maternal circulation through that villus territory. This leads in turn to ischemic damage and eventual collapse together of the villi. The dead twin's portion of the placentation delivered with the survivor is thus represented by a firm, pale, and sclerotic mass with avascular villi embedded in fibrin. It may be present as a separate mass or a residual portion of a single disk depending on the original pattern of placentation.[17]

An important and still unanswered question is whether the presence of a fetus papyraceous has any *implications for the surviving twin*. In the majority of cases it appears that the survivor is normal,[52] but there are case reports of a variety of abnormalities seen in twins delivered with a fetus papyraceous. The lesions reported in the survivor have included intestinal atresia,[56,67,68] congenital skin defects,[69,70] limb amputations,[65] gastroschisis,[61] brain damage,[70] and aortic stenosis.[71] The mechanism of these complications is not clear except in the case where the cord of the papyraceous fetus was wound around the leg of its monoamniotic co-twin, leading to amputation of the leg. It has been suggested that transanastomotic vascular complications such as disseminated intravascular coagulopathy (DIC) due to the death of the co-twin may be important.[72] Unfortunately, much of the literature in support of this interpretation contains little or no documentation of the presence of monochorionic placentation or vascular anastomoses that would be a sine qua non for such a mechanism. An evaluation of transchorionic DIC as a mechanism for fetal damage is presented in Chapter 9 following the discussion of intertwin vascular anastomoses and transfusion syndromes.

Examples of papyraceous fetuses from the Survey '91 cases of fetal death were not always clearcut. The term "fetus papyraceous" is usually considered to define a fetus who dies in the second trimester but who is delivered with the co-twin in the third trimester, but this category can become blurred at both ends of this time frame. A fetus who dies in the 10- to 13-week period but is not delivered until after 20 weeks may be classed as a fetus papyraceous. At the other end of the spectrum, in the late third trimester, an early fetal death may merge with the "retained macerated" stillbirth group depending on the gross description of the fetus. It has been suggested that it takes 10 weeks' retention to create a papyraceous fetus.[67] The timing of intrauterine fetal death, when known, was by ultrasonic and/or clinical data. Fetal length estimates to determine gestational age were made at postmortem examination in a manner analogous to those previously described that were used for aborted fetuses, with the same considerations regarding the diagnosis of intrauterine growth retardation. There were 16 cases that could be classified as fetus papyraceous, based on the gestational age at death. They ranged from 13 to 25 weeks of gestational age at fetal death and were delivered at 27 to 40 weeks of gestation after intervals of retention of 8 to 26 weeks. The papyraceous fetus was male in 37.5% of cases, female in 25%, and in the remainder the sex could not be determined due to the degree of degeneration. The placentation was dichorionic in 50% of the cases, both separate and fused examples being seen, monochorionic in 37.5% and undetermined in the rest. The cause was determined in three cases: the female twin died in one set of unlike-sex twins because of discordant response to anti-Kell antibodies; the cord of the dead twin was around the neck of the survivor in a female monoamniotic set; and a single umbilical artery velamentously inserted cord of a twin transfusion donor was wrapped around his ankle. In six other cases, there were cord anomalies that might have been important—marginally inserted in one, velamentous insertions in three, abnormally long by one-third in one, and a single artery velamentous cord in a fetus with discordant trisomy 21.

The survivor was well grown with no apparent clinical problems in the newborn period in 11 cases, did well after hyaline membrane disease in one, did well after resuscitation because of a nuchal cord in one, and no information was available in two cases. In one case, fetal death occurred at 10 to 14 weeks clinically, with the survivor delivered spontaneously at 29 weeks because of abruptio placenta. The only residue of the deceased twin was a plaque of involuted placenta in the membranes of the bilobed placenta of the survivor. The survivor, a female, died the day after birth with diffuse acute hypoxic damage of all viscera. In addition, there was complete atresia of the duodenum with separation of the ends of the bowel, and absence of the gallbladder. No other signs of chronic injury were identified. The involuted placental tissue was located in the isthmus of membranes between the lobes of the placenta of the survivor, but the survivor's vessels between the lobes were normal. The nature of the septum was not described. Neither the cause of the early fetal death nor the pathogenesis of the anomalies in the survivor were determined.

Some examples of the *patterns of pathology* with fetus papyraceous are shown in Fig. 5.9. In early second trimester fetal death, the degree of compression may preclude detailed analysis of the dead fetus as in Fig. 5.9a, although the nature of the placentation can be assessed histologically. If the fetus is hard to assess for developmental aging, an x-ray may be of assistance to provide an estimate of skeletal development (Fig. 5.9b). When fetal death occurs later (Fig. 5.9c), more detailed assessment is possible. The placental portion belonging to the dead twin may be a distinct portion of a single-disk placenta (Fig. 5.9d), more like a marginal plaque in the membranes (Fig. 5.9a), or a distinct separate mass (Fig. 5.9e). In occasional cases, the intertwin vascular anastomoses are so extensive, as in Fig. 5.9c, that the surviving twin takes over and maintains circulation to the entire placenta, and it may be difficult to define any involuted placenta at all.

FIGURE 5.9. Examples of fetal death in the second trimester with retention of the dead twin as a fetus compressus or fetus papyraceous within the placenta of the surviving twin, who was delivered 8 to 26 weeks later. The degree of analysis possible varies as shown in these cases. (a) This fetus died at 13 weeks by clinical ultrasound criteria. The fetal residue is easily seen and the crown–rump length and skeletal development were appropriate for the stated age. The placenta of the papyraceous twin is totally sclerotic and adjacent to the normal placenta of the survivor. The septum was dichorionic diamniotic. Fetal sex could not be determined in the residual twin. The female surviving co-twin was well grown and clinically normal when delivered at 35 weeks. (Reprinted with permission from Baldwin VJ, *Developmental Pathology of the Embryo and Fetus,* JB Lippincott, 1992:324.)

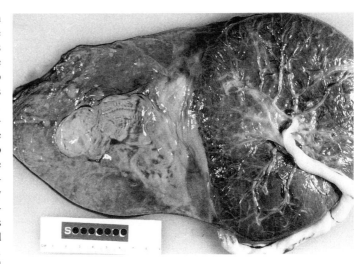

(a)

Elective Midtrimester Fetal Death

Elective or induced fetal death in the second trimester has been undertaken in twin pregnancies with discordant fetal compromise as an intermediate management option between termination of the entire pregnancy including the normal twin, or continuing the pregnancy with maternal and fetal risks from the abnormal twin.[73] The reported indications have been either discordant metabolic/structural/cytogenetic disorders, or cases with severe twin-to-twin transfusion syndrome. The discordant disorders have included Hurler's disease,[74] Tay-Sachs disease,[73] San Filippo A disease,[75] sialic acid storage disease,[76] thalassemia major,[77] male fetuses at risk for hemophilia[78,79] or Duchenne muscular dystrophy,[78] epidermolysis bullosa letalis,[78] craniospinal defects and anomalies,[22,75,78,80,81] limb/body wall anomaly,[22] nonsyndromic multiple anomalies with fetal hydrops,[82] and chromosomal anomalies, mainly trisomy 21.[22,73,75,83] The procedures used to cause the death of the abnormal twin have included exsanguination by cardiac aspiration[74]; air embolism into the umbilical vein[78,79]; intracardiac injection of sodium chloride,[80] calcium gluconate,[77] air,[22] or potassium chloride[22,82]; hysterotomy with removal of the affected twin[81]; pericardial tamponade with saline[22]; and most recently, intracardiac thrombogenic coils.[83] The effectiveness of the procedure, as determined by survival of the normal twin, is related in part to the technical aspects of the procedure chosen, but the results with monochorionic twins have not been encouraging,[22,84] attributed to complications affecting the unselected twin across placental anastomoses.

The pathologist's role in cases of selective survival or termination is to analyze the dead fetus and pattern of placentation at the time of delivery of the survivor, or to correlate the findings in both twins and the placenta in cases of failure of the procedure. The original diagnosis must be confirmed (or denied) where possible, and any complications explained. This analysis may be fairly straightforward with dichorionic sets, but can become more complex in cases of vascular complications in monochorionic sets.

There were no cases of selective termination of dichorionic twins in the Survey '91 Review. The cases of monochorionic twins with twin-to-twin transfusion syndromes that were subject to intervention are described in Chapter 9.

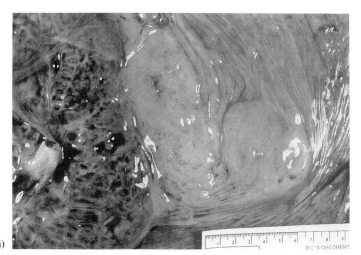

b(i)

FIGURE 5.9. *Continued.* (b) This was a dichorionic diamniotic twin placenta with fetal death of one twin documented at 15 weeks. As can be seen, the fetal residue is difficult to assess grossly (i), but has a well-defined skeleton when x-rayed (ii). The sex of the dead twin was not determined, nor the cause of fetal death. The surviving female co-twin was well grown and apparently normal when delivered at 41 weeks.

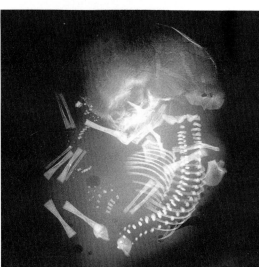

b(ii)

Late-Pregnancy Loss

In the literature, late fetal death is often discussed as part of an analysis of overall perinatal mortality of twins, but comparisons of the *patterns* of perinatal mortality suggest that considering twin stillbirth separately is also instructive. Late-pregnancy fetal death of twins usually presents in one of two patterns—concordant fresh stillbirth, or a stillborn co-twin delivered with the surviving twin, with the stillborn twin being more or less macerated depending on the interval of fetal death (Fig. 5.1f–h). Analysis of the characteristics of retained macerated and nonmacerated stillborn fetuses suggests that there are some interesting differences between

these groups, analogous to the situation with aborted twin fetuses in early pregnancy.

Twins are at greater *risk* for stillbirth than singletons with a 3- to 13-fold increase overall.[85–93] When risk of fetal death is compared by fetal weight, the increased risk for twins appears to be limited to the fetus greater than 2,500 g at birth, and the risk for fetal death of twins is equal to, or is less than, that of singletons for fetuses of 500 to 2,499 g, whether overall stillbirths rates are considered,[91,92] or just intrapartum deaths.[94] The reported rates of stillbirth of twins are 3% to 14%,[95–97] and there does not appear to have been much change in these rates in the last quarter century.[98] In a review of

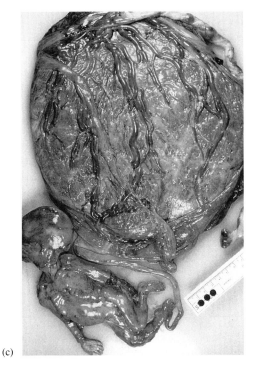

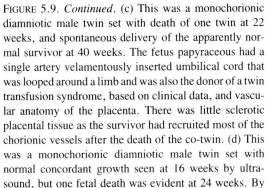

(c)

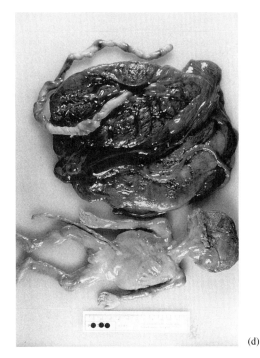

(d)

FIGURE 5.9. *Continued.* (c) This was a monochorionic diamniotic male twin set with death of one twin at 22 weeks, and spontaneous delivery of the apparently normal survivor at 40 weeks. The fetus papyraceous had a single artery velamentously inserted umbilical cord that was looped around a limb and was also the donor of a twin transfusion syndrome, based on clinical data, and vascular anatomy of the placenta. There was little sclerotic placental tissue as the survivor had recruited most of the chorionic vessels after the death of the co-twin. (d) This was a monochorionic diamniotic male twin set with normal concordant growth seen at 16 weeks by ultrasound, but one fetal death was evident at 24 weeks. By linear measurements, fetal death occurred at 20 to 21 weeks. The normally grown and apparently well co-twin was delivered at 38 weeks. There had been at least two surface intertwin vascular anastomoses that could be defined, one each arterial and venous, and one possible parenchymal shunt from the survivor to the fetus papyraceous. The dead twin had an abnormally long umbilical cord, twice the expected length for the gestational age at fetal death, and while the insertion into the placenta was normal, it was suggested that the abnormal length might have increased the risk of cord compression or fetal loops, although none was reported at delivery. No other cause for fetal death was determined.

10,204 pairs of twins, both twins were stillborn in 3% of the pairs, and in 4.2% of the pairs one twin was stillborn.[99] Of all twin deaths, 8.1% to 39.6% have been reported to be as stillbirths.[100–104] The risk for fetal death of twin B has been reported to be 1.6 times that of twin A overall, and seems to be constant at all birth weights.[93] Three-quarters of stillborn twins have been described as dying antepartum compared to less than half of stillborn singletons.[105] Of all the twin deaths in one series, 16% were fresh stillbirths, 18% were macerated stillbirths, and 2% were papyraceous fetuses.[104] The risk for stillbirth has been reported to be 1.5 times greater for like-sexed twins than unlike-sex pairs, with the majority attributed to complications of monochorionic placentation.[105]

The *causes* of fetal death of twins in late pregnancy are difficult to extract from the reported series on perinatal mortality of twins. Also, as with all reports of causes of death, it is not always possible to compare the information from different series because of differing classifications or interpretations of cause. In one survey of reported cause of death of 1,359 stillborn twins, "complications of placenta and cord" accounted for 34.3%, "maternal complications in pregnancy" for 29.2%, "congenital anomalies" for 10.2%, "intrauterine hypoxia and birth asphyxia" for 8.9%, "maternal conditions" for

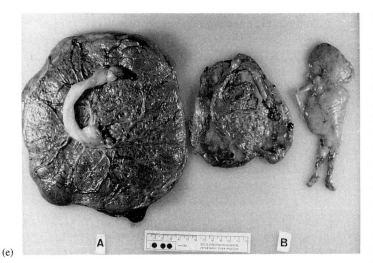

(e)

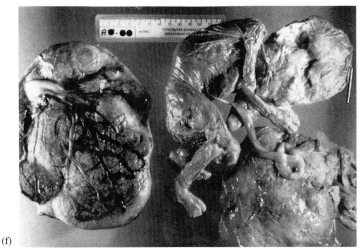

(f)

FIGURE 5.9. *Continued.* (e) This was a dichorionic diamniotic male twin pair. Amniocentesis at 16 weeks had identified discordant trisomy 21 in an hydropic twin with a nuchal hygroma. Fetal death of this twin occurred clinically at 23 to 26 weeks, but at autopsy the linear measurements were more appropriate for 14 to 15 weeks, suggesting severe fetal growth retardation. The co-twin was well grown and normal when delivered with the fetus papyraceous and both placentas at 38 weeks. The dead twin also had a single artery 1 cm velamentous cord of normal length and a separate placental mass. (f) Dichorionic male twins. Mother "knew" she had twins but no one believed her. Twin A, 2,040 g, was spontaneously live-born at 33 weeks. As the episiotomy was being sutured, the second fetus and placenta were delivered. By length measurements, the retained fetus was 25 weeks at death. There was histologic evidence of fetal asphyxia, but the cause was not identified.

8.3%, growth retardation for 1.8%, and "multiple pregnancy" for 26.5%.[90] In another review of perinatal death of twins, the percentage of twins that were stillborn in each category of cause of death was recorded.[106] The most important cause of stillbirth was fetal hypoxia, due to infarcted placentas, abruptio placenta or placenta previa, cord compression, or hypoxia of unknown cause affecting 46%. In 17%, obstetric complications consisting of incompetent cervix, premature rupture of membranes, and ascending infection were the causes of stillbirth. Twin transfusion syndrome in monochorionic twins accounted for just over 12%, and trauma to the mother or fetus was recorded in 5%. No cause was identified in 12.5% and a variety of other causes in the remainder, including congenital anomalies, in 4%.

In the Survey '91 Review of twin autopsies, 31.3% were stillborn twins. Of these, 34.9% were classed as "fresh" stillbirth, possibly equivalent to intrapartum death, although the exact time of death was not always known, 39.7% were defined as "macerated" with changes compatible with fetal death of less than 1 week prior to delivery, and 25.4% had been "retained" longer than 1 week after fetal death, based on clinical data and on the size and appearance of the fetus. In the overall autopsy review, there were 135 twin pairs that both came to autopsy, and of these pairs, both twins were stillborn in 29.6% and one twin was stillborn while the other died at varying intervals after birth in 12.6%.

A summary comparison of the characteristics of the stillborn twins overall and the same characteristics in the three patterns of stillbirth is presented in

FIGURE 5.9. *Continued.* (g) These were unlike-sex dichorionic twins. One twin was known to be growth retarded (26 weeks size at 30 weeks' gestation) before fetal death was documented at 32 weeks. Spontaneous delivery occurred at 37 weeks of a well 2,520-g male A and this macerated, growth retarded (by length) female B (i). The mode of death was asphyxial but the cause was not determined. Note the sclerotic appearance of the dead twin's placenta, both from the chorionic surface (i) and on section (ii).

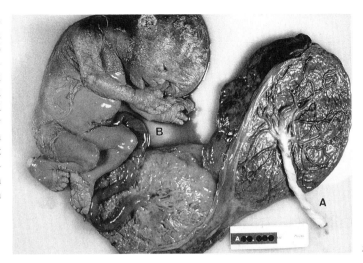

g(i)

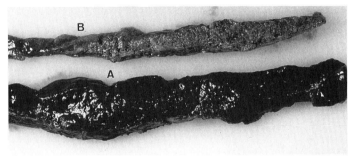

g(ii)

Table 5.3. There are some interesting differences observed, but not all can be explained as yet. The excess of male twins overall, both as single stillbirths and as like-sex male pairs, is not reflected in the retained group, where female twins predominate, but the reasons are not known. The stillborn twin is twin B at delivery overall, because of the marked excess in the retained group. This difference may be because the surviving twin becomes the presenting twin with loss of volume in the retained twin's sac, rather than there being any a priori increased risk for twin B for fetal death. The greater proportion of monochorionic placentation noted in the general discussion of twin mortality at the beginning of this chapter is noted in all groups, as well as overall. Concordant stillbirth was more frequent than individual stillbirth overall, but the ratios differed in each group. This may reflect the cause of fetal death, concordant causes such as complications of monochorionic placentation being represented in greater numbers in the fresh stillbirth group. Overall, there was a peak of stillbirths in the period of 20 to 24 weeks, with a sharp drop thereafter and similar numbers for each week from 25 to 36 weeks, and a further decline to term. This was true whether the gestational age of individual deaths, or of the sets represented, was considered. The majority of the early loss was as fresh stillbirths. Just over one quarter of the live-born co-twins of a stillborn twin also died at various times after birth, from minutes to 2½ years, represented mainly by the co-twins of fresh stillbirths. The details of causes of death are presented in the discussion that follows, but the role of complications of monochorionic placentation was quite evident and was usually associated with concordant stillbirth or stillbirth and perinatal death of a living co-twin. The greater proportion of cause unknown in the retained group likely reflects a masking of the cause by changes due to retention after fetal death.

Fresh Stillbirth

The freshly stillborn twins consisted of 18 pairs and 15 individuals, for a total of 51 twins. Of the total, 61% were male, 55% of the same-sex sets were

TABLE 5.3. Characteristics of late pregnancy fetal death (stillbirth).

	Total stillbirths	Fresh stillbirths	Macerated less than 1 week	Retained more than 1 week
Percent of all twin stillbirths	100%	35%	40%	25%
Males:females overall	1.4:1	1.5:1	2.6:1	1:2.3
Male pairs:female pairs:mixed pairs both stillborn	11.5:8:1	5:3:1	2.8:1:0	1:3:0
A:B when only one twin stillborn	1:1.3	2.8:1	1.2:1	1:9.5
Monochorionic:dichorionic:placentation not stated	5:2.8:1	4.5:2.8:1	9:5:1	3.2:1.4:1
Concordant:discordant stillbirth	2.4:1	2.4:1	1:1	1:1.3
Time of stillbirth (weeks gestation)	28% 20–24	84% ⩽28	48% ⩾33	Evenly spread
	55% 25–36			20–40+
	15% 37–40			
	2% >40			
Liveborn co-twins who died (%)	26	80	6	14
Lesions identified (%)				
Complications of monochorionicity	37.4	42	44.1	21
Cause not determined	25.2	20	20.3	39.5
Intrauterine asphyxia	23.8	14	30.5	26.3
Other anomalies	6.8	6	3.4	13.2
Ascending infection	6.8	18	1.7	0

male, and of the individual stillbirths, 73.3% were twin A. The majority, 58.8%, were stillborn at between 20 and 24 weeks' gestation, 84% were stillborn before 29 weeks, and no freshly stillborn twins were seen after 37 weeks. Monochorionic twin sets were seen in 54.5%, dichorionic sets in 33.3%, and the placental pattern in the remainder was not described. The majority, 80%, of the live-born co-twins of the individual stillbirths died, all of them within 5 days of birth, and 50% of them within an hour of birth. Although it has been suggested that twin B is at greater risk for perinatal mortality, in this group at least, in sets where the co-twin died after birth, the stillborn twin was twin A twice as often as twin B. This group of stillborn/perinatal death pairs were quite mixed when causes of death were considered and no pattern emerges; complications of prematurity were important in two-thirds of the live-born twins, but their stillborn co-twins had lesions of intrauterine asphyxia, multiple anomalies, or no obvious cause of death. Three sets had complications of monochorionic twinning, two chorangiopagus parasiticus pairs and one twin transfusion syndrome, and one set had concordant hydrops fetalis, cause unknown.

When the causes of death of freshly stillborn twins were considered, the largest number, 42%,

were due to complications of monochorionic twinning (see Table 5.3). These consisted of the twin transfusion syndrome across intertwin vascular anastomoses (see Chapter 9) in 71%, and the chorangiopagus parasiticus asymmetric twinning anomaly (see Chapter 10) in 29%, and in all cases the twins affected were concordantly stillborn, or a live-born co-twin died with lesions of prematurity. The category of intrauterine asphyxia refers to twins with aspiration of amniotic debris, with or without meconium, and visceral congestion with hemorrhages. The contributing factors included cord prolapse, obstructed labor, and an undiagnosed twin, but the underlying cause was not identified in the majority. In addition to the set with concordant hydrops fetalis, there were discordant anomalies in the stillborn twin, anencephaly in one and trisomy 18 in another, but the relationship between these anomalies and the fetal death is not known. A significant number of freshly stillborn twins, 18%, had signs of ascending infection with placental chorioamnionitis and aspiration of infected amniotic fluid, and in all cases there had been premature separation of the placenta with vaginal bleeding, although the underlying cause was not identified. In one-fifth of freshly stillborn twins, no cause of fetal death was identified at autopsy or from examination of the placenta.

Macerated Stillbirth

The macerated stillborn twins were defined as those who had died less than a week prior to delivery, based on clinical evidence and pathologic appearance (see Table 5.3). This was the largest group of stillborn twins, 58 fetuses from 14 pairs and 30 individual stillbirths. The majority, 72.4%, were male, and 73.3% of the like-sex stillborn pairs were male pairs. When only one twin was stillborn, it was as likely to be twin A as twin B. These twins were stillborn from 20 to 24 weeks in 22.4% of cases, all as concordant stillbirths, 48.3% were stillborn after 33 weeks of gestation, and the remainder evenly spread from 25 to 32 weeks of gestation. Monochorionic placentation was present in 59% of the twin sets represented in this group, 34% were dichorionic, and in 7% the placental pattern was not confirmed. Complications of monochorionic placentation were listed as the cause of death in 44.1%, consisting of the twin transfusion syndrome at 81% and chorangiopagus twinning in 19%, and 85% of these deaths were concordant stillbirths. Ascending infection was much less important in this group than with the fresh stillbirths, and there were only two fetuses with discordant abnormalities, one a neural tube defect and one rhesus isoimmunization. The proportion of cases with cause undetermined was the same as for the fresh stillbirths, one-fifth.

The macerated twins who were diagnosed as having signs of intrauterine asphyxia were a larger proportion of this pattern of late fetal death than in the other two patterns, and although no underlying cause was discerned in 44%, there were interesting associated findings in some others. In one case, there had been unspecified trauma to the maternal abdomen; in another case, one twin of a monochorionic set died from an acute fetomaternal hemorrhage for which no precipitating cause was identified, and in a third case one dichorionic twin died from the effects of a tight nuchal cord. In the remaining 39% of the asphyxiated macerated twins, many of their placental portions had discordant findings that suggested problems with placental development, with evidence of secondary effects on fetal blood flow[102] and fetal growth in some cases. These were encountered most often in dichorionic placentations, both separate and fused, and included the following combinations of findings: velamentous cord attachment to only one third of the chorionic volume; single artery umbilical cord attached to only one quarter of the chorionic volume; abnormally long umbilical cord (twice the mean for the gestational age) with 4-cm velamentous insertion attached to only one third of the chorionic volume with chorionic vessel thrombi and hemorrhagic endovasculopathy, with fetal growth retardation; marginally inserted umbilical cord and multiple calcified thrombi in the chorionic vessels; marginally inserted umbilical cord attached to one quarter of the total chorionic volume with chorionic artery thrombi and hemorrhagic endovasculopathy with fetal growth retardation. Other examples had multiple acute and chronic chorionic vessel thromboses with fetal growth retardation but no reported anomaly of development. While it might be argued that some fetal vascular changes could progress after fetal death, the asymmetric chorion and anomalous cord development would have been an important primary problem and probably contributed to the fetal death in these cases, particularly when the fetus was growth retarded. These cases are excellent examples of the value of placental assessment correlated with evaluation of fetal death.

Retained Stillbirth

Those stillborn infants who had been retained in utero for longer than 1 week merged with the fetus papyraceous group of the preceding section, and sometimes the distinction was not made clearly. Determination of the time of death of these twins was by a clinical history of lack of fetal movement, ultrasound findings, or fetal size at autopsy, although the limitations of the use of size as an assessment of maturity in cases where there might be intrauterine growth retardation is acknowledged. There were eight pairs and 21 single retained fetuses for a total of 37 fetuses (see Table 5.3). The sex ratio in this group was the complete opposite to that of the other two groups, just over two-thirds were female, 67.6%, and females outnumbered males in like-sex pairs by three to one. There was nothing in the data that suggested a cause for this difference. Although 90.5% of the individual stillborn twins were twin B, also a striking difference for the proportions noted in the other two groups, one wonders if that simply reflects a physical position change after fetal death, so that the survivor became the presenting fetus by the time of birth. There were not enough data in the records to assess the position of the dead twin prior to death in order to assess this possibility.

Retained twins were delivered with their living co-twin in equal numbers from 20 to 40 weeks' gestation. The interval from fetal death to delivery ranged from just over 1 week to 13 weeks, with 86% retained for 8 weeks or less, and 27% delivered after 2 weeks. The interval of fetal death was discordant in only one of the eight pairs of concordant still-birth, 6 weeks and just over 1 week in a monoamniotic pair with cord entanglement. The living co-twin was normal in 76% of sets with only one twin stillborn. One living co-twin in a monoamniotic pair had digital amputations from the amniotic bands that strangled the umbilical cord of her stillborn twin. There were three living co-twins who died, and two of these were from monochorionic pairs. In these two, there was significant brain damage in the survivor, which could be dated to the time of the death of the co-twin in one infant who died within 24 hours of birth, but could not be dated in a twin who died at 2½ years of age.

Monochorionic placentas were identified in 57% of the sets of twins represented by this group, but in 18% the membrane relationships were not clarified. An interesting note was that although only 21% of the deaths of the retained twins was attributed to complications of monochorionic twinning, all the Survey '91 cases of monoamniotic twinning with fetal death were seen in this group, and accounted for 13% of the deaths. Twin transfusion syndrome was confirmed far less often than in the other two groups of fetal death. There was a greater percentage of twins with other anomalies/disorders in this group, such as discordant hydrops fetalis, anti-Kell hemolysis, arthrogryposis, and multiple anomalies. Intrauterine asphyxia was important in this group and was of undetermined cause in 40% of the cases, associated with asymmetric chorion development with or without anomalous umbilical cords in 40%, and associated with a maternal septate uterus and premature separation in one and entanglement of the cord by an amniotic band in another. The largest category of causes of death with retained dead twins was the unknown group, nearly 40% of cases. This may be because of the changes that take place following retention after fetal death[107] that mask any clues as to the original cause.

Intragestational Fetal Loss—Summary

While there remains much to be learned about intrauterine death of twins, some general observations can be made from the preceding discussion. Male twins predominate in all categories except fresh fetal deaths at 12 to 20 weeks' gestation and late gestation fetal deaths retained for longer than 1 week, where two-thirds of the dead twins were female. No explanation for this observation was determined. There was no preponderance of A or B twins in sets where only one twin died except in the retained late gestational fetal death group, which were almost all B twins. This may reflect a physical readjustment of location within the uterus over the interval from death to delivery rather than any special risk for B twins. Documented embryo/fetal deaths peaked at 11 to 15 weeks' gestation, 80% of fresh stillbirths occurred at 20 to 28 weeks, and 48% of macerated stillbirths of less than 1 week of fetal death were delivered after 33 weeks' gestation. Monochorionic twins were represented far more frequently than the proportion seen with live-born twins, suggesting that complications of monochorionic monozygotic twinning or of monochorionic placentation are a significant source of fetal death of twins. Intrauterine death of one twin did not seem to have particular consequence for the surviving co-twin—81% of fetus papyraceus co-twins, 77% of macerated (<1 week) stillborn co-twins, and 76% of retained stillbirth co-twins had no apparent problems. In contrast, 80% of the living co-twins of the fresh stillbirth group died within the first 5 days after birth, possibly reflecting the greater rate of premature delivery in this group, related in turn to more frequent ascending infection and complications of twin-to-twin transfusion syndrome. The explanation for fetal death was not always complete. Developmental abnormalities were significant in embryos of less than 12 weeks gestational age and in macerated fetuses of 12 to 20 weeks' gestation. Complications of monochorionicity were important in concordant twin deaths at all stages of pregnancy. Obstetric complications were important in well-preserved twin fetuses and fresh stillbirths. Placental lesions were important in the macerated and retained late fetal death groups, but the longer the dead twin was retained, the less likely was a cause for fetal death identifiable.

TABLE 5.4. Patterns of concordant twin death.

	Stillbirth	<24 hours	1–7 days	8–28 days	>1 month
Stillbirth	43*	10	3	1	1
<24 hours	–	49	4	6	2
1–7 days	–	–	6	5	–
8–28 days	–	–	–	4	1
>1 month	–	–	–	–	5

*Number of affected twin sets in the cohort defined by the vertical and horizontal categories of age at death.

Perinatal and Postnatal Mortality

The increased mortality risk that twins face continues into the perinatal period and even later, contributing to rates of overall mortality that range from 4 to 11 times compared to singleton rates.[88,90,91,95,104,108–111] The excess mortality of twins that occurs antenatally has been described in the previous sections and the rest of this chapter discusses patterns of perinatal mortality and death of live-born twins. It is recognized, however, that patterns of perinatal mortality will include stillborn infants and that exclusive distinctions based on live birth or stillbirth are not always warranted. It is interesting to note that while the excess of twin stillbirth ranges from 3 to 13 times more frequent than singletons, depending on the study reported, neonatal death of twins is relatively uniformly reported to occur 6 to 7 times more often than of singletons,[85,90,91,112] although the exact definition of "neonatal" is rarely provided. It has been reported that 9.2% of all twins die in the neonatal period[100,101] and that neonatal deaths represent 60% to 70% of all twin deaths,[102–104] although none of these reports include consideration of the contribution of early fetal mortality to total twin deaths. Of all twin live births, 3% to 5% will die in the neonatal period,[90,91,111] the majority between 2 and 48 hours of age.[88,112]

Rates and Patterns

In many reports, the term "perinatal mortality" is used to connote a combination of stillbirth and neonatal mortality, although usually it is not defined as to gestational age or duration of survival of the fetuses/infants concerned. Reported rates of perinatal mortality of twins range from 2 to 11 times the rate for singletons, with most studies at the 4 to 5 times level.[90–92,113] As with reported neonatal death rates, reports of 14% to 17% perinatal mortality in twins overall do not appear to consider early fetal mortality.[85,100,101] Intrapartum mortality of twins, as a distinct component of perinatal mortality, has been reported as three times that of singletons.[94] Perinatal mortality of twins reportedly declined by 66% to 68% from 1956 to 1986, primarily due to an 80% reduction of preterm neonatal mortality, in parallel with improved outcomes for preterm singletons based on advances in obstetric and neonatal care.[98,114]

Reported rates of concordant twin death vary widely, 5.7% to 37%, without defining the time of death.[103,104] In one detailed analysis of the time of death, 3% of twin pairs were concordantly stillborn, both died neonatally in 4.4% of the twin pairs, 0.7% were stillbirth/neonatal death pairs, 0.1% were neonatal/postneonatal death pairs, and there were no concordant post neonatal deaths.[99]

In the Survey '91 autopsy review, concordant twin death occurred in nearly one-third, 31.3%, of the twin sets where one or both twins were autopsied (Table 5.4). Of these concordant deaths, 72.8% occurred as stillbirths or within the first 24 hours, representing over one fifth, 22.8%, of all twin sets in the autopsy series. The concordance in the stillbirth to <24 hours survival groups was associated with complications of monochorionic placentation in 40% and immaturity/prematurity in 35.3%, with intrauterine asphyxia and a variety of other conditions in the remainder. In the remaining concordant groups, the associated conditions included complications of prematurity or perinatal asphyxia and anomalies, both concordant and discordant, but all in small numbers. The concordant pairs over 1 month of age all had concordant disease, one set each of metachromatic leukodystrophy, Letterer-Siwe disease, and conjoined twins, and two sets with complications of prematurity.

TABLE 5.5. Interval of survival related to gestational age at delivery.

Gestational age at delivery (weeks)	Interval of life							N
	Stillbirth*	<1 hour	1–24 hours	1–7 days	8–28 days	1–12 months	>1 year	
20–24	41.0 / 36.6	23.0 / 50.0	30.0 / 33.7	1.7 / 2.7	2.6 / 6.4	1.7 / 8.3	– / –	117
25–28	18.4 / 19.1	7.4 / 18.5	33.8 / 44.2	23.5 / 43.8	11.8 / 34.0	4.4 / 25.0	0.7 / 7.7	137
29–32	20.3 / 11.5	6.7 / 9.3	18.9 / 13.5	24.3 / 24.7	14.9 / 23.4	12.2 / 37.5	2.7 / 15.4	74
33–36	39.1 / 19.1	9.4 / 11.1	10.9 / 6.7	21.8 / 19.2	14.1 / 19.2	4.7 / 12.5	– / –	64
37+	43.9 / 13.7	9.7 / 7.4	4.8 / 1.9	17.2 / 9.6	12.2 / 10.6	7.3 / 12.5	4.9 / 15.4	41
Unstated	– / –	14.3 / 3.7	– / –	– / –	21.4 / 6.4	7.1 / 4.2	57.2 / 61.5	14
N	133	55	105	75	47	23	9	447

Percentages above the diagonal line—read horizontally; percentages below the diagonal line—read vertically.
* Stillbirth category consists of fresh stillbirth plus fetal death of less than 1 week duration.
N, number of cases in each column.

A number of contributing factors to twin mortality have been examined including gestational age, birth weight, birth order, fetal sex, and race. There is general agreement on the importance of gestational age and birth weight, but less uniformity as to the significance of birth order or sex of the infants. It is difficult to separate the effects of low birth weight and prematurity as they so often occur together, and live-born twins are both smaller and more frequently premature than singletons.[94] In one report, up to 80% of twins born before 30 weeks of gestation and up to 93% of twins weighing less than 1,500 g at birth died in the neonatal period.[88] Even with advances in perinatal care, nearly three quarters of the mortality of live-born twins continues to be of the infant of less than 1,500 g[94,111] and the optimal birth weight category for twin survival appears to be 2,750 to 3,000 g, 700 g less than the range for singletons.[94] Twin sets with intrapair weight discordance of greater than 25% have been reported to be at 40% to 80% greater risk of concordant death than twin pairs with 10% or less weight discordance.[111] The reported low rate of twin survival after live birth at 26 weeks' gestation or less—no survivors at 25 weeks and only 12.5% at

25 to 26 weeks—has suggested to some that aggressive delivery at these gestational ages is not warranted.[7] In Table 5.5, the relationship of gestational age and duration of survival is presented for 447 twins from the Survey '91 autopsy review. As would be expected, the interval of survival of live-born twins varies with the gestational age at delivery. This table also indicates the load that premature twins represent for special care nursery facilities—57% of the twins that required intensive care for 8 to 28 days and 62% of the twins that needed intensive care for up to a year before death were born between 25 and 32 weeks' gestation. Premature delivery of twins is discussed in detail in Chapter 4, and growth of twins and problems of low birth weight are presented in Chapter 6.

The relationship of birth order, fetal sex, and race to twin mortality has been reported, but with inconsistent findings, so the significance of these relationships remains to be clarified. Perinatal mortality rates have been reported to be greater for twin B by one-third,[93] or no different for A and B.[92] In the Survey '91 autopsy series, one-third of the twin sets where only one twin died were represented by twin A and two thirds by twin B. The mortality risk for

TABLE 5.6. Causes of perinatal death of twins.

Cause	Year (source)								
	1964[+] (66)	1970 (100)	1975[+] (116)	1978 (88)	1978 (106)	1983 (117)	1987 (90)	1991 (111)	1991 (118)
Hypoxia/asphyxia	30.0†	8.0	13.0	17.0	19.7	21.9	6.5	2.3	2.9*/2.8**
HMD	8.0	37.0	47.8	52.0	N/S	29.3	19.7	21.0	19.9/14.2
Malformations	7.4	10.0	4.4	N/S	9.7	7.3	13.6	9.6	9.3/4.2
Infections	2.0	N/S	4.4	7.0	27.2	12.4	N/S	N/S	2.5/3.2
Prematurity/low birth weight	N/S	N/S	17.4	7.0	16.3	24.5	4.5	18.4	20.0/25.2
Birth trauma/injuries	3.6	N/S	N/S	N/S	1.8	N/S	N/S	N/S	2.8/1.9
Placenta/cord complications	N/S	N/S	N/S	3.0	N/S	N/S	10.4	1.7	2.4/1.7
Maternal complications	N/S	N/S	N/S	N/S	0.9	N/S	27.2	3.2	3.8/1.9
Other respiratory	N/S	N/S	N/S	N/S	N/S	2.4	7.8	13.5	12.6/14.1
Unknown	46.0	5.0	N/S	10.0	1.8	N/S	N/S	21.0	15.1/20.3
Other	3.0	40.0	13.0	4.0	22.6	2.2	10.3	9.3	8.7/10.5

"Other" includes erythroblastosis fetalis, necrotizing enterocolitis, twin transfusion, hydramnios, unspecified hemorrhage or circulatory disorders, sudden infant death syndrome, "multiple pregnancy," and unspecified causes.
[+] Stillbirth and live-birth data combined; the rest of the columns are all live birth only.
†Numbers are percentage of twin perinatal deaths due to each category of cause in each reported series.
*Whites.
**Blacks.
HMD, Hyaline membrane disease; N/S, not specified.

like-sex pairs is reported to be greater than unlike sex pairs with an excess of male pairs in some reports but not in others.[90,92,111,115] In the Survey '91 autopsy series, the proportions of male/female to female/female to male/male sets where both twins died was 1 : 2.8 : 3.7, supporting an excess risk of like-sex pairs, male pairs particularly. When only one twin came to autopsy, the ratio of males to females was 1.2:1, an equivalent excess risk for males. Reported differences in mortality of white and black twins appear to be related to lower birth weights of black twins.[111]

Causes of Death

Reports of causes of death of twins are sometimes difficult to compare because of differences in definitions of causes and groupings used. The choices of categories used are almost always a mixture of primary causes as well as mechanisms of death, and it is often difficult to decide how to classify a death. Should the death of a breech-presenting second twin with cord prolapse and signs of asphyxia be classed as a complication of being a breech presentation, or the second twin, due to a cord accident, or due to asphyxia? There is no easy answer. One way might be to classify the causes based on the point in the sequence at which diagnosis of the situation could lead to effective intervention and potential preven-

tion of the death. If diagnosis for intervention is not possible, then classification based on the underlying pathophysiology might be appropriate. Reported series tend to reflect the diagnostic/mechanistic biases of the authors, and even promulgated systems of classification of causes of death represent mixtures of causes and consequences. A selection of reported causes of death of twins is presented in Table 5.6. It is difficult to know if the variations reported are due to differences in definitions or to changes in the relative importance of the different causes over time.

In spite of these difficulties with classification of cause of death, all the studies emphasize the importance of prematurity and its complications as a major cause of perinatal and neonatal mortality, in contrast to anoxia or cause unknown in cases of stillbirth.[17,90,100–103,106,111,116–118] It has been suggested that the major obstetric factors related to perinatal loss of twins are the same as for singletons, but that they occur earlier in twin pregnancy.[119] The implication was that attention should be directed to preventing these obstetric complications that affect all pregnancies, rather than considering the causes of loss in twin pregnancies as a separate problem.

The suggestion that we should be looking at basic causes of perinatal mortality is helpful because it reminds us to look at why we classify causes of death. The value of classifying deaths is twofold—scientific and therapeutic—and the usefulness of any classification is dependent on the understanding of the pathophysiology of the events that led to the death, from the initial event in the sequence onward. The more detailed and accurate the knowledge of the sequence, the more appropriate the scientific analysis of potential contributing factors, such as genetic or environmental influences, and the more effective the therapeutic maneuvers, if any are possible. In a study by Keith et al.,[109] 26.6% of twin deaths were described as unavoidable and 59.4% as probably unavoidable, but the causes of death in these cases were not specified. Causes of death in the 13.9% of deaths considered avoidable were largely obstetric complications, such as prolapsed cord or vessels, interlocking of twins, and abruptio placenta, but also included the idiopathic respiratory distress syndrome. The problem of late diagnosis of twin gestations was discussed as more than one-third of the pregnancies in their series were not diagnosed as twins until the onset of labor. They also noted a bimodal risk for fetal loss related to maternal age and parity, with the lowest risk with maternal age in the 30s and in the third and fourth pregnancy, respectively.

Even considering the above suggestions as a basis for classifying causes of twin death, it was difficult to assign cases from the Survey '91 autopsy review to simple consistent categories. As a result, the eight groups chosen reflect a mixture of underlying causes and mechanisms based on the pathology reported in 422 autopsies (Table 5.7). A brief description of each group is presented first and then specific associations with mortality or patterns of mortality are examined in greater detail.

"Prematurity" category cause of death includes all infants with autopsy diagnoses of hyaline membrane disease, pulmonary interstitial emphysema, bronchopulmonary dysplasia, necrotizing enteropathy, and/or germinal matrix hemorrhages. Included are intrapartum and perinatal deaths with autopsy diagnoses of ascending infection. No attempt is made to subclassify these cases by cause of preterm delivery as causes of preterm labor and delivery are discussed in Chapter 4. The majority (77%) of these twins were delivered before 32 weeks' gestation, and 68.5% had died within the first week. However, complications of prematurity continued to contribute to twin mortality up to a year after birth. There was an excess of male and second born twins, and dichorionic twins occurred twice as often as monochorionic sets. One-third of the concordant twin deaths occurred in this group, with male sets seen three times as frequently as female sets or mixed sex sets.

The "asphyxia" category includes all perinatal and later deaths with autopsy diagnoses of aspiration of amniotic debris with or without meconium and hypoxic/ischemic visceral and neural pathology, whether or not the cause of the asphyxial insult was known. Causes of perinatal asphyxia are reviewed in Chapter 4. In this asphyxia group, there was an excess of male and second-born twins, and monochorionic placentations were more common than dichorionic. While all gestational ages were represented, 62.8% were stillborn and a further 20% died within the first 24 hours. All infants dying with lesions of asphyxia only had died by the end of the first month. The autopsy services that provided these cases have seen an occasional autopsy on an older child with evidence of birth- or gestation-associated brain damage, but in none of these cases were they identified as a twin. (It may be unnecessary to note that these data on asphyxial lesions in twins represent mortality cases only, with no esti-

TABLE 5.7. Causes of perinatal and later mortality of twins—Survey '91 autopsy series.

Category	Percentage of total mortality	Ratio of males to females	Ratio of first to second born	Monochorionic: dichorionic: unstated
Prematurity sequelae	30.4	1.5:1	1:1.3	1.3:3:1
Asphyxia	8.5	1.4:1	1:1.4	2.2:1.4:1
Prematurity/asphyxia	4.5	1:1.7	1:1.5	1:4:3.5
Immaturity	7.8	1.2:1	1:1	2:8.7:1
Anomalies	11.1	1.3:1	1:1.9	1:1:1
Monochorionic monozygosity	22.3	1:1	1:1.1	15.2:0:1
Other	5.0	1:2	1:1.6	1:1.2:1.6
Unknown	10.4	1.2:1	1:1	2:2:1

mate or assessment of the survivors of asphyxial insults who have continued morbidity.)

There was a smaller but distinct group of infants who had lesions of both "asphyxia" and "prematurity," and it was not possible to decide which was more important as a cause of death, although they could be classed with either. It was interesting that there were more females in this group than in the preceding two groups, although twin B was still more commonly affected. Dichorionic placentas outnumbered monochorionic, but there were a number of cases for which information on placentation was not available. The majority of these infants, 88.8%, were delivered between 25 and 32 weeks, a third died within 24 hours, and 77.8% had died by the end of the first week.

There was another small but distinct group of infants who died during or soon after birth, usually within 1 to 2 hours, who had no reported pathologic findings or minimal evidence of early bronchiolar epithelial necrosis or mild signs of ascending infection. It could be argued that these cases should be classified with the prematurity group, but they have been recorded separately as "immaturity," because they represent a group that is not a load on special care nursery facilities. In many of these cases a clinical decision had been made not to resuscitate, and the perinatal death occurred in the delivery room. There was a slight excess of males in this group, but A and B twins were equally represented. The majority of these twins were from dichorionic sacs and 10% of the concordant twin deaths were in this group. Nearly 80% were born between 20 and 24 weeks gestational age, 11.8% were intrapartum deaths, and all the remainder died within the first 24 hours after birth.

"Anomalies" accepted as a cause of death consisted of only those malformations that were lethal in the newborn period, and occasional rare anomalies that could explain fetal death. Anomalies are discussed further in Chapter 7, but this category included lethal neural tube defects, massive body wall defects, renal agenesis, and diaphragmatic hernias. In some of these cases, the defects were discordant, delivery occurred prematurely, and the normally developed co-twin died from complications of prematurity. The general excess of male and second born twins was seen in this group as well, with no excess of a particular placentation pattern. These tended to be more mature infants,

63% were born after 33 weeks' gestation, and while a third died within the first 24 hours, they represented a source of twin mortality up to a year and beyond. Interestingly, only 3.9% of the concordant twin deaths were in this group.

"Monochorionic monozygosity" represents a major category of problems of twinning leading to twin mortality and includes a number of conditions that are discussed in detail in Chapters 8, 9, and 10. The majority of the cases consists of problems of intertwin transfusion syndromes and anomalies of twinning. While it is true that the final mechanism of death in this group may vary, including asphyxial damage, hypovolemic shock, or lethal anomaly, the initial problem is the monochorionic placentation. The sexes were equally represented and A and B twins equally affected. The reported placentation was not 100% monochorionic because of lack of data or an inability to confirm the membranes because of fragmentation in a few cases. The majority, 62.9%, were delivered before 28 weeks' gestation, but they spanned the weeks until term. Half of these twins were fresh stillbirths or had died in utero less than a week before delivery, and another third died within the first 24 hours after birth, but deaths attributable to complications of monochorionic monozygosity were reported up to a year and beyond. One third of the concordant twin deaths occurred in this group, and male and female pairs were equally represented.

In the category of "other" diseases and disorders are those conditions not included in the six preceding categories. These include perinatal/neonatal disorders not related to prematurity or asphyxia or monochorionicity, such as nosocomial infections, hydrops fetalis of unknown cause, and metabolic disorders, as well as childhood illnesses and sudden infant death syndrome. These and other causes of morbidity in twins are discussed further in Chapter 6. These twins were delivered at 20 to 24 weeks (28.6%) and 33 to 36 weeks (50%), and they represented the majority of twin deaths beyond 1 month of age after infants with complications of prematurity. There was an excess of female twins in this group, and an excess of second-born twins. The patterns of placentation were not helpful as this was the group with the largest unstated category.

Finally, as always, there was an "unknown" group for which no adequate cause for perinatal, neonatal, or later mortality was determined. Con-

TABLE 5.8. Causes of death related to gestational age at delivery.

	20–24 weeks	25–28 weeks	29–32 weeks	33–36 weeks	37+ weeks	20–24 weeks	25–28 weeks	29–32 weeks	33–36 weeks	37+ weeks
Prematurity	20.4	56	39.4	5	–	17.5	59.5	20.6	2.4	–
Asphyxia	1.9	8.2	10.6	11.7	21.6	5.7	31.4	20	20	22.9
Prematurity + asphyxia	–	6	12.1	3.3	–	–	44.4	44.4	11.2	–
Immaturity	25	5.2	–	–	–	79.4	20.6	–	–	–
Anomalies	0.9	5.2	13.6	28.3	32.4	2.2	15.2	19.6	37	26
Monochorionic monozygosity	35.2	13.4	10.6	30	21.6	42.7	20.2	7.8	20.2	9.1
Other	3.6	–	3.1	11.7	2.8	28.6	–	14.3	50	7.1
Unknown	13	6	10.6	10	21.6	32.5	18.6	16.3	14	18.6
	(Numbers are percentage of each category of cause of death in the gestational age group column)					(Numbers are percentage of each age group within the diagnostic category)				
Percentage of total autopsied twins	26.7	33.1	16.3	14.8	9.1					

sidering that this autopsy review series includes cases from the late 1950s onward, the overall rate of 10.4% due to unknown cause is reasonable. The majority of these twins were stillborn (91%), but delivered all across the gestational time period from 20 weeks to term. There was a slight excess of males, but birth order was not important and no particular pattern of placentations was noted.

Causes of Death Related to Gestational Age and Duration of Survival

It has been noted at a number of points in this discussion of twin mortality, that *gestational age* is a critical consideration. An overall study of twins reported 80% mortality if delivered at less than 31 weeks gestational age, 20% between 31 and 33 weeks, and 6.7% mortality at 34 to 36 weeks.[116] Some years later, in a study trying to assess the value of maternal bed rest after 30 weeks of gestation with twin pregnancies, more than 70% of perinatal mortality of twins still occurred at less than 30 weeks' gestation, and was attributed almost entirely to complications of prematurity.[120] Perinatal mortality after 34 weeks of gestation was associated with intrauterine growth retardation, the twin-to-twin transfusion syndrome, fetal anomalies, or unknown causes. Puissant and Leroy[121] also note that twins die of different causes at different gestational ages. Of their cases of deaths of twins of 29 to 38 weeks of gestation, 17% died antepartum of unstated causes, 15% died intrapartum with low

birth weight and/or malformations, and 68% died as neonates from complications of prematurity. Those twins delivered after 38 weeks were stillborn for unstated reasons in 58%, succumbed to intrapartum obstetric complications in 19%, and died neonatally of a mixture of causes unrelated to prematurity in 23%.

In Table 5.8, the Survey '91 autopsy cases categories are compared to the gestational age at delivery. Nearly 60% of the deliveries were before 29 weeks' gestation and over 90% were delivered by 37 weeks. At 20 to 24 weeks, complications of monochorionic monozygosity were responsible for over one-third of the deaths, and immaturity/prematurity accounted for over 45%. Sequelae of preterm delivery were the main cause of death for twins who were born at 25 to 32 weeks of gestation. Complications of monochorionic monozygosity were important again at 33 to 36 weeks, as were lethal anomalies. Twins born after 37 weeks who died did so as a result of anomalies, complications of monochorionic monozygosity, or with asphyxial lesions. These data emphasize the importance of efforts to prevent premature delivery of twins and the contribution of perinatal asphyxia in the more mature twin. These are problems that are important with singletons as well, and progress with prevention of preterm labor and detection of causes of asphyxia can be applied to both single and twin gestations.[119] The other important point in this comparison is the prominence of complications of monochorionic monozygosity in early and late gestation, and lethal anomalies in the more mature twin, because the vast majority of these are not remediable, although attempts to intervene in twin transfusion syndrome are being made and are discussed in Chapter 9.

It is worthwhile to look at the *duration of survival* by diagnostic category to get an idea of the potential load of intensive care that twins represent before their death. In Table 5.9, the cause of death is related to the duration of survival. One-quarter of live-born twins who ultimately came to autopsy survived more than a week after delivery. As might be expected, complications of prematurity represented a major continuing need for care as they represented over half the infants who survived for 1 to 12 months before death. The anomalies group also consisted of conditions requiring ongoing care, but the cases in the "other" category were a mixture of ongoing problems, such as metabolic disorders, and acute events in otherwise well twins, such as myocarditis.

Causes of Death Related to Placentation and Zygosity

It was mentioned in Chapter 3 and illustrated in Fig. 3.20, that there was an excess of monochorionic placentations in the Survey '91 autopsy group compared with the surviving twin pairs, 51% compared with 32%. This has been noted before by a number of reviewers of twin death rates and *placental membrane patterns*.[17,85,100,101,103,122] Concordant twin death has been reported to be more frequent with monochorionic placentation, with death of

both twins in 13.6% of those with monochorionic placentas in contrast to no concordant deaths of twins with dichorionic placentas.[122] In the Survey '91 autopsy group, monochorionic placentas were seen in 50% of concordant death sets, 34% had dichorionic placentas, and the placentation in the remaining concordant death sets was not reported, although all the twin pairs in this unknown group were like-sex sets. Of the dichorionic concordant deaths, 42% were unlike-sex twins, but the zygosity of the 58% like-sex dichorionic sets was not known.

These data also raise the question of *zygosity* and twin mortality. Up to 25.3% of perinatal twin deaths have been attributed to problems associated with monozygosity,[63] and mortality rates of monozygotic twins have been reported as 2 to 3 times the rates of dizygotic twins.[100,101,103] It would appear that it is the monochorionic monozygotic twins that are at greatest risk, with reported death rates of 7.1% for monochorionic twins, 4.6% of dichorionic twins of like-sex, and 3.6% of dichorionic twins of unlike-sex.[123] The potential lethal complications of monochorionic monozygosity include cord entanglements with monoamniotic twins, and disturbed twinning or intertwin vascular connections with diamniotic twins.[124] There were few common causes in the perinatal deaths of dichorionic twins,[124] although it has been reported that concordant twin death is more frequent with separate than fused dichorionic placentas.[125] In the Survey '91 autopsy series, concordant twin deaths with dichorionic placentas had separate placentas

TABLE 5.9. Causes of death related to duration of survival.

	Still-birth*	<24 hours	1–7 days	8–28 days	1–12 months	>1 year	Still-birth*	<24 hours	1–7 days	8–28 days	1–12 months	>1 year
Prematurity	3.2	35.9	48.4	51.2	54.2	11.1	3.1	44.1	24.4	17.3	10.2	0.9
Asphyxia	17.5	4.5	4.7	7.1	–	–	62.8	20	8.6	8.6	–	–
Prematurity + asphyxia	–	3.8	12.5	4.6	8.3	–	–	33.3	44.5	11.1	11.1	–
Immaturity	3.2	19.2	–	–	–	–	11.8	88.2	–	–	–	–
Anomalies	4.8	10.9	15.6	20.9	12.5	22.2	12.8	36.2	21.3	19.1	6.4	4.2
Monochorionic monozygosity	38.9	21.8	9.5	11.6	12.5	11.1	50	34.7	6.1	5.1	3.1	1
Other	0.8	2.6	6.2	4.6	12.5	55.6	5.4	21	21	10.5	15.8	26.3
Unknown	31.6	1.3	3.1	–	–	–	91	4.5	4.5	–	–	–
	(Numbers represent percentage of deaths from each cause for the duration of survival shown)						(Numbers are percentage of each duration of the survival within the diagnostic category)					
% of total autopsied twins	29.9	37	15.2	10.2	5.7	2						

*Stillbirth includes intrapartum deaths and fetal death of less than 1 week duration.

TABLE 5.10. Causes of death related to placental membrane patterns and zygosity.

Category	Monochorionic (monozygotic)	Dichorionic Total	Dichorionic Separate	Dichorionic Fused	Unlike sex (dizygotic)	Chorionicity not stated
Prematurity sequelae	17.2	46.1	40.8	52.8	40.4	30.8
Asphyxia	8.3	6.5	8.4	3.8	–	9.0
Prematurity/asphyxia	1.1	5.2	5.6	1.9	9.6	9.0
Immaturity	3.3	17.0	16.9	20.7	7.7	3.8
Anomalies	7.8	10.4	12.7	3.8	17.3	19.2
Monochorionic monozygosity	50.6	–	–		–	7.7
Other	2.8	3.8	2.9	7.6	3.8	10.3
Unknown	8.9	11.0	12.7	9.4	21.2	10.2

Numbers are percentage of deaths from each cause for the pattern of placentation/zygosity noted.

1.7 times more often than fused placentas, but in 18% of the dichorionic placentas there was no comment whether they were fused or separate. The significance of this association is not clear as it did not seem to relate to zygosity, unlike-sex pairs had both fused and separate placentas. Also, there did not seem to be a particular relationship to cause of death. The separate dichorionic placentas were seen more commonly in all groups of causes of death, with a slightly greater excess in the anomalies group.

The relationship between placental membrane patterns and causes of death is represented in Table 5.7 by the ratio of monochorionic to dichorionic to unstated patterns and in Table 5.10 by the percentages of each cause of death in categories of membrane patterns and zygosity. The prominence of complications of monochorionic monozygosity with monochorionic placentations is obvious, while sequelae of prematurity are important in all other membrane patterns. The differential between separate and fused dichorionic placentation is seen in the asphyxia, prematurity/asphyxia, anomalies, and cause unknown groups, and anomalies and cause unknown are important with known dizygotic twins.

Causes of Death Related to Fetal Sex and Birth Order

While a *sex differential* is reported in perinatal deaths, the direction of the differential varies. The death rate has been reported to be greater for female twins[109] and yet another report recorded the male mortality rate at twice the female rate.[113] There seems to be greater agreement on an excess of male twins, with mortality rates of 11.7% for males and 9.4% for females,[17] representative of the overall observations. Also, like-sex twin pairs are more

susceptible than unlike-sex pairs, 12.2% and 7.3%, respectively,[17] with like-sex male pairs at greatest risk.[85,125] The increased risk for like-sex pairs is in the fetal and early neonatal period, and often both twins die.[108] After the neonatal period, equal rates are observed for like-sex and unlike-sex pairs.[108] These observations likely reflect the excess of monochorionic monozygosity complications as a cause of death in the stillborn/perinatal death groups.

In the Survey '91 autopsy group, male twins represented 54.7% of all twin autopsies, and as can be seen from the ratios in Table 5.7, there was an excess of male twins in five of the categories, male twins equaled female twins in complications of monochorionic monozygosity, while female twins were in excess in the prematurity/asphyxia and "other" groups. In the twin sets with concordant death, just over half (50.4%) were male sets, 38.5% were female sets, and the remainder were male/female pairs. This excess of male sets was almost entirely in the prematurity group. An interesting but unexplained observation is a change in the proportion of male and female twins in the complications of the monochorionic monozygosity group. At the time of the initial review of the twin autopsy data, there were 25% more female than male twins in this category, but additional cases in the following 5 years reduced the female predominance to the 1 : 1 ratio noted in Table 5.7. It will be interesting to see if there are further changes in this trend.

The concept of a differential mortality risk related to *birth order* has been discussed in Chapter 4, and it was pointed out that there are conflicting reports. Several authors have reported no difference in perinatal mortality for the second twin compared to the first,[86,104,113,126] others state that the death rates are greater for twin B, although stillbirth rates are equivalent,[102,127] and still others record greater mortality rates for twin B antenatally, but equal rates after birth.[100,101] When birth order differentials were correlated with birth weights and gestational age, the perinatal mortality rate of twin A of 9% and twin B of 11.4% was due to a greater differential in the 1,000- to 2,499-g weight group and 32 to 36 weeks gestation period.[17,112] Another report suggested that the greatest risk for twin B was in the 500- to 749-g range, and that mortality rates for twin A declined dramatically at 1,000-g birth weight, but that the same decline for twin B did not occur until 1,250-g. There are additional reports that suggest that the second twin is definitely at greater risk, although the consequences may not be fatal—using Apgar scores, umbilical venous pH, PCO_2 and PO_2 and umbilical artery PO_2.[128,129] A somewhat different measure of the greater risk for twin B was that A twins survived an average of 62.8 hours, while B twins survived an average of 34.2 hours.[125]

In the Survey '91 autopsy group, 55.6% of the twin autopsies of fresh stillbirths, perinatal deaths, and beyond were second-born twins. In sets where only one twin died, A and B twins were in equal numbers in the stillborn, 8 to 28 days, and over 1 year groups, but there were twice as many B as A twins in the <24 hours and 1 to 12 month groups, and nearly three times as many B as A twins in the 1 to 7 day survival group. Of the sets where both twins died, they died at or close to the same time in 84.2% of the pairs, 37.5% of these being stillborn sets, and in 47.9% both died within 24 hours of birth. In 15.8% of concordant twin deaths, there was a difference of time of death, ranging from stillbirth/perinatal death pairs to different durations of survival, such as 1 hour/24 days, or 3 months/4 months. Twin A survived longer than twin B in half the cases and the ranges of survival intervals were equal whether A or B survived longer. When this group was examined as to the reasons for the interval, no particular pattern emerged as the cases included discordant anomalies, twin transfusion sets, prematurity/asphyxia combinations, and a variety of other conditions.

The greater mortality risks for B twins are seen in most of the categories of causes of death (Table 5.7), with equivalent risks for A and B twins in the immaturity and "unknown" groups. Part of the excess of B twins is in the anomalies group particularly, and one wonders if there is a similar related but noncausal mechanism for this pattern as noted in fetal death. As noted in the previous discussion of fetal mortality, B twins were markedly overrepresented in the prolonged retention group and it was suggested that this observation might simply reflect physical alterations of the positions of the twins following fetal death, rather than any extra risk for twin B. Another review of relative risks of A and B twins based on diagnosis category also noted an increased relative risk for B twins for congenital anomalies (B/A = 1.24) and perinatal asphyxia (B/A = 1.27).[111]

Perinatal and Postnatal Mortality—Summary

It is difficult to be dogmatic about patterns of perinatal and postnatal twin mortality because of different approaches to the problems of definition and classification in the reported series. There is a consensus that twins are at greater risk than singletons with two categories of problems predominating—sequelae of prematurity and complications of monochorionic monozygosity. The considerations for prevention in the prematurity group are analogous to the problems with singleton gestations, but they occur earlier in pregnancy. While the majority of these twins die within the first week after birth, they continue to contribute to twin mortality up to a year after birth. These twins tend to be dichorionic male second born twins. Complications of monochorionic monozygosity are unique to the twinning situation and are largely unpreventable, although some remediation attempts are being made. These twins also die early, the majority before 1 day of age, but the rest contribute to twin mortality up to a year and beyond. The majority of concordant twin deaths occur in this group.

The other categories of twin mortality are less clear cut in their general characteristics, although a few patterns are noted. Twins with only asphyxial lesions at autopsy tend to be second-born monochorionic male twins delivered throughout gestation with a concentration after 37 weeks; the majority are stillborn or die in the first 24 hours, and all are dead by 1 month. Those twins with equally evident lesions of prematurity and asphyxia are more often females, although the reason for this reversal of the usual trend is not known. Lethal anomalies are more common among twins after 33 weeks and contribute to twin mortality up to a year and beyond.

Reported relationships of twin mortality to placental membrane pattern, fetal sex, and birth order are suggestive, but not conclusive, except for the consensus of the enhanced risk for the category of complications of monochorionic monozygosity. The degree of increased risk for male B twins varies considerably in different series, and probably also varies with different categories of cause of death, although the pathophysiologic explanation for the trend is not always evident.

Obstetric care of mothers with multiple pregnancies and perinatal care of the infants is becoming quite technically sophisticated, and it is possible that the patterns of mortality will change over the next decade. However, it is the pathologist who will continue to provide key information for the clinicopathological correlation that is essential for monitoring the new technology in order to select those procedures that truly enhance perinatal outcomes of twin pregnancies.

References

1. Guttmacher AF, Kohl SG. The fetus of multiple gestations. *Obstet Gynecol.* 1958;12:528–41.
2. Farr V. Prognosis for the babies, early and late. In: MacGillivray I, Nylander PPS, Corney G, eds. *Human Multiple Reproduction.* Philadelphia: WB Saunders; 1975:188–211.
3. Boklage CE. Survival probability of human conceptions from fertilization to term. *Int J Fertil.* 1990;35:75–94.
4. Bryan EM. The intrauterine hazards of twins. *Arch Dis Child.* 1986;61:1044–1045.
5. Millar C. *Second Self: Consequences of the Intrauterine Death of One of Twins.* Creswick, Australia: Holistikon Publishing; 1981.
6. Lewis E, Bryan EM. Management of perinatal loss of a twin. *Br Med J.* 1988;297:1321–1323.
7. Cetrulo CL. The controversy of mode of delivery in twins: the intrapartum management of twin gestation (Part I). *Semin Perinatol.* 1986;10:39–43.
8. Papiernik E, Keith LG. The cost effectiveness of preventing preterm delivery in twin pregnancies. *Acta Genet Med Gemellol.* 1990;39:361–369.
9. Livingston JE, Poland BJ. A study of spontaneously aborted twins. *Teratology.* 1980;21:139–148.
10. Galton F. The history of twins as a criterion of the relative powers of nature and nurture. *J Anthropol Inst. G Br Irel* 1876;5:391–406.
11. Benirschke K. The placenta in the litigation process. *Am J Obstet Gynecol.* 1990;162:1445–1450.
12. Schindler NR. Importance of the placenta and cord in the defense of neurologically impaired infant claims. *Arch Pathol Lab Med.* 1991;115:685–687.
13. Kalousek DK, Fitch N, Paradice BA. *Pathology of the Human Embryo and Previable Fetus. An Atlas.* New York: Springer-Verlag; 1990:37–60.
14. Kalousek DK, Baldwin VJ, Dimmick JE, Cimolai N, Andrews A, Paradice B. Embryofetal-perinatal autopsy and placental examination. In: Dimmick JE, Kalousek DK, eds. *Developmental Pathology of the Embryo and Fetus.* Philadelphia: JB Lippincott; 1992:799–824.
15. Baldwin VJ, Kalousek DK, Dimmick JE, Applegarth DA, Hardwick DF. Diagnostic pathologic investigation of the malformed conceptus. *Perspect Pediatr Pathol.* 1982;7:65–109.
16. Keeling JW. The perinatal necropsy. In: Keeling JW, ed. *Fetal and Neonatal Pathology.* Berlin: Springer-Verlag; 1989:1–43.
17. Potter EL, Craig JM. *Pathology of the Fetus and Infant.* 3rd ed. Chicago: Yearbook Medical Publishers; 1975:83–92.
18. Wigglesworth JS. Performance of the perinatal autopsy. In: Bennington JL, ed. *Perinatal Pathology. Major Problems in Pathology.* Philadelphia: WB Saunders; 1984;15(3):27–47.
19. MacPherson TA, Valdes-Dapena M. The perinatal autopsy. In: Wigglesworth JS, Singer DB, eds. *Textbook of Fetal and Perinatal Pathology.* Oxford: Blackwell Scientific; 1991:93–123.
20. Hellman LM, Kobayashi M, Cromb E. Ultrasonic diagnosis of embryonic malformations. *Am J Obstet Gynecol.* 1973;115:615–623.
21. Farquharson DF, Wittmann BK, Hansmann M, Ho Yuen B, Baldwin VJ, Lindahl S. Management of quintuplet pregnancy by selective embryocide. *Am J Obstet Gynecol.* 1988;158:413–416.
22. Golbus MS, Cunningham N, Goldberg JD, Anderson R, Filly R, Callen P. Selective termination of multiple gestations. *Am J Med Genet.* 1988; 31:339–348.
23. Levi S. Ultrasonic assessment of the high rate of human multiple pregnancy in the first trimester. *J Clin Ultrasound.* 1976;4:3–5.
24. Robinson HP, Caines JS. Sonar evidence of early pregnancy failure in patients with twin conceptions. *Br J Obstet Gynecol.* 1977;84:22–25.
25. Schneider L, Bessis R, Simonnet T. The frequency of ovular resorption during the first trimester of

twin pregnancy. *Acta Genet Med Gemellol*. 1979; 28:271–272.

26. Kurjak A, Latin V. Ultrasound diagnosis of fetal abnormalities in multiple pregnancy. *Acta Obstet Gynecol Scand*. 1979;58:153–161.

27. Varma TR. Ultrasound evidence of early pregnancy failure in patients with multiple conceptions. *Br J Obstet Gynecol*. 1979;86:290–292.

28. Brown BStJ. Disappearances of one gestational sac in the first trimester of multiple pregnancies—ultrasonographic findings. *J Can Assoc Radiol*. 1982;33:273–275.

29. Landy HJ, Keith L, Keith D. The vanishing twin. *Acta Genet Med Gemellol*. 1982;31:179–194.

30. Landy HJ, Weiner S, Corson SL, Batzer FR, Bolognese RJ. The "vanishing twin"; ultrasonographic assessment of fetal disappearance in the first trimester. *Am J Obstet Gynecol*. 1986;155:14–19.

31. Saidi MH. First trimester bleeding and the vanishing twin. *J Repro Med*. 1988;33:831–834.

32. Nakamura I, Uno M, Io Y, Ikeshita I, Nonaka K, Miura T. Seasonality in early loss of one fetus among twin pregnancies. *Acta Genet Med Gemellol*. 1990;39:339–344.

33. Abrams RH. Double pregnancy: report of a case with 35 days between deliveries. *Obstet Gynecol*. 1957;9:435–438.

34. Uchida IA, Freeman VCP, Gedeon M, Goldmaker J. Twinning rate in spontaneous abortions. *J Hum Genet*. 1983;35:987–993.

35. Evans MI, Fletcher JC, Zador IE, Newton BW, Quigg MH, Struyk CD. Selective first-trimester termination in octuplet and quadruplet pregnancies: clinical and ethical issues. *Obstet Gynecol*. 1988; 71:289–296.

36. Holder AR, Henifin MS. Selective termination of pregnancy. *Hastings Cent Rep*. 1988;February/March:21–22.

37. Howie PW. Selective reduction in multiple pregnancy. Legal confusion and ethical dilemmas. *Br Med J*. 1988;297:433–434.

38. Hobbins JC. Selective reduction—a perinatal necessity? *N Engl J Med*. 1988;318:1062–1063.

39. Editorial. Selective fetal reduction. *Lancet*. 1988;2:773–775.

40. Berkowitz RL, Lynch L, Chitkara U, Wilkins IA, Mehalek KE, Alvarez E. Selective reduction of multifetal pregnancies in the first trimester. *N Engl J Med*. 1988;318:1043–1047.

41. Evans MI, May M, Drugan A, Fletcher JC, Johnson MP, Sokol RJ. Selective termination: clinical experience and residual risks. *Am J Obstet Gynecol*. 1990;162:1568–1575.

42. Wapner RJ, Davis GH, Johnson A, Weinblatt VJ,

Fischer RL, Jackson LG, Chervenak FA, McCullough LB. Selective reduction of multifetal pregnancies. *Lancet*. 1990;1:90–93.

43. Gonen Y, Blankier J, Casper RF. Transvaginal ultrasound in selective embryo reduction for multiple pregnancy. *Obstet Gynecol*. 1990;75:720–722.

44. Lynch L, Berkowitz RL, Chitkara U, Alvarez M. First trimester transabdominal multifetal pregnancy reduction: a report of 85 cases. *Obstet Gynecol*. 1990;75:735–738.

45. Tabsh KMA. Transabdominal multifetal pregnancy reduction: report of 40 cases. *Obstet Gynecol*. 1990;75:739–741.

46. Porreco RP, Burke MS, Hendrix ML. Multifetal reduction of triplets and pregnancy outcome. *Obstet Gynecol*. 1991;78:335–339.

47. Melgar CA, Rosenfeld DL, Rawlinson K, Greenberg M. Perinatal outcome after multifetal reduction to twins compared with non-reduced multiple gestations. *Obstet Gynecol*. 1991;78:763–767.

48. Itskovitz J, Boldes R, Thaler I, Bronstein M, Erlik Y, Brandes JM. Transvaginal ultrasonography-guided aspiration of gestational sacs for selective abortion in multiple pregnancy. *Am J Obstet Gynecol*. 1989;160:215–217.

49. Birnholz JC, Dmowski WP, Binor Z, Radwanska E. Selective continuation in gonadotropin-induced multiple pregnancy. *Fertil Steril*. 1987;48:873–876.

50. Sulak LE, Dodson MG. The vanishing twin: pathologic confirmation of an ultrasound phenomenon. *Obstet Gynecol*. 1986;68:811–815.

51. Jauniaux E, Elkazen N, Leroy F, Wilkin P, Rodesch F, Hustin J. Clinical and morphological aspects of the vanishing twin phenomenon. *Obstet Gynecol*. 1988;72:577–581.

52. Yoshida K, Soma H. Outcome of the surviving co-twin of a fetus papyraceous or of a dead fetus. *Acta Genet Med Gemellol*. 1986;35:91–98.

53. Toor AH, Kidron D, Dische MR. Placental pathology in selectively reduced multiple pregnancies. (Abstract) *Pediatr Pathol*. 1989;9:800.

54. Chitayat D, Kalousek DK, McGillivray BC, Applegarth DA. A co-twin fetus papyraceous as a cause of elevated AFP and acetylcholinesterase in the amniotic fluid of the normal co-twin. *Pediatr Pathol*. 1991;11:487–491.

55. Stiller RJ, Lockwood CJ, Belanger K, Baumgarten A, Hobbins JC, Mahoney MJ. Amniotic fluid α-fetoprotein concentrations in twin gestations: dependence on placenta membrane anatomy. *Obstet Gynecol*. 1988;158:1088–1092.

56. Ottolenghi-Preti GF. Sopra un rarissimo caso di gravidanza gemellare con un feto papiraceo e con

inserzione velamentosa del funiculo del feto vivo. *Ann Ostet Ginecol Med Perinat*. 1972;93:173–199.

57. O'Regan JA, Craig RL. Fetus papyraceous—triplet pregnancy with one normal and two papyraceous fetuses. *Am J Obstet Gynecol*. 1941;43:343.

58. Roos FJ, Roter AM, Molina FA. A case of triplets including anomalous twins and a fetus compressus. *Am J Obstet Gynecol*. 1957;73:1342–1345.

59. Hommel H, Festge B. Drillingsschwangerschaft mit fetus papyraceus. *Zentralbl Gynakol*. 1979; 101:845–847.

60. Kindred JE. Twin pregnancies with one blighted. *Am J Obstet Gynecol*. 1944;48:642–682.

61. Baker VV, Doering MC. Fetus papyraceous: an unreported congenital anomaly of the surviving infant. *Am J Obstet Gynecol*. 1982;143:234–235.

62. Gilardi G, Giannone E. Ozzervazioni cliniche, morfologiche e patogenetiche su un caso di gravidanza gemellare con transformazione papiracea di uno dei feti. *Arch Ostet Ginecol*. 1972; 77:258–263.

63. Leroy F. Major fetal hazards in multiple pregnancy. *Acta Genet Med Gemellol*. 1976;25:299–306.

64. Nance WE. Malformations unique to the twinning process. In: Gedda L, Parisi P, Nance WE, eds. Twin Research 3: Twin Biology and Multiple Pregnancy. *Prog Clin Biol Res*. 1981;69A:123–133.

65. Balfour RP. Fetus papyraceous. *Obstet Gynecol*. 1976;47:507.

66. Desgranges M-F, De Muylder X, Moutquin J-M, Lazaro-Lopez F, Leduc B. Perinatal profile of twin pregnancies: a retrospective review of 11 years (1969–1979) at Hôpital Notre-Dame, Montreal, Canada. *Acta Genet Med Gemellol*. 1982;31:157–163.

67. Saier F, Burden L, Cavanagh D. Fetus papyraceous. (An unusual case with congenital anomaly of the surviving fetus.) *Obstet Gynecol*. 1975; 45:217–220.

68. Wagner DS, Klein RL, Robinson HB, Novak RW. Placental emboli from a fetus papyraceous. *J Pediatr Surg*. 1990;25:538–542.

69. Mannino FL, Jones KL, Benirschke K. Congenital skin defects and fetus papyraceous. *J Pediatr*. 1977;91:559–564.

70. Anderson RL, Golbus MS, Curry CJR, Callen PW, Hastrup WH. Central nervous system damage and other anomalies in surviving fetus following second trimester antenatal death of co-twin. *Prenat Diagn*. 1990;10:513–518.

71. Kaplan C. Isolated aortic stenosis with fetus papyraceous: a new vascular disruption anomaly. In: Ryder OA, Byrd ML, eds. *One Medicine*. Heidelberg: Springer-Verlag; 1984:77–83.

72. Clark DA. Hydrops fetalis attributable to intrauterine disseminated intravascular coagulation. *Clin Pediatr*. 1981;20:61–62.

73. Redwine FO, Hays PM. Selective birth. *Semin Perinatol*. 1986;10:73–81.

74. Aberg A, Mitelman F, Cantz M, Gehler J. Cardiac puncture of fetus with Hurler's disease avoiding abortion of unaffected co-twin. *Lancet*. 1978;2: 990–991.

75. Chitkara U, Berkowitz RL, Wilkins IA, Lynch L, Mehalek KE, Alvarez M. Selective second-trimester termination of the anomalous fetus in twin pregnancies. *Obstet Gynecol*. 1989;73:690–694.

76. Lake BD, Young EP, Nicolaides K. Prenatal diagnosis of infantile sialic acid storage disease in a twin pregnancy. *J Inherited Metab Dis*. 1989;12:152–156.

77. Antsaklis A, Politis J, Karagiannopoulos C, Kaskarelis D, Karababa P, Panourgias J, Boussiou M, Loukopoulos D. Selective survival of only the healthy fetus following prenatal diagnosis of thalassemia major in binovular twin gestation. *Prenat Diagn*. 1984;4:289–296.

78. Rodeck CH. Fetoscopy in the management of twin pregnancies discordant for a severe abnormality. *Acta Genet Med Gemellol*. 1984;33:57–60.

79. Daffos F, Capella-Pavlovsky M, Forestier F. Fetal blood sampling during pregnancy with use of a needle guided by ultrasound: a study of 606 consecutive cases. *Am J Obstet Gynecol*. 1985;153:655–660.

80. Papp Z, Csecsei K, Toth Z, Polgar K, Szeifert GT. Exencephaly in human fetuses. *Clin Genet*. 1986;30:440–444.

81. Bollmann R, Schilling H, Prenzlau P, Zienert A, Gust G, Leujak A, Warbanow R, Weihrauch P. Selektive Schwangerschaftsbeendigung durch Sectio parva in der 24. Schwangerschaftswache bei diskordanter Zwillingsgraviditat und Spontangeburt eines gesunden Kindes am Termin. *Dtsch Med Wochenschr*. 1988;113:383–386.

82. Still K, Kolatat T, Corbett T, Byrne P. Early third trimester selective feticide of a compromising twin. *Fetal Ther*. 1989;4:83–87.

83. Burke MS, Heyborne K, Bruno A, Porreco RP. Selective feticide in the second trimester: percutaneous ultrasound guided intracardiac placement of a thrombogenic coil (Abstract). *Am J Obstet Gynecol*. 1991;164:337.

84. Baldwin VJ, Wittman BK. Pathology of intragestational intervention in twin to twin transfusion syndrome. *Pediatr Pathol*. 1990;10:79–93.

85. Benirschke K, Kim CK. Multiple Pregnancy. *N Engl J Med*. 1973;288:1276–1284,1329–1336.

86. Koivisto M, Jouppila P, Kauppila A, Moilanen I, Ylikorkala O. Twin pregnancy neonatal morbidity and mortality. *Acta Obstet Gynecol Suppl*. 1975; 44:21–29.

87. Gedda L. Why can the study of twins be called Gemellology? In: Nance WE, ed. Twin Studies: Biology and Epidemiology. *Prog Clin Biol Res*. 1978;24B:1–8.

88. Manlan G, Scott KE. Contribution of twin pregnancy to perinatal mortality and fetal growth retardation; reversal of growth retardation after birth. *Can Med Assoc J*. 1978;118:365–368.

89. Layde PM, Erickson JD, Falek A, McCarthy BJ. Congenital malformations in twins. *Am J Hum Genet*. 1980;32:69–78.

90. Botting BJ, Davies IM, MacFarlane AJ. Recent trends in the incidence of multiple births and associated mortality. *Arch Dis Child*. 1987;62:941–950.

91. Fabre E, de Aquero RG, de Agustin JL, Perez-Hiraldo MP, Bescos JL. Perinatal mortality in twin pregnancy: an analysis of birth weight–specific mortality rates and adjusted mortality rates for birth weight distributions. *J Perinat Med*. 1988;16:85–91.

92. Ghai V, Vidyasagar D. Morbidity and mortality factors in twins. An epidemiologic approach. *Clin Perinatol*. 1988;15:123–140.

93. Spallacy WN, Handler A, Ferre CD. A case-control study of 1253 twin pregnancies from a 1982–1987 perinatal data base. *Obstet Gynecol*. 1990;75:168–171.

94. Kiely JL. The epidemiology of perinatal mortality in multiple births. *Bull NY Acad Med*. 1990;66:618–637.

95. Sehgal NN. Perinatal mortality in twin pregnancies (implications for clinical management). *Postgrad Med*. 1980;68:231–234.

96. Shah SB, Patel DN. Twinning and structural defects. *Indian Pediatr*. 1984;21:475–478.

97. Wharton B, Edwards JH, Cameron AH. Monoamniotic twins. *J Obstet Gynecol Br Cwlth*. 1968; 75:158–163.

98. Hartikainen-Sorri A-L, Rantakallio P, Sipila P. Changes in prognosis of twin births over 20 years. *Ann Med*. 1990;22:131–135.

99. Magnus P, Arntzen A, Samuelsen SO, Haldorsen T, Bakketeig LS. No correlation in postneonatal deaths for twins. A study of the early mortality of twins based on the Norwegian Medical Birth Registry. *Early Hum Dev*. 1990;22:89–97.

100. Myrianthopoulos NC. An epidemiologic survey of twins in a large, prospectively studied population. *Am J Hum Genet*. 1970;22:611–629.

101. Myrianthopoulos NC. Congenital malformations in twins: epidemiologic survey. *Birth Defects*. 1975; 11(8):1–39.

102. Ferguson WF. Perinatal mortality in multiple gestations. (A review of perinatal deaths from 1609 multiple gestations.) *Obstet Gynecol*. 1963;23: 861–870.

103. Potter EL. Twin zygosity and placental form in relation to the outcome of pregnancy. *Am J Obstet Gynecol*. 1963;87:566–577.

104. Bender S. Twin pregnancy (a review of 472 cases). *J Obstet Gynecol Br Cwlth*. 1952;59:510–517.

105. Bulmer MG. *The Biology of Twinning in Man*. Oxford: Clarendon Press; 1970:54–60.

106. Naeye RL, Tafari N, Judge D, Marboe CC. Twins: causes of perinatal death in 12 United States cities and one African city. *Am J Obstet Gynecol*. 1978;131:267–272.

107. Baldwin VJ. The placenta. In: Dimmick JE, Kalousek DK, eds. *Developmental Pathology of the Embryo and Fetus*. Philadelphia: JB Lippincott; 1992:271–319.

108. Hoffman HJ, Bakketeig LS, Stark CR. Twins and perinatal mortality: a comparison between single and twin births in Minnesota and Norway, 1967–1973. In: Nance WE, ed. Twin Research: Biology and Epidemiology. *Prog Clin Biol Res*. 1978; 24B:133–142.

109. Keith L, Ellis R, Berger GS, Depp R. The Northwestern University Multihospital twin study I. A description of 588 twin pregnancies and associated pregnancy loss, 1971–1975. *Am J Obstet Gynecol*. 1980;138:781–789.

110. Marivate M, Norman RJ. Twins. *Clin Obstet Gynecol*. 1982;9B:723–743.

111. Fowler MG, Kleinman JC, Kiely JL, Kessel SS. Double jeopardy: twin infant mortality in the United States, 1983 and 1984. *Am J Obstet Gynecol*. 1991;165:15–22.

112. Zahálková M. Perinatal and infant mortality in twins. In: Nance WE, ed. Twin Research: Biology and Epidemiology. *Prog Clin Biol Res*. 1978;24B: 115–120.

113. Chandra P, Harilal KT. Plural births—mortality and morbidity. In: Nance WE, ed. Twin Research: Biology and Epidemiology. *Prog Clin Biol Res*. 1978;24B:109–114.

114. Osbourne GK, Patel NB. An assessment of perinatal mortality in twin pregnancies in Dundee. *Acta Genet Med Gemellol*. 1985;34:193–199.

115. Jakobovits AA, Zubek L. Sex ratio in twin pregnancies (letter). *Am J Obstet Gynecol*. 1987;156:1360.

116. Ho SK, Wu PYK. Perinatal factors and neonatal morbidity in twin pregnancy. *Am J Obstet Gynecol*. 1975;122:979–987.

117. Khrouf N, Barkallah N, Miled SB, Bechr SB, Gastli H. Les grossesses gemellaires: frequence, developpment foetal et mortalite perinatale. *J Gynecol Obstet Biol Reprod (Paris)*. 1983;12:619–623.

118. Kleinman JC, Fowler MG, Kessel SS. Comparison of infant mortality among twins and singletons: United States 1960 and 1983. *Am J Epidemiol*. 1991;133:133–143.

119. Howarth GR, Pattinson RG, de Jong G. Total perinatal-related wastage in twin pregnancies. *S Afr Med J*. 1991;80:31–33.

120. Hawrylyshyn PA, Barkin M, Bernstein A, Papsin PR. Twin pregnancies—a continuing perinatal challenge. *Obstet Gynecol*. 1982;59:463–466.

121. Puissant F, Leroy F. A reappraisal of perinatal mortality factors in twins. *Acta Genet Med Gemellol*. 1982;31:213–219.

122. Sekiya S, Hafez ESE. Physiomorphology of twin transfusion syndrome: a study of 86 twin gestations. *Obstet Gynecol*. 1977;50:288–292.

123. Gruenwald P. Environmental influences on twins apparent at birth (a preliminary study). *Biol Neonate*. 1970;15:79–93.

124. Benirschke K. Twin placenta in perinatal mortality. *NY State J Med*. 1961;61:1499–1508.

125. Fujikura T, Froehlich LA. Twin placentation and zygosity. *Obstet Gynecol*. 1971;37:34–43.

126. McCarthy BJ, Sachs BP, Layde PM, Burton A, Terry JS, Rochat R. The epidemiology of neonatal death in twins. *Am J Obstet Gynecol*. 1981;141:252–256.

127. MacGillivray I. Twins and other multiple deliveries. *Clin Obstet Gynecol*. 1980;7:581–600.

128. Bender HG, Werner C. Functional aspects of placental maturation in twin pregnancies. In: Nance WE, ed. Twin Research: Clinical Studies. *Prog Clin Biol Res*. 1978;24C:147–150.

129. Young BK, Suidan J, Antoine C, Silverman F, Lustig I, Wasserman J. Differences in twins: the importance of birth order. *Am J Obstet Gynecol*. 1985;151:915–921.

6
Morbidity of Twins

Infants of multiple gestations are subject to all the diseases and disorders that singletons are, but with two additional levels of consideration—the degree of concordance of the abnormality, and the significance of the twinship to the pathophysiology or prevalence. The caveats surrounding twin studies and the interpretation of the significance of concordance of an observation in twins have been discussed in Chapter 1. However, it is worth restating the importance of careful pathologic documentation of placental findings and autopsy studies to the validity of any study of patterns of disease in twins.

In addition, the pathologist assessing a disease process in twins would do well to keep in mind at least five aspects of twinship that could be important to the interpretation. First, there are those disorders that are more frequent in twins because two individuals are located where there is usually only one. These include the complications of prematurity (because twins are more often delivered prematurely), and the problems of labor and delivery, both discussed in Chapter 4, and growth discordance discussed below. Second, there are those disorders that are unique to twins, such as the twin transfusion syndrome, discussed in Chapter 9. Third, some disorders may be modified in their expression because of the twin situation, such as discordance in the manifestations of blood group incompatibility in dizygotic twins, or possible variations in the manifestations of metabolic or infectious disease through vascular anastomoses or intrauterine position. Fourth, some studies suggest that the twinning stimulus/process may affect the potential for neoplasms, and concordance of leukemia in monozygotic twins is discussed later in this

chapter. Finally, there are social aspects, such as a fear of twins or the extra burden of caring for twins, that may contribute to pre- or postnatal abuse or neglect.

This chapter reviews the problems of impaired intrauterine growth of twins, infections, neoplasms, systemic morbidity and other disorders in twins. Anomalous development of twins is discussed in Chapter 7.

Low Birth Weight

Low birth weight of any infant is accepted as representing an increased risk for mortality and morbidity, but it has been suggested that low birth weight in twins is a different problem from low birth weight in singletons and should be considered separately.[1] However, the category of "low birth weight" is not a single entity, and three patterns of low birth weight of twins need to be described. First, twins may have low birth weights simply because they are premature. Second, twins may be growth impaired regardless of their gestational age at birth. Both these categories of low birth weight raise the question of what standards are appropriate for assessing growth of twins. Third, the relative weights of the twins in any one set have implications for survival, and discordant weights need to be explained.

Incidence, Definition, and Standards

Some of the variations in the reported observations from studies of fetal growth of twins arise from difficulties establishing what is "normal" growth of twins, and if it is in fact different from normal fetal growth of singletons. A difference in birth weights of twins compared to singletons has been noted for some time. In one study, just over 51% of twins, but only 6.5% of singletons, weighed less than 2,000 g at birth.[2] Another study compared percentages in different birth weight groups and reported that approximately 2% of singletons weighed less than 2,000 g at birth compared to 25% of twins.[3] At 2,000 to 3,000 g, the percentages were 19% and 60%; at 3,000 to 4,000 g, 68% and 15%; and over 4,000 g, 10% and <1% respectively. Alternatively, using comparative gestational age–matched singleton data, 19% of twin infants were identified as less than the 10th percentile using singleton birth weight standards.[4] In 27.5% of the twin sets, one twin was affected, and in a further 5%, both twins were affected. These observations suggest that if singleton criteria of fetal growth were applied to twins, up to a fifth of all twins would be considered undergrown.[5]

Such a high proportion of growth impairment raises the question whether it is valid to use singleton growth standards for twins—perhaps twins grow differently in utero. Based on an autopsy study of "normal" twin fetuses from induced abortions between 8½ and 21 weeks' gestation, it was reported that the body weight of twins compared to length was the same as observed in singletons, but that the average crown–rump length was "somewhat less" than that of singletons.[6] No explanation was apparent. Birth weights of live-born twins, excluding anomalous twins and twins with hemolytic disease, but not excluding antenatal complications, such as preeclampsia or polyhydramnios, were compared with those of singletons and reviewed by zygosity and birth order.[7] Birth weights of twins paralleled those of singletons to 32 weeks' gestation, but after that twin growth slowed markedly, more evident in monochorionic and second born twins. In dizygotic twins, like-sex female pairs weighed less than like-sex male pairs or unlike-sex pairs. No explanation was suggested. Other reports have also correlated low birth weights with placental pattern and sex of the infants. Monochorionic monozygotic twins had a slightly lower birth weight than dichorionic monozygotic twins,[8,9] and both were less than the weights for dizygotic twins of either like or unlike sex.[8] In

another report, 100% of monochorionic monoamniotic twins weighed less than 2,500 g at birth and 67% died; 60% of monochorionic diamniotic twins were less than 2,500 g and 18% died; 56% of dichorionic twins were less than 2,500 g and 6% died.[10] Male twins have been reported to weigh an average of 100 g more than female twins,[11] and male/female pairs tended to be heavier than male/male or female/female pairs.[12]

These observations of apparently different fetal growth patterns of twins can be assessed in utero, although not all examiners arrive at the same conclusion. Ultrasonographically determined biparietal diameters have been reported to indicate that intrauterine growth of twins was always below that of singletons.[13] However, another study reported that biparietal diameters of concordantly well growing twins were the same as appropriately growing singletons, verified by measurements of head circumference at birth.[14] These same twins were noted to be equally grown by length, but 300 g less in weight at birth than age-matched singleton controls. In other words, singleton standards for measurements of fetal linear growth and head size may be useful to assess twins, but twins can be expected to weigh less at birth without apparent detrimental effect. Another report also concludes that in the second trimester, the growth of twins can be treated like the growth of two singletons in the same mother.[15] Thus, the consensus seems to be that there is a different growth pattern for twins, represented mainly by a slower weight gain in the last trimester of pregnancy, barring any process that could affect fetal growth independent of twinning.

It is important, therefore, to consider the standards that are used when twin growth and development is assessed. The most commonly available newborn measurement of infants is still the birth weight. This is the one measurement that is the most readily altered by malnutrition or disease, but remains a universally accepted measure of fetal development. One of the largest series of reported birth weights of live infants from multiple conceptions is a report of just over 6,800 infants in 1980,[16] and the data are presented in Table 6.1. Keeping the caveats in mind of the use of fetal weights as the sole assessment of development, this table may serve as a useful reference if fetal weights are the only measure available. Naeye and Letts'[17] data consisting of body measurements and organ weights of

TABLE 6.1. Percentiles of birth weight for duration of pregnancy—Canada except Newfoundland, 1980: live-born multiple births.

Duration	Males							Females						
	Number	Mean	Median	P5	P10	P90	P95	Number	Mean	Median	P5	P10	P90	P95
20	2	340	340	340	340	340	340	–	–	–	–	–	–	–
21	4	316	350	199	199	365	365	6	424	411	396	396	496	496
22	11	379	360	170	183	538	560	7	471	453	280	280	730	730
23	10	583	575	425	430	723	725	10	492	505	340	342	716	730
24	19	654	670	453	480	814	819	9	543	490	453	453	679	680
25	21	963	907	683	727	1503	1943	14	727	720	450	450	984	1020
26	43	763	740	475	542	991	1095	26	722	795	192	376	1026	1100
27	33	1056	990	697	743	1612	2032	18	893	913	453	675	1034	1165
28	33	1088	1030	722	822	1305	1504	27	1116	1100	627	779	1373	2141
29	27	1277	1304	948	987	1531	1847	23	1150	1210	655	720	1414	1459
30	58	1511	1477	983	1070	1961	2120	42	1416	1340	1006	1133	1635	2272
31	54	1497	1500	1156	1244	1764	1827	44	1462	1442	910	1007	1869	2092
32	98	1802	1786	1216	1337	2212	2418	111	1750	1750	1077	1247	2261	2534
33	146	1908	1927	1425	1530	2239	2445	112	1860	1800	1428	1495	2320	2554
34	206	2088	2100	1556	1663	2477	2605	174	2027	2000	1556	1644	2443	2656
35	204	2190	2183	1557	1724	2608	2770	193	2179	2182	1484	1658	2715	2807
36	389	2396	2409	1680	1839	2969	3118	401	2309	2310	1630	1814	2825	2945
27	444	2576	2580	1904	2041	3100	3208	431	2505	2500	1924	2050	2976	3093
38	610	2755	2755	2012	2160	3320	3442	586	2651	2640	2000	2146	3147	3306
39	450	2890	2941	2089	2250	3458	3696	450	2738	2750	1956	2154	3298	3548
40	510	2920	2948	2115	2296	3537	3676	511	2842	2830	2142	2267	3430	3601
41	66	3004	3019	1946	2214	3728	3853	103	2933	2948	1929	2327	3535	3718
42	34	3095	3143	2033	2253	3699	4040	27	2969	2890	2251	2269	3687	3832
43	3	3184	3090	2863	2863	3600	3600	2	2778	2778	2466	2466	3090	3090
44	–	–	–	–	–	–	–	2	1940	1940	1900	1900	1980	1980
45+	1	3150	3150	3150	3150	3150	3150	1	3150	3150	3150	3150	3150	3150

From Effer.[16]

fetal and neonatal monozygotic and dizygotic twins by gestational age are presented in Table 6.2. It is always difficult to be sure that the fetuses and infants that are being used to create a normal range are in fact normal, but these authors describe their case material carefully. A review of the data from the Survey '91 autopsy-group cases that would be suitable to include in a "normal" table provided weights and measures that fell within the published ranges, and confirmed that they are indeed usefully representative. When these observations are compared with rigidly derived normals for singletons,[18] the differences between the dichorionic dizygotic and monochorionic monozygotic groups are more marked than the twins as a group compared to the singleton ranges.

It is important to note that any table of "normals" in a complex biologic system represents a relative value guide for comparisons only, and it is not a rigid "gold standard," above or below which equates with abnormality. The significance lies not only in comparing each measurement with the range of "normal," but also in noting the relative position of all the measurements of any one infant to the "normal" ranges. It is also important to remember that weight alone as a standard for growth failure is invalid when there is fetal maceration,[18,19] so that criteria used in studies of growth failure with fetal death must be examined carefully.[20]

Birth Weight and Mortality

The importance of low birth weight in twins is evident from mortality data, although the cohorts reported are often not well characterized. Low birth weight is reported to be a factor in 50%[21] to 85%[2] of the overall perinatal mortality of twins. Thirty percent of perinatal deaths of twins of more than 32 weeks gestational age have been associated with intrauterine growth retardation,[22] and 86% of twins dying of unknown causes weighed less than 2,000 g at birth.[23] The perinatal mortality of twins weighing

TABLE 6.2. Body and organ weights and measures of fetal and newborn twins by gestational age.

Twin pattern; gestational age (weeks)	Body weight (g)	Crown–rump (cm)	Crown–heel (cm)	Heart (g)	Lungs combined (g)	Liver (g)	Spleen (g)	Adrenal (g)	Kidneys combined (g)	Thymus (g)	Brain (g)
					Monochorionic monozygotic						
20–24 M	496	18.0	28.9	5.7	13.2	29.3	1.2	1.9	5.4	2.3	77.9
SD	148	5.4	2.0	3.0	5.6	11.7	0.6	0.7	3.0	1.0	17.6
24–28 M	813	22.4	33.8	7.3	19.2	36.4	1.8	2.7	8.6	2.7	120.0
SD	246	3.0	2.8	2.4	6.3	18.8	1.0	0.9	4.0	1.0	39.3
28–32 M	1291	26.4	39.4	10.2	28.9	51.8	3.5	3.5	13.3	6.0	185.0
SD	383	1.7	3.9	4.1	10.3	23.4	2.0	1.9	6.6	4.1	40.6
32–36 M	1660	28.9	44.3	13.7	42.3	70.3	4.9	5.4	16.0	7.5	251.0
SD	487	3.0	4.4	5.4	14.3	21.7	2.2	2.2	4.7	–	61.9
36–40 M	2542	31.4	46.4	18.6	49.8	89.9	9.9	7.1	22.5	10.4	308.3
SD	680	2.8	3.9	6.1	17.9	37.9	4.8	3.5	9.4	6.1	69.4
					Dichorionic dizygotic						
20–24 M	551	21.7	28.1	4.7	14.0	23.4	1.6	1.5	5.7	1.4	85.0
SD	154	2.0	2.8	1.7	6.2	9.0	0.2	0.2	2.5	0.2	30.5
24–28 M	896	22.5	34.8	6.6	20.6	35.5	2.0	2.5	8.8	2.8	131.2
SD	189	1.6	3.5	1.7	5.5	8.9	1.0	1.0	3.2	1.0	41.8
28–32 M	1354	26.5	39.4	10.5	30.6	53.4	3.7	3.6	13.6	6.2	199.2
SD	233	3.4	5.5	3.5	11.2	13.5	3.0	1.7	4.6	2.5	53.6
32–36 M	1660	27.0	40.3	12.6	40.8	59.0	5.2	4.4	14.3	7.4	218.0
SD	615	3.9	5.1	4.6	20.4	34.2	3.3	2.2	6.1	5.9	58.0
36–40 M	2689	32.2	47.8	18.0	39.1	103.2	10.4	5.6	19.5	8.0	385.8
SD	579	3.5	3.0	3.7	10.3	50.2	5.5	2.8	8.1	4.0	50.2

Modified from Naeye and Letts.[17]

M, mean; SD, one standard deviation.

less than 1,000 g at birth has been reported to be 44.6%, 19% between 1,000 and 2,400 g, and 1.7% of twins greater than 2,500 g.[24] In another review, 83% of neonatal deaths of twins occurred in infants who weighed less than 1,500 g at birth.[25] In this latter study, 55% of all the twins weighed less than 2,500 g at birth and 23.5% were small for gestational age. Twenty percent of A twins and 27% of B twins were growth retarded, and the mortality of the low birth weight infants was 13%.

While low birth weight is an important problem in multiple gestation, any discussion of it requires careful distinction between low birth weight due to prematurity and true intrauterine growth retardation, because the consequent risks are different.[5] One study that maintained this distinction reported perinatal death rates for small for gestational age preterm twins of 36%, small for gestational age term twins of 11%, appropriate for gestational age preterm twins of 6%, and appropriate for gestational age term twins of 0%.[10]

The low birth weight twin who is small because of *premature delivery* is a common finding, and prematurity is a problem for singletons as well as

twins. There is some suggestion that singletons who are going to be delivered prematurely grow more slowly than normal prior to the onset of preterm labor, but unfortunately, this observation was not confirmed in a study of preterm twins.[26] The factors contributing to morbidity and mortality of preterm twins have been reviewed in Chapter 4. It seems to be unclear whether twins are functioning physiologically at the same level as same-age singletons as regards complications of prematurity, although they appear susceptible to the same problems.

The low birth weight twin who is truly *growth impaired* may be different from a singleton with apparently the same degree of growth delay, in both cause and consequences,[5] although there are some similarities. As suggested above, there may be different standards required for the assessment of fetal growth of twins, so that indications for intervention can be more appropriate. It appears that a number of observations are needed to assess intrauterine growth impairment of twins, including a combination of sonographic measurement,[27] fetal blood flow studies,[28] flow studies combined with ultrasonography,[29] and possibly even magnetic resonance imaging.[30] Postnatal assessment by measurement has been discussed above. Assessing the developmental maturity of growth retarded infants using the Dubovitz system may provide falsely low values for the external criteria, but the neurological criteria should reflect the gestational age.[31] In fact, Dubovitz[32] commented that the observation of concordant neurologic scores, even when birth weights were very different, would argue against the interpretation of growth-discordant twins as representing examples of superfetation. The 2.4 times increased mortality risk for the growth-impaired twin is most marked in the lower weight ranges—at 500 to 999 g, small for gestational age (SGA) twins die 3.7 times as often as appropriate for gestational age twins (AGA); at 1,000 to 1,499 g, the increased risk is 3.4 times; at 1,500 to 1,999 g, it falls to 1.3 times, and over 2,000 g, there were no deaths in either group.[33] The smaller twin is also at increased risk for fetal asphyxia and neonatal morbidity,[33] as manifest by 16% with low 5-minute Apgar scores compared with 6.5% of appropriately grown twins.[34]

Causes

The causes of low birth weight in twins are the same as for singletons,[35] with possible additional factors related to placental site and development.[25] There is reportedly a 12% reduction in placental weight for gestational age compared to singletons,[21] and it has been reported that slowing of placental growth precedes slowing of fetal growth by up to 8 weeks.[36] It has been implied that placental crowding impairs placental growth with consequent limits to fetal growth,[36] but others suggest that in cases of low birth weight associated with placental abnormalities, such as anomalous insertions of the umbilical cord, there is a proportional reduction of fetal and placental mass, not that one leads to the other.[37] One study reported that placental weights did not vary with the sex of the infants, although male pairs were heavier on average.[38]

It has been suggested that the maternal circulatory adaptation to a twin-bearing uterus may be less than adequate, creating low-grade fetal hypoxia. In support of this are observations of elevated hemoglobin and red cell mass in twins,[21,39,40] and increased umbilical vascular resistance in normally grown twins compared to singletons.[41] Possibly related to placental perfusion is the observation that there is an increased risk for inadequate intrauterine growth of twins with mothers who are underweight or who smoke cigarettes.[42] An interesting study of energy metabolism in neonates from single and multiple gestation suggested that reduction of body growth led to a lower metabolic rate per neonate, although the energy metabolism of the total fetal mass was still higher than in singleton gestations.[43] This observation was the reason given for data describing a reduction of brain growth in twins as compared with singletons. However, this observation remains to be clarified as far as fetal growth overall and placental perfusion are concerned. An interesting observation of the umbilical cords of growth-impaired twins was a reduction in the volume of Wharton's jelly, and further studies relating this finding to blood flow were planned.[44]

Discordant Growth of Twins

Growth failure or impairment can affect one or both members of a twin pair, and some of the most striking examples of low birth weight are associated with marked intrapair discrepancies. There seems to be an increased risk of perinatal mortality when only one twin is growth retarded, particularly if its weight is less than 80% of the larger co-twin's weight, than if both twins are small, but more concordantly grown.[33] In contrast, there are other reports that suggest that prematurity and low birth weight for age present a greater threat to a twin than discordance of growth compared to its co-twin.[45,46] This discrepancy is probably more apparent than real because in twin sets where there is markedly discordant growth, the smaller twin is almost always small for gestational age, with all the risks that growth retardation entails. Of interest was a report that, along with an increased stillbirth rate, neonatal death rate, and incidence of intraventricular hemorrhage reported in a group discordant by 25% or greater, the larger twin was noted to be at increased risk for hyaline membrane disease, anemia, and hypoglycemia.[47] In contrast, what were termed "growth-promoted twins" did unusually well compared to macrosomic singletons.[48]

Part of the difficulty in assessing the increased risk of discordant development of twins is that there are a number of variables, such as birth order, fetal sex, and pattern of placentation, and thus this is not a homogeneous group. Unfortunately, the reported direction and magnitude of the effects of these contributing factors is somewhat varied. Twin A has been reported to average 100 g heavier than twin B,[11] be generally equivalent,[49] vary depending on gestational age,[7] or weigh less.[50] In this last report, 29% of singletons weighed less than 1,500 g at birth, compared to 54% of B twins and 66% of A twins. It has been suggested that in unlike-sex pairs, the female twin is at greater risk of being smaller if she is twin B, although no explanation is apparent.[51] Although female twins are reported to weigh less than male twins,[7] intrapair weight discrepancies of greater than 500 g are reported to occur with the same frequency in like-sex as in unlike-sex pairs.[11] Finally, intrauterine growth retardation and discordant weights are more common with monochorionic monozygotic twins than dichorionic monozygotic twins, suggesting that monochorionic placentation is a risk factor.[52] Of twins weighing <1,000 g at birth, 15% were monochorionic, 4% were same-sex dichorionic, and 3% unlike-sex dichorionic. Discordance of intrapair weights of greater than 25% was more frequent among monochorionic than dichorionic twins, particularly in the 26 to 36 week gestational age period.

Definition and Degrees

The definition and degree of intrapair weight discordance varies in the literature. The consensus seems to be that using the larger twin as 100%, growth discordance is deemed present if

$$\frac{\text{Weight of Larger Twin} - \text{Weight of Smaller Twin}}{\text{Weight of Larger Twin}}$$

is 20% to 25% or more. Usually, one twin is normally grown and one is small for gestational age, although differences of this magnitude can be encountered in heavier twins as well. These probably represent different groups. If the twins are growth discordant, but both within the normal range for age, there do not appear to be any increased risks for the smaller twin, although the reasons for the discordance were not discussed.[53] In contrast, in those cases where intertwin weight differences are greater than 20% and the smaller twin is small for age, the perinatal risks increase. From 20% to 25%, there is an elevated risk of perinatal death of 11.1%,

but the risk is even greater above 25%, with a perinatal death risk of 16.7%.[33] In a study of intrapair weight differences within 460 twin pairs, 8.9% varied more than 25% and 8.7% varied 20% to 24%. The risk for fetal death was 6.5 times greater, and the risk of perinatal death 2.5 times greater, for the over-25% group than for the 20% to 24% group.[54] Unfortunately, causes of death, placenta data, and zygosity were not described in the study. Identical increased risks for fetal and perinatal death of the smaller twin who was more than 25% smaller than the larger twin was reported associated with an increased risk for the presence of some developmental abnormality in the smaller twin.[55] It has been observed that if the twins are discordant by less than 20%, the smaller twin is as likely to be twin A as twin B. When the twins are discordant by more than 20%, the smaller twin is twice as likely to be twin B. It is not clear whether this represents an increased risk for twin B, or it is a function of gravity acting on the significantly heavier twin.[56]

The clinical and pathological significance of intertwin weight discordance depends therefore on the degree of the discrepancy. What has been termed grade 1 discordance of 15% to 25% occurs in 19% to 23% of twin pregnancies, grade 2 discordance of greater than 25% occurs in 4% to 9% of twin pregnancies,[57] and in this latter group the smaller twin is actually small for age more than 50% of the time.[34] As might be expected, the risks for perinatal morbidity and mortality are greatest for the smallest twin, and thus they are more likely encountered in sets with the greater degree of discordance. It was noted above that a number of measures of fetal growth are needed to identify the small twin, and it is the pathologist who is in a position to correlate the results of these investigations with actual measurements and gross and microscopic findings of at least the placenta, but also of any fetuses/infants who come to autopsy.

Causes of Discordant Growth

Although considerable clinical attention has been focused on discordant twins, most commentaries neglect any discussion of potential causes. This seems unfortunate as it is reasonable to suspect that different causes may explain the different risks and that some of these causes may be identifiable antenatally. It might also be helpful to know if one could identify causes that could be ameliorated before birth, or at least anticipated, so that more appropriate perinatal care could be planned.

It has been suggested above that fetal weight may be related to placental development, so that intertwin variations may reflect problems with placental implantation and growth. It has been observed that there was greater weight variation among twins with dichorionic fused than dichorionic separate placentas, so that whether the placentas were fused or separate was more important than chorion type or zygosity.[58] In the Survey '91 survivor group reviewed, there was a larger total placental volume by weight for dichorionic separate than dichorionic fused placentations over 36 weeks' gestation. Correlation of these data with fetal birth weights supported the concept that separately implanted placentas can grow larger and perhaps contribute to larger infants. This observation is modified when zygosity is considered as well.[59] There was greater intrapair variation when like-sex dichorionic twins were dizygotic than monozygotic, and disparities between dizygotic twins were similar for dichorionic fused and dichorionic separate placentas. This might argue for observed differences in dizygotic twins as being due to the different genetic constitution of the siblings.[57] Variations within monozygotic pairs were inversely associated with the degree of prenatal proximity of the pair members—greatest with monochorionic twins, less with dichorionic fused placentas, and least among twins with dichorionic separate placentas.[59] In addition, monochorionic monozygosity is a pattern of twinning that is prone to developmentally asymmetric twinning (see Chapter 10), as well as intertwin vascular anastomoses (see Chapter 9), both of which may be associated with dramatically discordantly grown twins. Thus, there are at least two aspects of placental development that are operative in discordant twins—monochorionic monozygosity in particular, and dichorionic placental fusion to a somewhat lesser extent.

There are two additional categories of placental findings that are important to discordant fetal growth—asymmetric placental development and discordant parenchymal disease. It was noted in Chapter 3 that discordant placental development can be associated with discordant growth of the twins, and this may be identified pathologically as

early as 37 days of gestation.[60] This placental asymmetry may consist of abnormalities of the umbilical cord, which occur more often with fused twin placentas, notably discordant volumes of placental tissue for each twin, seen with both fused and separate placental masses, and discordant placental disease, such as perivillus fibrin deposits. The increased incidence of abnormal cord insertions, especially velamentous, is likely a consequence of altered directions of placental growth because of closely implanted gestational sacs, and the abnormal cord may serve as a threshold factor for other forces affecting fetal growth. Single-artery cords are also increased and may reflect a more basic problem of placental development as decreased numbers of chorionic vessels are sometimes present as well. Asymmetries of chorionic volume may reflect differences in implantation sites and, theoretically at least, differences in the adequacy of maternal perfusion, or with monozygotic twins may reflect asymmetric twinning at a somewhat more subtle level than the gross distortions seen in some monochorionic twin fetuses. Discordant placental disease may reflect genetic diversity in responses to hematogenous infection or immunologic interactions, and in turn may be reflected in discordant growth of the twins.

In addition to these factors of placentation, there are other causes of intrapair weight variations. Anything that can cause growth retardation of a singleton can cause growth retardation in a twin. It has already been mentioned that the smaller twin is at risk for being developmentally abnormal and twins may be discordantly affected by genetically determined diseases that affect growth. In Fig. 6.1, the potential causes of intrapair variations in weight are summarized. It is worth remembering that virtually all of these potential influences on fetal growth are matters of degree, so that lesser degrees of twin discordance may be encountered with less severe examples of the underlying or associated abnormality.

Antenatal Considerations and Recovery Potential

The ability to identify potential causes for discordant growth of twins antenatally probably depends on the experience of the investigator and the level of sophistication of the tests available. Markedly ab-

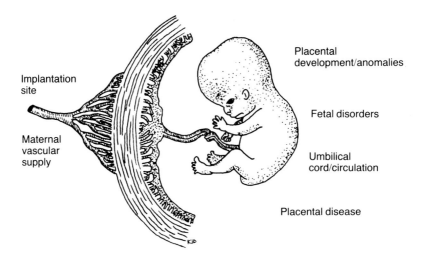

Implantation site

Maternal vascular supply

Placental development/anomalies

Fetal disorders

Umbilical cord/circulation

Placental disease

FIGURE 6.1. Potential sources of growth variation of twins. Fetal growth can be affected by disturbances in the categories shown. Problems of maternal vascular supply are well recognized, and it may be important whether the placenta is fundal or in the lower uterine segment. Disorders of placental development include possible constitutional features of the blastocyst, asymmetric twinning, crowding at the implantation site that affects development of the chorionic mass, and fetal chorionic circulations. Fetal disorders influencing growth are well recognized and include anomalies, chromosomal errors, infections, and genetic disease. Disorders of the umbilical cord and fetal circulations include anomalies of cord insertion, single-artery cords, and the effects of anastomoses. Disorders of placental parenchyma such as perivillus fibrin or infection can affect one or both fetuses.

normally developed monozygotic twins, such as the chorangiopagus parasiticus twin, and major developmental lesions, such as with dwarfing disorders or some of the chromosomally abnormal twins, can be detected by careful ultrasonic studies.[61] The chorionicity of the membrane between the twins can be determined ultrasonically, and occasionally abnormalities of the umbilical cord are detectable. Identification of a "thin" membrane between the twins can predict monochorionic diamniotic placentation in 86% of cases, but if no membrane is seen, that observation may be predictive of a monoamniotic placenta in only 25%.[62] Absent end diastolic flow in the smaller twin may identify a subset of discordant twins at greater risk for perinatal morbidity and mortality.[63] Discordant disorders may be reflected by other secondary clues, such as alterations of amniotic fluid volume or the presence of fetal edema. Cordocentesis or amniocentesis may provide evidence of fetal anemia or chromosomal anomaly. A useful observation was that when the growth discrepancy was evident in the

second trimester, it reflected potentially severe problems such as twin transfusion syndrome, while onset in the third trimester was related to intrauterine malnutrition, and these twins were less severely affected.[14] Also, significantly growth retarded twins were small in all three measures of growth—head circumference, length, and weight. Discordant placental form or disease, and the details of intertwin anastomoses require pathologic evaluation after delivery.

It is probable that except for the twin transfusion syndrome and some other complications of monochorionic monozygosity, intervention to alter the situation of growth failure of twins is not a consideration. However, a better idea of the probable cause of the impaired growth of the smaller twin will allow more appropriate management of labor and delivery. For example, if it is known that the smaller twin is twin B and that it has a lethal chromosomal error, management of delivery may be quite different if fetal distress is noted after delivery of the first twin.

An important final consideration is the long term significance of low birth weight, but the reports are conflicting. It has been noted that when one twin dies in utero, the other fetus attains normal singleton standard growth, including weight, if there are no anomalies or other problems.[5] This would suggest that each twin has a full potential for growth that is inhibited only by the intrauterine environment. Catch-up growth might be expected in those cases where antenatal growth retardation was due to a subnormal amount of cytoplasm in individual cells.[39] However, some monozygotic twins that are less than 75% of the expected value for singleton infants of the same gestational age are also deficient in cell numbers, so catch-up growth would be unlikely.[39]

Twins overall have been reported to reach singleton norms before the teenage years, attributed to dissipation of perinatal influences on birth size as each twin converged on his or her genetic growth curve.[64] Monozygotic twins became progressively more concordant, while dizygotic twins became less concordant. Monozygotic twins that differed by >750 g birth weight, were still discordant in weight at 6 years, although linear growth was nearly equivalent and IQ scores matched. This was interpreted as suggesting "a high degree of buffering for intelligence against the effects of nutritional deficit in the prenatal period."[64] In another study, monozygotic twins who differed in birth weight by an average of 36% were more concordant in head circumference than height and weight by 18 years of age, and some equalization of school performance was observed, although the small twin continued to lag.[65] Another review of twin sets discordant by 25% or more, with a mixture of zygosity patterns and no discussion as to causes of discordant growth, found no statistically significant differences in weight, height, or head circumference at a mean age of 9.4 years. No differences were found in gross motor performance or mean school grades, but in fine motor performance, balance, coordination, and visuomotor perception there was a statistically significant difference favoring the larger twins.[66] It is probable that the long-range outcome depends at least in part on the underlying cause, and until comparisons are available on that basis, the prognosis for the smaller twin after the newborn period will not be definable, aside from the prognosis of whatever perinatal or neonatal complication he or she overcame.

Survey '91 Growth-Discordant Twins

The Survey '91 twin data were examined to assess the patterns of discordant-twin growth in an attempt to define this observation more clearly. As was suspected, the data from the survivor group were somewhat different from the autopsy group, so they are described separately.

Survivor Group

In the survivor group of twin placentas, where both twins were live born and survived the newborn period at least, there were 1,075 twin placentations with adequate information on birth weights. Of these, 284 twin sets, or 26.4%, consisted of twins discordant in weight by 15% or greater. Of these, 35.2% differed by 15% to 19.9% (mild), 23.9% differed by 20% to 24.9% (moderate), 30.3% differed by 25% to 39.9% (marked), and 10.6% differed by more than 40% (severe). These categories were chosen on the basis of the categories used in the literature with the additional severe category because it did seem to be a different group. The major observations are reported in Table 6.3 and a number of additional comments follow.

There are several observations that can be made from the data in Table 6.3. In this group of surviving twins, discordant birth weights were surprisingly frequent, over one-quarter of the sets, and just under half of these differed by more than one-quarter of the weight of the larger twin. The percentage of the small twins that were actually small for gestational age increased with the magnitude of the discrepancy, as might be expected. There were 5 of the 284 sets where both twins were small for age, two each in the mild and marked groups and one in the severe group. There were two sets where the larger twin was large for gestational age, both in the marked group. The gestational age refers to the age at delivery, and it can be seen that discordant growth was observed throughout the third trimester. It is not known how many of these discordant twins were identified antenatally, nor if so, when. Male pairs were more frequent in the groups with the smallest and largest differences, while unlike sex pairs were fairly uniformly represented at all levels. As the discrepancy in the weight increased, the smaller twin was more likely the second born. This may reflect more a physical positioning effect than a pathophysiologic phenomenon. The proportion of

TABLE 6.3. Patterns of discordant growth of twins.

	Degree of discordance and study group							
	Mild (15–19.9%)		Moderate (20.0–24.9%)		Marked (25.0–39.9%)		Severe (>40%)	
	S	A	S	A	S	A	S	A
Percentage of study group	35.2	18.5	23.9	29.2	30.3	38.5	10.6	13.8
Gestational ages (weeks)								
Range	27–40	23–33	28–40	22–39	28–42	20–38	28–39	23–38
Mean	35.1	25.3	36.2	29.7	35.3	27.5	32.6	28.3
% Smaller twin also SGA	10.0	16.7	17.6	21.0	52.3	68.0	96.7	89.9
Sex distribution								
% unlike	26.0	16.7	26.5	15.8	25.6	4.0	20.0	22.2
Male:female pairs	1.4:1	2.3:1	1:1.1	1.6:1	1.1:1	1.2:1	1.8:1	1.3:1
Smaller twin A:B	1:1.2	1:1.4	1:1.4	1:2.8	1:2.3	1:1.8	1:2.8	1:3.5
Placentation (%)								
Monochorionic	37.0	33.3	38.2	52.6	34.9	68.0	36.6	44.4
Dichorionic	63.0	66.7	61.8	31.6	65.1	20.0	63.4	55.6
Dichorionic fused:separate	1.4:1	1:1.7	1:1.4	1.5:1	2.3:1	1:1	3.8:1	1:2
Possible causes (%)								
No cause determined	26.0	66.7	35.3	26.3	16.3	4.0	3.3	–
Major fetal anomaly	–	–	–	5.3	1.2	32.0	–	33.3
Twin transfusion	23.0	16.7	26.0	31.6	22.1	56.0	26.6	44.4
Placental development*	62.0	25.0	50.0	26.3	53.6	12.0	120.0*	11.1
Umbilical cord	24.0	20.0	16.2	26.3	36.1	8.0	40.0	–
Disk	38.0	5.0	33.8	–	17.5	4.0	80.0	11.1
Placental disease	10.0	8.3	16.2	15.8	41.8	–	60.0	22.2
Multiple possible	15.0	16.7	25.0	15.8	36.0	8.0	66.7	11.1

% recorded are within each degree for each study group.

*Placental developmental abnormalities include a number of lesions (see text) and some placentas had more than one.

S, survivor group; A, autopsy group; SGA, small for gestational age.

monochorionic twins was slightly higher when there was growth discordance than in the group of live-born twins as a whole, where 32% of placentas were monochorionic. In the live-born group as a whole, dichorionic separate placentas were more common than dichorionic fused by a ratio of 1.2 : 1. Not only was this ratio reversed in all but the moderate group, but fused dichorionic placentas were the majority of all patterns in the last two groups, increasing with the degree of discordance. This suggested that there might be significant findings in the placenta, particularly in the severe group.

The *placental findings* were assessed to look for associated lesions that might have pathogenetic significance. There were more abnormalities detected as the degree of discordance increased, although in more than a third of the cases in the moderate group there was not only no discordant placental abnormality, there was no abnormality of note described at all. These "cause undetermined" cases are described in more detail further in the

discussion. The term "placental development" refers to a number of findings that suggest a developmental influence on the placenta that might have significance for fetal growth. In 19% of the mild group, 17.6% of the moderate group, 7.0% of the marked group, and 6.7% of the severe group, the only difference was a concordant difference in placental volume, by weight or measure, in all patterns of placentation, that ranged from 17% to 50% (Fig. 6.2a,b). There were no other abnormalities in these placentas. This raises the question of whether the placenta was small for some reason and so the fetus was small secondarily, or whether placenta and fetus were smaller than the co-twin for the same primary reason. This question cannot be resolved from the information available.

The percentage of the placentas with more than one abnormality present on the placental portion of the smaller twin was impressive (Fig. 6.2c–i), and explains why the percentages of the observed abnormalities totals more than 100%. These combinations encompassed all the potential permutations and combinations of the abnormalities possible, but the majority were combinations of smaller chorionic volume with unilateral abnormalities of the umbilical cord and/or discordant parenchymal pathology, with superposition of twin transfusion in monochorionic cases. It was noted in Chapter 3 that abnormalities of the umbilical cord are more frequent with twins, and it is an important observation that umbilical cord anomalies are frequently associated with the smaller twin in discordant pairs.[67] The observed abnormalities were single umbilical artery to marginal insertion to velamentous insertion in ratios up to 1 : 3 : 7, with combinations such as single artery velamentous cords seen. Whether the anomaly causes the growth impairment by affecting blood flow, or it contributes to growth impairment by presenting a threshold, or it is simply a coincidental abnormality accompanying the growth failure remains to be determined. It is possible that any one of these three mechanisms could be operative under different circumstances. The frequent association of anomalies of the cord with small chorionic volume and reduced chorionic vessel numbers, particularly in the severe group, suggest a major detrimental influence to placental development for that one twin, but again, the underlying cause is undetermined.

The presence of *intertwin vascular anastomoses* is significant in all categories, but it is worth noting the difference between the percent of the twin sets in each group who have monochorionic placentas and the percent for whom twin transfusion is considered possible or probable. The interpretation "probable" was made when there were detailed injection studies with a pattern of anastomosis that could have been associated with the direction of weight discordance observed. The "possible" interpretation was used where anastomoses were mentioned as being present, but not enough details were provided to assess the potential direction of flow (see Chapter 9 for further discussion). In none of these cases was there any mention of differential volumes of amniotic fluid, nor was there a reported clinical concern of twin transfusion syndrome, so the degree to which these anastomoses were important to the growth discordance is conjectural. The remaining monochorionic placentas could be divided into two categories. In each discordant group there were two to three monochorionic placentas with anastomoses described that could not be rationalized with the reported birth order and birth weights. No other lesion was present to explain the discordance and these remain unsettled, although the possibility of mislabeling of the cords cannot be excluded. There were nine sets in the mild and marked groups, four in the moderate, and two in the severe group that had no anastomoses described. In the mild group, four had no placental abnormality, four had anomalies of the cord or chorionic vessel numbers, and one had discordant villitis. In the moderate group, two had no placental abnormality, one had a combination of increased villus fibrin and a velamentous cord, and in one there was a true knot of the cord. In the marked group, three had velamentously inserted cords, two had reduced numbers of chorionic vessels, one had a smaller but otherwise normal placental portion, and three had discordant parenchymal disease, villitis in one and villus fibrin in two. In the severe group, one had a marginally inserted cord and in the other the villus tissue of the smaller twin had a number of abnormalities compared to the villus tissue of his co-twin, but the underlying problem was never clarified. These cases are mentioned in some detail to emphasize the point that not all monochorionic discordantly grown twins can be assumed to be the result of the twin transfusion syndrome—28% to 58% may be due to something else.

The importance of discordant *placental parenchymal pathology* to asymmetric growth of twins is suggested by the dramatic increase in these diagnoses as the degree of asymmetry increased. Discordant ischemic changes might be expected with separately implanted placentas, suggesting that one was less advantageously implanted, but 70% of the discordantly ischemic placentas were dichorionic fused, 7.4% monochorionic, and the remainder separate disks. There was no way of confirming implantation sites in the majority of these cases, so the cause of the asymmetry remains unexplained. Whether this lesion was sufficient cause for the growth discordance is uncertain as it was often in a smaller placental mass, and coupled with excessive perivillus fibrin or fibrinosis. Fibrinosis too was more common in the dichorionic fused placenta, 53%, (Fig. 6.2f,g), and in 14.7% it was discordant in monochorionic placentas. As the pathogenesis of this lesion is not known, its significance in the twin context cannot be discussed further except to note that maternal floor infarction, the pattern of fibrino-

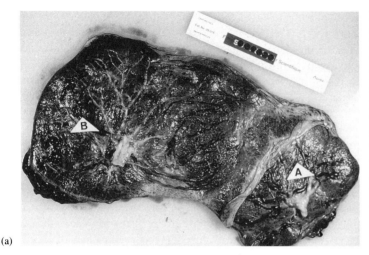

(a)

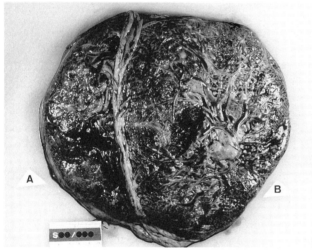

(b)

FIGURE 6.2. Placental findings with discordantly grown surviving twins. (a,b) Parallel discrepancy of chorionic volume only, no histologic differences. (a) Discordant size of dichorionic diamniotic separate disks with shared overlapping membranes, A = 220 g, B = 390 g; female twins (zygosity undetermined) discordant by 54.8% at 32 weeks' gestation (A = 975 g, B = 2160 g); the small twin is also growth retarded for age; the cause of discordant growth was not determined. (b) Discordant areas of dichorionic diamniotic fused placenta; unlike-sex twins discordant by 35.4% at 37 weeks' gestation (female A = 2,350 g, male B = 3,640 g); the cause of discordant growth was not determined. (Reprinted with permission from Baldwin VJ, *Developmental Pathology of the Embryo and Fetus*, JB Lippincott, 1992: 330.)

sis that recurs, was seen in only one case. It was surprising to note that 87.5% of the discordant nonspecific villitis was seen in monochorionic placentas (Fig. 6.2i). This was not a common lesion in the discordant twin placentas overall, and the explanation for the asymmetric distribution in what should theoretically be a homogeneous organ remains unexplained. In two cases, it was the only lesion identified, but in the others, there were a number of additional lesions that could have been more important as contributions to the growth discordance.

In the discordant twins in whom no placental lesions were found, there were some interesting differences from the group as a whole. While like-sex female twins were 30% to 38% of the whole group, they were only 18.8% of the cause

unknown group, with the remainder equally divided between unlike-sex pairs and like-sex male pairs. There was no obvious reason for this difference except that female sets were more represented in monochorionic pairs and only 6.3% of the unknown group were monochorionic. Of the 93.7% dichorionic twins, fused placentas were half again as frequent as separate placentas. In the 40.6% that were presumed dizygotic by virtue of unlike sex, the growth discordance may represent different genetic programs for growth. The zygosity of the 9 dichorionic female pairs and the 23 dichorionic male pairs is not known, but some of them may be dizygotic with different hereditary growth potentials. The remainder are unexplained.

When the unlike-sex twins are considered, in 38% there was no placental lesion identified. In

FIGURE 6.2. *Continued*. (c–e) Parallel discrepancy of multiple gross features of placentation. (c) Discordant areas of monochorionic placenta (A = 2/3, B = 1/3), discordant degrees of velamentous cord insertions (A = 2 cm, B = 24 cm), single umbilical artery in cord B, both sides with decreased numbers of chorionic vessels; female twins discordant by 16.0% at 36 weeks (A = 2,440 g, B = 2,050 g). (No intertwin anastomoses were identified.) (d) Discordant areas of monochorionic placenta (A = 2/3, B = 1/3) with one arterial, one venous, and bidirectional parenchymal (arteriovenous) anastomoses; female twins discordant by 43.2% at 33 weeks (A = 1,250 g, B = 710 g). (e) Discordant areas of dichorionic fused placenta (A = 1/3 with fewer vessels), with abnormal septal intramembranous cord insertion for twin B; male twins (zygosity undetermined) discordant by 32.8% at 35 weeks (A = 1,860 g, B = 1,250 g); note that asymmetry of chorionic volume favors smaller twin but appears offset by abnormal umbilical cord; no microscopic differences. (Reprinted with permission from Wiggelsworth and Singer, *Textbook of Fetal and Perinatal Pathology*, Chapter 8, Blackwell Scientific Publications, 1991:235.)

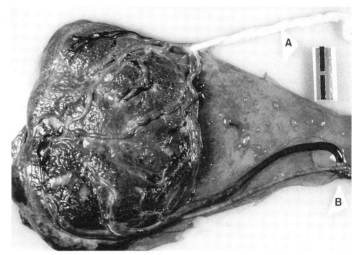

(c)

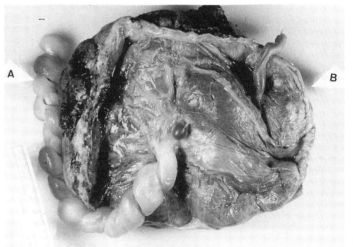

(d)

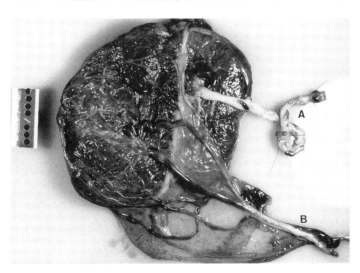

(e)

FIGURE 6.2. *Continued.* (f–i) Combinations of gross and microscopic differences. (f,g) Discordant volume of dichorionic fused placenta (A = 2/5, B = 3/5) with discordant extent of perivillus fibrin. Note differential pallor of parenchyma grossly (f) and differential entrapment of villi in fibrin (g); male twins (zygosity undetermined), discordant by 53.2% at 28 weeks (A = 1,080 g, B = 2,310 g). (Reprinted with permission from Wiggelsworth and Singer, *Textbook of Fetal and Perinatal Pathology,* Chapter 8, Blackwell Scientific Publications, 1991:235.)

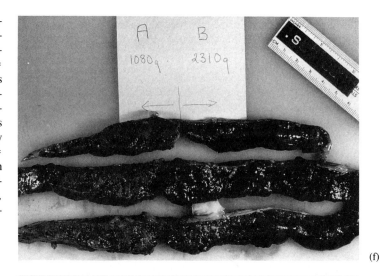

(f)

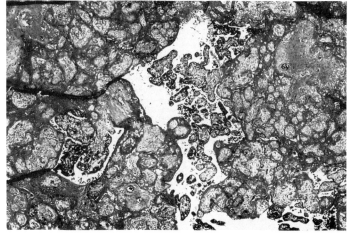

g(

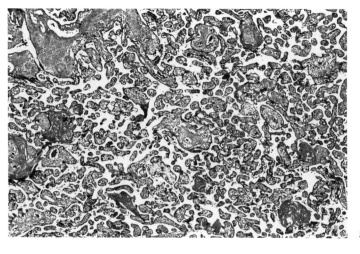

g(

FIGURE 6.2. *Continued*. (h) Dichorionic fused placenta with portion B deeply invaginated into portion A coupled with villus ischemic changes in portion B microscopically and normal histology portion A. Female twins (zygosity undetermined) discordant by 38.0% at 31 weeks (A = 1840 g, B = 1140 g). (i) Decreased numbers of chorionic surface vessels on smaller twin's side but also more widespread involvement by nonspecific villitis. Monochorionic placenta with no intertwin anastomoses. Twins discordant by 24.8% at 38 weeks (A = 2,380 g, B = 1,790 g). (Reprinted with permission from Wiggelsworth and Singer, *Textbook of Fetal and Perinatal Pathology,* Chapter 8, Blackwell Scientific Publications, 1991:235.)

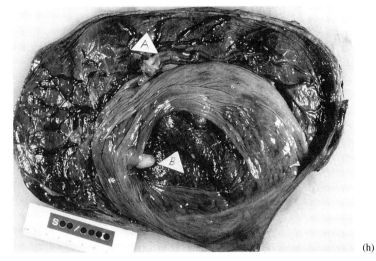

(h)

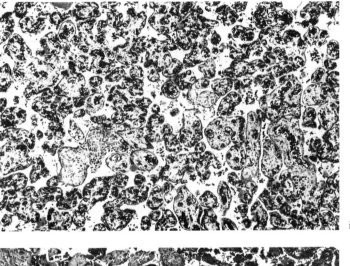

i(A)

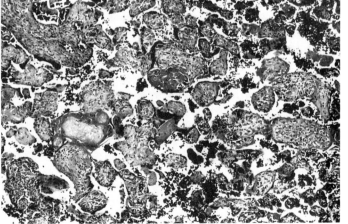

i(B)

40% of those with placental findings, the only abnormality was a concordantly smaller placental mass, mainly in the mild and moderate groups; in 16.7% there was an umbilical cord abnormality; in 35.7% there was parenchymal disease; and in the remainder there were mixtures of findings. How many of these differences were genetically determined in these presumably dizygotic twins and how many were due to other influences is not determined.

Finally, there are some additional comments and observations worth noting. The importance of correct identification of the umbilical cords at delivery and careful attention to birth order assignments in the pathologic examination and description should be obvious from the results of this analysis. There were few cases with pathologic evidence of fetal vascular perfusion problems, such as mural thrombi in chorionic or deeper vessels or hemorrhagic endovasculopathy, five cases in all, across the groups. There were two monoamniotic pairs, one each in the mild and marked groups, both female sets, with a velamentous cord for the smaller twin and one artery to artery anastomosis in the mild group case, and fewer chorionic vascular units but no anastomoses identified in the case in the marked group. In one of the moderate group sets, the portion of the dichorionic placenta for the smaller twin of the female pair had an unusual number of trophoblastic cysts, an observation of unknown significance. In both the marked and severe group were several cases where the sac and chorionic tissue of the smaller twin was almost completely encircled by the larger twin and this encircled chorionic tissue was ischemic (Fig. 6.2h). This too remains unexplained. In 4 of the 15 known in vitro fertilization–embryo transfer pregnancies in the Survey '91 Review, the twin sets were discordant by 15.7% to 44.5%. All were dichorionic fused placentas with no lesions in the two unlike sex sets, discordant perivillus fibrin in the female pair, and in the fourth there was a smaller chorionic volume with decreased chorionic vascularization and parenchymal ischemic changes with fibrinosis in a female pair. In the nine known cases of Clomid- induced live-born twins, there were two discordant sets, 22.4% and 40%, both dichorionic fused placenta male pairs with ischemic changes on the smaller twin's side in both.

In summary, a number of abnormalities of placentation have been observed in these cases of growth discordant surviving live-born twins, and many of them may be significant as causal factors in the impaired growth of the smaller twin. Caution is warranted, however, as these findings are all seen with normally grown twins, and the element of degree of influence, particularly when there is more than one abnormality, may not be determinable. It is important to note that while many of these cases could be detected antenatally, probably none of these conditions is preventable and the majority are likely a result of the fact that the conception is twins instead of a singleton. Amelioration of the discordance does not seem to be a consideration in this group, although appropriate perinatal care of the very small fetuses would be facilitated by antepartum diagnosis and investigations to rule out other causes of discordant growth. It is noteworthy that in only one of these 284 sets was there discordant fetal pathology, a monochorionic set with discordant Wiedemann-Beckwith syndrome. This might suggest that the absence of detectable fetal anomaly is a favorable prognostic sign with growth discordant twins.

From this same group of live-born surviving twins, there were an additional 13 sets with one or both twins (total 21) growth retarded, but with concordant or minimally divergent growth. There were three times as many female twins in this small group, eight sets were monochorionic, three sets with dichorionic fused placentas, and two with dichorionic separate placentas. Nine sets were female pairs, three monochorionic sets were male pairs, and the unlike-sex pair had a dichorionic separate placentation. None of these twins were much less than a week delayed in growth and the associated pathology in the placenta mirrored the distribution noted above. It is not known why these 13 sets were more concordantly grown than the others except that they probably represent the left hand tail of the normal curve.

Autopsy Group

A number of difficulties were encountered during the review of the Survey '91 autopsy series for growth-discordant twins, and this has led to two important recommendations regarding procedures to be followed in reporting twin autopsies. This series spanned 33 years of reporting and the awareness of these requirements obviously increased in the latter years, but they still should be emphasized. The most important observation is that twin mortality cannot be assessed adequately in the absence of information about the co-twin or the placenta. This comment will be self-evident to those with a special interest in twins, but is not appreciated fully by many investigators. The degree to which twins are equally affected by a disorder in question may have significance for interpretation and counseling. For example, concordantly growth-retarded twins may be due to a different problem than when only one twin is affected. This in turn has a direct relationship to the type of twinning. It was noted in Chapter 3 that if the sex of both twins and the pattern of placentation are known, zygosity can be assigned in just over 50% of cases. Also, the importance of monochorionic monozygosity as a source of difficulties for twins is emphasized throughout this book. Determining that twin mortality is attributable to some factor within the twin set has considerably different counseling impact than detecting a lesion that may recur, such as a recessive hereditary disorder. Finally, the importance of the gross and microscopic findings in the placenta to the analysis of fetal growth has been demonstrated amply by the preceding discussion, and it is no less important when analyzing twin death.

It is suggested therefore that any report of a twin autopsy include details of the placental findings and a description of the co-twin, with interpretations of these details as they relate to the death under investigation. Only then can the autopsy findings be placed in perspective. These recorded details should include the respective birth observations—weight, length measurements, Apgar scores, blood gas studies, and any other relevant information—and comments on the perinatal course of the survivor. This is true whether the twins died perinatally or as infants, because the details of their condition at birth may be related to what happened neonatally and later on prior to their death. If the co-twin was autopsied, the twins can be reported as a combined report if they were autopsied together. Alternatively, information should be provided in the later report about the twin reported first, if they are autopsied at different times. It is best if the placental examination is part of the autopsy, but this is not reasonable if the twins survive more than a few hours. In that case, the findings must be reiterated in the autopsy report and correlated with the autopsy

results. Accurate identification of the portions of the placentation for each twin and careful designation of the sides in the report are essential to meaningful interpretation of any findings. Just what details are relevant will depend on the individual case, but the significance of some observations may not be apparent at first review, so the selection of what data to include should be generous. It is true that reports of co-twin autopsies or placental findings may be in "the system" somewhere, but it surely makes more sense to all concerned to have the relevant data in one place.

The other recommendation for twin autopsy reporting relates to the assessment of fetal growth. Measurements of linear growth and weight are not always concordant in a growth-impaired twin and are always modified by maceration. Fetal weight can fluctuate widely without comparable effects on linear measurements, such as crown–heel, crown–rump, or foot length. Thus, linear measurements are more valid standards in those cases of excessive weight due to fetal edema, for example, or when there is tissue loss (and therefore weight loss) with maceration. Better still, all measures of linear growth and body and visceral weights should be assessed as a unit. For example, the heart of an hydropic twin may seem to be normal in weight if compared to the body weight, but will be seen to be excessive when compared to the expected weight for the twin's linear growth. This becomes an important pathologic finding in the context of the hydropic twin, and would have been missed if the proper comparisons were not made. Similarly, a liver that is the expected weight for a twin of a certain crown–heel length, may be abnormal if that twin is macerated. With maceration, there is tissue loss, and an organ that seems to be of normal weight was likely heavier than the normal before death, and that observation needs to be explained. These considerations are also critical when one tries to assess the time of death of a long dead co-twin—retained macerated or fetus papyraceous. The problems differentiating sudden fetal death with appropriate growth for age at death and fetal death superimposed on growth retardation are discussed in Chapter 5.

The Survey '91 autopsy cases were reviewed to assess growth impairment in a manner analogous to the review of the survivor group. Cases excluded from the analysis were conjoined or asymmetrically duplicated twins, fetus papyraceous, and retained macerated twins. The caveats noted above further limited the number of cases suitable for analysis to 165 sets where one or both twins came to autopsy, but information was available on both twins, and an additional 73 twins were assessable individually for the presence of growth retardation. From these, there were 65 pairs with growth discordance greater than 15%, eight pairs with one or both growth retarded but more concordantly grown, and another eight growth-retarded twins. The discordant sets were analyzed like those in the survivor group and are reported in Table 6.3 for comparison. As might be expected, the autopsy group contained greater discrepancies with the twins delivered earlier in gestation and a higher proportion of actual growth retardation of the smaller twin. Like-sex pairs were more frequent in the autopsy group, likely reflecting the higher proportion of monochorionic sets. The ratio of dichorionic fused to separate placentas in the autopsied group was the opposite of the ratio in the survivor group, but no pattern emerged from which to suggest an explanation. While problems of placental development and the presence of placental parenchymal disease were noted in a number of cases, twin transfusion syndrome and fetal anomalies were far more important in the autopsy series. Even so, except for the severe group, the number of monochorionic placentas exceeded the number of cases of twin transfusion syndrome by 18% to 50%, a discrepancy already noted in the survivor group. In one set, both twins were small for gestational age, but no cause was identified, in one set the larger twin was large for age, and both these sets were in the mild group. In two cases, it was the larger co-twin who died, and the smaller twin died twice as often as both twins died.

In the autopsy group of discordant twins, the associated placental findings mirrored those in the survivor group. Abnormalities such as those shown in Fig. 6.2 were seen with additional examples in Fig. 6.3. Virtually all of the associated anomalous cord insertions were velamentous, and discordant chorionic volumes were seen. There were two sets with discordant placental involvement with cytomegalovirus, a fused dichorionic unlike-sex pair at 23 weeks and monochorionic female twins at 22 weeks with superimposed twin transfusion findings, both in the moderate group. Perivillus fibrin was reported much less frequently in the autopsy

group, and ischemic changes somewhat less often.

The anomalies in the autopsy group that were considered important as a cause for growth discordance consisted of discordant major abnormalities. Two-thirds were dichorionic sets—trisomy 18, renal agenesis with neural defects as well, anal agenesis, and anencephaly. The placentation was not recorded in cases with diaphragmatic hernia or lumbosacral meningomyelocele. Caudal regression was present in one of monochorionic twins, and microcephaly with Werdnig-Hoffmann lesions in one of monoamniotic twins. The anomalies of twins are discussed in Chapter 7.

The autopsy cases of growth retardation without discordant growth greater than 15% consisted of 24 individuals. The degree of growth impairment ranged from just below the 10th percentile for age to delays of up to 8 weeks. As noted with the survivor twins, the small twin was female twice as often as male, compared to the male predominance in the discordant group. The other characteristics of this group were not appreciably different from the findings in the concordant group of survivor twins.

Survey '91 Twins—Summary

In summary, intrauterine growth impairment of twins is common, even using twin-derived standards, but it is not a homogeneous condition. Growth discordance of greater than 15% is often associated with discordant placental developmental abnormalities and parenchymal disease, particularly in the survivor group, although the pathophysiologic connection remains to be determined. Fetal anomalies and twin transfusion syndromes are more important in cases of growth discordance with twin mortality, but in neither the survivor nor the autopsy series are all discordantly grown monochorionic twins affected by the twin transfusion syndrome. Prevention does not seem to be a reasonable avenue to pursue as many of the associated pathologies are features of the twin conception, but antepartum identification of the presence and degree of growth impairment may influence perinatal care of the mother and infants. From the data, it would appear that the earlier the growth impairment is identified and the greater the discordance, the more likely it is to be associated with fetal or perinatal death. Finally, any pathologic evaluation of twins at autopsy

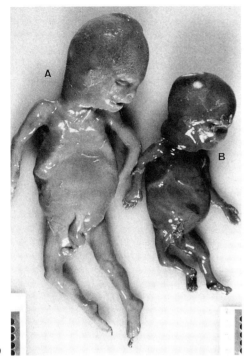

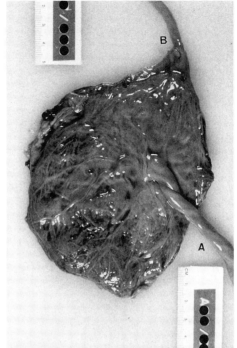

FIGURE 6.3. Placental findings in discordantly grown autopsied twins. (a,b) Discordant placental volume with possible twin transfusion, acute on chronic. Monochorionic female twins stillborn at 21 weeks, 2 weeks after clinical fetal death. Growth discordance by linear measurements equivalent to 5 weeks (A = 21 weeks, B = 16 weeks) (a). Asymmetric placental vascularization with cord A serving 9/10 and cord B 1/10 of chorionic surface

(b). One arterial anastomosis is discernible; injection was not successful due to postmortem changes. Discordant heart size for body size suggested chronic twin transfusion but the relative pallor of the larger twin suggested acute reversal before death. The relative role of discordant placental volumes and twin transfusion is difficult to establish.

is best done with consideration of the details of the placentation and findings in the co-twin.

Infection

Infections in twins can be considered in three patterns—acquired in utero, acquired perinatally or neonatally and twin related, and postnatal infections unrelated to twinning. The pathology of the infection is no different because it is in a twin. The importance is whether the infection is concordant or not, and what that may indicate about pathogenesis. Twins are reported to die as a consequence of infection in the newborn period at a rate equivalent to singletons.[50] A 6% rate of perinatal death due to infection has been reported, with twin B succumbing four times as often as twin A, although twin A

was described as being septicemic more often than twin B.[49] Congenital infection is said to be more often discordant when ascending and concordant when hematogenously acquired,[68] although there are striking exceptions that may be related to placental or fetal factors.

Infections In Utero

Infections that must have been acquired in utero can have different manifestations in multiple pregnancies, patterns that do not fit with the usual concepts of pathophysiology. Infections accepted as being hematogenously spread from the mother would theoretically be the same risk to the placenta of either twin. However, there are well recognized cases where only one twin is affected, or both are infected but only one has clinical disease. Alterna-

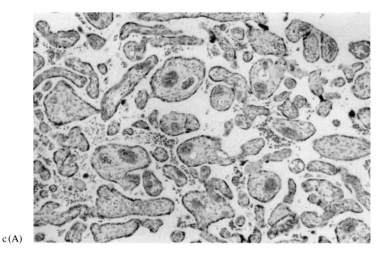

c(A)

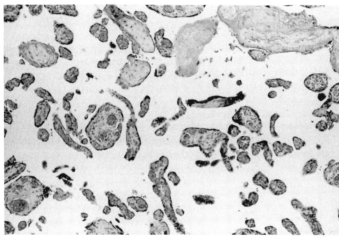

c(B)

FIGURE 6.3. *Continued.* (c) Discordant placental volumes and maternal perfusion. Dichorionic fused placenta (A = 3/4, B = 1/4) with marked villus hypotrophy and ischemic changes in B's portion, but normal villi on side A. Male twins of undetermined zygosity at 26 to 28 weeks, discordant by 53.7% (A = 1,080 g, B = 500 g). Twin A died at 6 hours of age from hyaline membrane disease with barotrauma, including left tension pneumothorax; growth retarded twin B died at 55 minutes of age. (Hematoxylin and eosin, original magnification ×12.5.) (Reprinted with permission from Baldwin VJ, *Developmental Pathology of the Embryo and Fetus,* JB Lippincott, 1992:330.)

tively, those infections considered to have ascended into the uterus and thereby affecting the presenting infant may be shown to affect both infants. Genetically based differences in fetal resistance or the placental barrier to infection could explain discordant fetal response to infection, but other explanations may be needed in some cases. Unfortunately, much of the literature makes little or no reference to placental pattern or histology in many of these cases. The following reports exemplify these comments.

Transplacental Infections

Hematogenously derived transplacental infection can have several patterns. Concordant fetal infection as evidenced by immunologic methods, but with clinically discordant disease, has been reported for rubella,[69,70] toxoplasmosis,[71,72] cytome-galovirus,[73,74] and echovirus 11.[75] Discordant infection and disease, leaving one twin ill or dead and the other twin normal, has been reported for cytomegalovirus,[76-78] syphilis[79] and *Listeria.*[80] Most of these twins were assumed dizygotic because they were of unlike-sex. Unfortunately, the placental histology was not reported in the majority of cases, so that there was no indication whether there was discordant placental involvement as well. Toxoplasmosis is reportedly concordant in monozygotic twins and discordant in dizygotic twins.[81] All three female infants of a triplet set were described as being equally infected, but unfortunately there was no mention of placental morphology nor any indication of zygosity.[82] There is an intriguing report of a maternal death due to systemic coccidioidomycosis 24 hours after delivery.[83] There was no demonstrable infection of the uterus or placenta, but

FIGURE 6.3 *Continued* (d,e) Discordant placental volumes and microscopic features, underlying problem not clarified. Monochorionic placenta with asymmetric U-shaped parenchymal mass, both cords marginal; larger cord with vessels limited to larger mass, smaller cord with vessels to smaller mass and through membranes to larger mass (d). No vascular anastomoses were detected by injection and while heart of the small twin was small for age, the heart of the larger twin was normal for age, both observations suggesting twin transfusion was not a factor. Female twins were freshly stillborn and discordant by 20% in crown–heel length and weight at 23 weeks (e). Villi of the larger lobe of placenta were mature for age with sclerosis of fetal vessels, while villi of the smaller lobe were immature with villus edema and intravillus hemorrhage.

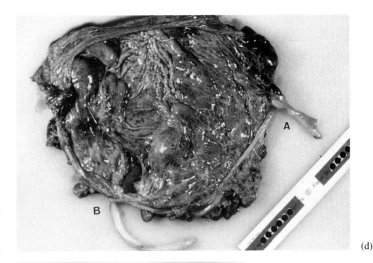

(d)

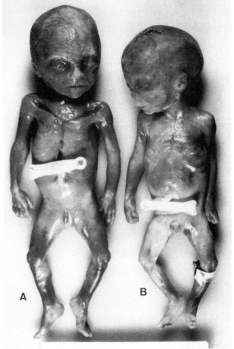

(e)

obvious congenital infection of both females who died of the disease; zygosity was not indicated.

One report reviewed cytomegalovirus infection related to chorionicity and zygosity.[78] Monochorionic monozygotic twins were regularly concordantly infected. Known dizygotic twins with separate dichorionic placentas were all discordantly infected. These two patterns are readily explained by genetic factors influencing resistance to infection, concordantly in monozygotic twins and dis-

cordantly in dizygotic twins. Monozygotic twins with dichorionic placentas, fused or separate, could not be identified from the literature. Dizygotic twins with fused placentas had a mixed pattern of infection, some pairs concordant and some discordant. It was suggested that the less resistant placenta and fetus was infected, and then perhaps the infection spread within the placenta to the adjacent fetus. These authors emphasized the importance of including adequate data on placental morphology in any report of infections in twins. In their review, they noted that uninfected infants had uninflamed placentas, and most infected infants had infected placentas, but not all. In a dichorionic dizygotic pair with separate placentas, the male twin was infected and died, the female twin was normal, and no signs of placental infection were found in either placenta.[76] A fused dichorionic placenta of male twins (zygosity not reported) was histologically normal, although one twin died of cytomegalovirus infection and the other twin was also infected, but less severely affected and it survived.[74] These observations remain unexplained unless mitotic crossing-over can lead to differential resistance to infection in the fetus and placenta after the twinning event has determined the pattern of placentation.[84]

Twins infected with the human immunodeficiency virus (HIV) have attracted special interest. Vertical (hematogenous) transmission of HIV is well recognized and the general rate is estimated to be 24% to 33% with an estimated rate of 25% with twins.[85] Studies of rates of fetal infection and birth order in 66 sets of twins suggest that while some infants may be infected in utero before labor, a substantial proportion of HIV-1 transmission occurs as the first twin encounters the cervix and birth canal.[86] In this review, 50% of first-born twins delivered vaginally, and 38% of first-born twins delivered by section were infected, compared to 19% of second-born twins by either route. Concordance of HIV-1 infection status was greater in monozygotic (82%) than dizygotic (60%) sets, but frequency and clinical signs of HIV-1–related disease were similar in only 3 of the 10 sets with both children infected. In another review of 11 twin gestations of 10 HIV-positive mothers, all infants were seropositive at birth, but 75% seroreverted. All infected same-sex twin pairs and half the infected unlike-sex pairs were concordant for infection. One study observed an unexpected number of twins in a cohort of pediatric acquired immunodeficiency syndrome (AIDS) due to vertical transmission.[87] While it was suggested that the mothers might have a propensity for bearing twins, or that twins are somehow more likely to become infected, it was concluded that twins may be more severely affected at an early age due to prematurity and low birth weight, and were thus overrepresented in the early years of surveillance. Postnatal acquisition of AIDS that could be attributed in part to the twinning

occurred in a second twin delivered at term by section.[88] The infant was asphyxiated at birth and had a prolonged hospital course requiring 18 blood transfusions for iatrogenic blood loss. One of the donors had been asymptomatic at the time of donation, but developed the disease later.

Ascending Infection

Infection that gains access to the uterine contents from the maternal vagina/cervix is often called ascending infection, and the accepted pattern is that the lowest or first-presenting twin is the only one infected, or the more severely affected if both are infected.[89] An analysis of preterm twin labor with intact membranes found positive cultures of amniotic fluid taken by amniocentesis from eight sacs in five patients, 10.8%.[90] The presenting sac was involved in all cases, but in three of the five cases both sacs provided positive cultures, although the colony count in the second sac was considerably lower than from the first sac. In two of these three patients, there were polymicrobial cultures from the first sac. Four of these five patients had dichorionic placentas, one was monochorionic, but the sex and zygosity of the infants was not mentioned. Only the two cases with *Fusobacterium nucleatum* isolates had clinical chorioamnionitis, but no placental histology was reported. Without these details, it is difficult to assess the reported results. An interesting case was that of quintuplets with five separate chorionic gestational sacs.[91] Group B streptococci were grown from the maternal cervix during labor, and the organisms ascended through intact membranes. Not only was quint A infected with mild chorioamnionitis as well, so were the other four infants. It might be suspected that infection of the second sac would occur across the common membranes if the infection in the first sac was of sufficient intensity. Transmembrane infection of all five sacs, with only mild histologic chorioamnionitis in all sacs, may speak for the virulence of the organism, although all five infants survived after mild illness.

Survey '91 Congenital Infections

In the Survey '91 autopsy series, there were 8 twins with congenital infection, 11 with infection in the perinatal/neonatal period or later that represented complications of being a twin, and 6 twins with

TABLE 6.4a. Infections in twins from the Survey '91 autopsy series: congenital infections.

Case	Organism	Lesion	Affected twin*	Placental findings**	Co-twin†
1	Coxsackie B4	Encephalomyocarditis	37/F/A ? F/B	DF—uninfected	–
2	Cytomegalovirus	Systemic infection	22/F/A MZ F/B	M—both portions infected	–
3	Cytomegalovirus	Systemic infection	23/M/A DZ	DF—side A infected	F—questionable infection
4	Not identified	Pneumonia	21/M/A DZ	DF—chorioamnionitis A >> B	F—not infected
5	*Listeria*	Systemic infection	28/M/A ?	?	M—survived ? infected

*Gestational age in weeks/sex/birth order/zygosity; F, female; M, male; MZ, monozygotic; DZ, dizygotic; ? = not stated.
**Placental form/histology; DF, dichorionic fused; DS, dichorionic separate; M, monochorionic.
†Sex/outcome; F, female; M, male; D, died.
Case comments:
1. Emergency section for acute maternal abdominal pain and fever. Twins well until day 3 (B) and 4 (A), died within 48 hours. Organism cultured from mother and both infants.
2. Preterm delivery because of twin transfusion syndrome. Concordant involvement of viscera and placenta at death at 4 hours age.
3. Cause of preterm delivery not stated; both died at age 2 hours. Only possible sign of infection in co-twin was very focal positive immunoperoxidase staining in brain.
4. Preterm delivery due to premature rupture of membranes with ascending infection. Both died within 2 hours with early bronchiolar cell necrosis.
5. Mother ill and treated for listeriosis 1 week before delivery; twin A positive culture at birth, lived 12 days.

other infections. All these infections were considered central to the cause of death. This represents 5.5% of all autopsied twins in the series and 5.9% of all twin sets, and this incidence agrees with the majority of the reported series. The details of these cases are summarized in Table 6.4.

The patterns of congenital infection seen follow the reported cases. Viral infections were the most common, 75%, and least concordant with the known dizygotic pair. Although 10% of sets of preterm twins have been reported to have positive cultures from amniotic fluid,[90] unequivocal congenital pneumonia in twin A associated with discordant chorioamnionitis was diagnosed in only one pair of the autopsy series. This diagnosis was accepted only if the aspirated polymorphonuclear leukocytes were accompanied by pulmonary interstitial acute inflammation.

Perinatal/Neonatal Infections

In the 11 cases of perinatal/neonatal or later infection, the infection was the final insult after various problems that arose from complications associated with being a premature twin. The infected twin was sometimes small and/or asphyxiated, both problems potentially contributing to decreased resistance to infection. In others, the infection was superimposed on lungs already badly damaged by the sequelae of the idiopathic respiratory distress syndrome. In infants with bronchopulmonary dysplasia, there were often focal clusters of acute inflammatory cells, but even in the few with more marked acute inflammation, postmortem cultures were negative. Most of these infants were on a variety of antibiotics during life for positive cultures from the endotracheal tube and this likely limited successful cultures of lung tissue. Also, it was sometimes several days before the parents were prepared to grant autopsy permission when the neonatal course had been so complex, and this delay also reduced the success of cultures. The source of the infecting agent was not known in the majority of cases, although it was considered likely to be nosocomial because of the interval since birth.

There was no particular pattern to the details of the twins with other infections. These were considered to be complications not directly related to the twin status and were infections acquired postnatally.

Neoplasia

While neoplasia seems to have a lower prevalence in twins than in singletons,[68,92] perhaps particularly in male twins,[93] a variety of relationships between

TABLE 6.4b. Infections in twins from the Survey '91 autopsy series: perinatal/neonatal infections.

Case	Organism	Lesion	Affected twin*	Contributing factors**	Co-twin†
1	*Staphylococcus aureus*	Necrotizing pneumonia	29/F/B/8d ?/DF	LBW/PA	F—no problems
2	*Staphylococcus aureus*	Pneumonia with abscesses	25/M/B/23d DZ/NR	BPD	F—D2 days; HMD; PIE; PT; GEH
3	Not identified	Bronchopneumonia	24/M/A/9mo DZ/DS	BPD	M—D17½hrs; HMD; PIE; PT
4	Not identified	Pneumonia; aspiration	37/F/A/16d ?/DS	PA; severe HIE	F—no problems
5	*Candida*	Systemic infection	24/F/A/17d MZ/M	NEC with peritonitis	F—D9 hrs; HMD; PIE; PT
6	*Candida*	Septicemia	30/F/A/9d ?/DF	SGA	F—D37 hrs; HMD; GEH
7	*Pseudomonas*	Bronchopneumonia	30/M/B/40 hrs DZ/DS	Unknown	F—D; no autopsy
8	Hemolytic streptococcus	Septicemia	28/M/B/2d ?/?	Unknown	?—no information
9	*Escherichia coli*	Meningitis	29/F/B/53d ?/?	PA	"survived"—no details
10	*Klebsiella pneumoniae*	Septicemia	28/M/B/30d ?/DS	Not identified	–
11	*Candida*	Systemic	28/M/A/7 mo ?/DS	Uncertain	–

*Gestational age (weeks)/sex (F, female; M, male)/birth order/age at death. Zygosity (DZ, dizygotic; MZ, monozygotic; ?, not stated)/placental form (DF, dichorionic fused; DS, dichorionic separate; M, monochorionic; NR, not reported).

**LBW, low birth weight; PA, perinatal asphyxia; BPD, bronchopulmonary dysplasia; HIE, hypoxic ischemic encephalopathy; NEC, necrotizing enterocolitis; SGA, small for gestational age.

†F, female; M, male; D, died; HMD, hyaline membrane disease; PIE, pulmonary interstitial emphysema; PT, pneumothorax; GEH, germinal eminence hemorrhage.

Case comments:

1. Cause of perterm delivery not stated. Reasons for low birth weight and asphyxia not identified.
2. Cause of preterm delivery not stated.
3. Twins dizygotic by blood groups. Cause of preterm delivery not stated.
4. Undiagnosed second twin delivered by emergency section after cord prolapse. Repeated aspiration attributed to severe hypoxic ischemic encephalopathy and caused diffuse alveolar damage. Lung cultures negative but gram-positive cocci seen in gastrointestinal tract.
5. Cause of preterm delivery not stated.
6. Growth discordant by 27%, with 50% smaller chorionic volume and marginal cord. Cause of preterm delivery not stated.
7. Cause of preterm delivery not stated.
8. Cause of preterm delivery not stated.
9. Meningitis in first week of life led to aqueductal gliosis and hydrocephalus. At death also had necrotizing enteropathy, patent ductus arteriosus, oxygen retinopathy, and hepatic changes of intravenous alimentation. Cause of preterm delivery not stated.
10. Cause of preterm delivery not stated. Predisposing factors uncertain as lung findings minimal in both. Longer lived twin had hypoxic ischemic encephalopathy, nondiagnostic hepatomegaly and nephromegaly.
11. Cause of preterm delivery not stated.

twinning and tumors have been assessed and reported.

A variety of tumors have been associated with some malformation syndromes, congenital functional defects (particularly immunologic), and chromosomal errors (especially trisomy 21).[94,95] It is possible that these tumors could be encountered if the associated disorder was present in one or both twins, but this relationship has not been addressed specifically in references to cancer and twins. There is one report of a cerebral tumor in the twin of an infant with hereditary microcephaly,[96] and a report of concordant cardiac rhabdomyomas, although other signs of tuberose sclerosis were not identified and zygosity assessment was questionable.[97]

The occurrence of sacrococcygeal teratomas has been related to twinning.[98] It was noted that 7.5% of those affected were one of twins, and twinning

TABLE 6.4c. Infections in twins from the Survey '91 autopsy series: other infections.

Case	Organism	Lesion	Affected twin(s)*	Comment
1	Coxsackie B2	Myocarditis and meningoencephalitis	35/F/A/recovered F/B/8d ?/DS	Mother not ill; placentas not infected; predisposing factors unknown; source of infection unknown
2	Escherichia coli	Meningitis	31/F/B/6d ?/DF	Mother, placenta, and co-twin uninfected; predisposing factors and source unknown
3	Staphylococcus aureus	Meningitis	?/M/?/8years ?/?	"Premature"; meningitis age 5 weeks with postmeningitic hydrocephalus; predisposing factors and source not stated
4	Bacteroides	Colitis with intramesenteric abscess	?/M/B/17mos ?/?	"Premature"; had colonic aganglionosis with three operations; reason for ulcer in transverse colon not known; status of co-twin not stated

*Gestational age (weeks)/sex (F, female; M, male)/birth order/age at death. Zygosity (?, not stated)/placentation (DS, dichorionic separate; DF, dichorionic fused).

occurred in the families of 50% of those responding to a follow-up questionnaire. The significance of these observations is not known, but they are thought-provoking. Teratomas are tumors and caudal duplications are anomalies of twinning—occasionally it is not easy to be sure where the borderline exists between tumorous and teratomatous growth.[99,100] Anterior cervical teratomas are rare, but one has been reported in a dizygotic dichorionic male twin with a normal female co-twin.[101] Ovarian mature teratomas (cystic dermoids) have been reported in twins and triplets but the relationship to twinning of these tumors encountered in the third and fourth decade of life remains to be determined.[102,103]

The degree to which tumors affect both members of the twin pair seems to depend on the type of study as well as the tumor. Single-case reports of neoplasia in twins suggest that there is an increased risk of concordance for the same or similar tumors at nearly the same time. Reported tumors have included cystic ovarian dermoids,[102,103] neuroblastoma,[104] Wilms' tumor,[105] neurofibromatosis,[106,107] cardiac rhabdomyomas,[97] and gliomas.[108] Some congenital tumors have a strong genetic component, perhaps indicating a special class of malformation, and these could be expected to appear simultaneously in monozygotic twins.[99] Unfortunately, in many of the single case reports, the basis for statements of monozygosity is not given. Discordant congenital giant pigmented nevus in twins identified as "identical" by DNA studies, or blood group and human leukocyte antigen (HLA) system findings, has suggested a role for nongenetic factors in the production of this tumor.[109,110] Tumors could be discordant in monozygotic twins if they were concordant for a first mutation that conferred cancer proneness, but the second promoting mutation depended on intrauterine or postnatal "environmental" exposures.[111]

Broad-based population studies do not support an increased risk for concordance of tumors in twins, with the possible exception of leukemia and renal cancer, but agreement is not universal even on these.[92,93,112] A review of 440 children with Wilms' tumor in 1964 identified only one example of concordant tumor in twins,[113] but another study 12 years later identified a rate of Wilms' tumors that was four times the expected rate in twins and 80% of such tumors occurred in concordant monozygotic pairs.[92] The subject of leukemia in twins has received considerable attention and it has been suggested that if leukemia is diagnosed in one twin under a year of age, the other twin should be examined. Concordance for leukemia has been reported as high as 10 : 1 in monozygotic pairs, and the leukemia in the concordant twin was diagnosed within a month in 75% of such twin pairs.[112] Concordance was also identified in early childhood leukemia, late childhood leukemia, and adult-onset leukemia in monozygotic twins, but the greatest concordance was in the perinatal-congenital period. This concordance pattern has suggested that there may be genetic or environmental factors unique to monozygosity that are important to the instigation of leukemia—possibly a carcinogen or cancer cell exchange across anastomotic vessels, or disturbances of the genome secondary to the monovular origin of the twins.[114] One potential factor in concordant carcinogenesis in twins may be radiation—a 2.4 times greater risk of childhood cancer was noted in twins who had been subject to prenatal x-ray examination. The use of ultrasound instead of conventional x-rays may reduce the significance of this factor.[115]

Neither grossly visible nor microscopic in situ tumors were recorded in any of the twins in the Survey '91 autopsy series.

System-Related and Other Disorders

Twins are vulnerable to the same diseases as singletons, but some reported cases of concordant or discordant disease in twins are instructive regarding the pathophysiology of the disorder in question. However, the number of examples of each disorder is small, so biases of ascertainment and reporting must be kept in mind when reviewing these reports. Those conditions with a known hereditary component would be expected to be concordant in monozygotic twins and discordant in a variable number of dizygotic twins, depending on the inheritance pattern and genetic contribution. Discordant manifestations in apparently monozygotic twins may be due to phenomena such as dispermic monovular twinning (see Chapter 2), mitotic crossing-over,[84] or somatic mutation.[116] This section includes clinically evident functional disturbances that may have microscopic structural abnormalities, but excludes those disorders that are manifest mainly as structural malformations because these are discussed in Chapter 7. The reported problems are discussed in six groupings—endocrine, neuromuscular, cardiovascular, and miscellaneous disorders, sudden infant death syndrome, and neglect/abuse.

Endocrine

Endocrine-related disorders in twins have been described for the adrenal, thyroid, parathyroid, and pancreatic islet glands.

Microcystic changes of the outer adrenal cortex have been reported concordant in five out of nine twin pairs of less than 35 weeks gestational age.[117] In the one discordant set, the twin who had the lesion died just after delivery, while the twin who died at 17 days did not have the lesion, which suggests that the lesion might be due to some systemic disorder that can affect both twins, but may be reversible if the child survives. Alternatively, it may simply represent the state of immaturity, or the stress-related pseudofollicular pattern, either of which could be expected in stressed preterm twins, and both of which might resolve with time. Discordant genital manifestations of *congenital adrenal hyperplasia* in dichorionic separate female twins was initially attributed to dizygosity.[118] However, concordance of blood groups and subtypes, as well as rare heteromorphic markers on chromosomes confirmed monozygosity. The explanation of the dissimilar degree of virilization was not determined, although it was noted that the postnatal serum concentration of 17-OH progesterone was twice as high in the less-affected twin. This report suggests that monochorionic and dichorionic monozygotic twins may have differences that are more related to environment than genetics.

Discordant congenital *hypothyroidism* has been documented in 10 like-sex twin pairs (8 female), but monozygosity on the basis of monochorionic placentation or concordant blood cell antigens was established in only 6 pairs.[119] Discordant athyrotic hypothyroidism in one monochorionic set with possible twin transfusion syndrome is an example of a discordant metabolic/endocrine abnormality, in which the twin status may have influenced the manifestation of the disorder. It was the anemic and therefore possible donor twin who was hypothyroid, raising the possibility that thyrotropic hormones were lost across the anastomoses to an extent that deficiency of thyroid function was manifest postnatally. The co-twin was normal. Concordant congenital *hyperthyroidism* was reported in female twins that were termed "identical," but without any information as to how that was determined.[120] The condition resolved with residual brain damage in both girls. The cause was not identified because although the mother had a history of thyroid disease, this pregnancy was not affected.

A mother who had hypoparathyroidism delivered male twins of unstated zygosity who were concordant for congenital *hyperparathyroidism*.[121] One twin died at birth and the other twin died at 3 months of age, possibly of the sudden infant death syndrome or hydrocephalus secondary to intracranial hemorrhage that had occurred in the newborn period. When the findings in the two autopsies were compared, a notable improvement in bone growth and parathyroid abnormalities had occurred in the 3 months that the second twin survived. Discordant *neonatal rickets* was reported in monochorionic female twins with the affected twin manifesting a transient delay of maturation of renal 25-hydroxy-cholecalciferol-1-alpha hydroxylase enzyme.[122] The affected twin was normal by 20 weeks of age, while her co-twin never had any evidence of rickets or detectable enzyme abnormality. No cause for the differential maturation was apparent.

The potentially complex interaction of genetic predisposition and environmental influences is evident in studies of *diabetes mellitus* in twins.[123] When diabetes was manifest before 40 years of age, concordance in proven monozygotic twins (blood cell and serum protein studies) was less than 50%, but approached 100% when diabetes was first manifest after 40 years of age. However, diabetes mellitus, particularly the juvenile-onset form, is not a homogeneous disorder, and there are probably a number of factors to consider in assessing its distribution in twins.

Neuromuscular

Most of the attention to neuromuscular disorders in twins has focused on brain damage, particularly *cerebral palsy*. It has been pointed out that brain growth and development in twins is subject to environmental circumstances that may begin in utero and affect the twins unequally.[124] For example, the length of the umbilical cord may be a marker for in utero influences on neurologic development.[125] When the cord lengths of full-term same-sex siblings differed by more than 20 cm, those with the shorter cords more often had low IQ values and neurologic abnormalities than did their paired siblings. It is not yet known whether this same differential exists for siblings in utero together, as cord lengths are rarely mentioned in reports of twins with neurologic impairment.

The incidence of twins in any group of individuals afflicted with cerebral palsy is greater than in the normal population. In such twin sets, the first born has been reported to have cerebral palsy twice as often as the second born, but with increased mortality among the second born. In a detailed correlation of the type of cerebral palsy with birth order, there was discordance in all types.[126] It was concluded that the first twin suffered trauma as it dilated the cervix, leading to spastic diplegia, while the second twin was anoxic and either died or survived with tetraplegia, spastic, or athetoid. However, not all studies suggest an enhanced risk for brain damage in the second twin[127–129] (see Chapter 4 for discussion of perinatal asphyxia), and one report documented an increased risk for neurologic morbidity in larger twins.[128] Also, an analysis of genetic contributions to cerebral palsy noted that the motor handicaps in each concordant pair were very similar.[129] All concordant pairs were monozygotic and it was suggested that genetic factors could contribute to an individual's susceptibility to adverse environmental conditions. An important environmental condition unique to some twins is the presence of intertwin anastomoses on the placenta, and detrimental consequences of intertwin placental vascular anastomoses have been suggested as a mechanism for some types of brain damage in twins.[130–132] Unfortunately, reports of cerebral palsy in twins rarely include the anatomy of the placenta of the affected twins, so this concept of transvascular etiology for the lesions of cerebral palsy cannot be assessed.

Congenital *myasthenia gravis* was reportedly concordant in six like-sex female twin pairs, but discordant in three like-sex male twin pairs.[133] All pairs were called monozygotic, but in only one female pair was it stated to be by blood group studies. This distribution suggested a sex related differential that might be important to an understanding of the disorder, but no placental details were provided.

Cardiovascular

There are some diseases for which the cause is not known. Until the pathophysiology of such disorders is clarified, it is worthwhile to examine cases in twins carefully. For example, *idiopathic arterial calcification* of infancy is a rare condition of unknown pathogenesis. There are two reports of concordant involvement of like-sex twin sets, one male and one female, but in neither report is there a discussion of zygosity assignment or a description of placental findings.[134,135] The males were growth discordant by 35% and there was discordant hydrops in the female twins, suggesting some additional pathophysiology, but without information on the placentation further interpretations are not possible.

Carefully documented monozygotic female twins were concordant for severe *systemic hypertension,* retrospectively symptomatic in the perinatal period, but diagnosed at 10 months of age.[136] There was no relevant family history or definable cause for the hypertension, although both went on to have interstitial nephritis with severe medial hypertrophy of renal arterioles.

Miscellaneous System Disorders

Sometimes, when *nephrotic syndrome* occurs in infants, it is due to diffuse mesangial sclerosis. The pathophysiology has not been determined and familial instances are not common, but when mesangial sclerosis has been reported in twins, monozygotic concordance was high.[137] Unfortunately, the basis for the designation of monozygosity was not given, a recurring problem in twin literature. Male monozygotic twins studied at 18 years of age and concordant by erythrocytic antigens, were discordant for *paroxysmal nocturnal hemoglobinuria,* thought possibly to be on the basis of toxin exposure.[138] *Cystic fibrosis* is a known hereditary condition, but reports in twins are rare. Concordant meconium ileus was the presenting problem in discordantly grown (40%) twin girls delivered from a woman with cystic fibrosis, but there was no mention of zygosity or placental studies.[139]

Sudden Infant Death Syndrome

Sudden infant death syndrome (SIDS) has been reported to be twice as common in twins, with rates in all infants of 1.81/1,000 births, compared to all twins of 3.56/1,000,[140] and a relative risk of twin/singleton of 1.97.[141] The risk to second-born twins is debated. First-born twins have been reported to have a rate of 1.53/1,000, while second-born twins have nearly four times that risk, with a reported rate of 5.6/1,000.[140] Another report suggested the rela-

tive risk was less, twin B/twin A of 1.03.[142] No mention is made of concordance or zygosity, but the differential raises the question of the significance of the "second-twin syndrome," particularly in relation to perinatal asphyxia. An assessment of concordant SIDS suggested either a shared environment that could include exposure to pathogenetic organisms,[143] or coincidental trauma, either intentional or otherwise,[144] rather than concordant susceptibility on a genetic basis to the pathophysiologic events leading to sudden death.

Neglect/Abuse

In some societies, twins inspire fear, and for some families twins may simply be too much of a burden to care for, so that neglect and abuse may be encountered.[5] In one study, the predicted cases of abuse of twins based on the percentage of twins in the at-risk group under the age of 4 years was 6.2, but there were 16 cases observed, 2.6 times greater than expected.[145] In a study from India, twins died of malnutrition with 90 times greater frequency than singletons.[2] A study of abuse of twins in Japan found that both twins were abused when there were serious psychosocial or socioeconomic problems in the family, but that when only one twin was abused it was the one with medical problems, who was more difficult to care for.[146] Abuse of one twin was five times more common than abuse of both.

The Munchausen syndrome has been reported in a set of dizygotic twins who had repeated hospital admissions at age 5 months, with a history given of vomiting blood.[147] The source of the bleeding was never found. Some of the blood on the infants' bibs was maternal and, on one occasion, the mother was proven to have injured the lip of the female twin with a safety pin. It was suggested that the demands of caring for twins were too much for this mother, who created an apparent reason for the twins to be admitted to hospital, thus avoiding the burden temporarily.

Survey '91 Autopsy Cases

Infants with other diseases/disorders reported in the Survey '91 autopsy series were not numerous after fetomaternal interactions, complications of prematurity, and complications of monochorionic

TABLE 6.5. Other diseases/disorders in twins—Survey '91 autopsy series.

Disease/disorder	Twin involvement	Comment
Letterer-Siwe disease	Concordantly affected females; zygosity not known	Disease course and severity nearly identical; death at 12 mos and 15 mos
Generalized eczematoid ulcerative dermatitis with secondary infection and visceral venous thrombosis	Concordantly affected females; zygosity not known; one twin died age 4 mos; outcome other twin not known	Strong family history of allergies with skin manifestations; no diagnosis recorded, immunologic deficit not mentioned
Congenital nephrotic syndrome	Concordantly affected males; zygosity not known; one died at 2 mos; other died, findings not known	Microcystic kidneys with gonadal dysplasia in reported autopsied twin
Metachromatic leukodystrophy	Concordantly affected females; said to be "identical," but criteria not stated	Disease course and severity nearly identical; death at 6yr 3mos and 6yr 7mos
Hirschsprung's disease (aganglionic rectum)	Affected male; sex, zygosity and status co-twin not stated	Affected twin died age 17 mos with colitis and septicemia
Ideopathic pituitary hypoplasia	Affected male twin; female dichorionic (dizygotic) co-twin normal	Testes small, adrenals 1/10 normal with no fetal cortex; 5/10 sibs died as neonates, 1 at 20 mos with liver tumor; no other information
Idiopathic serous effusions without cutaneous edema	Unilaterally affected dichorionic male; sex of co-twin not stated, apparently normal	Lungs 1/2 expected weight; no underlying problem identified
Hydrops fetalis—cause not determined—? lymphatic disorder	Discordantly affected monochorionic female B; co-twin mildly growth retarded (velamentous cord and 1/3 placental volume) but no excess fluid	No evidence acute or chronic twin transfusion; hydropic twin anemic with extensive intravillus hemorrhage in placenta; serous effusions with high lymphocyte counts
Hydrops fetalis—with unequal growth and congenital heart disease	Discordantly affected monochorionic females; hydropic twin anemic with endocardial fibroelastosis of right ventricle, died 10½ hours; co-twin small for gestational age, died at 18 days of bronchopulmonary dysplasia	Growth discordance possibly due to twin transfusion syndrome but relative hematocrits not typical (fetomaternal hemorrhage from hydropic twin not ruled out)
Hydrops fetalis—cause undetermined	Concordant in monochorionic males; no cause found, one twin slightly more edematous	No signs of chronic or acute twin transfusion syndrome
Hydrops fetalis with idiopathic arterial calcification	Discordant monochorionic males; hydropic twin with arterial calcification, macerated stillbirth; mildly edematous co-twin with no vessel pathology died <24 hours with hyaline membrane disease and barotrauma	Possibility of chronic twin transfusion leading to vascular injury and calcification in recipient not separable from possibility of discordant vessel disease causing hydrops with vascular anastomoses incidental
Hydrops fetalis—cause undetermined	Discordant monochorionic males; cause of hydrops not determined; co-twin mildly small for age possibly on basis discordant placental disease (perivillus fibrin and infarcts), cords not identified, not edematous	Both twins growth impaired from midpregnancy (placenta ischemia); both twins with low albumin and low platelets; no explanation of differential hydrops

monozygosity were excluded. Twelve sets of twins were identified in the series and they are summarized in Table 6.5. The most interesting findings relate to the twin sets that had hydrops fetalis/serous effusions—a rather remarkable 50% of the cases.

Five of the six pairs were discordantly affected monochorionic sets, and in none of these was twin-to-twin transfusion syndrome considered an adequate explanation, or even possible, considering the placental vascular anatomy. This is an important observation, as it is typically described that the recipient of a chronic twin-to-twin transfusion syndrome is hydropic. These cases point out that not all hydropic monochorionic twins can be considered to be the result of imbalances across intertwin vascular anastomoses; in occasional cases, there may be other pathophysiologic processes involved, although the underlying problem may not be identified, even after a thorough autopsy. (See Chapter 9 for a further discussion of twin transfusion syndrome.)

One curious microscopic observation was adrenal cytomegaly. This was noted in four sets of twins without the usual associated Wiedemann-Beckwith syndrome.[148] All twins were live- born (20–27 weeks' gestation) and all had died by 10 hours of age. The lesion was discordant in two dichorionic unlike-sex sets, one male and one female, and associated with cytomegalovirus infection in the former but only prematurity in the latter. In two sets, both twins had the lesion but it was discordant in degree. In monochorionic twin girls with ascending infection, twin A had more infection and bilateral diffuse cytomegaly, while the lesion was focal in the co-twin. In a dichorionic male twin set (zygosity not established) the infants were 21% discordant by weight and the lesion was diffuse and bilateral in the larger twin and focal in the smaller. These may be examples of differences in stress and pituitary/steroid responses, but more cases are needed.

Summary

Many of the causes of morbidity in twins described in this chapter will not be reflected in an autopsy series as reported here, but the pathologist has an important contribution nonetheless. Growth impairment of twins is a major problem and the importance of detailed placenta examination correlated with the twins' growth is as important for live-born surviving twins as it is for assessment of twins who come to autopsy. Correlating placental findings with perinatal infections in twins is also important to an understanding of the pathophysiology. Zygosity assessment for any set of twins with a disease/disorder of any sort, whether potentially congenital, genetic or acquired, begins with adequate reporting of the pattern of placentation in order to reduce the number of twin sets for whom other studies are required. Discordant manifestations of diseases/disorders may relate as much to the patterns of placentation as to genetic predisposition because the environment of the twins truly begins in utero.

References

1. Gedda L, Brenci G, Gatti I. Low birth weight in twins versus singletons: separate entities and different implications for child growth and survival. *Acta Genet Med Gemellol.* 1981;30:1–8.

2. Chandra P, Harilal KT. Plural births—mortality and morbidity. In: Nance WE, ed. Twin Research: Biology and Epidemiology. *Prog Clin Biol Res.* 1978;24B:109–114.

3. Gedda L. Why can the study of twins be called Gemellology? In: Nance WE, ed. Twin Research: Biology and Epidemiology. *Prog Clin Biol Res.* 1978;24B:1–8.

4. Marivate M, Norman RJ. Twins. *Clin Obstet Gynecol.* 1982;9:723–743.

5. Secher NJ, Kaern J, Hansen PK. Intrauterine growth in twin pregnancies: prediction of intrauterine growth retardation. *Obstet Gynecol.* 1985; 66:63–68.

6. Iffy L, Lavenhar MA, Jakobovits A, Kaminetsky HA. The rate of early intrauterine growth in twin gestation. *Am J Obstet Gynecol.* 1983;146:970–972.

7. Fliegner JR, Eggers TR. The relationship between gestational age and birth weight in twin pregnancy. *Aust NZ J Obstet Gynecol.* 1984;24:192–197.

8. Corney G. Twin placentations and some effects on twins of known zygosity. In: Nance WE, ed. Twin Research: Biology and Epidemiology. *Prog Clin Biol Res.* 1978;24B:9–16.

9. Hrubec Z, Robinette CD. The study of human twins in medical research. *N Engl J Med.* 1984;310:435–441.

10. Sekiya S, Hafez ESE. Physiomorphology of twin transfusion syndrome: a study of 86 twin gestations. *Obstet Gynecol.* 1977;50:288–292.

11. Hoffman HJ, Bakketeig LS, Stark CR. Twins and perinatal mortality: a comparison between single and twin births in Minnesota and in Norway, 1967–1973. In: Nance WE, ed. Twin Research: Biology and Epidemiology. *Prog Clin Biol Res.* 1978;24B:133–142.

12. Alexander S, Leroy F. Gestational length and intrauterine growth in twin pregnancy. In: Nance WE, ed. Twin Research: Clinical Studies. *Prog Clin Biol Res.* 1978;24C:129–136.

13. Schneider L, Bessis R, Tabaste J-L, Sarramond M-F, Papiernik E, Baudet J, Pontonnier G. Echographic survey of twin fetal growth: a plea for specific charts for twins. In: Nance WE, ed. Twin Research: Clinical Studies. *Prog Clin Biol Res.* 1978;24C:137–141.

14. Crane JP, Tomich PG, Kopta M. Ultrasonic growth patterns in normal and discordant twins. *Obstet Gynecol.* 1980;55:678–683.

15. Stefos T, Deter RL, Hill RM, Simon NV. Individual growth curve standards in twins: prediction of third-trimester growth and birth characteristics. *Am J Obstet Gynecol.* 1989;161:179–183.

16. Effer S. Personal communication. All births in Canada except Newfoundland, 1980. Stats Canada, Ottawa, 1986.

17. Naeye RL, Letts HW. Body measurements of fetal and neonatal twins. *Arch Pathol.* 1964;77:393–396.

18. Kalousek D, Baldwin VJ, Dimmick JE, Cimolai N, Andrews A, Paradice B. Embryofetal-perinatal autopsy and placental examination. In: Dimmick JE, Kalousek D, eds. *Developmental Pathology of the Embryo and Fetus.* Philadelphia: JB Lippincott; 1992:799–824.

19. Manlan G, Scott KE. Contribution of twin pregnancy to perinatal mortality and fetal growth retardation; reversal of growth retardation after birth. *Can Med Assoc J.* 1978;118:365–368.

20. Desgranges M-F, De Muylder X, Moutquin J-M, Lazaro-Lopez F, Leduc B. Perinatal profile of twin pregnancies: a retrospective review of 11 years (1969–1979) at Hôpital Notre-Dame, Montreal, Canada. *Acta Genet Med Gemellol.* 1982;31:157–163.

21. Leroy F. Major fetal hazards in multiple pregnancy. *Acta Genet Med Gemellol.* 1976;25:299–306.

22. Hawrylyshyn PA, Barkin M, Bernstein A, Papsin PR. Twin pregnancies—a continuing perinatal challenge. *Obstet Gynecol.* 1982;59:463–466.

23. Ferguson WF. Perinatal mortality in multiple gestations (a review of perinatal deaths for 1609 multiple gestations). *Obstet Gynecol.* 1963;23:861–870.

24. Potter EL. Twin zygosity and placental form in relation to the outcome of pregnancy. *Am J Obstet Gynecol.* 1963;87:566–577.

25. Ho SK, Wu PYK. Perinatal factors and neonatal morbidity in twin pregnancy. *Am J Obstet Gynecol.* 1975;122:979–987.

26. Smith APM, Campbell DM, Lemon J. Growth patterns in preterm and term twin deliveries. *Acta Genet Med Gemellol.* 1990;39:413–416.

27. Chitkara U, Berkowitz GS, Levine R, Riden DJ, Fagerstrom Jr RM, Chervenak FA, Berkowitz RL. Twin pregnancy: routine use of ultrasound examinations in the prenatal diagnosis of intrauterine growth retardation and discordant growth. *Am J Perinatol.* 1985;2:49–54.

28. Farmakides G, Schulman H, Schneider E, Mesogitis S, Coury A. Umbilical artery velocimetry in multiple pregnancy. *Clin Obstet Gynecol.* 1989; 32:687–691.

29. Divon MY, Girz BA, Sklar A, Guidetti DA, Langer O. Discordant twins—a prospective study of the diagnostic value of real-time ultrasonography combined with umbilical artery velocimetry. *Am J Obstet Gynecol.* 1989;161:757–760.

30. Brown CEL, Weinreb JC. Magnetic resonance imaging appearance of growth retardation in a twin pregnancy. *Obstet Gynecol.* 1988;71:987–988.

31. Woods DL, Malan AF. Assessment of gestational age in twins. *Arch Dis Child.* 1977;52:735–737.

32. Dubowitz V, Dubowitz LMS. Inaccuracy of Dubowitz gestational age in low birth weight infants (letter). *Obstet Gynecol.* 1985;65:601–602.

33. Guaschino S, Spinillo A, Stola E, Pesando PC. Growth retardation, size at birth, and perinatal mortality in twin pregnancy. *Int J Gynecol Obstet.* 1987;25:399–403.

34. O'Brien WF, Knuppel RA, Scerbo JC, Rattan PK. Birth weight in twins: an analysis of discordancy and growth retardation. *Obstet Gynecol.* 1986; 67:483–486.

35. Brar HS, Rutherford SE. Classification of intrauterine growth retardation. *Semin Perinatol.* 1988;12:2–10.

36. Bleker OP, Oosting J, Hemrika DJ. On the cause of retardation of fetal growth in multiple gestations. *Acta Genet Med Gemellol.* 1988;37:41–46.

37. Shanklin DR. The influence of placental lesions on the newborn infant. *Pediat Clin North Am.* 1970;17:25–42.

38. Bleker OP, Hemrika DJ. Gestational age according to fetal sex in twins. *Am J Obstet Gynecol.* 1985;151:830–831.

39. Naeye RL. Organ abnormalities in a human parabiotic syndrome. *Am J Pathol.* 1965;46:829–842.

40. Bulmer MA. *The Biology of Twinning in Man..* Oxford: Clarendon Press; 1970:52.

41. Farmakides G, Schulman H, Saldana LR, Bracero LA, Fleischer A, Rochelson B. Surveillance of twin pregnancy with umbilical artery velocimetry. *Am J Obstet Gynecol.* 1985;153:789–792.

42. Newman RB, Ellings JM, Campbell BA, Eller DP, Miller MC. Factors affecting intrauterine growth in

twin gestations (Abstract). *Am J Obstet Gynecol.* 1991;164:319.

43. Hofman MA. Energy metabolism and relative brain size in human neonates from single and multiple gestations. *Biol Neonate.* 1984;45:157–164.

44. O'Neill JP, Nimrod C, Okum N, Narbitz R, Mikhael N. Discordant twin growth is associated with diminished Wharton's jelly. *J Soc Obstet Gynecol Can.* 1990;12:54,56.

45. Patterson RM, Wood RC. What is twin birthweight discordance? *Am J Perinatol.* 1990;7:217–219.

46. Bronsteen R, Goyert G, Bottoms S. Classification of twins and neonatal morbidity. *Obstet Gynecol.* 1989;74:98–101.

47. Maher JE, Khoury AD, Moretti ML, Shaver DC. Twin discordance: ultrasound prediction and perinatal outcome (Abstract). *Am J Obstet Gynecol.* 1991;164:370.

48. Blickstein I, Weissman A. "Macrosomic" twinning: a study of growth promoted twins. *Obstet Gynecol.* 1990;76:822–824.

49. Koivisto M, Jouppila P, Kauppila A, Moilanen I, Ylikorkala O. Twin pregnancy neonatal morbidity and mortality. *Acta Obstet Gynecol Suppl.* 1975;44:21–29.

50. Zahálková M. Perinatal and infant mortality in twins. In: Nance WE, ed. Twin Research: Biology and Epidemiology. *Prog Clin Biol Res.* 1978; 24B:115–120.

51. Blickstein I, Weissman A. Birth weight discordancy in male-first and female-first pairs of unlike-sexed twins. *Am J Obstet Gynecol.* 1990;162:661–663.

52. Gruenwald P. Environmental influences on twins apparent at birth (a preliminary study). *Biol Neonate.* 1970;15:79–93.

53. Blickstein I, Shoham-Schwartz Z, Lancet M. Growth discordancy in appropriate for gestational age twins. *Obstet Gynecol.* 1988;72:582–584.

54. Erkkola R, Ala-Mello S, Piiroinen O, Kero P, Sillanpää M. Growth discordancy in twin pregnancies: a risk factor not detected by measurements of biparietal diameter. *Obstet Gynecol.* 1985;66:203–206.

55. Newton ER. Antepartum care in multiple gestation. *Semin Perinatol.* 1986;10:19–29.

56. Blickstein I, Shoham-Schwartz Z, Lancet M, Borenstein R. Characterization of the growth-discordant twin. *Obstet Gynecol.* 1987;70:11–15.

57. Blickstein I, Lancet M. The growth discordant twin. *Obstet Gynecol Survey.* 1988;43:509–515.

58. Buzzard IM, Uchida IA, Norton JA, Christian JC. Birth weight and placental proximity in like sex twins. *Am J Hum Genet.* 1983;35:318–323.

59. Corey LA, Nance WE, Kang KW, Christian JC. Effect of type of placentation on birth weight and its variability in monozygous and dizygous twins. *Acta Genet Med Gemellol.* 1979;28:41–50.

60. Boyd JD, Hamilton WJ. *The Human Placenta.* Cambridge: W. Heffer; 1970:313–334.

61. Hansmann M, Hackelöer B-J, Staudach A, Wittmann BK. *Ultrasound Diagnosis in Obstetrics and Gynecology..* Berlin: Springer-Verlag; 1985:71–79,188–324,352.

62. Watson WJ, Valea FA, Seeds JW. Sonographic evaluation of growth discordance and chorionicity in twin gestation. *Am J Perinatol.* 1991;8:342–344.

63. Baker E, Crowley J, Wilkes KH, D'Alton M. The perinatal significance of absent end diastolic flow in discordant twins (Abstract). *Am J Obstet Gynecol.* 1992;166:334.

64. Wilson RS. Twin growth: initial deficit, recovery, and trends in concordance from birth to nine years. *Ann Hum Biol.* 1979;6:205–220.

65. Babson SG, Phillips DS. Growth and development of twins dissimilar in size at birth. *N Engl J Med.* 1973;289:937–940.

66. Ylitalo V, Kero P, Erkkola R. Neurological outcome of twins dissimilar in size at birth. *Early Hum Dev.* 1988;17:245–255.

67. Leung AKC, Robson WLM. Single umbilical artery. A report of 159 cases. *Am J Dis Child.* 1989;143:108–111.

68. Benirschke K, Kim CK. Multiple pregnancy. *N Engl J Med.* 1973;288:1276–1284,1329–1336.

69. Forrester RM, Lees VT, Watson GH. Rubella syndrome: escape of a twin. *Br Med J.* 1966; 1:1403.

70. Montgomery RC, Stockdell K. Congenital rubella in twins. *J Pediatr.* 1970;76:772–773.

71. Warkany J (1971). *Congenital Malformations.* Chicago: Year Book Medical Publishers; 1971:80.

72. Miller MJ, Seaman E, Remington JS. The clinical spectrum of congenital toxoplasmosis: problems in recognition. *J Pediatr.* 1967;70:714–723.

73. Sehgal NN. Perinatal mortality in twin pregnancies (implications for clinical management). *Postgrad Med.* 1980;68:231–234.

74. Duvekot JJ, Theewes BAM, Wesdorp JM, Roumen FJME, Bouckaert PXJM. Congenital cytomegalovirus infection in twin pregnancy: a case report. *Eur J Pediatr.* 1990;149:261–262.

75. Bose CL, Gooch WM, Sanders GO, Bucciarelli RL. Dissimilar manifestations of intrauterine infection with Echovirus 11 in premature twins. *Arch Pathol Lab Med.* 1983;107:361–363.

76. Shearer WT, Schreiner RL, Marshall RE, Barton

LL. Cytomegalovirus infection in a newborn dizygotic twin. *J Pediatr*. 1972;81:1161–1165.

77. Morton R, Mitchell I. Neonatal cytomegalic inclusion disease in a set of twins, one member of whom was a hydropic stillbirth, the other completely uninfected. Case report. *Br J Obstet Gynecol*. 1983;90:276–279.

78. Alfors K, Ivarsson S-A, Nilsson H. On the unpredictable development of congenital cytomegalovirus infection. A study in twins. *Early Hum Dev*. 1988;18:125–135.

79. Penrose LS. Congenital syphilis in a monovular twin. *Lancet*. 1937;1:322.

80. Bigrigg A, Chissell S, Swingler GR. Listeriosis in a twin pregnancy. *Br J Hosp Med*. 1991;45:171.

81. Remington JS, Desmonts G. Toxoplasmosis. In: Remington JS, Klein JO, eds. *Infectious Diseases of the Fetus and Newborn Infant*. Philadelphia: WB Saunders; 1976:209,257.

82. Wiswell TE, Fajardo JE, Bass JW, Brien JH, Forstein SH. Congenital toxoplasmosis in triplets. *J Pediatr*. 1984;105:59–60.

83. Shafai T. Neonatal coccidioidomycosis in premature twins. *Am J Dis Child*. 1978;132:634.

84. Côté GB, Gyftodimou J. Twinning and mitotic crossing-over: some possibilities and their implications. *Am J Hum Genet*. 1991;49:120–130.

85. Viscarello RR, DeGennaro NJ, Capobianco L, Hobbins JC. Perinatal transmission of human immunodeficiency virus (HIV) in twin gestations (Abstract). *Am J Obstet Gynecol*. 1991;164:300.

86. Goedert JJ, Duliege A-M, Amos CI, Felton S, Biggar RJ. The International Registry of HIV-exposed Twins (1991). High risk of HIV-1 infection for first born twins. *Lancet*. 1991;338:1471–1475.

87. Thomas PA, Ralston SJ, Bernard M, Williams R, O'Donnell R. Pediatric acquired immunodeficiency syndrome: an unusually high incidence of twins. *Pediatrics*. 1990;86:774–777.

88. Cox F, Wray B, Chaudhary T, Karlson K, Sherwood B, Greenberg M. Transfusion-associated acquired immunodeficiency syndrome in a twin infant. *Pediatr Infect Dis*. 1985;4:106–108.

89. Benirschke K. Routes and types of infection in the fetus and the newborn. *J Dis Child*. 1960;99:28–35.

90. Romero R, Shamma F, Avila C, Jiminez C, Callahan R, Nores J, Mazor M, Brekus CA, Hobbins JC. Infection and labor VI. Prevalence, microbiology, and clinical significance of intra amniotic infection in twin gestations with preterm labor. *Am J Obstet Gynecol*. 1990;163:757–761.

91. Neri A, Wielunsky E, Friedman S, Ovadia J.

Group B Streptococcus amnionitis with intact membranes associated with quadruplet delivery. *Eur J Obstet Gynecol Reprod Biol*. 1984;17:29–32.

92. Windham GC, Bjerkedal T, Langmark F. A population-based study of cancer incidence in twins and in children with congenital malformations or low birth weight, Norway, 1967–1980. *Am J Epidemiol*. 1985;121:49–56.

93. Inskip PD, Harvey EB, Boica JD, Stone BJ, Matanoski G, Flannery JT, Fraumeni JF Jr. Incidence of childhood cancer in twins. *Cancer Causes Control*. 1991;2:315–324.

94. Miller RW. Relation between cancer and congenital defects in man. *N Engl J Med*. 1966;275:87–93.

95. Miller RW. Relation between cancer and congenital defects: an epidemiologic evaluation. *J Natl Cancer Inst*. 1968;40:1079–1085.

96. Koch G. Genetics of microcephaly in man. *Acta Genet Med Gemellol*. 1959;8:75–85.

97. Scariano N. Rhabdomyoma of the heart in both of a set of twins. *Acta Genet Med Gemellol*. 1962;11:124–128.

98. Gross RE, Clatworthy HW, Meeker IA. Sacrococcygeal teratomas in infants and children (a report of 40 cases). *Surg Gynecol Obstet*. 1951;92:341–354.

99. Willis RA. *The Borderland of Embryology and Pathology*. 2nd ed. London: Butterworths; 1962:442–462.

100. Potter EL, Craig JM. *Pathology of the Fetus and the Infant*. 3rd ed. Chicago: Year Book Medical Publishers; 1975:180–197.

101. Hitchcock A, Sears RT, O'Neill T. Immature cervical teratoma arising in one fetus of a twin pregnancy. Case report and review of the literature. *Acta Obstet Gynecol Scand*. 1987;66:377–379.

102. Feld D, Labes J, Nathanson M. Bilateral ovarian dermoid cysts in triplets. *Obstet Gynecol*. 1966;27:525–528.

103. Simon A, Ohel G, Neri A, Schenker JG. Familial occurrence of mature ovarian teratomas. *Obstet Gynecol*. 1985;66:278–279.

104. Lee CM. The surgical significance of tumors in identical twins. (A short review of the literature and a report of sympathicoblastoma occurring in monozygotic twins.) *Ann Surg*. 1953;19:803–811.

105. Gaulin E. Simultaneous Wilms' tumor in identical twins. *J Urol*. 1951;66:547–550.

106. Vaughn AJ, Bachman D, Sommer A. Neurofibromatosis in monozygotic twins: a case report of spontaneous mutation. *Am J Med Genet*. 1981;8:155–158.

107. Eeg-Olofsson O, Lindskog U. Congenital neurofibromatosis (multiple subcutaneous tumors with

spontaneous regression in twins). *Acta Pediatr Scand*. 1983;72:779–780.

108. Warkany J (1971). *Congenital Malformations*. Chicago: Year Book Medical Publishers; 1971: 1213.

109. Amir J, Metzker A, Nitzan M. Giant pigmented nevus occurring in one identical twin. *Arch Dermatol*. 1982;118:188–189.

110. Morganroth GS, Taylor RS, Izenberg PH. Congenital giant pigmented nevus presenting in one identical twin. *Cutis*. 1991;48:53–55.

111. Gericke GS. Genetic and teratological considerations in the analysis of concordant and discordant abnormalities in twins. *S Afr Med J*. 1986;69:111–114.

112. Keith L, Brown E. Epidemiologic study of leukemia in twins (1920–1969). *Acta Genet Med Gemellol*. 1971;20:9–22.

113. Miller RW, Fraumeni JF, Manning MD. Association of Wilms' tumor with aniridia, hemihypertrophy and other congenital malformations. *N Engl J Med.*. 1964;270:922–927.

114. MacMahon B, Levy MA. Prenatal origin of childhood leukemia. (Evidence from twins). *N Engl J Med*. 1964;270:1082–1085.

115. Harvey EB, Boice JD, Honeyman M, Flannery JT. Prenatal x-ray exposure and childhood cancer in twins. *N Engl J Med*. 1985;312:541–545.

116. Kastern W, Kryspin-Sorensen I. Penetrance and low concordance in monozygotic twins in disease: are they the results of alternations of somatic genomes? *Mol Reprod Dev*. 1988;1:63–75.

117. Damjanov I, Janculjak I. Microcystik change in the outer fetal adrenal cortex in twins (author's trans). *Zentralbl Allg Pathol*. 1974;118:494–496.

118. Kanjilal D, Verma RS, Glass L, Babu A, Ramazanoglu F, Popescu S. Congenital adrenal hyperplasia in monozygotic twins with variable clinical manifestations. *Jpn J Hum Genet*. 1989;34:231–234.

119. Rettig KR, Vargas A, Reiter E, Root AW. Discordance for congenital athyrotic hypothyroidism in one monozygotic twin. *Clin Pediatr*. 1980; 19:63–65.

120. Kopelman AE. Delayed cerebral development in twins with congenital hyperthyroidism. *Am J Dis Child*. 1983;137:842–845.

121. Stuart C, Aceto T, Kuhn JP, Terplan K. Intrauterine hyperparathyroidism (postmortem findings in two cases). *Am J Dis Child*. 1979;133:67–70.

122. Kovar IZ, Mayne P, Wallis J. Neonatal rickets in one of identical twins. *Arch Dis Child*. 1982;57: 792–794.

123. Johansen K, Soeldner JS, Gleason RE, Gottlieb MS, Park BN, Kaufmann RL, Tan MH. Serum insulin and growth hormone response patterns in monozygotic twin siblings of patients with juvenile-onset diabetes. *N Engl J Med*. 1975;293:57–61.

124. Norman MG. Mechanisms of brain damage in twins. *Can J Neurol Sci*. 1982;9:339–344.

125. Naeye RL. Umbilical cord length: clinical significance. *J Pediatr*. 1985;107:278–281.

126. Griffiths M. Cerebral palsy in multiple pregnancy. *Dev Med Child Neurol*. 1967;9:713–731.

127. Amato M, Howald H, Schneider H. Neurosonographic assessment of twin pairs in the perinatal period. *Eur Neurol*. 1990;30:9–13.

128. Ghai V, Vidyasagar D. Morbidity and mortality factors in twins. An epidemiologic approach. *Clin Perinatol*. 1988;15:123–140.

129. Petterson B, Stanley F, Henderson D. Cerebral palsy in multiple births in western Australia: genetic aspects. *Am J Med Genet*. 1990;37:346–351.

130. Melnick M. Brain damage in survivor after in-utero death of monozygous cotwin. (Letter) *Lancet*. 1977;2:1287.

131. Jung JH, Graham JM, Schultz N, Smith DW. Congenital hydrancephaly/porencephaly due to vascular disruption in monozygotic twins. *Pediatrics*. 1984;73:467–469.

132. David TJ. Vascular basis for malformations in a twin. *Arch Dis Child*. 1985;60:166–167.

133. McLean WT, Toole JF. Congenital myasthenia gravis in identical twins with crises in the newborn period. *Am Neurol Sci Trans*. 1971;96:155–157.

134. Chen H, Fowler M, Yu CW. Generalized arterial calcification of infancy in twins. *Birth Defects*. 1982;18:67–80.

135. Van Reempts PJ, Boven KJ, Spitaels SE, Roodhooft AM, Vercruyssen ELJ, Van Acker KJ. Idiopathic arterial calcification of infancy. *Calcif Tissue Int*. 1991;48:1–6.

136. Bergstein JM, Fangman J, Fish AJ, Herdman R, Good RA. Severe hypertension in identical twin infants. *Am J Dis Child*. 1971;122:348–352.

137. Kikuta Y, Yoshimura Y, Saito T, Ishihara T, Yokoyama S, Hayashi T. Nephrotic syndrome with diffuse mesangial sclerosis in identical twins. *J Pediatr*. 1983;102:586–589.

138. Freeman H, Hill JR, Edwards AM, Wolowyk MW. Paroxysmal nocturnal hemoglobinuria in an identical twin. *Can Med Assoc J*. 1973;109:1002–1009.

139. Chawls WJ, Lally KP, Mahour GH. Neonatal surgical casebook: meconium ileus in premature twins. *J Perinatol*. 1987;7:62–64.

140. Getts A. SIDS: increased risk to second born twins. *Am J Public Health*. 1981;71:317–318.

141. Kleinman JC, Fowler MG, Kessel SS. Comparison

of infant mortality among twins and singletons: United States 1960 and 1983. *Am J Epidemiol.* 1991;133:133–143.

142. Fowler MG, Kleinman JC, Kiely JL, Kessel SS. Double jeopardy: twin infant mortality in the United States, 1983 and 1984. *Am J Obstet Gynecol.* 1991;165:15–22.

143. Roberts SC. Vaccination and cot deaths in perspective. *Arch Dis Child.* 1987;62:754–759.

144. Bass M. The fallacy of the simultaneous sudden infant death syndrome in twins. *Am J Forensic Med Pathol.* 1989;10:200–205.

145. Nelson HB, Martin CA. Increased child abuse in twins. *Child Abuse Negl.* 1985;9:501–505.

146. Tanimura M, Matsui I, Kobayashi N. Child abuse of one of a pair of twins in Japan. *Lancet.* 1990;2:1298–1299.

147. Lee DA. Munchausen syndrome by proxy in twins. *Arch Dis Child.* 1979;54:646–647.

148. deSa DJ. The adrenal glands. In: Wigglesworth JS, Singer DB, eds. *Textbook of Fetal and Perinatal Pathology.* Boston: Blackwell Scientific; 1991: 1057–1077.

7
Anomalous Development of Twins

As we learn more about the human genome and develop more sophisticated ways of studying diseases, disorders, and disturbed development, the borders between these abnormalities become harder to define. For example, as we learn more about the underlying biochemical defects in dwarfing syndromes such as thanatophoric dysplasia, this "malformation" becomes more like an inborn error of metabolism—a genetic defect or alteration with a specifically altered or absent product, leading to a predictable set of consequences depending on the role of that product. Considering this concept, it is perhaps somewhat artificial to discuss developmental/morphologic/structural anomalies separate from the sorts of diseases and disorders reviewed in Chapter 6. However, we are still a long way from defining the underlying molecular mechanisms in most structural variations from "normal," so there is probably more we can learn from reviewing them in a broader context. Careful analysis of patterns of malformations and associated epidemiologic characteristics may help define where the basic defect could be looked for, and examinations of malformations in twins may provide particularly useful data.

Patterns of Anomalous Development of Twins

Infants of multiple conceptions can have anomalies that fall into one of two main categories: those that are seen in singletons, and those specially related to the twinning process and subsequent situation.

Anomalies that are encountered in singletons have the same morphologic manifestations when they are seen in twins. The importance in twins is the degree to which the anomaly is present in both twins, how that correlates with the type of twins affected, and what that correlation may reveal about the pathophysiology of the anomaly. Anomalies in twins can have four classes of concordance/discordance: (1) both twins with the same kind of anomaly and of the same severity, (2) both twins with the same kind of anomaly but of differing severity, (3) both twins with an anomaly but of a different kind in each, and (4) one twin with an anomaly but none in the other. Details of concordance/discordance must therefore be supplemented with accurate descriptions of the pattern of placentation and documentation of zygosity assignment or, ideally, genetic congruity. If the anomaly in question is observed more frequently in twins than in singletons, the next question is, What is the role of the twinning process or the "twinship" circumstance in the pathophysiology of that anomaly?

Anomalies related to twinning are those that are seen more commonly in twins and consist of four classes of defects: (1) anomalies that may be related to the twinning process, particularly monovular monozygotic twins, (2) anomalies that are only seen with disturbed monovular/monozygotic twinning, (3) anomalies due to or influenced by the different patterns of placentation possible with twins, and (4) anomalies related to other aspects of the "twinness" of the conception and gestation. In this category of anomalies, the patterns of placentation and relevant genetic studies are essential to any useful assessment of underlying pathophysiology.

Sources of Developmental Variation in Twins

Many early reviews of malformations were an attempt to categorize malformations within a "nature versus nurture" dichotomy, but our concepts of the sources of influence on human development are changing. Potential sources of variation among twins have been discussed in relation to twin studies (Chapter 1) and mechanisms of twinning (Chapter 2). These are enlarged upon here in order to emphasize the factors that need to be considered when assessing anomalous development of twins. While it is true that the same concepts can be applied equally to diseases and disorders in twins, malformations are a more concrete end point, so the choice was made to have this review precede the discussion of anomalies.

As represented in Fig. 7.1, there are at least five different ways that a set of twins may develop with different genetic programs or instructions in each twin. The first way is the most obvious—the classic polyovular/polyspermic dizygotic pattern of twinning and the more recently documented dispermic monovular twinning mechanisms, both of which lead to twins with distinct genomes, as described in Chapter 2. When twinning of the monovular/monospermic zygote takes place, the embryos have generally been considered to be genetically identical, but as more examples of discordant development of what were thought to be monozygotic twins have been identified, it has become apparent that the source of these variations might be very early and based in the genome and its expression.[1]

One early source of variation in monozygotic twins may be due to symmetry problems. Development is not identical in both sides of the singleton embryo, as shown by the lateral asymmetry that is evident in everyone, such as in facial features, visceral situs, or handedness. It has been suggested that the developing embryonic cell mass expresses preliminary determinants of spatial relationships or body symmetry quite early, so that if the mass divides along a line between these fields, the embryos will consist of cells with different commitments and this may influence development significantly, such as the mirror imaging reported in twins.[2] This early laterality may actually originate in an inhomogeneous distribution of genetically

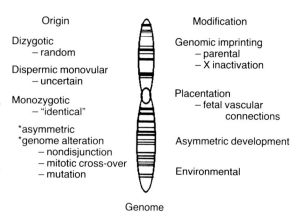

FIGURE 7.1. Sources of variation in the origin and expression of the genetic program in twins. The genetic program or genome can originate from different sources as in the random combination of dizygotic twinning or the uncertain but probably less random combination in dispermic monovular twinning. Monozygotic twinning theoretically leads to identical copies, but these may be modified by postzygotic genomic alterations, such as nondisjunction, mitotic cross-over, and mutation, as well as by asymmetric division of the embryonic blastomeres. The genomic program can be modified by forces of genomic imprinting, depending on the parental source of the genetic information and which X chromosome is inactivated. Patterns of placentation can have a significant influence on the modification of the genetic potential as can factors that lead to asymmetric embryonic development. Finally, environmental influences may create significantly discordant individuals from potentially genetic identical sources.

active components in the cytoplasm of the ovum prior to fertilization.[3] Another possible source of different genetic instructions may depend on the degree of development of the embryonic blastomeres when twinning takes place, because there may be more or less asymmetry of division of the embryonic cell mass and/or placental cell mass. This could lead to asymmetric twins and/or asymmetric placental development. Some cases of chorangiopagus and other parasitic twins may well be extreme examples of unequal twinning—the affected twin is usually smaller, is certainly malformed, and has no placenta of its own at all (see Chapter 10). Even if the twins were equal and only the placental mass was unevenly divided, there could be secondary effects on the development of the associated twins.

Alternatively, even if the twinning process creates symmetric embryonic and placental masses, three chromosomal changes could affect the twins differently. Chromosomal rearrangements or deletions (see discussion on heterokaryotic twins below), mitotic crossing-over,[4] or exogenous sources of postzygotic mutations could create genetically dissimilar embryos and/or placentas with developmental differences as a consequence.[5] In fact, it has been suggested that postzygotic mitotic crossing-over may represent the stimulus for twinning in the first place.[4] It has been proposed that somatic mutation can be the source of more localized variations within an ostensibly genomically identical twin pair.[6]

Even if the twins have an identical genome, there are potential sources of variation in the expression or manifestation of that genome. In the purest or most straightforward expression of genetic instructions, the genetic program is "read" and a specific factor/function/component results. A specific error in the program could lead to a specific product error that may have recognizable functional and/or morphological effects, often with measurable biochemical effects, such as the absence of an enzyme or cell product. However, the expression of the genetic potential may depend on which parent provided the genetic material. This phenomenon is called genomic imprinting and has been documented for whole genome sets in triploidy[7] and for portions of chromosomes,[8] and may explain sex-related variations in expression of mutant genes.[8] The source of this influence is not fully defined, but may relate to gene transcription[8] as affected by factors on the X chromosome, and discordance may relate to nonrandom inactivation of X chromosomes, which may in turn be related to the twinning process.[9] This has been termed "sex-dependent developmental penetrance," as opposed to sex linkage.[3]

Even if the genetic instructions are read appropriately, the effect of the "product" may be influenced by "environmental" factors. As the most immediate environment of twins is the pattern of placentation, this can have a significant modifying influence on the expression of genetic potential.[10] This includes the effect of aberrantly inserted umbilical cords,[11] which may act as an enhancing or enabling influence, the effect of hemodynamically imbalanced blood flow across intertwin vascular anastomoses in monochorionic placentas (see Chapter 9), and the

effects of cord entanglements in monoamniotic twins (see Chapter 8). Differential responses to teratogens (e.g. drugs, infections) may be due to slight differences in the rate of development with differing patterns of susceptibility,[12] and these in turn may be due to minor differences in the genetic program or be related to placental factors of implantation or development.

As well as the potential sources of variation in development of twins described above, there are three additional general concepts that need to be kept in mind when assessing anomalies in a fetus or infant. First, it is important to be aware that the constellation of abnormalities may vary with the age of the fetus or infant. The progression of phenotypic features in infancy and childhood is documented for many syndromes, and this evolution can be seen even earlier in some conditions, e.g., the classic phenotype of trisomy 21 is minimal in the fetal period.[13] Second, it is also important to be able to recognize those anomalies that are primary and those that are simply a complication of, or secondary to, the primary lesion, e.g., pulmonary hypoplasia or facial dysmorphism as part of the oligohydramnios phenotype in cases with renal/urinary tract lesions that prevent urine production or excretion.[14] While these secondary anomalies may have more immediate clinical significance, questions related to underlying mechanisms must focus on the primary defect. Finally, there are two additional patterns of pathogenesis that may have very indirect genomic connections, but need to be recognized specifically because they seem to be primarily environmentally induced. The category of anomalies referred to as "deformations" consists of aberrant position or shape of a fetal part on the basis of physical pressures in utero.[8,12,15] The category of anomalies referred to as "disruptions" consists of the destruction of previously formed normal tissues by physical forces such as the amnion disruption complex (see below), or on a vascular basis.[16]

Even with current concepts of sources of variation in twins, research into anomalies might still be considered to be concerned with "nature versus nurture," but on a considerably more refined and complex scale. It may be time now to move from large general surveys of anomalies in twins to focused investigations of particular defects, especially those that are increased in twins, or unexpectedly concordant or discordant. This chapter reviews the general topic of anomalies in twins and then looks at selected specific types of abnormalities.

Population-Based Studies

There have been a number of general reviews of anomalies in twins. From a series of reports that span the past 30 years, the consensus is that twins have more anomalies of some types compared to singletons, although the degree of excess reported varies; but there does not seem to be agreement on whether twins overall have more anomalies than singletons.[17–33] The differences reported result from varying biases in the different reviews, including biases of ascertainment such as exclusion of stillbirth data, lack of pathologic confirmation, and, in many cases, little or no information about placental morphology or zygosity assignment. A limited selection from the reported series of malformations in twins is summarized in Table 7.1. Most of these are retrospective studies from registry data—from birth reports and malformation reporting systems—so that the data available are limited. In the absence of placentation or zygosity data, the information is often analyzed by like-sex/unlike-sex patterns, with statistical assignments of zygosity in the like-sex groups. Some authors group the anomalies by systems to try to get larger numbers to analyze, as the rates for individual anomalies are low. These studies represent considerable work on the part of the reviewers, but it is difficult to draw conclusions from the collated data. It is also important to note that all these reports refer to anomalies in twin births compared with singleton births. It is well recognized that a number of anomalies are identifiable in embryonic or fetal singletons,[13] but the load of embryonic or fetal malformations with twin conceptions has been assessed by only a few.[32]

One of the most extensive analyses of malformations in twins was from the data collected by the Collaborative Perinatal Project in the United States.[24] Congenital malformations were defined as any gross anatomic developmental anomaly present at birth or detected during the first year of life. Where possible, zygosity was determined by sex, gross and microscopic placental morphology, and nine blood group systems. The study reviewed 187 monozygotic pairs, 308 dizygotic pairs, and 87 pairs (15%) where zygosity could not be deter-

mined, as well as 33 individuals from incomplete pairs, 31 of whom were of undetermined zygosity. While malformations were reportedly associated with 6.6% of all twin deaths in the study, twins usually died in the neonatal period of causes other than the consequences of malformations. The commonest malformations were in the musculoskeletal system, followed by skin lesions, gastrointestinal abnormalities, ear anomalies, cardiovascular anomalies, upper respiratory anomalies, central nervous system lesions, and genitourinary anomalies. Major malformations occurred most commonly in the gastrointestinal and musculoskeletal systems, followed by cardiovascular, central nervous system, skin, upper respiratory and genitourinary. Minor anomalies were commonest of the skin, the ear, and the musculoskeletal system, followed by upper respiratory, gastrointestinal tract, and genitourinary tract. Most of the malformations of the central nervous system or cardiovascular system were multiple. No relation to birth order was identified.

In this same study, twins had an overall greater rate of malformations than singletons, both of malformations and numbers of twins with malformations, but not of multiple malformation complexes or individuals with multiple malformations. Twins had twice the rate of cardiovascular or gastrointestinal anomalies, and central nervous system and related skeletal anomalies were also increased, but to a lesser extent—almost all of these anomalies were major ones. Also greater in twins were mixtures of major and minor anomalies of the ear, upper respiratory tract, and mouth. Almost all specific malformations were increased in twins, but the numbers were too small for statistical comparisons with singletons in most cases. Major malformations particularly increased were macrocephaly, encephalocele, cleft lip, cleft palate, diaphragmatic anomalies, tracheoesophageal fistula, intestinal malrotation, inguinal and umbilical hernias, and cystic kidneys. Minor anomalies of the ear were also increased. Interestingly, hypospadius was not reported in twins. Black twins had an increase in polydactyly and branchial cleft anomalies. Male twins had more major malformations and more malformations overall than singleton males, while female twins and singletons had the same rates.

The increased rate of anomalies in twins was attributed to the increased occurrence of anomalies

TABLE 7.1. Incidence and patterns of malformations in twins as reported from selected series.

Ref/year	Population studied	Malformation rate reported	Zygosity relationships		Placentation relationships		Specific malformations/groups malformations		Comments
			Methods	Rate	Methods	Rate	Increased in twins	Decreased in twins	
17/1963	300 twin perinatal deaths (Canada)	1.8× rate in all perinatal deaths	--------NR--------		--------NR--------		--------NR--------		Malformations studied as cause of death; 36% autopsy rate
18/1970	2,000 live-born twins, birth certificate data (United States)	LS higher than US, which equaled singletons	Only LS/US differentiation		--------NR--------		Anencephaly, hydrocephaly, CHD, positional foot defects	Down syndrome	No data on twin deaths; anomalies not detected at birth not included
20/1971	2,498 twin pairs, clinical and postmortem records (Czechoslovakia)	2X rate in single births	--------NR--------		------NR------	DC rate = 1.8 × MC rate	--------NR--------		Twins more likely to have multiple malformations affecting more systems than singletons
21/1972	258 twin pair births (Taiwan)	Not increased over singletons	Genotype	------NR------	--------NR--------		NR—only six sets reported anomalous, four sets conjoined twins, two sets aneuploid		Tabulated only major or lethal malformations, omitted CHD, autopsy data
23/1975	335 twin pair births perinatal data (Finland)	5.7% all twins; "higher" than general incidence	--------NR--------		--------NR--------		Twin B more CNS, GIT, GUT anomalies, twin A more CVS, bone and joint anomalies; overall incidence A = B		Malformations reported to cause 4.5% of all twin deaths
24/1975	581 twin pairs + 33 twin individuals up to 1 year (Collaborative Perinatal Project— United States)	18.3% of all twins, 1.2× number of malformations and numbers twins with malformations over singletons	Sex; placentation; 9 blood groups	All anomalies MZ = 2× DZ; concordance greater MZ	Gross and microscopic examination	Only specified monoamniotic— 33.4% major + minor anomalies	Almost all, but especially CVS, GIT; also encephalocele, cleft lip, cleft palate, pre-auricular skin tags	CDH, clubfoot; hypospadius	Most complete analysis to date; zygosity of 17% study group undetermined; no increase of twins with multiple malformations compared to singletons; males more affected than females

TABLE 7.1. *Continued.*

Ref/year	Population studied	Malformation rate reported	Zygosity relationships		Placentation relationships		Specific malformations/groups malformations		Comments
			Methods	Rate	Methods	Rate	Increased in twins	Decreased in twins	
25/1978	409 twin pairs—data at delivery (Ghana)	NR	NR		NR		Extra digit—always discordant	NR	Assessed visible birth defects only; no details provided
26/1978	345 twin deliveries (India)	2.4% of all twins	NR		NR		NR		Majority reported anomalies were of CNS
27/1980	4,490 twin infants; Defects Registry (Atlanta)	Increased risk in twins due to LS pairs	Statistical only	Most anomalies more common in LS twin sets	NR		CHD, GIT, lung, genital; omphalocele/ gastroschisis	Spina bifida, pyloric stenosis, clubfoot	Autopsy data for CNS anomalies only; no zygosity assignment—ranked LS pairs using Weinberg's formula
28/1983	657 twin pairs—neonatal examination records (Scotland)	8.4% of twin pairs, 4.3% twin individuals	Placentation; blood and placental genetic markers	MZ:DZ = 1.3:1	NR	MC:DC = 1.7:1 for MZ twins; DZ—NR	Numbers considered too small to analyze, only two pairs concordant for any anomaly		Zygosity assignment not determined in 16.9% of pairs and 19.3% of malformed individual twins
29/1983	1,424 twin pairs; prospective (Belgium/England)	2.9% of 2,848 twins	Sex; 6 blood groups; placental enzymes; placental structure; red blood cell isoenzymes	MZ:DZ = 2:1	Gross and microscopic examination	DZ:MZDC:MZMC = 4:1:4 for CHD	Commonest malformation in MZ twins was discordant CHD		Most detailed zygosity testing to date; analysis focused on monozygotic twins—discordant: concordant malformations = 3.5:1
30/1984	7,660 twin pairs; birth registration (Norway)	Twins = singletons; LS slightly higher than US	Only LS/US differentiation	See comment	NR		CNS; CVS	CDH	Both malformed—LS:US = 3:1, same malformation—LS:US = 4.4:1

#/Year	Sample	Findings	LS/US data	LS/US result		Malformations increased in twins	Malformations decreased in twins	Comments
31/1986	15,427 twin infants; birth registry (Sweden)	6% of all twins had malforma-tions 1.3% concordant	LS/US groups and statistical estimates	No difference in rates LS/US pairs; males higher rates	------NR------	Hydrocephaly; CHD, SUA, esophageal, anal atresias; intersex; severe renal anomalies; spine malformations	Hypospadius; hydrocoele; CDH; Down syndrome; nevi	Relates 42 malformations to sex of twins and birth order; neural tube defects increased in male twins, CHD in female twins, compared to sex distribution in singletons
33/1990	76,000 twin births; birth and anomaly registers (to 7 days) (England/Wales)	Overall rates malformed twins = singletons; more twins with multiple anomalies	------NR------	------NR------	------NR------	Intersex; anencephaly; PDA; exomphalos; hydrocephalus; SUA; esophageal/ anorectal atresias	Polydactyly, syndactyly; CDH; branchial arch/cleft; Down syndrome	Compares reported rates 51 different anomalies in twins and singletons

DZ, dizygotic; MZ, monozygotic; NR, not reported; US, unlike-sex twin pairs; LS, like-sex twin pairs; DC, dichorionic; MC, monochorionic; CHD, congenital heart disease; CNS, central nervous system; GIT, gastrointestinal tract; GUT, genitourinary tract; CVS, cardiovascular system; SUA, single umbilical artery; PDA, patent ductus arteriosus; CDH, congenital dislocated hip.

in monozygotic twins, and applied to both major and minor malformations. Chorionicity was not related to the malformations except to note the high rate of malformations in monoamniotic twins— 16.7% with major anomalies and another 16.7% with minor anomalies.

Because of the small number of some of the anomalies in this study, analysis of concordance of specific anomalies was limited. Monozygotic concordance was consistently greater than dizygotic concordance, but was only statistically significant with musculoskeletal malformations. All concordant dizygotic pairs had at least one similar malformation, but only 69% of concordant monozygotic pairs had a similar anomaly; 31% of concordantly anomalous monozygotic pairs had different anomalies. Concordance for central nervous system, cardiovascular system, and gastrointestinal tract anomalies was low overall.

One of the most thorough assessments of zygosity and malformations also reported a rate of malformations that was higher in monozygotic (3.7%) than dizygotic (2.5%) twins, and that two thirds of the anomalies in monozygotic twins were discordant.[29] The authors observed that concordance in monozygotic twins might suggest a genetic origin, but nongenetic teratogenic factors, such as drugs or maternal disease, could affect both twins equally, and discordant responses in dizygotic twins may be due to genetic factors. They emphasized the importance of zygosity and placentation data and recommended multicenter studies using an adequate protocol.

There are five conclusions that can be drawn from these broad reviews of malformations in twins. First, observed increased rates of anomalies in twins appear to be due to an excess load in monozygotic twins, although the importance of chorionicity was not assessed in detail. It may be that monochorionic monozygosity should be considered in a class by itself, as suggested by the data presented in this volume. Second, some groups of anomalies appear to be increased in twins, but without adequate data on placentation and zygosity it is difficult to assess the significance of this observation to concepts of pathogenesis of the anomalies as they relate to twins. Third, a few specific anomalies are seen less frequently in twins, and these warrant closer scrutiny as well. Fourth, concordance or discordance can only be assessed

with full diagnosis including genetic and placental studies. Fifth, the value of broad-based surveys is probably limited by the depth of analysis possible. Registries of anomalies are helpful for detecting trends and frequencies of the more visible defects, but pathophysiologic studies of mechanisms of anomalies that use twin studies as a resource must have more detailed data than population based reporting schemes provide.

Survey '91 Autopsy Review of Anomalies

Anomalies in the Survey '91 Review of autopsied twins were encountered from the embryonic period onward. Anomalies that were associated with embryo/fetal and perinatal/neonatal/infant death are discussed in Chapter 5 and summarized here. In the embryonic period, lethal chromosomal errors with an excess of monochorionic female twin sets were seen. Well-preserved fetal deaths of less than 20 weeks' gestation were occasionally associated with induction of delivery because of prenatal diagnosis of a lethal fetal anomaly. Fifty percent of the macerated fetuses delivered at less than 20 weeks had a malformation and these are summarized in Table 5.2. In twin sets with a fetus papyraceous, 50% of the dead fetuses had abnormalities of the umbilical cord. Anomalies exclusive of abnormalities of monozygotic twinning were found in 6.8% of all stillborn twins: 6% of freshly stillborn twins, 3.4% of twins who died within the week before delivery, and 13.2% of retained macerated twins. In 39% of the asphyxiated twins who had died in the week before delivery, the dead twin's placental portion had discordant findings suggesting problems with placental development, especially abnormalities of the umbilical cord. Finally, anomalies that were considered a sufficient cause of death, excluding anomalous monozygotic twinning, accounted for 11.1% of the perinatal and later twin mortality. These twins were more likely to be males, second born, and more mature, 63% were born after 33 weeks. One-third died of their anomaly within the first 24 hours, but the rest lived up to a year and beyond. There was no predominating pattern of chorionicity, and anomalies accounted for only 3.9% of concordant twin deaths.

Not all developmental abnormalities are major or

lethal lesions, and the autopsy review also recorded other anomalies, many of which might not have been identified without autopsy. The following comments exclude those 5.5% of twins with malformations attributed solely to anomalous monozygotic twinning (chorangiopagus and conjoined twins) because these are discussed in Chapter 10. They are discussed separately because they seem to represent a pathophysiologically distinct group that should not be combined with discussions of malformations that also occur in singletons, although there may be some conceptual crossover possible. Also excluded are those occasional cases with anomalies considered secondary to unrelated events, consisting mainly of features of the oligohydramnios phenotype after prolonged premature rupture of membranes.

Patterns of Anomalies

As with singletons, the anomalies in the autopsied twins occurred in a variety of patterns, and at least one anomaly was reported in 22.5% of the cases autopsied from 20 weeks' gestation onward, liveborn and stillborn (macerated, retained, and fresh). Only one anomaly was reported in 44.4% of twins with anomalies. In 21.2% of the anomalous twins, there were multiple individual but related malformations (multiple-related). These anomalies were either all within one system, such as the features of the hypoplastic left heart syndrome or lumbosacral meningomyelocele with Arnold-Chiari malformation and hydrocephalus, or represented a related constellation with a primary defect and secondary findings, such as pulmonary hypoplasia with renal agenesis or diaphragmatic hernia. It seemed reasonable to identify these separately, as they were more obviously connected than some other combinations of anomalies. Recognized syndromes, although they might have varied manifestations, were also classed as a separate group and were seen in 8.0% of the anomalous twins. These included autosomal trisomy, asplenia isomerism, Noonan's syndrome and Smith-Lemli-Opitz syndrome. The last group of 26.4% were nonsyndromic constellations of multiple malformations that ranged from a combination of small ventricular septal defect and cryptorchidism to major malformations in three or four organ systems in one patient. In keeping with the philosophy of this chapter, that a large table with

small numbers of cases is less helpful than a closer look at specific cases when considering causes of anomalies, comments here are general with more specific points in the relevant sections that follow.

The malformations were categorized as either major or minor and the patterns assessed. Major malformations were those that were lethal or life threatening, potentially affected function significantly, or would have required major surgical correction. Examples of major malformations were anencephaly, pulmonary hypoplasia, coarctation of the aorta, intestinal atresia, hydronephrosis, and cleft lip/palate. Minor malformations were those that were easily remedied, unlikely to be detected without autopsy, or served as a potential marker for other anomalies. Examples of minor anomalies were low-set ears, Meckel's diverticulum, and transverse distal palmar creases. Growth retardation alone (see Chapter 6) was not considered an anomaly because only structural malformations were being assessed. Also if a single-artery umbilical cord was the only finding, it was not recorded because it is discussed in Chapter 3. Finally, a persistent patent ductus arteriosus was not recorded if it was the only anomaly in a premature infant with respiratory distress syndrome. Of those twins with only one malformation, 68% were minor and most frequently in the gastrointestinal and genitourinary systems. Of the major anomalies presenting in twins with only one malformation, two-thirds were in the cardiovascular and central nervous systems. Of the multiple-related anomalies, 43% were cardiovascular and over three quarters were major constellations, such as the hypoplastic left heart syndrome. All the multiple-related combinations in the central nervous system, urinary, and musculoskeletal system were major defects. The twins with nonsyndromic multiple malformations were analyzed to see if any patterns could be found. Combinations of major anomalies of the cardiovascular, gastrointestinal, and central nervous systems were noted and combinations of minor lesions of the genitourinary and gastrointestinal systems as well. No other particular combinations occurred. Examples of major combinations were large body wall defects with multiple visceral lesions, amnion disruption complex with involvement of the head and body, and cloacal exstrophy with neural tube defect and short gut; examples of minor combinations were mild hypospadius and a Meckel's diverticulum.

An attempt was made to assess concordance or discordance of the anomalies in the four categories noted previously. This was not helpful, as there was often no comparable data on the co-twin, who either survived or did not have an autopsy. Some major features, such as anencephaly, could be assessed from the records, but proven concordance or discordance in most cases was only possible when both twins were autopsied. Of those sets where concordance could be assessed accurately, 8.9% were concordant for the same lesion(s), 13.3% had the same system(s) involved, but with varying severity or different manifestations, 4.4% were each anomalous but with different systems affected, and the majority were discordant with a normal co-twin, 51.1% when the lesion was single or in a single system, and 22.3% for multisystem defects.

The importance of placental morphology and zygosity/genetic studies to complete assessment of twins is exemplified by a set of female twins at 35 weeks who lived only 3 hours. Both were similarly growth retarded. One twin had a Dandy Walker malformation, horseshoe kidney, bronchogenic cyst, and congenital heart disease with a ventricular septal defect, atrial septal defect, small left ventricle, and coarctation of the aorta. The other twin had microcephaly, horseshoe kidney, pulmonary hypoplasia, hypoplastic left heart with a ventricular septal defect, bicuspid aortic valve and coarctation of the aorta, bilateral eventration of the diaphragm, hypertelorism, right simian crease, and accessory spleen. The only reported placenta-related finding was that the second twin had only one umbilical artery, the placenta itself was not processed. Both were chromosomally 46,XX, but not otherwise characterized. The malformation cluster and the similarities and differences are remarkable, but unfortunately could not be assessed any further without additional placental and genetic data.

Both major and minor malformations were noted to be discordant in monochorionic twins, representing a particularly interesting group and ranging from persistent left superior vena cava to cloacal exstrophy. These are discussed in the relevant sections that follow.

In the 30-year span represented by the Survey '91 and the general reviews discussed above, the level of sophistication available in genome analysis has increased dramatically. Thus, while broad monitoring of anomalies in twins will continue to be important, detailed studies of specific malformations in twins may provide more precise information about the relative roles of genomic and environmental factors. In the following discussion, individual malformations or groups of related malformations are described in more detail, followed by comments on those malformations that seem to be related to twinning.

Specific Malformations and Malformation Groups

A number of specific malformations and groups of malformations have been reported in twins in an attempt to derive information about mechanisms that can produce developmental anomalies. This section reviews major groups of anomalies with selected specific examples to see what the pattern of occurrence in twins might suggest about the malformation.

Cardiovascular System

Reports of anomalies in the cardiovascular system (CVS) have focused mainly on structural lesions of the heart [congenital heart disease (CHD)] and great vessels.[34–38] This has been a difficult group to assess because of the problems of accurate diagnosis and the incomplete genetic/placentation data. Population surveys have suggested that twins have more CVS anomalies than singletons, although the magnitude of the increase varies, that monozygotic twins are overrepresented among twins with heart defects, and that the majority of anomalies are discordant even in monozygotic twin sets.

A wide variety of cardiac anomalies have been reported in twins, but it has been suggested that because many of these anomalies appear to be developmentally related, looking at *embryonic mechanistic groups* might be instructive.[38] The mechanistic groups consist of the following: (1) conotruncal malformations, such as tetralogy of Fallot and transposition of the great vessels; (2) hemodynamic abnormalities, such as membranous septal defects, valvular stenoses or atresia, coarctation of the aorta, hypoplastic left heart syndrome, and patent ductus arteriosus; (3) extracellular matrix abnormalities, such as atrioventricular canal; (4) excessive cellular death, such as Ebstein's anomaly and muscular septal defect; and (5) a group of unverified categories—(5a) looping abnormalities, such as levocardia; (5b) targeted growth abnormalities, such as total anomalous pulmonary venous return; and (5c) a miscellaneous group with anomalies of pulmonary veins and cardiomyopathy, for example.

In an analysis of 2,303 live-born infants less than 1 year of age with confirmed CHD, compared to a control group of 2,793 without CHD, twins were nearly twice as common in the affected group— 2.8% versus 1.5% in case versus control groups, respectively.[38] Female twins were overrepresented in the case group by a factor of 1.7, compared to the control twins. The distribution of the anomalies observed in the twins is presented in Table 7.2. The different numbers and distribution in male and female twins are unexplained unless affected males die as embryos or fetuses. The authors noted the increased numbers of looping abnormalities in twins compared to singletons and suggested that these were more common in monozygotic twins, but zygosity assignment in this report was by hearsay only. Hemodynamic anomalies were increased in male twins, but there was no information on placentation patterns. It has been suggested that heart development is particularly sensitive to disturbances of situs or laterality,[37] so that asymmetric division of a monozygotic-derived cell mass may create variations in expression of the cardiac genome based on altered spatial influences. Concordance of cardiac defects was noted in 6.2% of affected twin pairs, for the same mechanistic group, but not necessarily for the specific anatomic defect. A number of extracardiac anomalies were noted in 23.1% of the case twins, but they presented no particular pattern.

Two specific cardiac lesions are worth considering because they seem to be rare in twins, and one wonders what this observation may mean regarding the pathogenesis. *Truncus arteriosus* (TA) was not one of the anomalies mentioned in the surveys of CHD reviewed, so its occurrence in twins would appear to be rare. The relative role of genetic and subsequent events is not known for this anomaly, although genetic factors seem important based on reports in families. Three of the four reported concordant cases of TA have been in monozygotic or monochorionic twin sets, two with multiple other cardiac and extracardiac anomalies. The fourth set was apparently dizygotic, concordantly hydropic ultrasonically dichorionic twin females with isolated TA.[39] Although these twins had cytogenetic chromosomal differences in kilobase pair segments from three loci, the possibility of aberrant monozygotic or monovular twinning was not considered. *Endocardial fibrosis/fibroelastosis* (EFE) is a morphologic lesion of cardiac chamber endomyocardium, usually of the left ventricle, of uncertain cause or pathogenesis. EFE is often complicated by congenital heart block (CHB), and CHB may be immunologically mediated,[40] so maternally derived immunologic damage might be considered. This lesion is not mentioned in the general surveys of CHD in twins, so it also appears to be rare in twins. Three case reports exemplify the problems of analysis of this lesion in twins: (1) isolated biventricular EFE (right greater than left) with CHB in male twins said to be identical, but no criteria for identity provided[41]; (2) isolated EFE of the right ventricle was found in two of three monochorionic triplets, while the third survived without signs of

TABLE 7.2. Congenital cardiovascular malformations in twins and singletons.

Mechanistic group of defects	Twins, number (%)			Singletons: number (%)	Survey '91 autopsy series: number (%)
	Male	Female	Total		
Conotruncal	1 (5.3)	5 (10.9)	6 (9.2)	399 (17.8)	5 (15.7)
Hemodynamic	14 (73.7)	27 (58.7)	41 (63.1)	1,332 (59.5)	24 (75.0)
Extracellular matrix	2 (10.5)	4 (8.7)	6 (9.2)	195 (8.7)	1 (3.1)
Cellular death	0	3 (6.5)	3 (4.6)	81 (3.6)	0
Looping	2 (10.5)	3 (6.5)	5 (7.7)	88 (3.9)	0
Targeted growth	0	1 (2.2)	1 (1.5)	56 (2.5)	0
Miscellaneous	0	3 (6.5)	3 (4.6)	87 (3.9)	2 (6.2)

From Berg et al.[38]

heart disease but with possible cerebral palsy, and although placental vascular anastomoses between the triplets were present, there was no discussion of possible hemodynamic imbalances[42]; (3) isolated four-chamber EFE was present in one of a female twin pair who was hydropic, but placentation/ zygosity was not reported.[43]

The vascular component of CVS anomalies is rarely reported in twins other than anomalies of the great vessels. Generalized arterial calcification of infancy in twins is mentioned in Chapter 6, as it suggests more a disease process than true malformation.

An extensive review of *absence of one umbilical artery* recorded a three to four times greater incidence of single umbilical artery among members of multiple gestation, but the affected infants had associated malformations at the same rate as singletons and there was no consistent pattern to these malformations.[44] Most twins were discordant for single umbilical artery and the infant with the single umbilical artery was the smaller of the two in 82.4% of the cases where the weights of both were known. Concordance was greater in monozygotic twins than dizygotic twins, but 37% of the twins with single umbilical artery were monozygotic and 63% dizygotic. Cases of chorangiopagus twins (acardia) were excluded. The conclusion was that the presence of only one umbilical artery denotes a greater risk of perinatal mortality beyond that due to any associated malformation.

In the autopsied twins from Survey '91, there were 7 with solitary CVS anomalies, 9 with multiple anomalies limited to the CVS, 12 had CVS defects as part of non-syndromic combinations, and five as part of syndromes. The sexes were equally affected. The anomalies were grouped mechanistically and the distribution of cases is listed in Table 7.2 for comparison with the reported series. When there were several lesions in one twin that fell into one group, such as atresia of the aortic valve and ventricular septal defect (VSD), they were recorded as one case in that group, but if a twin had several lesions that belonged to different groups, they were recorded separately, in order to convey an idea of the frequency of the mechanistic groups. Other than the constellation of lesions with the hypoplastic left heart syndrome, there were no patterns in the combinations of multiple anomalies limited to the CVS, nor was there any pattern in the combinations

of nonsyndromic multiple lesions, either the type of cardiac defect or the other systems affected. The minor lesions included persistent left superior vena cava to the coronary sinus, and fenestrated atrial septum operculum. The major lesions included coarctation of aorta, valve atresias, tetralogy of Fallot, truncus arteriosus, endocardial fibroelastosis, aorticopulmonary window, and hypoplastic left heart syndrome.

There were three proven concordantly affected sets: persistent left superior vena cava to the coronary sinus in monochorionic female twins with twin transfusion syndrome; truncus arteriosus with growth retardation but no other system affected in twin females of undefined chorionicity or zygosity; and hypoplastic left heart syndrome with minor variation in twin females, also of undefined chorionicity or zygosity. One monochorionic set was discordantly affected—the recipient of a twin transfusion syndrome was hydropic with EFE of the right ventricle and a duplex left ureter, while her co-twin was normal at autopsy.

There were two cases with associated placental findings. In one case there was persistent left superior vena cava to the coronary sinus with ventricular septal defect and coarctation in the aorta in the smaller of two dichorionic male twins of unknown zygosity, associated with a velamentously inserted single artery umbilical cord. In the other case, persistent left superior vena cava to the coronary sinus was combined with crossed fused renal ectopia and Meckel's diverticulum in one of female twins of unknown zygosity or placentation, who also had a single umbilical artery cord. Unfortunately, placenta information was not provided with a number of the earlier cases in the survey. The mechanistic approach to anomalies in the CVS is a useful one and may be made more valuable in twins in future cases with the inclusion of details of placental vascular anatomy.

Central Nervous System

Anomalies of the central nervous system (CNS) have been reported to be increased in twins in the broad surveys, but there is little agreement on which are increased, and reported concordance/ discordance is rarely coupled with genetic/ placentation data. The concept of an embryonic "midline" as a developmentally unstable region has been suggested as a source for midline defects in singletons.[45] Whether this can be related to midline anomalies in monozygotic twins is not clear, nor whether it could explain discordant lesions in monozygotic twins.

Concordant severe *microcephaly* has been reported in monochorionic female twins from consanguineous parents with additional blood group and dermatoglyphic analyses, supporting autosomal recessive inheritance.[46]

Holoprosencephaly/synotia was grossly discordant in a set of monochorionic female twins spontaneously aborted at 15 weeks.[47] Although grossly quite distinct, there were "some subtle histologic features that are associated with holoprosencephaly" in the apparently normal twin. There was differential size and color suggesting twin transfusion, but vascular anastomoses were not described, so the role of hemodynamic factors as a threshold for severity cannot be assessed. The larger plethoric twin was the one that was grossly anomalous. Another report of holoprosencephaly in one of triplet female fetuses used chromosome polymorphisms to confirm monozygosity of the two surviving triplets (the third was a fetus papyraceous).[48] Again, there was differential size and hematocrit with the anomaly in the smaller anemic twin, but details of fetal membranes or fetal vessel anastomoses were not given.

Of all the CNS anomalies reported in twins, the greatest attention has been to *neural tube defects* (NTD), anencephaly in particular.[49–51] As with other surveys of twins with anomalies, the earlier literature on twins and NTD is inconclusive. Anencephaly and encephalocele are often lethal perinatally, so studies that do not include stillbirth or autopsy data may be incomplete. A large survey of 16,888 twin pairs that included fetal deaths or stillbirths over 20 weeks' gestation, found that twin pairs represented 3.4% of cases of anencephaly, 1.4% of spina bifida cases and 9.7% of encephalocele cases, although twin pairs were only 1.95% of all births.[50] Both anencephaly and encephalocele had a statistically significant increased relative risk in twins over singletons, but spina bifida did not. All defects were more common in like-sex twins, but zygosity assignment was not stated. Like-sex female twins were at highest risk for NTD and fetal death, with a significant excess of female twins with encephalocele compared to male twins.[51] Concor-

dance was observed only in like-sex pairs at a rate of 5.3%. The underlying mechanisms of NTD remain to be determined. The apparent concurrence of NTD with female genotype and monozygotic twinning may suggest a common associated process, such as an early "insult" causing duplication and additional morphologic abnormalities.[49,51] The occurrence of anencephaly with female incomplete twinning (diprosopus) would also support this association.[52] The fact that most anencephaly is discordant remains to be explained, and may relate to factors of placentation. The association between sirenomelia and anencephaly has been noted, with discordant sets reported in monochorionic female twins[53] and dichorionic female twins.[54] The latter were said to be dizygotic, but the basis for this was not provided. Whether myelocystocele with cloacal exstrophy in female twins is part of this spectrum is not clear.[55] A set of monoamniotic twins were concordant for the defect, but the paler twin was more severely affected. Discordant congestion of the placenta was reported but no further details of fetal vascular anatomy were provided, so the role of vascular thresholds could not be assessed.

An interesting side issue related to fetal anomalies in twins is the possibility of intervention when the anomaly is identified antenatally. Selective termination of one of anomalous twins was discussed in Chapter 5. Selective treatment of affected twins might be considered based on the nature of the defect and has been reported for discordant hydrocephalus.[56] The cause of the hydrocephalus was not discussed nor was zygosity or placentation reported.

Malformations identified in the CNS in the autopsied Survey '91 twins were all major defects except for one case of unilateral hypoplasia of the left cranial nerve I. The major defects were midline in 72% (anencephaly, encephalocele, and lumbosacral meningomyelocele in equivalent numbers), microcephaly in 22%, and associated with amnion disruption in 6%. The distribution by sex affected was equal with 80% of the anomalies in twins of like-sex pairs. Chorionicity was known in 65% of the cases—just over half were monochorionic and 60% of these were monoamniotic, an unusual distribution not seen in any other group of anomalies. In 72% of cases with additional nonsyndromic anomalies in other systems, the defect was renal agenesis or other renal malformation. The significance of this observation is not known. Concordantly affected twins with discordant CNS lesions were seen in two sets of unknown zygosity/chorionicity: Dandy-Walker/microcephaly in twin females; and aqueduct stenosis with thalamic fusion, agenesis corpus callosum and septum pellucidum, and hydrocephalus/anencephaly in female twins. These major defects were quite evident grossly, and it was noted that in six sets of monochorionic twins no similar lesion was reported in the co-twin, although minor related defects were not ruled out as none of the co-twins came to autopsy. Two of these were monoamniotic twin sets. In four of these discordant monochorionic twin sets, there were placental findings that could be interpreted to represent a disadvantage to the affected twin—a marginally inserted single artery cord with microcephaly, an abnormally short single artery cord with anencephaly/iniencephaly, a single artery cord and smaller placental mass with a closed neural tube defect with cloacal exstrophy, and vascular anastomoses with the donor of the twin transfusion being anencephalic. Whether these are causal, coincidental, or contributing factors remains to be determined but the concurrence is noteworthy and supports the value of placental findings in cases of anomalous development.

Gastrointestinal Tract

The third group of anomalies reported to occur more commonly in twins in the large literature series is in the gastrointestinal tract (GIT). For purposes of this review, that group is taken to include associated viscera, particularly the liver.

The commonest abnormalities of the gastrointestinal tract reported in twins were *atresias or stenoses* of various types. Twins were four times as frequent in cases of *esophageal atresia* as the general population, and the majority (89%) had other malformations, particularly cardiac.[57] Zygosity and placentation were not mentioned and the possibility that affected twins had the VATER constellation of anomalies[58] was not discussed. *Pyloric stenosis* was reported in all three of monochorionic male triplets, and this observation tends to support the importance of genetic factors in this condition.[59] Cases of *jejunal atresia* included an excess of twins, and while vascular causes were potentially important, placentation was not usually

discussed. The observation in one series that jejunal atresia in twins was most common in nonidentical sets appears to be based on the erroneous interpretation that separate placentas means nonidentity.[60] A suggested relationship of atresias of jejunum and ileum in twins with advanced maternal age and use of intra-amniotic methylene blue injections for prenatal diagnosis remains to be clarified.[61] The etiology of *small left colon syndrome* is not known, but genetic or intrauterine environmental factors are suggested by two sets of twins: discordantly affected monochorionic female twins, and concordantly affected twins of unstated sex and placentation.[62] Discordant *anal atresia/agenesis* is part of the sirenomelia anomaly and has been reported in one of monoamniotic twins associated with renal agenesis but normal limbs.[63] The influence of vascular/hemodynamic factors to the discordant anomalies is suggested by the fact that the umbilical cords of these latter twins were extensively intertwined and the cord to the anomalous twin had only one artery. It may be argued that absence of one artery was simply part of the anomaly complex, but entanglement of the cords could have a greater effect on the circulation in the single artery cord.[64]

Aganglionosis of the intestine (Hirschsprung's disease) may have a postmigration destructive cause in some cases, and reports of discordantly affected monozygotic [by blood group and human leukocyte antigen (HLA) typing] twins have been used in support of this theory.[65] The placentas were "common," but no reference was made to fetal vascular patterns, so that possible hemodynamic factors contributing to "perinatal environmental insults" cannot be assessed.

Extrahepatic *biliary atresia* has not been reported to be concordant in any twin pair and the suggestion is that it is an acquired lesion due to perinatal regional ischemia or congenital infection. The reported twin sets are almost all same-sex pairs, but placentation was not discussed and zygosity assignment is uncertain.[66]

The majority of the anomalies (79%) in the GIT identified in the Survey '91 autopsy series were minor lesions consisting of Meckel's diverticulum in 29%, minor degrees of malrotation of the bowel in 25%, and accessory nodules of pancreatic/splenic tissues in the remainder. Atresia was seen in 14.3%, involving the esophagus (with tracheal fistula), duodenum (with absent gallbladder), colon (ileocecal valve to rectum), or anus. The infant with cloacal exstrophy had a short intestine. In half the twins with GIT anomalies, it was the only defect found. When the GIT anomaly was associated with defects in other systems, the associated defects were all minor except for the tracheal fistula with esophageal atresia. Males were affected 1.6 : 1. Two monochorionic male twin sets were discordant for malrotation of the ascending colon, a monochorionic male twin set was concordant for Meckel's diverticulum, and a monoamniotic male twin set was discordant for short gut associated with cloacal exstrophy and a shorter single artery umbilical cord.

In this group of autopsied twins, anomalies of the GIT did not represent a major burden and the majority were incidental. This is an interesting observation, as the intestine is perhaps as much a midline structure as the neural tube, and yet it appears to be disturbed far less—endodermal and ectodermal "midlines" do not seem to be comparable entities—and the most serious defects, atresias, are perhaps acquired in utero from vascular causes.

Genitourinary System

Anomalies of the urinary tract are less commonly reported in twins, but a few particularly interesting studies are worth noting. One exemplary report of discordant malformations in male monochorionic twins discussed the potential role of placental morphology and fetal hemodynamics.[67] The twin with sacral agenesis, anal atresia, and urethral atresia, with related findings in the bladder, ureters, kidneys, and abdominal wall, also had an abnormally long umbilical cord that was velamentously inserted and had only one umbilical artery. It was suggested that interference with adequate placental development in early embryogenesis could affect embryonic development, and that a potential source of that interference was the other twin's placental mass. This case is an excellent example of the concept that even if twins are genetically identical, their intrauterine environment is not identical, because the environment of each is the other twin, and that environment may not be identical based on factors of placentation.

The possible interaction of environmental factors affecting genomic expression is suggested by reports of several other anomalies. Based on family studies, bilateral *renal agenesis* may have a genetic component and may be related to unilateral renal agenesis and total renal dysplasia, but concordance in twins is rarely reported.[68] It has been suggested that bilateral renal agenesis in both monochorionic female twins could be on the basis of a common environmental factor during fetal life, as well as on a genetic basis.[68] The *absence of recognizable proximal tubules* in the nondeformed fetal/neonatal kidney is rare, but has been associated with monochorionic placentation and evidence of disturbed intertwin hemodynamics.[69] The affected twins were possible donors of twin transfusion syndromes and a chorangiopagus twin, suggesting that the lesion in these cases was a secondary, degenerative change on the basis of chronic renal hypoperfusion. Whether hypoperfusion can explain this anomaly in nontwin cases is not yet certain, but the association of renal tubular dysgenesis with certain antihypertensive therapy of the mother is supportive.[70] The observations in this anomaly example are evidence of the value of careful analysis of specific defects in twins with a view to suggesting possible avenues of further investigation. The fact that zygosity must be supplemented with placenta data is evident from a report of three sets of monozygotic (by HLA and blood group) but discordantly affected twins with *valves and reflux*.[71] Environmental differences were invoked as a potential explanation, but placentation was not described. It was pointed out that anomalies of the urinary tract in one twin should prompt investigation of the entire urinary tract of the other twin, as they may actually have concordant involvement in the system, but of a different pattern.

Genital anomalies have been most commonly reported with chromosomal errors as discussed below, while isolated hypospadius has been specifically mentioned as being decreased in twins, although why this might be so is not known.

Genitourinary (GU) anomalies in the Survey '91 autopsy series are considered together, as they often coexist, particularly in males. There were twice as many urinary anomalies as genital defects reported, with an excess of males of 1.4:1 in both categories. Nearly two-thirds of the GU anomalies were isolated lesions and 75% of these were minor, such as focal renal blastema, müllerian cysts in the prostate, and ectopic adrenal tissue in the testis. All the multiple-related anomaly cases had major defects as did the majority of the cases of nonsyndromic multiple anomalies that had GU malformations. Most of the major urinary defects consisted of unilateral or bilateral renal agenesis, or obstructive uropathy of various patterns. Only minor genital defects were reported in males while all the genital defects in females were major with agenesis of portions of the internal genitalia, but there were few cases in either category. There was no pattern of associated defects outside the GU system in the nonsyndromic multiple anomaly twins with GU anomalies.

It is difficult to derive conclusions from the concordance/discordance of the observed GU anomalies as placenta/zygosity data were not always provided. There were three concordantly affected twin sets: (1) both twin females had horseshoe kidneys among a number of other major lesions of the CNS, CVS, and respiratory tract, but placentation and zygosity was not stated; (2) dichorionic male twins of unknown zygosity were concordant for system affected, but one had hypospadius and the other mild hydronephrosis with undescended left testis plus minor malrotation of the cecum; and (3) monochorionic male twins both had posterior urethral valves with bilateral megacystis, hydroureter, and renal cystic dysplasia. In this last set, there were variations in severity, but no contributing factor identified. There were three discordantly affected monochorionic sets: (1) caudal regression with renal agenesis in one male twin with cleft lip and palate in the co-twin; (2) unilateral duplex ureter in a female twin with EFE and hydrops; and (3) cystic dysplastic right kidney in the recipient of a twin transfusion syndrome in a female twin.

In five cases of renal malformation, there were potential contributing placental findings. (1) In a monochorionic twin girl (details of co-twin not known), there was a 3-cm velamentous insertion of a single artery cord with the persistent vessel on the right. Interestingly, it was the right kidney and ureter that were missing, along with the uterus, cervix, and upper vagina, although the ovaries were normal. She also had a Meckel's diverticulum and agenesis of cranial nerve I. (2) The donor of a twin transfusion syndrome had renal hypoplasia, as well as a velamentous cord insertion. (3) The discordant caudal regression/facial cleft twin set mentioned above had a peculiar insertion of the umbilical

cords, each in odd folds of membranes from the separating diamniotic wall between the twins, and the insertion of the cord of the anomalous twin was actually within the sac containing the less anomalous twin (Fig. 7.2). (4) A recipient twin with twin transfusion syndrome had a cystic dysplastic right kidney. (5) A dichorionic separate twin placentation of a boy/girl pair had a velamentously inserted single artery umbilical cord (side of persistent vessel not stated) for the male twin who had agenesis of the left kidney and multiple other minor anomalies of extremities, spine, and ribs, and a Meckel's diverticulum. In these cases of associated renal/ placental findings in multiple anomaly infants, the cord lesions may be simply another reflection of the more general defect, but the potential hemodynamic augmentation of the defects is not ruled out.

The phenotypic secondary effects of oligohydramnios due to fetal anuria on the basis of agenesis/obstructive lesions of the urinary tract include pulmonary hypoplasia, facial and extremity deformations, and amnion nodosum.[14] These manifestations are sometimes modified when they occur in twins. In Fig. 7.3, the amnion nodosum on side A is easily seen, consistent with the consequences of bilateral renal agenesis, and twin A also had pulmonary hypoplasia (one-third the expected weight), but no limb deformation and minimal facial anomalies. The lack of face and limb lesions usually attributed to compression was thought due to the less constrictive intrauterine environment because he was one of twins, with a "cushioning" effect of the normal twin's sac. Why the lung hypoplasia was so severe under this theoretically less constrictive environment was not explained.

Body Wall Defects

Defects of the abdominal wall and diaphragm are sometimes associated with gastrointestinal and renal anomalies, and are occasionally reported in twins. Discordant male twins of unknown zygosity/ placentation had different patterns of urinary tract anomalies with deficiencies of the abdominal muscles, the typical prune belly in one and a large omphalocele in the other.[72] The influence of vascular factors on morphogenesis was suggested by an observed association of bowel atresias and twinning in patients with amyoplasia, with localized defects of the trunk muscles and gastroschises.[73] Mono-

FIGURE 7.2. This infant (a) was one of monochorionic male twins, discordant by 31.5% at 34 weeks' gestation. The co-twin had unilateral cleft lip and alveolus, restricted extension of the left elbow, and minor positional anomalies of the fingers, and did well. This twin had sacral agenesis, with agenesis of right leg, left femur and fibula, growth retardation (31 weeks' size), and bilateral renal agenesis with the oligohydramnios phenotype including pulmonary hypoplasia (14% of expected volume) and amnion nodosum on the placenta. The attachment of the diamniotic septum was Y-shaped, with the V pattern demarcating one-quarter of the chorionic surface of side A (b). The "I" of the attachment contained the first 5 cm of each umbilical cord, and the insertion site of the cord of the anomalous twin A was actually into the chorionic surface within the amniotic sac of twin B. There were two anastomoses, a direct 3 mm arterial connection between the 5 cm separate cord insertions and a peripheral 1 mm parenchymal shunt from B to A. The role of the odd cord insertion pattern to the discordant anomalies remains undetermined. No other differentiating feature was noted. Both cords had three normal vessels.

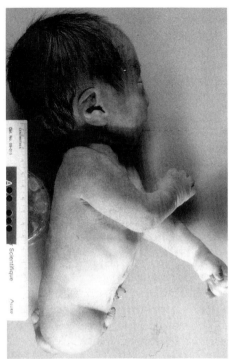

(a)

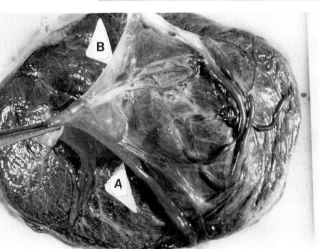

(b)

chorionic twins were overrepresented in cases of amyoplasia alone, and discordant involvement was the rule, but placental details, such as umbilical cord and fetal vascular anatomy, were not provided.[74] Mitotic crossing-over has been suggested as another explanation for these observations of discordantly affected twins.[4] Concordantly affected male twins with gastroschisis were monochorionic, but no other placental details were provided.[75] Defective formation of the diaphragm has been reported concordant in twins—bilateral eventration

in male twins, possibly monozygotic by chromosomal analysis,[76] and symmetric left diaphragmatic hernias in female twins, monozygotic by red cell antigens.[77] It is not clear how these observations relate to the defects as the lesion seems to be rare in twins.

Because few diaphragmatic hernias are reported in twins, the Survey '91 autopsy cases are presented in Table 7.3, along with three other cases related to body wall defects. Two-thirds of the cases are male, and other than the case with trisomy 18 and the

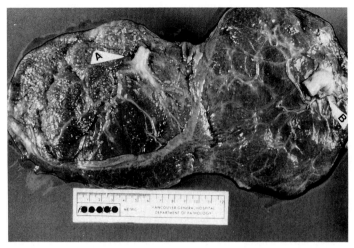

FIGURE 7.3. This dichorionic fused placenta was from twins discordant for bilateral renal agenesis. The amnion nodosum on side A (the affected twin) is evident as one of the components of the oligohydramnios phenotype. Twin A also had significant pulmonary hypoplasia, 6.5 g versus 21.6 g expected, but minimal facial dysmorphism and no limb deformations. The sex and zygosity of the co-twin were not reported. The presence of an adjacent twin sac with normal amounts of amniotic fluid was construed as representing a buffering influence on the normal constrictive phenotypic features of the oligohydramnios phenotype.

major body wall defect case, the associated abnormalities in the other systems, other than pulmonary hypoplasia, are minor. At least two cases are probably discordant in monochorionic twins, but no other placental factors were noted.

Miscellaneous

The twin literature contains a number of case reports of other anomalies in twins, with varying degrees of completeness of zygosity assignment and placental morphology. A few selected examples of special interest are reviewed here.

Facial anomalies, such as clefts of lip or palate and preauricular skin tags, have been reported to be more common in twins.[24] Vascular factors have been suggested as important in oroacral malformations, but reports of discordantly affected twins did not provide details of placentation.[78] Full concordance has never been reported for the facial asym-

TABLE 7.3. Diaphragmatic hernias and body wall defects in twins—Survey '91 autopsy series.

Defect	Additional defects	Sex	Placentation/ probable zygosity	Co-twin/comment
Hernia left diaphragm	PH; patent foramen ovale	M	--------------NS--------------	--------------NS--------------
Hernia left diaphragm	PH; trisomy 18	F	Dichorionic/DZ	M—SUA, distal palmar crease, survived
Hernia left diaphragm	PH	F	Dichorionic separate/NS	F—said to have congenital heart disease; one prior sib in family also with diaphragmatic hernia
Hernia left diaphragm	PH; hydropic	M	Monochorionic/MZ	M—
Hernia left diaphragm	PH; bicuspid pulmonary valve; donor twin transfusion	M	Monochorionic/MZ	M—
Hernia right diaphragm	PH; severe IUGR	M	Single disk/NS no other comment	M—IUGR
Eventration right diaphragm; attenuated muscle in left	PH; artrial septal defect	M	--------------NS--------------	M—clinically the same but survived
Left inguinal hernia	Nil	F	--------------NS--------------	F—
Major right body wall defect	Multiple visceral and lower spine anomalies	M?*	?Dichorionic/?DZ	F—

*External genitalia looked male but testes not found and cytogenetic culture failed. Placenta in fragments but said to be dichorionic clinically.

PH, pulmonary hypoplasia; DZ, dizygotic; MZ, monozygotic; NS, not stated; IUGR, intrauterine growth retardation; SUA, single umbilical artery; M, male; F, female; —, no similar defect reported but twin still alive.

FIGURE 7.4. This monochorionic placenta was from twin girls with discordant Wiedemann-Beckwith syndrome. The affected twin had the edematous cord. The weight discordance of 70% at 35 weeks may have been due in part to the effects of twin transfusion. There were chorionic vascular anastomoses compatible with this interpretation consisting of an arteriovenous shunt from the smaller to the larger twin, and an arterial anastomosis with the vessel from the smaller twin four times the diameter of the vessel from the larger twin. The hematocrits also differed at birth, 0.637 in the larger twin and 0.297 in the smaller twin.

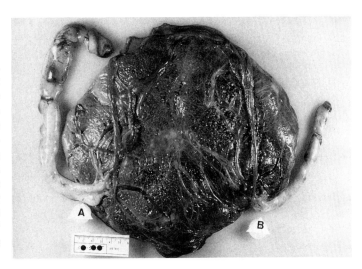

metry of the Goldenhar complex, although a number of cases in twins have been reported.[79] A vascular cause for the discordance was considered ruled out because not all discordantly affected monozygotic pairs had monochorionic placentas. Arguments for abnormalities of the egg with increased risks for mitotic crossing-over, perhaps related to twinning, have been suggested as explanation for these cases as well.[4] Facial anomalies, other than deformations associated with oligohydramnios were rarely noted in the autopsied twins from the Survey '91. One monochorionic twin female had a low set right ear but no other anomalies, and the co-twin was normal. A male twin of an unlike-sex dichorionic-separate disk pair had a velamentously inserted two vessel cord with multiple nonsyndromic anomalies including low-set ears, abnormal left auricle and preauricular tag, beaked nose, and large tongue. Unless associated with other causes of death or other major malformations, facial defects are unlikely to be found in an autopsy series.

Several *syndromes* have been observed to be discordant in apparently monozygotic twins. Monochorionic twin girls with concordant red blood cell antigens, plasma proteins, HLA testing, and hematocrits were discordantly affected with the Russell-Silver syndrome.[80] The affected twin had a velamentous insertion of the umbilical cord and the possibility of intrauterine events contributing to the expression of genetic information was discussed along with the alternative possibility that the syndrome is etiologically heterogeneous.

The Wiedemann-Beckwith syndrome has been of particular interest because monozygotic twins with the syndrome have all been female and discordantly affected.[4] Although placental vascular factors were suggested as a cause of this variability, placental morphology was not described.[81] Current investigation seems to suggest a combination of mitotic crossing-over with loss of heterozygosity in chromosome 11p,[4] followed by disrupted imprinting.[9,82] In the Survey '91 survivor series, one placenta (Fig. 7.4) was from a monochorionic discordantly affected set of twin girls. The 70% discrepancy in twin size may have been augmented by an element of chronic twin transfusion. There was one concordantly affected monochorionic male twin pair that came to autopsy. The first twin was stillborn and quite macerated but had adrenal cytomegaly, pancreatic islet cell hyperplasia, and Leydig cell hyperplasia and cytomegaly. The second twin had an omphalocele and facial features of Wiedemann-Beckwith syndrome, lived for 2½ months, and died from the effects of perinatal asphyxia. Both twins were concordantly large for gestational age at birth by linear measurements. The macerated twin was intensely congested and the survivor pale and hydropic at birth, suggesting an acute twin transfusion syndrome as a potential cause for these findings. There were appropriate vascular anastomoses on the delivered placenta, a 2-mm-diameter venous shunt, and bidirectional parenchymal anastomoses. Although DNA studies in the macerated twin were unsuccessful, the 11p chromosomal finding was absent from the surviving twin.

Many of the infants with the various forms of *osteochondrodystrophy* are thought to be the result of new mutations, and concordance in monochorionic twins may help decide when this mutation took place.[83] Components of the bony abnormalities may be modified by being a twin, as for example discordant kleeblattschädel (cloverleaf skull) anomaly in monochorionic twins with thanatophoric dysplasia, although whether "crowding" is a sufficient explanation remains to be determined.[83]

In the *Survey '91* autopsy series, there were a few additional anomalies reported in the respiratory tract (RT), musculoskeletal system (MS), and limbs. There were few respiratory tract anomalies other than pulmonary hypoplasia. The majority (85%) of significant *pulmonary hypoplasia* (lungs less than half the expected weight and/or histologically hypoplastic) were associated with oligohydramnios due to anuric renal malformations or the intrathoracic space-occupying effects of anomalies of the diaphragm. In three cases no cause for the hypoplasia was defined because it was a solitary finding in discordantly affected male twins of unknown chorionicity/zygosity, discordantly affected monoamniotic male twins with marked entanglement of the umbilical cords (lungs were one-fourth the expected weight), and a third set with an affected male twin but no other data. There was complete *agenesis* of the right lung in a monochorionic female twin with tracheoesophageal fistula, vertebral anomalies, focal renal blasteme, and a velamentous cord insertion. The co-twin also had a velamentous insertion of the umbilical cord, but no other information was given. A female twin of a like-sex pair of unstated chorionicity/zygosity had a small multilocular *bronchogenic cyst* as a minor anomaly with other major lesions in the brain, heart, and kidney, and the co-twin had related nonsyndromic multiple anomalies in the same systems, but with pulmonary hypoplasia due to eventration of the diaphragm bilaterally. Minor variations in lobation were reported occasionally without any apparent pattern.

MS and limb anomalies were uncommon other than deformations of foot position in cases with oligohydramnios, or vertebral and rib anomalies in twins with major malformations in multiple systems. Arthrogryposis of unknown origin was associated with microcephaly, abnormal facies, and growth retardation in a discordantly affected mono-

chorionic twin who also had a marginally inserted single artery umbilical cord. Unilateral or bilateral transverse palmar (simian) creases were seen as isolated findings in five discordant sets (females affected in four), and minor vertebral anomalies, mild scoliosis, pectus excavatum, and 11 pairs of overtubulated ribs (in a monoamniotic set) in one each.

Amniotic Band/Fetal Disruptions

The patterns of amniotic band/fetal disruptions in twins have received considerable attention, because the cause of premature disruption of the amnion is not known, nor is it agreed whether the fetal disruptions are purely secondary or part of the underlying problem. The spectrum of reported observations in twins includes a small residual sac of amnion around the insertion of the umbilical cord with no fetal disruptions[84]; entanglements of the umbilical cord, concordant and discordant[85]; digital/limb constrictions/amputations only, concordant[86] and discordant[87]; major body wall defects with limb and related visceral anomalies, also concordant[88] and discordant[89]; and severe craniofacial defects, although these were less often reported with twins and usually combined with body wall defects.[89,90] Involvement of reportedly monochorionic twins has been both concordant and similar[86,88,91] and discordant with affected and normal.[87,89,90,92] There was no discernible pattern of antenatal history or maternal disorder reported and no apparent male/female predisposition to occurrence or pattern.

What may be important to consider in these cases is the location of the disruption of the amnion. The amnion covering of the umbilical cord seems to be immune from disruption as the residual sacs or strands are firmly attached at the site of insertion of the cord and the cord surface is always intact. A number of reports described strands of amnion coming off the fetal surface of the placenta on the side of the affected twin.[86,87,91,92] One report stated that amnion was missing from the fetal surface and reflected membranes on both sides of the placenta with concordantly affected twins, but with an intact dividing septum in a monochorionic diamniotic placenta.[88] The histology of the membrane layer between the twins was not displayed. If in fact the separating membranes were two layers of amnion

FIGURE 7.5. Amniotic band disruptions in female monochorionic twin pair. The residual collar of amnion encircles the two umbilical cords (a), (b, heavy arrows), and there was no residual amnion elsewhere. The stillborn twin died from constriction of the cord (a) and had no amputations or other defects—note the pallor of its portion of the placenta after 4 weeks of fetal death. The surviving co-twin had digital amputations but did well. Confirmation of the monoamniotic nature of the placenta is seen in (b, small arrows), with a uniform layer of amnion between the cord insertions.

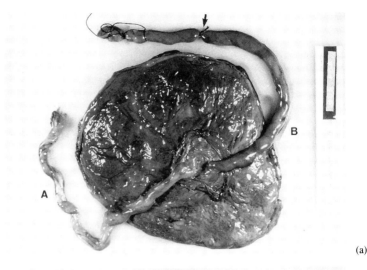

(a)

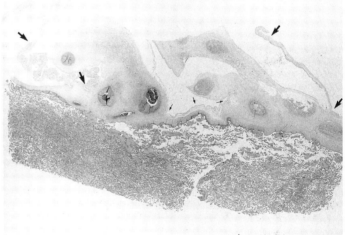

(b)

only, it is striking that they remained intact in the face of disruption of the rest of the amniotic lining layer. If this is indeed the pattern of amnion disruption in monochorionic twins, that is, sparing of the intervening membranes, an explanation is needed and may be important to the pathogenesis of premature rupture of amnion. Thus, it is suggested that any history of fetal adherences, constrictions, or amputations in twins should prompt a particularly careful pathologic analysis of the location of persistent amnion and the areas where it has become disrupted, documenting the extent of loss of amnion. It would also be worth noting the insertion of the umbilical cord because in more than a third of the cases cited above (36.8%), abnormal insertions were depicted or described—marginal insertions in three cases and passing in the separating mem-

branes in four cases. The significance of this observation remains to be determined.

There were two sets of twins in the Survey '91 autopsy series with amniotic bands as a cause of anomalies. In a female monochorionic monoamniotic set the umbilical cords inserted 1.5 cm apart in the center of the disk, surrounded together by a residual collar of amnion (Fig. 7.5a). The stillborn twin B died as a result of severe constriction of the umbilical cord (Fig. 7.5a), by a strand of amnio/chorial connective tissue 22 cm above the placental surface. There was no residual amnion layer on the chorionic surface, or on the inside of the reflected membranes. The section through the cord insertion site contained the residual collar of amnion (Fig. 7.5b), and an intact surface layer of amnion between the cords, confirming the monoamniotic pattern. The live-born co-twin had multiple digital amputations of both hands sparing the thumb, with tissue strands attached, but no other signs of amniotic bands, and she did well. The pregnancy had been uneventful until intrauterine fetal death was identified during a routine follow-up (for twins) ultrasound examination at 28 weeks.

In the second case, a dichorionic (separate disks) set of female twins were dizygotic by ABO blood groups (AB+/A+), and one twin was entirely normal. The other twin had an aberrant facial cleft from the upper lip to the inner canthus of the right eye, absence of the first cranial nerve bilaterally, stenosis of the aqueduct with hydrocephalus and a number of microscopic abnormalities of the brain, digital amputations and fusions of fingers and toes, simian crease of the right hand, a slight varus deformity of the right foot, and congenital heart disease consisting of tetralogy of Fallot with a right aortic arch and ductus arteriosus. The facial cleft and digital features are pathognomonic of the amniotic band syndrome, and aqueduct stenosis with hydrocephalus have been seen in these cases, but the connection is not known. Congenital heart disease is not usually a feature unless there is ectopia cordis, so the connection in this case is not clear. The umbilical cord of the affected twin had a marginal insertion and amnion was missing from the chorionic surface of the placenta and the lining of the reflected membranes in this twin's sac.

Teratogens

Discordant phenotypic effects of teratogens have been reported in twins and higher multiples, and have been attributed to differing genetic susceptibility on the basis of dizygosity, although how zygosity was assigned is not always clear and placental data are not provided. Cases reported have included the effects of alcohol,[93] hydantoin,[94] and thalidomide.[95] Discordant involvement of reportedly monozygotic twin girls with fetal alcohol syndrome (both affected but with different severity) was cited to suggest intrauterine modifiers of the teratogenic effects,[93] but the basis for monozygosity and the pattern of placentation was unclear.[96] An association of congenital anomalies among monozygotic twins conceived within 3 months of cessation of oral contraceptives did not specify the pattern of

placentation or the anomalies observed, but said that no abnormality appeared to be more common.[97] There were no anomalies attributable to teratogens in the Survey '91 autopsy series.

Chromosomal Anomalies—Monozygotic Heterokaryotic Twins

It has been suggested that there is an increased risk of chromosomal abnormalities in twin gestations[98] and studies of the association of chromosomal anomalies with twinning has provided some particularly interesting findings. Both numerical and structural aberrations have been described with discordant manifestations in some sets of apparently monozygotic twins, referred to as monozygotic heterokaryotic twins (MZHT). A migration error, occurring during an early postzygotic cell division before the emergence of the primitive streak, has been suggested as the origin of MZHT. Depending on the timing of this event in relation to the twinning process, the twins will each be more or less mosaic for the defect.[99] In monochorionic placentations there may be shared chorionic circulations, and MZHT twins may be hematopoietic mosaics due to chimerism.[100]

The commonest reported abnormality in MZHT is discordance for phenotypic sex with a variety of chromosomal combinations. The most common of these is a female phenotype with *Ullrich-Turner syndrome* in one of a twin pair. In 25 affected twin pairs, the co-twin was similarly affected in 7, was a phenotypically normal female in 10, a phenotypically normal male in 7, and an infant with intersex in 1.[99,101] The cytogenetic makeup of cells cultured from blood, skin, fascia, gonads, and bone marrow varied. Nearly two-thirds of the affected infants were mosaics with different mixtures of normal and abnormal cell lines in blood, skin, or other tissues, or different karyotypes from different tissues. In six of the seven concordantly involved sets, the cytogenetic patterns were the same. Three of the seven normal female co-twins were mosaics in blood and skin, as were three of the normal male co-twins. The phenotypic intersex co-twin was mosaic 45,X/ 46,XY in all cultures. The problem of assessing mosaicism in blood lymphocytes was mentioned, based on fetal vascular connections in monochorionic placentas, but while zygosity was considered confirmed in all cases, the pattern of placentation was not stated in most. Although mosaicism is difficult to rule out in any one case, a number of investigations suggested that one discordantly affected normal male twin pair were in fact nonmosaic.[99] This might mean that the nondisjunction occurred after the twinning process, and after differentiation of cells intended for the embryo and for the placenta. However, the placental tissues on the side of the affected twin were distinctly hydropic, suggesting the presence of abnormal tissues there as well, possibly embryo-derived mesenchyme. Cytogenetic analysis of chorionic villus components would be needed to clarify this observation.[5] A report of lymphocytic nonmosaic chromosomally identical [45,X,inv(9)(p13;q13)], but phenotypically discordant twins mentioned that the placenta was monochorionic, but provided no further assessment of potential hemodynamic influences on the discordant severity.[102]

The association of distribution discrepancies of the X chromosome is not limited to MZHT with Turner's syndrome. There is also an association of twinning with *Klinefelter's syndrome* (47,XXY), with a reported incidence of 7.1% compared to 0.1% in singletons.[103] Also, there is an increase in the incidence of twinning in sibships with Klinefelter's or Turner's syndrome.[104,105] It has been noted in Chapter 3 that a higher proportion of monozygotic twins are females and there is an even greater excess of females among conjoined twins. The associations remain unexplained except for unverified suggestions of greater unidentified mortality of males early in gestation, or qualities of the X chromosome that predispose to migration errors or monozygotic twinning.

Determining the zygosity of twins with *autosomal discordance* can be a bit confusing on occasion. The commonest autosomal aneuploidy reported has been trisomy 21, or Down syndrome, in spite of the fact that Down syndrome has been reported to be less frequent in twins than singletons in the population surveys (Table 7.1). It has been generally observed that monozygotic twins were concordant and dizygotic twins discordant for the syndrome. Discordant apparently monozygotic twins raise some interesting questions. In one set, discordant twin boys were nonmosaic 46,XY and 47,XY,+

21, respectively in skin and by clinical appearance, but were lymphocytic mosaics.[106] The placenta was monochorionic with intertwin anastomoses. The twins were identical in 4 blood group antigens, 5 HLA haplotypes, and 13 protein polymorphisms. The explanations offered included the loss of the trisomic cell line in the one twin, or a mitotic nondisjunction after twinning with loss of the monosomy 21 cell line. Chimerism of the serum proteins and blood antigens studied was not ruled out. A second set, discordant for trisomy 21, consisted of monochorionic twins also discordant for sex, but with normal sex chromosome patterns in skin fibroblasts with mixoploidy of blood lymphocytes and identical blood groups.[107] There were vascular anastomoses, so chimerism was concluded, and dizygosity further confirmed by discordant α_1-antitrypsin phenotypes, a serum enzyme of hepatic origin. Dispermic monovular twinning could explain these observations (see Chapter 2).

These cases of MZHT, with trisomy 21 and the anomalies of X chromosome distribution described above, are examples that serve to refute the dogma that the problem of proving zygosity does not arise in the case of twins of opposite sex. It is investigation of precisely these cases that "don't fit" that provide the possibility of extending our knowledge about twinning. Concordance of trisomy 21 in twins reportedly dizygotic because of unlike sex thus may have several explanations.[108]

Discordant phenotypes with concordant autosomal aneuploidy in twins has been described, with both twins having the chromosomal error but with different manifestations. Monozygosity has been assigned by various means, but although contributions from intrauterine environmental influences were suggested for the differences, placental data were not often presented. This pattern of discordance has been reported for trisomy 13[109] and trisomy 18,[110] and in a set of monoamniotic twins, the more severely anomalous twin had a single artery umbilical cord and the twins' cords were entwined several times.[111]

Other chromosomal anomalies are less commonly reported in twins. Karyotypic discordance in chorangiopagus twins is discussed in Chapter 10. Triploidy and choriomas related to twins are discussed in Chapter 3. Twins have been reported to be no more frequent among triploid conceptions, whether aborted, stillborn, or live-born.[112] Monochorionic twins have been reported to be discordant for partial trisomy 1,[113] partial monosomy 10[114] and monozygotic twins discordant for 22 : 22 translocation with normal phenotypes.[101] The placentation described with the discordant deletion of chromosome 10 was unusual—monochorionic diamniotic with separate disks connected by membranes and no vascular anastomoses—but was not commented on further.[114]

In the Survey '91 autopsy series, the only chromosomal anomaly identified in twins autopsied after 20 weeks' gestation was trisomy 18 and all three twin sets were discordant and dichorionic with unlike sex pairs in two sets.

Malformations Related to the Twinning Process

In the introduction to this chapter, it was suggested that there are four classes of defects potentially related to twinning. (1) Anomalies that are seen only with disturbed monovular or monozygotic twinning are discussed in Chapter 10. (2) Crowding of two infants in a uterus that is meant ideally for one may result in fetal deformities, or affect placental development with secondary consequences for the fetuses. (3) The chorionicity of placentation may influence the manifestations of a malformation, particularly if there are intertwin vascular connections. (4) Finally, the process that leads to monovular or monozygotic twinning may itself influence the further development of each twin. The evidence for this is the greater frequency of anomalies in monozygotic twins than can be explained by hereditary influences alone, and the fact that rates of malformations increase with increasing proximity of monozygotic twins. A number of the examples already discussed make reference to these relationships, but a brief expansion is warranted.

An excess of *midline malformations,* such as symmelia, cloacal exstrophy, and neural tube defects, has been reported associated with monozygotic twinning.[115] It is not understood yet what the relationships might be between the forces that lead to the formation of two sets of embryonic axes and the genetic/spatial programs that would have affected the development and separation or fusion of midline structures in the original zygote or cell mass.[3,45] Symmelia (sirenomelia) and neural tube

defect have been reported in the same twin with a normal co-twin in three female sets, monochorionic,[53] dichorionic but zygosity assignment unspecified[54] and without placenta/zygosity details,[116] and similarly affected but with discordant severity in monoamniotic male twins.[117] All these sets may be monozygotic and may reflect a twinning process that went awry with an "injury" to one twin,[118] or "dizygotic" in the sense of "tertiary oocyte" (polar body) twinning.[3] A search for evidence of a "vanishing twin" may be worthwhile in these cases.[118] Reference has already been made to the association of female twins with neural tube defects[51] and abnormalities of monozygotic twinning, such as conjoined twins, but the nature of the relationship is not known.

Related to midline malformations and twinning is the concept of body symmetry and mirror imaging in twins. *Mirror imaging* can be considered to be of four types: anatomical, external and visceral; functional, mainly dominance in voluntary muscle action, such as handedness; pathological, sides affected with concordant disorders, such as in the teeth; and psychological, complementary characteristics.[2] Visceral mirror imaging is described more commonly in conjoined twins than in monozygotic twins that are completely separate, and is more often situs inversus than isomerism syndromes.[119] The orientation in conjoined twins may be affected by the proximity of the twins, or the state of the symmetry program of the original embryonic cell mass at the time of twinning. Whether orientation disturbances in separate monozygotic twins can be explained similarly is not certain.[3]

A number of accounts of discordant malformations have mentioned that there might be factors of the *intrauterine environment* that influence the expression of a defect. The intrauterine environment of a twin is first its placenta, second its co-twin, and third its mother (see Fig. 4.1). Thus each twin has a different intrauterine environment. It has been suggested throughout this chapter that the pattern of placentation may be very important to the expression of an abnormality, and the pattern of placentation relates to the pattern of twinning and implantation. The observation that velamentous insertions of the umbilical cord were correlated with cleft palate and anencephaly in discordant monozygotic twins was interpreted to mean that the cord anomaly might have functioned as a threshold for the malformation.[120] Some anomalies that are polygenic with a threshold for expression may have that threshold provided by a particular pattern of placentation that arises because of twinning.

Conclusion

We still have much to learn about the relationships of malformations and twinning based on the discussion above, and the pathologist has a key contribution to make. Any description of anomalies in twins must be correlated with detailed placental morphology that includes the cord insertions, numbers of disks, patterns of membrane relations, and details of intertwin vascular anastomoses. In addition, cytogenetic/zygosity/DNA investigations would include analysis of several tissues including the placenta. Placental and genetic findings are then correlated with autopsy and/or clinical investigation results, preferably for the twins together in a single report. While this may seem to be a daunting load of work for a general service pathologist, it actually takes less time than expected and the payoff is far more valuable information. As can be seen from the comments in this chapter, the cases with the greatest value are those with anatomic/placental/genetic data correlated with the other twin, and twin studies using such cases may be one of the keys to future studies of anomalies and their pathogenesis.

References

1. Nielsen J. Inheritance in monozygotic twins. *Lancet*. 1967;2:717–718.
2. Farber SL. *Identical Twins Reared Apart. A Reanalysis*. New York: Basic Books; 1981:10–13.
3. Boklage CE. Invited editorial essay: twinning, nonrighthandedness, and fusion malformations: evidence for heritable causal elements held in common. *Am J Med Genet*. 1987;28:67–84.
4. Côté GB, Gyftodimou J. Twinning and mitotic crossing-over: some possibilities and their implications. *Am J Hum Genet*. 1991;49:120–130.
5. Kalousek DK. The role of confined placental mosaicism in placental function and human development. *Growth Genet Horm*. 1986;4:1–3.
6. Kastern W, Kryspin-Sorensen I. Penetrance and low concordance in monozygotic twins in disease: are they the results of alterations in somatic genomes? *Mol Reprod Dev*. 1988;1:63–75.
7. Szulman AE, Surti U. The syndromes of partial and complete molar gestation. *Clin Obstet Gynecol*. 1984;27:172–180.
8. Graham JM. Clinical approach to human structural defects. *Semin Perinatol*. 1991;15(suppl 1):2–15.
9. Lubinsky MS, Hall JG. Genomic imprinting, monozygous twinning, and X inactivation. *Lancet*. 1991;337:1288.
10. Benirschke K, Kaufmann P. *Pathology of the Human Placenta*. 2nd ed. New York: Springer-Verlag; 1990:717.
11. Robinson LK, Jones KL, Benirschke K. The nature of structural defects associated with velamentous and marginal insertion of the umbilical cord. *Am J Obstet Gynecol*. 1983;146:191–193.
12. Gruenwald P, Mayberger HW. Differences in abnormal development of monozygotic twins. *Arch Pathol*. 1960;70:685–695.
13. Kalousek DK, Fitch N, Paradice BA. *Pathology of the Human Embryo and Previable Fetus. An Atlas*. New York: Springer-Verlag; 1990:181–185.
14. Jones K. *Smith's Recognizable Patterns of Human Malformations*. 4th ed. Philadelphia; WB Saunders; 1988:572–573.
15. Graham JM. *Smith's Recognizable Patterns of Human Deformation*. 2nd ed. Philadelphia; WB Saunders; 1988:102–105.
16. Van Allen MI. Fetal vascular disruptions: mechanisms and some resulting birth defects. *Pediatr Ann*. 1981;10:219–233.
17. Ferguson WF. Perinatal mortality in multiple gestations. (A review of perinatal deaths from 1609 multiple gestations.) *Obstet Gynecol*. 1963;23:861–870.
18. Hay S, Wehrung DA. Congenital malformations in twins. *Am J Hum Genet*. 1970;22:662–678.
19. Warkany J. *Congenital Malformations*. Chicago; Year Book Medical Publishers; 1971.
20. Onyskowova Z, Dolezal A, Jedlicka V. The frequency and character of malformations in multiple birth (a preliminary report) (Abstract). *Teratology*. 1971;4:496–497.
21. Emanuel I, Huang S-W, Gutman LT, Yu F-C, Lin C-C. The incidence of congenital malformations in a Chinese population: the Taipei collaborative study. *Teratology*. 1972;5:159–169.
22. Benirschke K, Kim CK. Multiple pregnancy. *N Engl J Med*. 1973;288:1276–1284,1329–1336.
23. Koivisto M, Jouppila P, Kauppila A, Mailanen I, Ylikorkala O. Twin pregnancy neonatal morbidity and mortality. *Acta Obstet Gynecol Suppl*. 1975; 44:21–29.

24. Myrianthopoulos NC. Congenital malformations in twins: epidemiologic survey. *Birth Defects*. 1975; 11:1–39.

25. Bonney GE, Walker M, Gbedeman K, Konotey-Ahulu FID. Multiple births and visible birth defects in 13,000 consecutive deliveries in one Ghanaian hospital. In: Nance WE, ed. Twin Research: Biology and Epidemiology. *Prog Clin Biol Res*. 1978;24B:105–108.

26. Chandra P, Harilal KT. Plural births—mortality and morbidity. In: Nance WE, ed. Twin Research: Biology and Epidemiology. *Prog Clin Biol Res*. 1978;24B:109–114.

27. Layde PM, Erickson JD, Falek A, McCarthy BJ. Congenital malformations in twins. *Am J Hum Genet*. 1980;32:69–78.

28. Corney G, MacGillivray I, Campbell DM, Thompson B, Little J. Congenital anomalies in twins in Aberdeen and Northeast Scotland. *Acta Genet Med Gemellol*. 1983;32:31–35.

29. Cameron AH, Edwards JH, Derom R, Thiery M, Boelaert R. The value of twin surveys in the study of malformations. *Eur J Obstet Gynecol Reprod Biol*. 1983;14:347–356.

30. Windham GC, Bjerkedal T. Malformations in twins and their siblings, Norway, 1967–79. *Acta Genet Med Gemellol*. 1984;33:87–95.

31. Källén B. Congenital malformations in twins: a population study. *Acta Genet Med Gemellol*. 1986;35:167–178.

32. Bryan E, Little J, Burn J. Congenital anomalies in twins. *Baillieres Clin Obstet Gynecol*. 1987;1:697–721.

33. Doyle PE, Beral V, Botting B, Wale CJ. Congenital malformations in twins in England and Wales. *J Epidemiol Community Health*. 1990;45:43–48.

34. Ross LJ. Congenital cardiovascular anomalies in twins. *Circulation*. 1959;20:327–342.

35. Nora JJ, Gilliland JC, Sommerville RJ, McNamara DG. Congenital heart disease in twins. *N Engl J Med*. 1967;277:568–571.

36. Anderson RC. Congenital cardiac malformations in 109 sets of twins and triplets. *Am J Cardiol*. 1977;39:1045–1050.

37. Burn J, Corney G. Congenital heart defects and twinning. *Acta Genet Med Gemellol*. 1984;33:61–69.

38. Berg KA, Astemborski JA, Boughman JA, Ferencz C. Congenital cardiovascular malformations in twins and triplets from a population-based study. *Am J Dis Child*. 1989;143:1461–1463.

39. Lang MJ, Aughton DJ, Riggs TW, Milad MP, Biesecker LG. Dizygotic twins concordant for truncus arteriosus. *Clin Genet*. 1991;39:75–79.

40. Rosenberg HS, Donnelly WH. The cardiovascular system. In: Wigglesworth JS, Singer DB, eds. *Textbook of Fetal and Perinatal Pathology*. Boston: Blackwell Scientific; 1991:757.

41. Rios B, Duff J, Simpson JW. Endocardial fibroelastosis with congenital complete heart block in identical twins. *Am Heart J*. 1984;107:1290–1293.

42. Seibold H, Mohr W, Lehmann WD, Lang D, Spanel R, Schwarz J. Fibroelastosis of the right ventricle in two brothers of triplets. *Pathol Res Pract*. 1980;170:402–409.

43. Alpan G, Gottschalk S, Glick B, Eyal F. Endocardial fibrosis and hydrops fetalis in a premature infant. *Helv Paediatr Acta*. 1985;40:69–73.

44. Heifetz SA. Single umbilical artery. A statistical analysis of 237 autopsy cases and review of the literature. *Perspect Pediatr Pathol*. 1984;8:345–378.

45. Opitz JM, Gilbert EF. Editorial comment: CNS anomalies and the midline as a "developmental field." *Am J Med Genet*. 1982;12:443–455.

46. Fried K, Micle S, Goldberg MD. Genetic microcephaly in a pair of monozygous twins. *Teratology*. 1984;29:177–180.

47. Machin GA, Sperber GH, Wootliffe J. Monozygotic twin aborted fetuses discordant for holoprosencephaly/synotia. *Teratology*. 1985;31:203–215.

48. Suslak L, Mimms GM, Desposito F. Letter to the editor: monozygosity and holoprosencephaly: cleavage disorders of the "midline field." *Am J Med Genet*. 1987;28:99–102.

49. James WH. Twinning and anencephaly. *Ann Hum Biol*. 1976;3:401–409.

50. Windham GC, Sever LE. Neural tube defects among twin births. *Am J Hum Genet*. 1982;34:988–998.

51. Windham GC, Bjerkedal T, Sever LE. The association of twinning and neural tube defects: studies in Los Angeles, California, and Norway. *Acta Genet Med Gemellol*. 1982;31:165–172.

52. Riccardi VM, Bergmann CA. Anencephaly with incomplete twinning (diprosopus). *Teratology*. 1977;16:137–140.

53. Rodriguez JI, Palacios J, Razquin S. Sirenomelia and anencephaly. *Am J Med Genet*. 1991;39:25–27.

54. Schwaibold H, Oehler U, Helpap B, Böhm N. Sirenomelia and anencephaly in one of dizygotic twins. *Teratology*. 1986;34:243–247.

55. McLaughlin JF, Marks WM, Jones G. Prospective management of exstrophy of the cloaca and myelocystocele following prenatal ultrasound recognition

of neural tube defects in identical twins. *Am J Med Genet*. 1984;19:721–727.

56. Goldstein P, Taylor WS, Zisow D, Carson B, Shuster E, Brodner R. Ventriculoamniotic shunt for treatment of hydrocephalus in one of twins: medical, ethical and legal considerations. *Fetal Diagn Ther*. 1990;5:84–91.

57. German JC, Mahour GH, Woolley MM. The twin with esophageal atresia. *J Pediatr Surg*. 1979;14:432–435.

58. Jones KL. *Smith's Recognizable Patterns of Human Malformation*. 4th ed. Philadelphia: WB Saunders; 1988:602–603.

59. Janik JS, Nagaraj HS, Lehocky R. Pyloric stenosis in identical triplets. *Pediatrics*. 1982;70:282–283.

60. Moorman-Voestermans CGM, Heij HA, Vos A. Jejunal atresia in twins. *J Pediatr Surg*. 1990;25:638–639.

61. Lancaster PAL, Pedisich EL. High risk of intestinal atresia among twins born to older mothers (Abstract). *Teratology*. 1992;45:330.

62. Cohen MD, Beck J, Weber T, Harper J. Neonatal small left colon in twins. *Gastrointest Radiol*. 1982;7:283–286.

63. Berry SA, Johnson DE, Thompson TR. Agenesis of penis, scrotal raphe, and anus in one of monoamniotic twins. *Teratology*. 1984;29:173–176.

64. Kaplan C, August D, Mizrachi H. Single umbilical artery and cord accidents (Abstract). *Mod Pathol*. 1990;3:4P.

65. Hannon RJ, Boston VE. Discordant Hirschsprung's disease in monozygotic twins: a clue to pathogenesis? *J Pediatr Surg*. 1988;23:1034–1035.

66. Schweizer P, Kerremans J. Discordant findings in extrahepatic bile duct atresia in 6 sets of twins. *Z Kinderchir*. 1988;43:72–75.

67. Johnstone BH, Benirschke K. Monozygotic twins discordant for urinary tract anomalies and presenting as hydramnios. *Obstet Gynecol*. 1975;47:610–615.

68. Yates JRW, Mortimer G, Connor JM, Duke JE. Concordant monozygotic twins with bilateral renal agenesis. *J Med Genet*. 1984;21:66–67.

69. Genest DR, Lage JM. Absence of normal-appearing proximal tubules in the fetal and neonatal kidney: prevalence and significance. *Hum Pathol*. 1991;22:147–153.

70. Barr M Jr, Cohen MM Jr. ACE inhibitor fetopathy and hypocalvaria: the kidney-skull connection. *Teratology*. 1991;44:485–495.

71. McCandless SE, Uehling D, Friedman AL. Urinary tract malformation in identical twins. *J Urol*. 1991;146:145–147.

72. Petersen DS, Fish L, Cass AS. Twins with congenital deficiency of abdominal musculature. *J Urol*. 1972;107:670–672.

73. Reid COMV, Hall JG, Anderson C, Bocian M, Carey J, Costa T, Curry C, Greenberg F, Horton W, Jones M, Lafer C, Larson E, Lubinsky M, McGillivray B, Pembry M, Popkin J, Seller M, Siebert V, Verhagen A. Association of amyoplasia with gastroschisis, bowel atresia, and defects of the muscular layer of the trunk. *Am J Med Genet*. 1986;24:701–710.

74. Hall JG, Reed SD, McGillivray BC, Herrmann J, Partington MW, Schinzel A, Shapiro J, Weaver DD. Part II amyoplasia: twinning in amyoplasia—a specific type of arthrogryposis with an apparent excess of discordantly affected identical twins. *Am J Med Genet*. 1983;15:591–599.

75. Gorczyca DP, Lindfors KK, Giles KA, McGahan JP, Hanson FW, Tennant FP. Prenatally diagnosed gastroschisis in monozygotic twins. *J Clin Ultrasound*. 1989;17:216–218.

76. Elberg JJ, Brok KE, Pedersen SA, Kock KEF. Congenital bilateral eventration of the diaphragm in a pair of male twins. *J Pediatr Surg*. 1989;24:1140–1141.

77. Watanatittan S. Congenital diaphragmatic hernia in identical twins. *J Pediatr Surg*. 1983;18:628–629.

78. Robinow M, Marsh JL, Edgerton MT, Sabie H, Johnson GF. Discordance in monozygotic twins for aglossia-adactylia, and possible clues to the pathogenesis of the syndrome. *Birth Defects*. 1978;14(6A):223–230.

79. Boles DJ, Bodurtha J, Nance WE. Goldenhar complex in discordant monozygotic twins: a case report and review of the literature. *Am J Med Genet*. 1987;28:103–109.

80. Samn M, Lewis K, Blumberg B. Monozygotic twins discordant for the Russell-Silver syndrome. *Am J Med Genet*. 1990;37:543–545.

81. Olney AH, Buehler BA, Waziri M. Wiedemann-Beckwith syndrome in apparently discordant monozygotic twins. *Am J Med Genet*. 1988;29:491–499.

82. Hall JG. Genomic imprinting: review and relevance to human disease. *Am J Hum Genet*. 1990;46:857–873.

83. Horton WA, Harris DJ, Collins DL. Discordance for kleeblattschadel anomaly in monozygotic twins with thanatophoric dysplasia. *Am J Med Genet*. 1983;15:97–101.

84. Yang SS. Intrauterine amniotic rupture with innocent amniotic bands and amniotic band syndrome (Abstract). *Mod Pathol*. 1990;3:10P.

85. Heifetz SA. Strangulation of the umbilical cord by

amniotic bands: a report of 6 cases and literature review. *Pediatr Pathol.* 1984;2:285–304.

86. Zionts LE, Osterkamp JA, Crawford TO, Harvey JP Jr. Congenital annular bands in identical twins. A case report. *J Bone Joint Surg.* 1984;66A:450–453.

87. Kancherla PL, Untawale VG, Gabriel JB Jr, Chauhan PM. Intrauterine amputation in one monozygotic twin associated with amniotic band: a case report. *Am J Obstet Gynecol.* 1981;140:347–348.

88. Herva R, Karkinen-Jääskeläinen M. Amniotic adhesion malformation syndrome: fetal and placental pathology. *Teratology.* 1984;29:11–19.

89. Pysher TJ. Discordant congenital malformations in monozygous twins. The amniotic band disruption complex. *Diagn Gynecol Obstet.* 1980;2:221–225.

90. Bieber FR, Mostoufi-zadeh M, Birnholz JC, Driscoll SG. Amniotic band sequence associated with ectopia cordis in one twin. *J Pediatr.* 1984;105:817–819.

91. Fiedler JF, Phelan JP. The amniotic band syndrome in monozygotic twins. *Am J Obstet Gynecol.* 1983;146:864–865.

92. Lockwood C, Ghidini A, Romero R. Amniotic band syndrome in monozygotic twins: prenatal diagnosis and pathogenesis. *Obstet Gynecol.* 1988;71:1012–1016.

93. Abel EL. Consumption of alcohol during pregnancy: a review of effects on growth and development of offspring. *Hum Biol.* 1982;54:421–453.

94. Bustamante SA, Stumpff LC. Fetal hydantoin syndrome in triplets. A unique experiment of nature. *Am J Dis Child.* 1978;132:978–979.

95. Mellin GW, Katzenstein M. The saga of thalidomide. Neuropathy to embryopathy with case reports of congenital anomalies. *N Engl J Med.* 1962;267:1184–1193,1238–1244.

96. Palmer RH, Ouellette EM, Warner L, Leichtman SR. Congenital malformations in offspring of a chronic alcoholic mother. *Pediatrics.* 1974;53:490–494.

97. Macourt DC, Stewart P, Zaki M. Multiple pregnancy and fetal abnormalities in association with oral contraceptive usage. *Aust NZ J Obstet Gynecol.* 1982;22:25–28.

98. Rodis JF, Egan JFX, Craffey A, Ciarleglio L, Greenstein RM, Scorza WE. Calculated risk of chromosomal abnormalities in twin gestations. *Obstet Gynecol.* 1990;76:1037–1041.

99. Perlman EJ, Stetten G, Tuck-Muller CM, Farber RA, Neuman WL, Blakemore KJ, Hutchins GM. Sexual discordance in monozygotic twins. *Am J Med Genet.* 1990;37:551–557.

100. Benirschke K, Kaufmann P. *Pathology of the Human Placenta.* 2nd ed. New York: Springer-Verlag; 1990:718–720.

101. Dallapiccola B, Stomeo C, Ferranti B, DiLecce A, Purpura M. Discordant sex in one of three monozygotic triplets. *J Med Genet.* 1985;22:6–11.

102. Lin AE, Garver KL. Monozygotic Turner syndrome twins—correlation of phenotype severity and heart defect. *Am J Med Genet.* 1988;29:529–531.

103. Flannery DB, Brown JA, Redwine FO, Winter P, Nance WE. Antenatally detected Klinefelter's syndrome in twins. *Acta Genet Med Gemellol.* 1984;33:51–56.

104. Nielsen J. Twins in sibships with Klinefelter's syndrome and the XYY syndrome. *Acta Genet Med Gemellol.* 1970;19:399–404.

105. Uchida IA, deSa DJ, Whelan DT. 45,X/46,XX mosaicism in discordant monozygotic twins. *Pediatrics.* 1983;71:413–417.

106. Rogers JG, Voullaire L, Gold H. Monozygotic twins discordant for trisomy 21. *Am J Med Genet.* 1982;11:143–146.

107. Gilgenkrantz S, Marchal C, Wendremaire Ph, Seger M. Cytogenetic and antigenic studies in a pair of twins: a normal boy and a trisomic 21 girl with chimera. In: Gedda L, Parisi P, Nance WE, eds. Twin Research 3: Twin Biology and Multiple Pregnancy. *Prog Clin Biol Res.* 1981;69A:141–153.

108. Avni A, Amir J, Wilunsky E, Katznelson MBM, Reisner SH. Down's syndrome in twins of unlike sex. *J Med Genet.* 1983;20:94–96.

109. Naor N, Amir Y, Cohen T, Davidson S. Trisomy 13 in monozygotic twins discordant for major congenital anomalies. *J Med Genet.* 1987;24:502–504.

110. Schlessel JS, Brown WT, Lysikiewicz A, Schiff R, Zaslav AL. Monozygotic twins with trisomy 18: a report of discordant phenotype. *J Med Genet.* 1990;27:640–642.

111. Mulder AFP, van Eyck J, Groenendaal F, Wladimiroff JW. Trisomy 18 in monozygotic twins. *Hum Genet.* 1989;83:300–301.

112. Uchida IA, Freeman VCP. Triploidy and chromosomes. *Am J Obstet Gynecol.* 1985;151:65–69.

113. Watson WJ, Katz VL, Albright SG, Rao KW, Aylsworth AS. Monozygotic twins discordant for partial trisomy 1. *Obstet Gynecol.* 1990;76:949–951.

114. Juberg RC, Stallard R, Straughen WJ, Avotri KJ, Washington JW. Clinicopathologic conference: a newborn monozygotic twin with abnormal facial appearance and respiratory insufficiency. *Am J Med Genet.* 1981;10:193–200.

115. Nance WE. Malformations unique to the twinning process. In: Gedda L, Parisi P, Nance WE, eds. Twin Research 3: Twin Biology and Multiple Pregnancy. *Prog Clin Biol Res*. 1981;69A:123–133.

116. Young ID, O'Reilly KM, Kendall CH. Etiologic heterogeneity in sirenomelia. *Pediatr Pathol*. 1986;5:31–43.

117. Pfeiffer RA, Becker V. Comments on Schwaibold's "Sirenomelia and anencephaly in one of dizygotic twins." *Teratology*. 1988;38:497–498.

118. Kapur TP, Mahony BS, Nyberg DA, Resta RG, Shepard TH. Sirenomelia associated with a "Vanishing Twin." *Teratology*. 1991;43:103–108.

119. Wilkinson JL, Holt PA, Dickinson DF, Jivani SK. Asplenia syndrome in one of monozygotic twins. *Eur J Cardiol*. 1979;10:301–304.

120. Benirschke K. The origin and clinical significance of twinning. *Clin Obstet Gynecol*. 1972;15:220–235.

8
The Pathology of Monochorionic Monozygosity

One of the major concepts espoused in this volume is that placental form can be as important to the outcome of a twin conception as the genetic derivation of the conceptuses. The most clear-cut evidence for this concept is in monochorionic monozygotic twinning. Except for genetic considerations, monozygotic twins with dichorionic placentas have similar developmental and gestational risks as dizygotic twins. Monochorionic monozygotic twins, however, have two additional potential sources of problems—vascular anastomoses between the fetuses and/or abnormalities of duplication.[1,2] The consequences of aberrations of monochorionic twinning may be a pair of remarkably different so-called identical twins—an argument for avoiding the term as it is not only inaccurate but potentially confusing when counseling affected families. Some of the most bizarre anomalies of human reproduction are seen in these cases—as Antonio asks of Sebastian "How have you made division of yourself?" (Shakespeare, *Twelfth Night,* V, i).

The mechanisms of monozygotic twinning, and the potential sources of variations and abnormalities of that process, have been described in more detail in the preceding chapters, but are summarized briefly here. Monozygotic twins begin as a single zygote from fertilization of one egg by one sperm. Just what factors make the multiplying cell mass develop into two embryos instead of one are not known, nor how that force or forces might be exerted, nor what determines when twinning will take place. Twinning is probably a process rather than an event, and one of the key factors may be the genetic makeup of the zygote, particularly the influence of the extra X chromosome prior to its

inactivation in the female zygote (Hall JG, 1991, personal communication).

Theoretically, if twins have arisen from a single cell, that should mean that the twins are truly identical. However, the previous discussions have pointed out that the potential sources of variation are numerous and can affect not only the genome, but the transcription of the genome (see Chapter 7), so that what started out as a cluster of identical cells may become two embryos with potentially quite different genetic programs. Then, the actual visible or identifiable manifestations of those programs can be influenced by environmental factors, particularly related to the pattern of placentation and fetal vascular development especially, creating further discrepancies between the twins.

The pattern of placentation appears to be established by the timing of the process of twinning—generally, the longer the interval from fertilization to twinning, the fewer the barriers between the twins (dispermic monovular twinning perhaps represents an exception, see Chapter 2). Thus, monochorionic monozygotic twins arise when twinning occurs in the inner cell mass after some of the cells of the morula have committed to becoming the outer cell mass or trophoblast, days 3 to 4 after fertilization.[3,4] These twins will be separated by a bilaminar layer of amnion with the two amniotic sacs surrounded by a single layer of chorion. If twinning takes place after some cells are committed to amniogenesis, days 8 to 9, then both twins are in the same amniotic sac and are monochorionic monoamniotic. In this context, it has been noted in one series that all monoamniotic conceptions were spontaneous, while 5.2% of diamniotic twins occurred after ovulation induction.[5] Even later twinning that overlaps the development of the bilaminar disk/primitive streak of the embryo leads to incomplete separation of the embryos and conjoined twins.

Monozygotic Mortality and Morbidity

Monozygotic twinning has been considered to be an anomaly itself, and the observation of greater rates of morbidity and mortality of monozygotic twins would support such a concept. It was noted in Chapter 4 that monozygotic twins were more likely to be prematurely delivered, and in Chapter 6 that monozygotic twins were more likely to be significantly growth discordant. Monozygotic twins are more likely to have developmental anomalies (Chapter 7) and monozygotic twins are overrepresented in cases of twin mortality throughout gestation (Chapter 5). When this excess of monozygotic twins is looked at in more detail, the excess is almost all accounted for by increased morbidity and mortality of monozygotic twins with monochorionic placentation. This is why monochorionic monozygosity has been considered as a separate category of twins throughout this text. This chapter discusses monochorionic monozygosity in general and monoamniotic twins in particular. The magnitude of the morbidity and mortality attributed to complications of monochorionic monozygosity has necessitated two additional chapters—complications of intertwin vascular anastomoses (Chapter 9) and anomalies of monozygotic duplication including asymmetric twins and conjoined twins (Chapter 10).

Monochorionic placentas represent 5% (Africa[6]) to 71% (Japan[7]) of all twin placentas depending on the relative rates of monozygotic/dizygotic twinning in the population. Looked at another way, two-thirds[8] to nearly three-quarters[9] of monozygotic twins will have monochorionic placentas. In the Survey '91 Review, 32% of the survivor-group placentas were monochorionic, but monochorionic placentation was seen in 51% of the autopsy group (see Fig. 3.20). Fifty percent of the aborted twin embryos from the survey were monochorionic; 40% of well-preserved and nearly 64% of macerated aborted twin fetuses were monochorionic; and 37.5% of placentas with a fetus papyraceous were

monochorionic. Monochorionic placentation was twice as common as dichorionic in all patterns of stillbirth, and complications of monochorionic monozygosity were considered to have contributed to death in 21% of retained, 42% of fresh, and 44% of macerated stillbirths for a rate of 37.4% overall. Perinatal and postnatal twin mortality was attributed to complications of monochorionic monozygosity in 22.3% of cases, due mainly to problems of intertwin transfusion syndromes and anomalies of twinning. The sexes were equally affected and birth order was not a factor. The majority, 63%, were delivered before 28 weeks' gestation, half were stillborn, and a third died within the first 24 hours after birth. One third of concordant twin deaths were monochorionic twins, both male and female sets in equal numbers. (Chapter 5 can be consulted for further details of monochorionic mortality.)

Monoamniotic placentas represent 6% to 12% of monochorionic placentas and they require special consideration. Table 8.1 contains the details of the Survey '91 cases of nonconjoined monoamniotic twins. Of the total, 26 monoamniotic sets reviewed from both the survivor and autopsy groups, seven cases or 27% were conjoined twins. These are discussed in Chapter 10 and the remaining 19 cases form part of the discussion that follows.

Monoamniotic Twins

Twins contained within the same amniotic sac were first described in 1612 (cited in Pauls[10]) and still represent a reportable twinning anomaly because of unusual features of the feto-fetal interaction (see Fig. 4.1e). There are two aspects to consider—the biology of monoamniotic twinning and the potential complications.

Developmental Considerations

Monoamniotic placentas are the least common pattern of placentation, found in 1% to 2% of twin sets. Monoamniotic twinning appears to take place after amniogenic-committed cells have emerged in the developing embryo, days 8 to 9 after fertilization. The stimulus and mechanism of twinning at this time are unknown, but the patterns of amnion distribution related to the umbilical cords support the concept of a process over time. Rarely, a remnant of a bilaminar amnion membrane is noted between the closely adjacent cord insertions, suggesting that amniogenesis was in progress but was interrupted by the twinning process.[11] Also rarely, the cords may insert side by side and be bound together for a short distance by a fold of amnion (Fig. 8.1), but without any other evidence of a septum. This pattern could arise a bit later than cases with a residual plica.[11] In most cases, there is no sign of a septum between the cord insertion sites, simply a continuous sheet of amnion, suggesting that twinning occurred after amnion development could be altered (Fig. 8.2). If the process is delayed until days 12 to 13, there may be incomplete separation of the umbilical cords (fused cords), or embryos (conjoined twins—see Chapter 10). It has been observed that some cases of monoamniotic placentation are not developmental, but are acquired due to disruption of the dividing membranes, perhaps on the basis of fetal or external trauma or infection.[12] This raises the problem of correct diagnosis of monoamnionic placentation. The amnion tends to separate readily from the underlying chorion, to which it is apposed but not adherent in the more mature placentas, and absence of a septum between the cords must be documented carefully.

Related to the discussion of the process of monoamniotic twinning is the observation that virtually all monoamniotic multiples are twins. Single amniotic sacs containing two fetuses of a dichorionic diamniotic triplet set are well known,[13] but monoamniotic triplet sets are rare.[14] Monoamniotic triplets in quadruplet sets have been reported in reviews of older European literature, as has a case of monoamniotic quintuplets.[13] If one assumes that the diagnosis of monoamnioticity was accurate in these cases, it is difficult to imagine what forces might have been acting to create such incredible embryonic divisions in such a short time without affecting fetal development. The most recent monoamniotic triplets were normal,[14] but there is no comment on the other sets, so it is not certain that the other high multiples were normal. The difficulty of accurate diagnosis of truly monoamniotic gestation (not ruptured or artifactually separated at delivery) must be considered as well, although the diagnosis with the triplets seems unequivocal.[14] Case 9 in Table 8.1 was a monoamniotic twin pair in a dichorionic diamniotic triplet set. All the rest were twins.

The other developmental consideration in monoamniotic placentas is the *pattern of fetal vessels* (see Table 8.1). In most cases, the umbilical cords inserted immediately adjacent to, or within 6 cm of, each other. They were usually eccentrically placed on the common chorionic surface, although central and marginal or velamentous pairs were seen (Fig. 8.3). Single artery cords occurred, most often with major anomalies, as in case 16. As the cords are usually close together and there is no intervening septum, vascular anastomoses might be expected and two patterns were seen. There were large diameter surface artery–artery and vein–vein anastomoses running more or less directly between the cord insertion sites, as in Fig. 8.4, and more conventional surface and deep arteriovenous anastomoses, as in Fig. 8.2. Within the limits imposed by formalin fixation or specimen fragmentation, it is probable that all monoamniotic placentas have intertwin vascular anastomoses, with large caliber vessel connections always present when the cords are adjacent. In the cases in Table 8.1, where anastomoses are not described, the placentas were fixed, fragmented, or the twins were macerated.

One final comment related to the biology of monoamniotic twins concerns the sex ratios. It was noted in Chapter 2 that in twins overall the proportion of female like-sex pairs increases with proximity of the twins. When the sex distribution is reported, the female to male like-sex pairs ratio is usually of the order of 1.6 : 1[15,16] in monoamniotic twins, although there is one reported unexplained exception with a ratio of 1 : 1.4.[5] Whether the increased frequency of female sets observed in most series reflects the effect of the mass of the X chromosomes on rates of cell division, or is due to some genetic factors on the as yet inactivated X chromosome is not known, but it would seem that some connection will be determined eventually. If all 26 cases of monoamniotic twins from Survey '91 are considered, the female to male ratio is 1.6 : 1. However, if the 6 : 1 ratio of conjoined twins is removed and the double survivor and autopsied twins considered, the ratio changes to 2 : 1 in the double survivors' group and 1 : 1.2 in the group of one or both deceased. Thus, the sex ratio may depend on the group being assessed, particularly whether conjoined twins are included in the statistics.

TABLE 8.1. Survey '91 Review: cases of nonconjoined monoamniotic twins.

Case #	Sex	Cord–cord insertion distance	Placenta/cords			Twins		
			Anastomoses	Entanglement	Other findings	Size	Anomalies	Other findings
1	F	6 cm	U/A	–	–	N/R	One has CHD–no details known	N/R
2	F	19 cm	One a-a	–	Velamentous insertion of cord of smaller twin	w = 17%	N/R	N/R
3	M	SXS	a-a at insertion; bi-directional a-v	–	Cords joined by fold of amnion	equal	N/R	N/R
4	F	5.5 cm	N/R	–	Only three major vascular units on one side	w = 28%	N/R	Bilateral candidiasis
5	M	5 cm	Ba-Av	+	–	w = 7%	N/R	–
6	F	3 cm	a-a v-v 2(Aa-Bv)	–	Asymmetric chorion vascularization 1/3–2/3; only three major vascular units from each cord	w = 7.4%	N/R	–
7	M	SXS	a-v v-v a-a	–	Few major vascular units both sides; multiple thrombi in cord vessels both sides	N/R	N/R	Both stillborn; autopsy data not available
8	M	4 cm	a-a	+	100-cm long cord with SUA of anomalous twin	N/R	Microcephaly with microgyria, neuronal heteropia; undescended testes; focal renal dysplasia; pulmonary hypoplasia; 11 ribs and spinal anomalies	Anomalous twin also had hepatomegaly with old infarcts, multifocal acquired ischemic gliosis of brain, Werdnig-Hoffmann disease; co-twin normal
9	M	"Close"	Large v-v between cords	+	Monoamniotic set of dichorionic diamniotic triplets	Twins died at different stages	–	Both stillborn
10	F	N/R	N/R	–	Cord of stillborn twin compressed by amniotic band	N/R	Surviving co-twin had digital amputations	–

11	M	N/R	"Present"	—	—	Organ weight differential compatible with chronic twin transfusion	—	Both died of prematurity/HMD
12	F	3 cm	"Multiple" and all patent	+	Cord of stillborn twin twice around neck of co-twin	N/R	—	Co-twin well; no signs of DIC
13	F	3 cm	a-a	+	—	N/R	—	Both stillborn and died at different ages; both with healed myocardial ischemic lesions
14	F	SXS	Large a-a with mural thrombi	—	Both velamentous cord insertions	Stillborn twin 18-weeks size at 27 weeks when died	—	Co-twin normal at 33 weeks
15	M	N/R	"Multiple"	+	Stillborn twin with long cord 51 cm (32 exp)	Stillborn twin growth retarded	—	Co-twin normal
16	M	6 cm	"Multiple"	—	SUA cord of smaller anomalous twin with 1/3 chorionic area	w = 27%	Cloacal exstrophy and related lesions	Co-twin normal
17	F	N/R	"Multiple"	—	Long cord—75 cm	SGA	Encephalocele and related anomalies	Co-twin normal
18	F	2.5 cm	Bidirectional a-v 2(v-v) a-a	+	"Long cords"	—	—	Co-twin normal
19	M	N/R	N/R	+	N/R	Both SGA	Both secundum ASD	Both stillborn

F, female; M, male; U/A, unable to assess due to fixation or fragmentation; N/R, not reported; —, not present; SXS, immediately adjacent cord insertions; a-a, artery to artery anastomosis on placental surface; v-v, vein to vein anastomosis on placental surface; a-v, arteriovenous anastomosis through parenchyma; direction indicated when reported, A = twin A, B = twin B; +, present; SGA, small for gestational age; SUA, single umbilical artery in cord; w, weight discordance; CHD, congenital heart disease; HMD, hyaline membrane disease; DIC, disseminated intravascular coagulation; ASD, atrial septal defect.

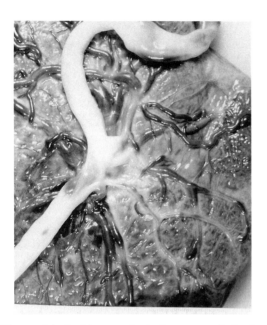

FIGURE 8.1. In this monochorionic monoamniotic placenta (case 3 in Table 8.1), the cord insertions are adjacent and bound together by a fold of amnion for a short distance above the insertion site, perhaps reflecting the timing of the twinning process in relation to amniogenesis.

Pathology

The pathology of monoamniotic twins consists of increased risks for many of the complications described in this volume plus specific problems, based on the fact of both twins being contained in the same sac. The reported obstetric profiles and rates of complications, such as prematurity and low birth weight, compared to diamniotic twins, vary somewhat depending on the population studied.[5,17] Premature contractions were reported in 50% of mothers with monoamniotic twins and preterm delivery occurred in 70% of cases.[5] In one report, monoamniotic pregnancies were more than four times as likely than diamniotic pregnancies to be delivered before 34 weeks' gestation, perhaps in part due to a fourfold increase in the incidence of polyhydramnios with monoamniotic twins, cause not stated. However, another report suggested that preterm labor was not more frequent in monoamniotic pregnancies and that polyhydramnios was rare.[17] Low birth weight was noted to be more frequent with monoamniotic than diamniotic twins, 91% were less than 2,500 g, and 27% less than 1,500 g,

compared with 41% and 5%, respectively, although possible causes seen to excess in monoamniotic twins were not discussed.[5] Monoamniotic twins were delivered abdominally twice as often as diamniotic twins, but the reasons were not stated. Finally, perinatal mortality of monoamniotic twins was five to six times as common as of diamniotic twins, due in part to a three times increase of major malformations, but also due to the increased prematurity and respiratory distress syndrome.[5]

Part of the reported increased rate of 15% to 20% malformations in monoamniotic twins is due to aberrations of monozygotic twinning, particularly conjoined twins (see Chapter 10), but other anomalies are also mentioned, most frequently anencephaly and hydrocephaly.[5,11,13,18] However, many series of monoamniotic twins do not report anomalies in detail, so the relative load of lethal/major/minor anomalies is not known and it is possible that the actual pattern of malformations, other than major anomalies of the twinning process itself, may not differ significantly from that seen with diamniotic twins. Specific reports of anomalies in nonconjoined monoamniotic twins are usually completely discordant, with one normal and one affected twin, or both with a disorder but discordantly affected.

The factors in concordance/discordance of anomalies in twins have been presented in Chapter 7, with a discussion of the importance of the details of placental development, especially the fetal vascular component. The importance of the placenta in discordant anomalies in monoamniotic twins is suggested by the following cases. There is an interesting report of a discordant major midline perineal anogenital malformation in one twin that was associated with entwined cords, but with a single umbilical artery in the cord to the affected male twin.[19] Unfortunately, a report of remarkably parallel discordant anomalies in a female twin set did not describe the placentation, but did make the important observation that an anuric anomaly in a monoamniotic twin was not associated with the classic oligohydramnios phenotype, because of the contribution of urine from the normal co-twin in the same sac.[20] Discordant phenotypes in monoamniotic twins with trisomy 18 were associated with entwined umbilical cords, but the more malformed twin also had only one umbilical artery in his cord.[21] Four of the five sets with anomalies in Table 8.1 were discordant, and three of the four were

FIGURE 8.2. In this monochorionic monoamniotic placenta (case 16 in Table 8.1), there is no remnant of intervening septum between the cord insertions, suggesting that the twinning process occurred after amniotic development was committed. Note absence of direct anastomoses between cord insertion sites but presence of more peripheral connections (arrows).

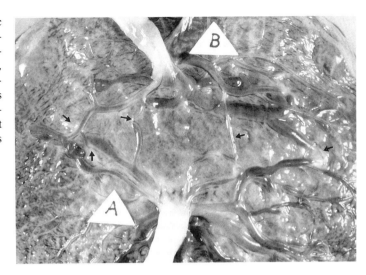

reported to have associated abnormally long and/or single-artery cords on the affected side. Also, three cases of growth discordance were associated with developmental abnormalities of the fetal circulation including velamentous insertion of the cord, decreased numbers of chorionic vessels, and an abnormally long umbilical cord (Fig. 8.5).

The pathologic complications specific to nonconjoined monoamniotic twins consist of problems with the umbilical cords and the consequences of feto-fetal transfusion across shared vessels. One might expect that twins in the same sac would be at risk for becoming interlocked, but this does not appear to have been reported.

Umbilical Cord Complications

The umbilical cord complications seen with monoamniotic twins consist of anomalies that may have significance to fetal growth and development, cord entanglements of several types, and cord prolapse during labor and delivery. It has been suggested above that single-artery cords may be associated with discordant malformations, but it is not known whether that lesion represents a coincidental, causally related, or threshold anomaly. The same applies to observations of abnormally long cords and velamentous insertions. When there is no membrane between the twins, there is a risk of cord

FIGURE 8.3. Bilateral adjacent velamentous cord insertions with monoamniotic twins (case 14 in Table 8.1). It was not determined why one twin was so growth retarded before fetal death at 27 weeks, 6 weeks before labor and delivery.

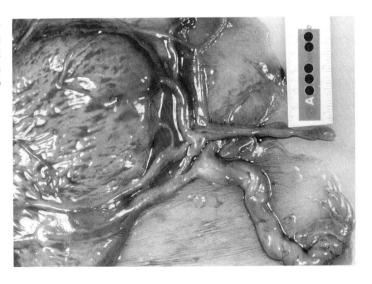

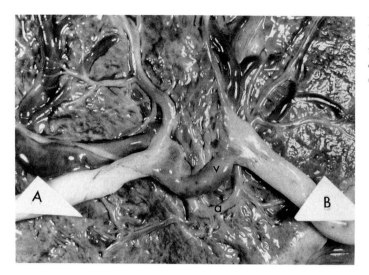

FIGURE 8.4. Large caliber direct arterial (a) and venous (v) anastomoses between the cord insertion sites in a monoamniotic placenta with closely inserted cords (case 6 in Table 8.1).

prolapse from the second twin, and this has been reported in 21.4% of vaginally delivered patients.[5] Cord entanglements consist of rare cases of amniotic bands (Fig. 8.5), entanglements of one cord about the other twin (Fig. 8.6), or the cords together (Fig. 8.7). Fetal entanglements of the cord around the neck or other parts of the body, often of the other twin, have been reported in up to 21.7% of cases of monoamniotic twins, and a true knot of an individual cord has also been reported.[5] The importance of the fetal entanglements is not only compression of the cord, but the risk that the loop of cord may be cut in order to deliver the first twin, only to find that it was actually the cord of the second twin, who must be delivered promptly.[22]

Much of the focus in reports of monoamnionic twins has been the potential for entanglements of the two cords together and the resultant risk of fetal morbidity and mortality. Identifying the tangled cords is easier than assessing the significance to the fetuses. The complexity of entanglement can be truly remarkable, with near-Gordian knot proportions in some reported cases.[13] A relatively minor example of this is shown in Fig. 8.7. It is not known when entanglements occur, but one suspects that the fetal activity necessary would be easier with smaller fetuses at a time when there is proportionately more amniotic fluid to fetal mass. To date, the occurrence of tangles has not been correlated with cord length, although at least one quarter of the tangles in Table 8.1 were with identifiably abnormally long cords. This might be expected if cord length relates to fetal activity. The proximity of

cord insertions does not appear to be related to whether or not they become entangled.[11] The entanglements seem to be of two basic kinds—equally intertwined or "knotted" cords with varying sites of compression in both, and one cord variably wound around the second cord which passes through the loops of the first cord with no alteration except possibly sites of compression along the length contained within the loops as in Fig. 8.7. If one cord has been compressed for some time, it may be quite thin.[11] The potential significance of these cord entanglements is difficult to assess. In theory, it is compression of the cord by the entanglement that compromises the fetal circulation and can lead to fetal death or death during labor and delivery. This seems a reasonable interpretation in cases such as depicted in Fig. 8.8, where fetal death is associated with distinct pathology in the umbilical cords. It becomes much more difficult to assess the contribution that tangled cords may make to fetal distress/perinatal asphyxia, when there is perinatal morbidity or mortality.

The difficulty of assigning significance to cord entanglements where there is no obvious residual pathologic sign of obstruction is analogous to assessing the importance of true knots seen in singleton cords.[23] The association of knots (entanglements) with unusually long cords supports a role for fetal activity as a factor. True knots in singleton umbilical cords are far more frequent than unfavorable clinical consequences that can be attributed to them. Perinatal mortality rates of 8% to 11% were due to stillbirth in the majority and neonatal com-

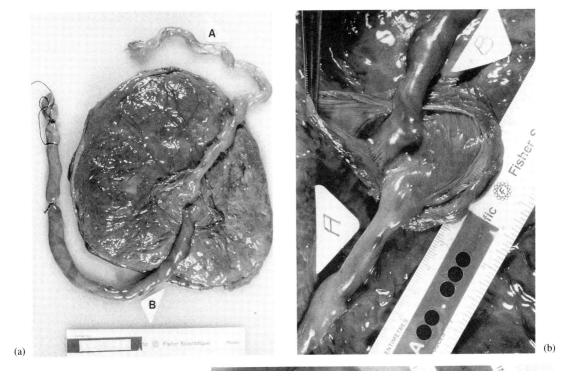

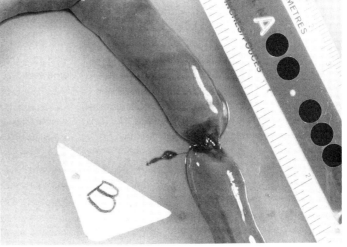

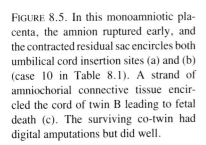

FIGURE 8.5. In this monoamniotic placenta, the amnion ruptured early, and the contracted residual sac encircles both umbilical cord insertion sites (a) and (b) (case 10 in Table 8.1). A strand of amniochorial connective tissue encircled the cord of twin B leading to fetal death (c). The surviving co-twin had digital amputations but did well.

(a)

(b)

(c)

plications after live birth were not increased.[23] There are several physical characteristics of the umbilical cord that might protect against compression by a knot—the surface of the cord is low friction, Wharton's jelly may act as a malleable cushion, and the presence of three turgid vessels may resist kinking and compression.[24] In order to determine whether a true knot might have been tight enough to affect fetal blood flow, secondary effects, such as focal grooving, narrowing, edema, or thrombosis in the cord, or marked congestion of the cord between the knot and the placenta must be identified.

These observations of true knots in singleton cords must be kept in mind when reviewing the literature on cord entanglements with monoamniotic twins. The impression from some reports is that monoamniotic twin mortality is high and due largely to cord entanglements. One early report described 53.2% of monoamniotic twins with en-

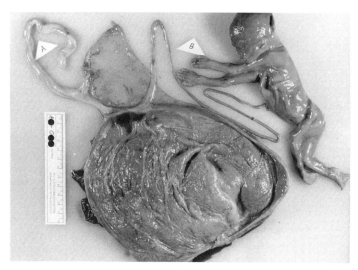

FIGURE 8.6. This monoamniotic male twin B was growth retarded by 3 weeks when he died in utero at 21 weeks (case 15 in Table 8.1). He was retained until delivery of the normal survivor at 32 weeks. The umbilical cord was abnormally long, 51 cm observed versus 32 expected for age, and was around the body and cord of twin A. Both cords were marginally velamentous 5 cm apart with large direct arterial and venous anastomoses and a number of other circulatory connections, with the result that no definite area of involuted placenta could be identified and assigned to the long dead twin.

tangled cords and a 68% mortality, apparently attributed to the cord abnormality.[13] A more recent report noted entangled cords in 71.4% of monoamniotic twins, but a 42% mortality in those cases of entangled cords, 61% of which were concordant deaths.[15] Another review found cord twisting or knotting in only 17% of cases and did not attribute any of the 28% perinatal mortality of monoamniotic twins to this finding, although fetal distress leading to section delivery was attributed to cord entanglements in 8.7%.[5] Fetal death associated with cord entanglements is often associated with retention in utero and maceration of the affected twin, suggesting that clinically significant obstruction of the cords requires a degree of fetal activity and this is more likely in middle than late pregnancy.[11,15,23]

Thus, the rates of mortality attributed to cord entanglements may depend on the case material being reviewed. In addition, the criteria for diagnosing cord compression within entangled cords need to be defined clearly and applied thoughtfully in order to arrive at a reasonable estimate of the risks of cord entanglements to the twins involved. In the eight cases (42.1%) in Table 8.1 with cord entanglements, the mortality rate was 62.5%. In six of the seven cases where one or both twins died, the twins were stillborn and there was significant pathologic evidence to implicate the entanglements. This evidence consisted of grooving of the cord (Fig. 8.8, cases 9, 13, and 19), evidence of impaired fetal blood flow, such as growth retardation (cases 15 and 19), or ischemic lesions in viscera (case 13), a groove in the neck of the surviving co-twin related

to entanglement by the cord of the dead twin (Fig. 8.9, case 12), and in one case the dead twin had a single-artery cord that was potentially more compressible (case 8). In the remaining case, the twins were live-born, but one died neonatally with evident hypoxic ischemic encephalopathy. In that placenta (Fig. 8.7, case 18), one cord was surrounded by convoluted turnings of the other cord, but it was difficult to be certain of the degree of obstruction that might have been possible, and the cords had not been identified as to the twin of origin. It has been suggested that entangled cords might not be a problem until labor and delivery, with the cord of the second twin caught in the knot of the first twin and compressed by the descent of the first twin.[13] Alternatively, the forces of labor on a very complex entanglement may lead to relatively acute obstruction of venous return to one twin, with resultant "placental transfusion" and a fetus in shock.[25]

It is worth summarizing the mortality of the Survey '91 monoamniotic twins as it relates to cord entanglements. Cord entanglements were reported in 42.1%, and 62.5% of those twins died, almost all before delivery. However, nearly as many monoamniotic twins died of other causes. The total mortality in the 19 cases of monoamniotic survivor-group and autopsy-group infants was 47.4%, and 55.5% of this was attributable to cord entanglements, but 44.5% was due to other causes, such as multiple anomalies, prematurity, or cause undetermined (see Table 8.1). Thus, cord entanglements are unquestionably a risk factor for monoamniotic

FIGURE 8.7. An example of moderately entangled umbilical cords of monoamniotic twins (case 18 in Table 8.1). The second twin was asphyxiated at birth at 38 weeks and although she responded to resuscitation initially, support was discontinued at 2 days of age when the degree of brain damage was documented. While the gross appearance is one of intertwining of both cords (a), careful examination identified that it was one cord wound around itself and the other cord, which passed straight through the coils (b). The cords had not been identified in the case room so it could not be determined whether the coiling and compression were more important than the loops surrounding the through-passing cord. F, fetal ends; P, placental ends.

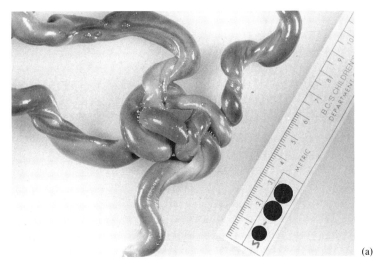

(a)

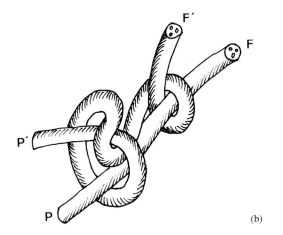

(b)

twins, but the magnitude of that risk for mortality and morbidity remains to be clarified.

Intertwin Vascular Anastomoses

The second major potential source of complications with monoamniotic twins is the presence of intertwin vascular communications, anastomoses between chorionic vessels on the surface and within the parenchyma of the placenta. It was suggested above that they are probably always present, so the concern is the occurrence of imbalanced blood flow across them. Feto-fetal transfusion, or twin transfusion syndrome is discussed at length in the next chapter, but a few comments specific to monoamniotic twins are presented here. Reports of evidence of acute or chronic twin transfusion syndrome are

scanty in the literature on monoamniotic twins: one report specifically noted that it was not identified in 18 cases reviewed,[16] and another made the diagnosis in only one of 23 cases.[5] A contrasting report was of "an astonishing frequency of transfusion syndrome fatalities during earlier gestation" (cited in ref. 11), but without further definition provided, so that no comments are possible. There is an interesting case of an acute reversal of a chronic twin transfusion syndrome in monoamniotic twins, analogous to those described in Chapter 9.[26]

Two of eight cases with secondarily monoamniotic gestational sacs were diagnosed as twin transfusion syndrome.[12] As this prevalence is unusually high compared to other series of monoamniotic twins, one wonders if fetal vascular development and blood flow is different depending on whether the twins are in one sac or two. The sequence might

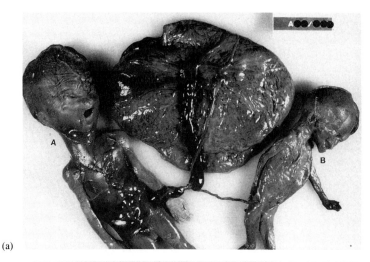

(a)

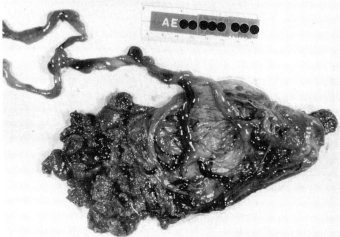

(b)

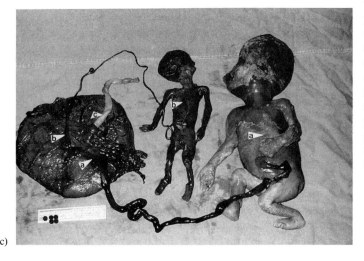

(c)

FIGURE 8.8. Fetal deaths due to entangled monoamniotic cords. (a) Twins delivered at 25 weeks after fetal death of twin A at 24 weeks and twin B at 19 weeks (case 13 in Table 8.1). Twins equally grown by ultrasound examination at 18 weeks. Note the relative sizes of umbilical cords and the constriction produced in the larger cord due to encirclement by the smaller cord. There were extensive intertwin anastomoses so the regressive changes in the placenta were relatively homogeneous. The larger twin had ischemic renal lesions and healed subendocardial myocardial necrosis. The smaller twin had subendocardial calcification. These findings suggested ischemic injury prior to death, reasonably attributable to the cord entanglement. (b) Twins delivered at 19.5 weeks after the diagnosis of fetal death by ultrasound examination for polyhydramnios (case 19 in Table 8.1). Bilateral marginal/velamentous cords with a long intertwined segment and complex knot. Both babies were small for age (16.5 weeks size) and each had a secundum atrial septal defect. (c) Monoamniotic twins from dichorionic diamniotic single-disk male triplet set (case 9 in Table 8.1). The cords of these twins were intertwined when the triplets were delivered by section at 34 weeks. Triplet A was appropriately grown for 33 weeks when it died. Triplet B was more appropriate for 24 weeks but the time of its death was not certain, triplet C was normal. Note the unusual length of the cords—triplet A, 65 cm; triplet B, 60 cm. Triplet B appeared to have died first, based on size and maceration, and most of the A/B chorionic surface appeared to be supplied from cord A, perhaps by recruitment through the vein to vein anastomosis between the cord insertions after the death of triplet B.

FIGURE 8.9. This monoamniotic fetus papyraceous was delivered at 27 to 28 weeks with a well-grown and normal co-twin (case 12 in Table 8.1). There had been normal equal fetal growth at 13 weeks, but by 21 weeks, one twin was slightly smaller. At delivery, twin B was 20 to 21 weeks' size with no anomalies. The length of cord B was not recorded but the delivery note described that it was looped twice around the neck of the surviving twin. The chorionic circulations were connected by sufficient arterial and venous anastomoses that no area of involuted placental tissue could be defined—the surviving twin had recruited the entire placenta without apparent detrimental effect.

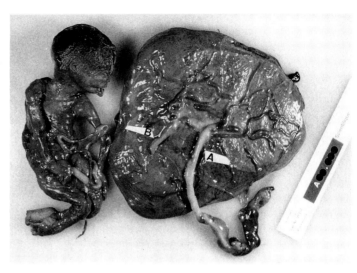

be as follows. Depending on the vascular anatomy of the placenta and fetal hemodynamics, a small net feto-fetal transfusion may be established between a set of monochorionic diamniotic twins. This may lead to changes in fetal fluid dynamics that affect volumes of amniotic fluid. When the twins are in separate amniotic sacs, changes may develop in intra-amniotic pressure that may influence the feto-fetal transfusion differentially. This would not be a factor in monoamniotic twins and in fact the single cavity may serve as a buffer for intertwin differences. It is not clear when the septal disruption occurred in the two cases of twin transfusion with secondarily monoamniotic sacs, but it may be that the hemodynamic imbalance was well established and persisted, as fluid flow tends to follow established paths (Green SI, 1991, personal communication). Thus, in the secondarily monoamniotic twin transfusion cases, the hemodynamic imbalance may have been established when they were diamniotic and because they were diamniotic it simply persisted.

In the Survey '91 Review of monoamnionic twins, chronic twin transfusion was identified in one case where both twins died of complications of prematurity, with linear measurements and organ weight differentials compatible with that diagnosis, a rate of 5.2%, which is consistent with other reports of incidence.[5] Based on the presence of large diameter vessels connecting the cord insertion sites (as in Fig. 8.4), simple acute twin transfusion might be a risk, but other than the case reports of cutting the wrong umbilical cord,[13,22] this has not been mentioned specifically in relation to monoamniotic twins.

A frequent topic in literature related to the risks of twin transfusion has been the potential risk for damage to the surviving twin after intrauterine death of one twin, when they share vascular anastomoses. This is discussed in detail in Chapter 9, as it has important medicolegal implications, but several comments are warranted here. First, case reports suggesting transchorionic coagulopathy as a cause of survivor damage need to be read with care to make sure that there is adequate documentation of monochorionicity and intertwin vascular anastomoses. This seems self-evident, but it is not always provided. Second, one must consider the possibility that lesions in the survivor that have the appearance of being due to a coagulopathy, could be due to an episode of shock that killed the co-twin, but that the survivor was able to overcome after its own in situ shock-induced coagulopathy.[27] Third, and related to the second, is the possibility that the death of one twin, for whatever reason, allowed it to become a "vascular sink," so that the survivor essentially hemorrhaged into its co-twin's blood vessels that now had no resistance, creating hypovolemic shock with potential visceral consequences if the twin survived the hemorrhage.[12,28]

A random example of these considerations is the case of monoamniotic twins where one died in utero and the survivor was born with organ damage, anasarca, anemia, and coagulopathy. There was no reference to intertwin vascular anastomoses, but the umbilical cords were said to be intertwined, and there was no reference to the color of the deceased twin who was macerated.[29] The findings in the survivor were attributed to transchorionic coagulopathy from the dead to the live twin, but based on the information provided, an alternative explanation is possible. If it is assumed that there were anastomoses, as the report implies by postulating transchorionic coagulopathy, it is possible that one twin died from the effects of the cord entanglement, and that the survivor bled into the circulation of the dead co-twin, leading to shock, visceral damage, anemia and heart failure, and hydrops. While it is true that the end result is the same, a dead twin and a damaged twin, and that the pathology in the surviving twin is related to aspects of the twin condition—specifically the intertwin vascular anastomoses—it is important to be clear about the possible mechanisms involved. This requires careful assessment of each circumstance of bad outcome suspected to be due to complications of vascular anastomoses with full documentation of placental findings, emphasizing the fetal vasculature.

Antepartum Diagnosis

The foregoing discussion of the increased risks with monoamniotic twins leads to consideration of possible prevention of mortality and morbidity. Monoamniotic twins are sufficiently infrequent that a management consensus has not been established.[30] As noted in Chapter 4, there is agreement that antepartum diagnosis of the fact of any twin gestation allows more specifically appropriate monitoring and management. Determining the absence of an intervening membrane to diagnose a monoamniotic pregnancy is not always easy ultrasonographically,[31] unless combined with additional markers, such as dye or air,[32] perhaps augmented with computed tomography.[33] One specific consideration is related to amniocentesis in monochorionic diamniotic twin pregnancies. There are several reports of disruption of diamniotic membranes following puncture during amniocentesis, when the second sac was sampled by passing through the separating membranes.[12,34] It has been suggested, therefore, that to prevent these secondarily monoamniotic sacs with their attendant complications, that puncture of the separating membranes during

amniocentesis be avoided.[34] It has been suggested that elective early delivery of twins might avoid much of the preventable mortality of monoamniotic twins, but other studies suggested that this was not warranted as fetal mortality in monoamniotic twins was not increased after 30 to 32 weeks, and risks of elective prematurity could be avoided.[17,30]

Summary

The excess mortality and morbidity of monozygotic twinning is due largely to the complications of monochorionic placentation with intertwin vascular anastomoses, and developmental anomalies of monochorionic twinning. Monoamniotic twins have additional problems because of the potential for intimate intertwin entanglements, although the complications of intertwin vascular anastomoses would appear to be less frequent than with diamniotic twins. The actual risk of cord entanglements remains to be determined and presentations of twins with circulatory complications requires complete documentation of placental anatomy.

References

1. Schinzel AAGL, Smith DW, Miller JR. Monozygotic twins and structural defects. *J Pediatr.* 1979;95:921–930.
2. Burn J. Monozygotic twins. In: Chamberlain G, ed. *Contemporary Obstetrics and Gynecology.* London: Butterworth; 1988:161–176.
3. Kalousek DK, Fitch N, Paradice BA. *Pathology of the Human Embryo and Previable Fetus. An Atlas.* New York: Springer Verlag; 1990:3–4.
4. Benirschke K, Kaufmann P. *Pathology of the Human Placenta.* 2nd ed. New York: Springer Verlag; 1990:648.
5. Lumme RH, Saarikoski SV. Monoamniotic twin pregnancy. *Acta Genet Med Gemellol.* 1986;35:99–105.
6. Nylander PPS. The value of the placenta in the determination of zygosity—a study of 1052 Nigerian twin maternities. *J Obstet Gynecol Br Cwlth.* 1969;76:699–704.
7. Soma H, Yoshida K, Tada M, Mukaida T, Kikuchi T. Fetal abnormalities associated with twin placentation (Abstract). *Teratology.* 1975;12:211.
8. Leroy F. Major fetal hazards in multiple pregnancy. *Acta Genet Med Gemellol.* 1976;25:299–306.

9. Cameron AH. The Birmingham twin survey. *Proc Soc Med.* 1968;61:229–234.

10. Pauls F. Monoamniotic twin pregnancy—a review of the world literature and a report of two new cases. *Can Med Assoc J.* 1969;100:254–256.

11. Benirschke K, Kaufmann P. *Pathology of the Human Placenta.* 2nd ed. New York: Springer Verlag; 1990:662–676.

12. Gilbert WM, Davis SE, Kaplan C, Pretorius D, Merritt TA, Benirschke K. Morbidity associated with prenatal disruption of the dividing membrane in twin gestations. *Obstet Gynecol.* 1991;78:623–630.

13. Quigley JK. Monoamniotic twin pregnancy. A case record with review of the literature. *Am J Obstet Gynecol.* 1935;29:354–362.

14. Sinykin MB. Monoamniotic triplet pregnancy with triple survival. *Obstet Gynecol.* 1958;12:78–82.

15. Salerno LJ. Monoamniotic twinning. A survey of the American literature since 1935 with a report of four new cases. *Obstet Gynecol.* 1959;14:205–213.

16. Wharton B, Edwards JH, Cameron AH. Monoamniotic twins. *J Obstet Gynecol Br Cwlth.* 1968; 75:158–163.

17. Tessen JA, Zlatnik FJ. Monoamniotic twins: a retrospective controlled study. *Obstet Gynecol.* 1991; 77:832–834.

18. James WH. The sex ratio of monoamniotic twin pairs. *Ann Hum Biol.* 1977;4:143–153.

19. Berry SA, Johnson DE, Thompson TR. Agenesis of the penis, scrotal raphe, and anus in one of monoamniotic twins. *Teratology.* 1984;29:173–176.

20. van der Harten HJ, van Velzen D. Transport of squamous cells from the peritoneal cavity to axillary lymph nodes in an infant with multiple malformations. *Pediatr Pathol.* 1986;5:319–324.

21. Mulder AFP, van Eyck J, Groenendaal F, Wladimiroff JW. Trisomy 18 in monozygotic twins. *Hum Genet.* 1989;83:300–301.

22. McLeod F, McCoy DR. Monoamniotic twins with unusual cord complication (case report). *Br J Obstet Gynecol.* 1981;88:774–775.

23. Naeye RL. *Disorders of the Placenta, Fetus, and Neonate: Diagnosis and Clinical Significance.* St. Louis: Mosby Year Book; 1991:102–104.

24. Kaplan C, August D, Mizrachi H. Single umbilical artery and cord accidents (Abstract). *Mod Pathol.* 1990;3:4P.

25. Golan A, Amit A, Baram A, David MP. Unusual cord intertwining in monoamniotic twins. *Aust NZ J Obstet Gynecol.* 1982;22:165–167.

26. Bendon RW, Siddiqi T. Clinical pathology conference: acute twin-to-twin in utero transfusion. *Pediatr Pathol.* 1989;9:591–598.

27. Norman MG. Mechanism of brain damage in twins. *Can J Neurol Sci.* 1982;9:339–344.

28. Baldwin VJ, Wittmann BK. Pathology of intragestational intervention in twin to twin transfusion syndrome. *Pediatr Pathol.* 1990;10:79–93.

29. Clark DA. Hydrops fetalis attributable to intrauterine disseminated intravascular coagulation. *Clin Pediatr.* 1981;20:61–62.

30. Carr SR, Aronson MP, Coustan DR. Survival rates of monoamniotic twins do not decrease after 30 weeks gestation. *Am J Obstet Gynecol.* 1990;163: 719–722.

31. Watson WJ, Valea FA, Seeds JW. Sonographic evaluation of growth discordance and chorionicity in twin gestation. *Am J Perinatol.* 1991;8:342–344.

32. Tabsh K. Genetic amniocentesis in multiple gestation: a new technique to diagnose monoamniotic twins. *Obstet Gynecol.* 1990;75:296–298.

33. Perkins RP, Terry JD. Exclusion of monoamniotic twinning by contrast-enhanced computed tomography. *Obstet Gynecol.* 1992;79:876–878.

34. Megory E, Weiner E, Shalev E, Ohel G. Pseudoamniotic twins with cord entanglement following genetic funipuncture. *Obstet Gynecol.* 1991;78:915–917.

9
Intertwin Vascular Anastomoses

One of the less well characterized aspects of the pathophysiology of twin pregnancies is the clinical and pathological significance of intertwin vascular anastomoses. These can be associated with marked intertwin growth discordancy, and may contribute to severe fetal compromise or death, or perinatal disability or death. These possible consequences are not only clinically important but also have been the subject of concern in disputes over poor perinatal outcome of twins. Thus, it is worthwhile to devote an entire chapter to a discussion of these anastomoses and their importance. In the first part of the discussion, intertwin anastomoses are defined as to their genesis, location and appearance, and anatomic and functional assessment. In the second part, potential patterns of pathologic hemodynamics are described, with their natural history and complications, diagnosis, and possible treatments. The pathologist has an extremely important contribution to make to the assessment of intertwin vascular anastomoses, in close collaboration with clinical colleagues caring for the mother and fetuses/infants, as will be noted throughout the discussion.

The simplest *definition* of intertwin vascular anastomoses is that they are blood vessels that connect the circulation of one twin to the circulation of the other twin. While it is true that conjoined twins have interconnected circulations through their common body portions (see Chapter 10), this chapter refers only to intertwin vascular anastomoses on the surface or through the parenchyma of the placenta. A special pattern of placental vascular anastomoses occurs in some cases of asymmetric twinning, where one twin has no placenta of its own and

survives only because of direct umbilical artery and vein connections to an artery and vein of the normal co-twin, either of the umbilical cord or placental surface. These are the chorangiopagus parasiticus twins, discussed in Chapter 10.

The *historical background* of intertwin vascular anastomoses dates back at least to the late 1600s, with reports of vascular connections between twins proven by injection studies, and discussion of the possibility of exsanguination of an undelivered twin out the cut cord of the first delivered twin.[1] The meticulous anatomic studies of Hyrtl and Schatz from 1870 to 1900 are still instructive, although they could only speculate on the functional significance of the anastomoses they found.[1,2] An appreciation of the potential clinical consequences as related to the anatomy of the anastomoses was expanded by the work of Herlitz in 1942,[2] and many case reports followed. These were collated by Benirschke in 1961 who added a discussion of the possible effects of disseminated intravascular coagulation (DIC) in one twin after intrauterine fetal death of the co-twin.[3] Morphologic details of the effects of shunting asymmetry in the twins themselves was contributed by Naeye[4,5] in 1963 and 1965. In 1965, Rausen et al.[6] delineated the spectrum of the syndrome and gave specific criteria for its diagnosis, and in 1968, Aherne et al.[7] described the morphological details of the placental villus morphology. Much of the literature since has simply expanded on these previous reports and has dealt particularly with the potential role of transanastomotic DIC as a source of anomalies, disease, or death in the surviving twin after intrauterine fetal death of one of the pair.

Development and Anatomic Patterns

When twins share the same chorionic sac, the potential exists for vascular anastomoses to form between the developing *embryonic circulations* that are sprouting all over the inner surface of the primitive chorionic membrane.[8] When embryonic cardiac activity begins, these fine vascular precursors fill with blood, and the developing vascular linkages allow circulation to occur. The number and pattern of anastomoses that form which connect the circulations of the twins, as opposed to the vascular linkages that are limited to each twin individually, is probably initially a matter of chance, influenced further by subsequent events. For example, whether the vessels become arteries or veins will be determined by the direction of blood flow and its pressure. Also, whether the anastomoses remain patent or atrophy may depend on the volume and velocity of flow. It has been suggested that if the twinning process led to embryos with initially unequal cell numbers, that the embryonic hearts might differ in time of onset of beating or strength of contraction, and this could influence the direction of flow in anastomoses in the early more "plastic" period of vessel development.[8]

An appreciation of the anatomic complexity of the *fetal circulation* in the placenta is necessary in order to consider the potential hemodynamic patterns. In the chorionic circulation radiating from the umbilical cord, the arterial (and parallel venous) branching occurs in one of two main patterns: disperse type, with small branching vessels radiating from the cord insertion site like umbrella struts, and magistral type, with fewer larger longer vessels that provide branches along their course. These patterns are seen in singleton placentas in 62% and 38%, respectively, although the factors underlying the formation of the different patterns are not known, nor do they appear to be correlated with any particular fetal outcome or other placental feature, except possibly the cord insertion site.[9] Each umbilical artery provides eight or more terminal chorionic plate arteries that disappear at the inner boundary of the placental marginal zone, by perforating the plate to become the stem arteries of the peripheral trunci chorii to the fetal villus cotyledons.[10] The branching of the arteries provides other collat-

eral perforating vessels that penetrate the chorionic plate to become the arteries of the central trunci chorii to the fetal villus cotyledons of the placenta. Most of these collateral vessels branch off at varying angles and have a short course on the surface of the chorionic plate before they disappear, while a few others arise from the inferior surface of the artery and penetrate directly (Fig. 9.1). These perforating vessels, or first order branches in the trunci chorii, have an average length of 5 to 10 mm, although there are considerable variations, and the artery is an average of 1.5 mm in diameter, with the accompanying vein about 2 mm.[10,11] These truncal vessels divide into four to eight horizontal cotyledonary or ramal vessels of the second order, with an average diameter of 1 mm. The horizontal distance varies with the size of the cotyledon, and as they curve toward the basal plate, they begin branching into the third-order villus branches of the ramuli chorii. A total of 29 to 60 ramal branches have been noted in each cotyledon, with calibers of 0.1 to 0.6 mm and lengths of 15 to 25 mm.[11]

There are four additional observations of value to consideration of the vessels in twin placentas. First, with all this vascular branching, it is important to note that meticulous studies have suggested that virtually all cotyledons have only one truncal arterial supply and only one truncal draining vein.[9–11] Second, direct vascular anastomoses are limited to the chorionic surface. No direct vascular connections have been demonstrated between arterial or venous vessels below the chorionic plate, nor any anastomoses of capillaries between branches of the villus tree.[11] Third, visual identification of the vessels on the chorionic surface is aided by the observation that arteries are generally the superficial vessels, passing over veins,[12,13] although occasional peripheral branches may reverse this pattern.[11] Fourth, each artery has a more or less parallel venous branch and they usually penetrate the chorionic plate within millimeters of each other.

Occurrence

The description of the genesis of intertwin vascular anastomoses implies that they occur only in monochorionic placentas, and this would appear to be the general experience, although the existence of vascular anastomoses in dichorionic fused placentas has been debated for some time. One study sug-

FIGURE 9.1. This chorionic surface has a disperse type of vessel branching (a) with the arteries passing over the veins. When one artery is unroofed (b), the collateral vessels can be seen more readily (white arrows) as well as openings for penetrating branches (black arrows), going directly into the parenchyma from the inferior surface of the artery.

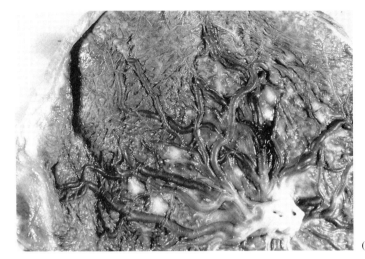

(a)

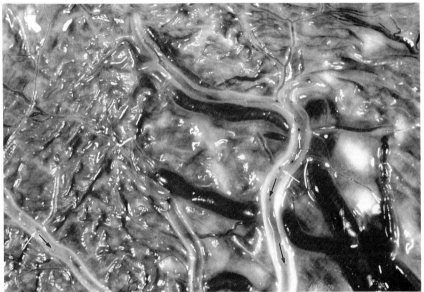

(b)

gested that nearly 5% of dichorionic placentas had arteriovenous shunts and that two-thirds of all intertwin arteriovenous shunts were in dichorionic placentas,[14] but this is in direct contrast to most descriptions, which maintain that dichorionic placentas do not have vascular anastomoses. It is recognized that in some fused dichorionic placentas, the respective villus territories of the twins may appear to be intimately related at their junction zone, but injection studies have failed to demonstrate any vascular connection between the intermingled villi.[8]

A few carefully documented exceptions of intertwin vascular anastomoses in dichorionic placentas have been described. One was reported in monozygotic dichorionic twins,[15] and another placenta was described that was partially monochorionic, with a vascular anastomosis across the surface under the diamnion-only portion of the septum on the chorionic plate.[16] In a third example, several "superficial" artery to vein anastomoses were described in diamniotic dichorionic twin girls (zygosity not further defined), with apparent hemodynamic imbalance, but it is not clear whether the septum was dichorionic at the site of the anastomoses—the illustration suggests it was not.[17] While unequivocal anatomic vascular anastomoses in dichorionic placentas are rarely documented pathologically, they must be inferred to have been present occasionally, at least transiently, because of the demonstration of rare cases of blood chimerism in dichorionic twins.[18–20]

It is interesting to speculate on why vascular anastomoses are seen so rarely in dichorionic fused placentas. Observation of the chorionic surface of such placentas notes that the peripheral vessels bend down into the parenchyma at the septum, analogous to their pattern at the periphery of the disk. Is there some chemical or mechanical message at the evolving margin of the chorion frondosum, as it becomes demarcated from the chorion laeve, that directs the tips of the marginal chorionic vessels to stop growing and anastomose with the villus vessels? If so, this message may be active at the junctional zone of the fused dichorionic placenta as well, because that junctional zone represents simply a zone of intimately adjacent peripheral chorion frondosum. One might speculate that in those cases where anastomoses are adequately documented in dichorionic fused placentas, that something interfered with that message, allowing the vessels to grow close enough to anastomose. Such might be the case in monozygotic twins with genetic identity,[15] or in regions where the chorionic tissue was missing from the septum for some unknown reason.[16] Also, it was suggested in Chapter 7 that chimeras may have other explanations than intertwin vascular anastomoses.

Reported experience indicates therefore that with rare exceptions, placental vascular communications between twins are present only in monochorionic placentas. Nearly 100% of such placentas have been reported to have vascular anastomoses, but there is marked variation in the number, size and direction of these haphazardly formed connections.[20] In any series, the demonstrable anastomoses may vary depending on their suitability for injection, since demonstration may be difficult or impossible if there is placental fragmentation or previous formalin fixation. Also, it is possible that some of the anastomotic vessels may regress in later pregnancy and therefore not be demonstrable by injection of the delivered placenta. Reported instances of demonstrable anastomoses varied from 76%[21] to 85%[12] to 98%.[22]

Reported Patterns of Anastomoses

The reported patterns of intertwin anastomoses are quite variable. Artery-to-artery connections on the chorionic surface are the commonest and have been identified in up to 64% of injected monochorionic placentas.[23] Vein-to-vein anastomoses on the chorionic surface have been identified in 19% of such placentas. These direct surface connections can be imagined to occur as chorionic plate vessels grow, with happenstance meetings of the ends of developing vessels, one from each embryo. Indirect anastomoses that involve the capillary bed of the villus tissue create a so-called common villus district or third circulation.[2] These involve the connection of an artery of one twin to the vein of the other twin through the intervening villus capillaries, and these have been identified in up to 58% of injected placentas. The actual anatomy of these arteriovenous parenchymal connections can be appreciated best by remembering that the fetal circulation in the placenta develops by differentiation from, and growth within, regional mesenchyme, with eventual connections formed between the two developing systems of villus and chorionic surface vessels.[10,24] The pattern of these connections may relate to trophic or mechanical (pressure) forces, as well as regional variations in the developing embryonic circulation.[9] Thus, for an arteriovenous anastomosis to occur, the returning truncal venous vessel from the developing villus tree of a cotyledon must anastomose with a developing chorionic vessel that has become connected to the umbilical cord vein of the other twin, instead of the vessel returning to the cord that the arterial supply came from. The forces underlying this process are unknown and may be quite arbitrary. For example, it may be that for some reason no parallel venous or arterial vessel was available to connect back to the cord of the ipsilateral twin, or it was damaged or otherwise ineffective.

Isolated anastomoses and various combinations have been identified with the following frequencies: an artery-to-artery connection plus an artery-to-vein connection is the commonest reported combination and has been noted in 28% of cases; an artery-to-artery connection alone, 21%; artery-to-vein alone, 19%; and the remaining possible combinations in 3% to 5% each.[23] One vessel may be demonstrated to have several connections, occasionally in both directions.[25] For example, a branch from one artery may connect to the other twin in an artery-to-artery pattern, while a nearby branch from the same artery connects through the parenchyma to a vein from the other twin, and maybe even with a vein returning to its own twin as well. Virtually any theoretical permutation or combination can be encountered.

The type of vascular anastomosis has been related to the placental membrane pattern. In monoamniotic placentas, artery-to-artery, artery-to-vein, and vein-to-vein anastomoses were seen in equal numbers.[26] In contrast, in diamniotic placentas, artery-to-artery shunts were seen in 75%, vein-to-vein in 46%, and artery-to-vein anastomoses in 49%.

Finally, the quantitative pattern of vascular anastomoses can vary as much as the qualitative pattern. The actual number of anastomoses in any one placenta is highly variable, and there can be numerous connections, even when the cord insertions are far apart. Generally, however, the further apart the cord insertions are, the smaller the anastomotic vessels.[27]

Patterns of Anastomosis in Survey '91 Placentas

The reports of monochorionic placentas from both the survivor and the autopsy groups in the Survey '91 were reviewed to characterize the patterns of vascular anastomoses observed. The data derived from the Survey '91 Review should be interpreted as probably representing an underestimate of intertwin anastomoses. Not all twin placentas could be assessed adequately because of formalin fixation or fragmentation, and the value of recording some of the details of the anastomoses was not always appreciated. One of the most frequent problems in the interpretation of the findings was an inability to assign a direction for arteriovenous anastomoses because of absence of delivery room identification of the umbilical cords as to twin of origin. This is still a problem, unfortunately, and can be solved only by those who assist the delivery of twins. The relevant anatomic information was better detailed in the more recent cases because of the enhanced understanding of the significance of the findings. However, as the consequences of problems due to these anastomoses are being studied more carefully, it is becoming evident that even more detailed characterization of the vascular anatomy is required for valid clinicopathologic assessments. Injection techniques have been presented in Chapter 3, and a discussion of anatomic assessment follows this summary of the data available from the Survey '91 material.

The patterns of fetal vessels on the chorionic surface of monochorionic twin placentas are difficult to categorize into rigid subsets, but two descriptive approaches are helpful: the overall appearance and the anastomotic details. In the overall appearance of the surface vessels from each twin, there were three main distributions observed—separated, adjacent, and overlapping (Fig. 9.2). In the "separated" distribution, the vessels from each twin seemed to be separated by a zone of apparently avascular chorionic surface that was 2 to 5 cm wide and sometimes occupied the entire vascular equator between the two circulations (Fig. 9.2a). Anastomoses were infrequent in these cases, and when present were most often at the margins of the disk and of threadlike vessels, usually artery to artery or arteriovenous. In the "adjacent" pattern (Fig. 9.2b), the terminal branches of the chorionic surface vessels from each twin were near each other, and all patterns of anastomoses were documented across this narrow vascular equator, although no connection could be documented by injection in rare cases. In the "overlapping" pattern (Fig. 9.2c), the vessels from each twin were so intermingled that it was quite a challenge to sort out which vessels belonged to which twin. All patterns of anastomoses were identified in these cases as well, sometimes numerous, with larger diameter vessels documented more frequently. Overall, the commonest observation was the "adjacent" pattern, although mixtures of degrees of proximity of the circulations were also described. Relative frequencies cannot be provided from this series, as the patterns were not recorded in enough detail. Occasional remarkable cases were seen, such as in Fig. 9.2d.

The specific anatomic connections described are diagrammed in Fig. 9.3. In addition to the simple direct surface vessel communications of artery to artery (arterial), or vein to vein (venous), and the single artery-to-vein intraparenchymal connection (parenchymal), that could be present in either direction, there were compound connections. These consisted of arteriovenous connections in either direction arising from anastomosing surface vessels, mainly artery to artery, and arterial vessels with arteriovenous connections in two directions, across to the co-twin and back to the twin of origin. Occasionally, one arterial branch would divide with a cluster of thin branches, which anastomosed in various patterns to arterial and/or venous branches of the co-twin. The size of the anastomotic vessels

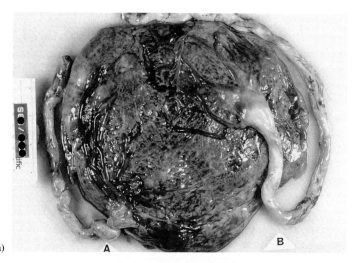

(a)

FIGURE 9.2. The overall pattern of distribution of fetal vessels from each cord insertion site has three main forms. In one, (a), the circulations seem to be separated by a zone of chorionic plate devoid of vessels and are "separated"; in another, (b), the circulations approach each other, and are "adjacent";

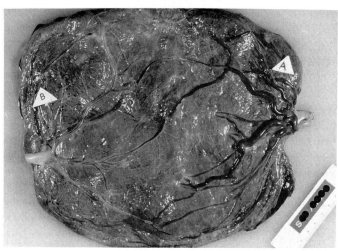

(b)

reported in the survey cases ranged from threadlike (<1 mm) to 7 mm in diameter, and the anastomosing vessels were sometimes reported to be of different caliber, most frequently in the arteriovenous connections. The volume of shared villus territory in arteriovenous anastomoses was evident occasionally on the basis of villus pallor after air injection forced fetal blood out of villus tissue, and while usually 1 to 2 cm in size was occasionally as much as 5 cm in diameter.

Survivor Group

Of the 430 reports of placentas of monochorionic twin survivors spanning 18 years, 86.7% were reported to have anastomoses. There was no mention of vascular anastomosis in 8.8%, anastomoses

were said to be "present" but no details provided in 3.7%, the specimens were too fragmented or otherwise unsuitable for demonstration of anastomoses in 2.6%, and the phrase "no surface anastomoses" was used without reference to injection studies in 1.9%. The following data are derived from 357 cases (83%), which had sufficient reported detail to assess.

The *number of anastomoses* reported in each case was correlated with the distance separating the cord insertion sites (Table 9.1). The reported insertion sites ranged from 1 cm to 28 cm apart, with one unusual case of anastomoses between the vessels from a near marginally inserted cord and a 33-cm distant, 11-cm velamentously inserted cord across a 22-cm-wide placental surface. While the majority were from 8 to 20 cm apart, there were noteworthy peaks at 12 cm, 15 cm, and 16 cm distances,

FIGURE 9.2. *Continued.* and sometimes the vessels from each twin seem to overlap considerably, and are "overlapping" (c); rarely, there are connections between the circulations within the fetal membranes between velamentous vessels (d—white arrows).

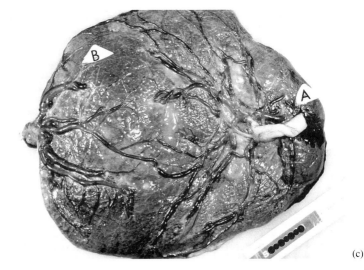

(c)

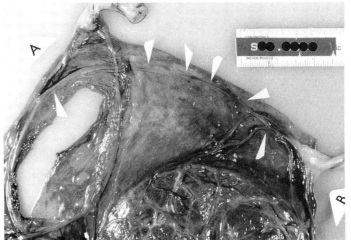

(d)

suggesting that these might represent an optimum for intertwin anastomoses. Within the 8 to 20 cm range, there did not seem to be any unusual relationship between the distance and number of anastomoses. While up to 11 anastomoses were reported in any one placenta, the majority had 1 to 4. The number of anastomoses was assessed in relation to the sex of 274 twin pairs and the data are presented in Table 9.2. There were 137 each of male pairs and female pairs, but the total number of anastomoses described was 372 in the female pairs and 422 in the male pairs. This was because 78% of the female pairs had three or fewer anastomoses, while 69% of the male pairs had three or fewer. These data would suggest that male twins tend to have more vascular anastomoses than female twins, but this remains to be confirmed and its significance determined.

The *patterns of anastomosing vessels* were assessed and also correlated with the cord insertion distances. There were 296 placentas with adequate descriptions of the vascular anastomoses, and the relative numbers of the four types of anastomoses are presented in Table 9.3. The general distribution of the types of anastomoses agrees with the reported patterns, with most placentas having one or more arterial shunts, followed by parenchymal and then venous shunts. The pattern of compound anastomosis has been described before,[25] but not analyzed separately as is being done here. It is interesting to note that when the total number of all anastomoses is examined for the different types, that the parenchymal pattern is actually more common. This is because while fewer placentas have parenchymal anastomoses, there were more of them per placenta,

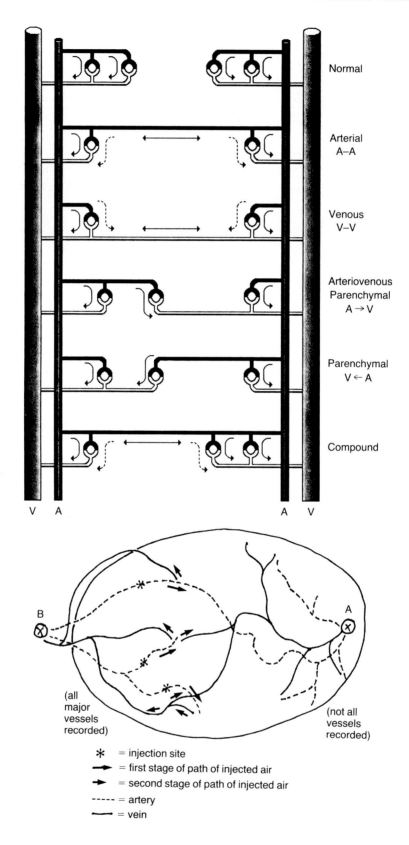

TABLE 9.1. Number of intertwin anastomoses related to cord insertion distances from Survey '91 Review survivor group.

	Distance between cord insertion sites (cm)																													Total cases
---	1	2	3	4	5	6	7	8	9	10	11	12	13	14	15	16	17	18	19	20	21	22	23	24	25	26	27	28	33	
# 0								2	3			1	2	4	3	2	3	2	2	1	3		1		1	1				31
1			1			1		2	1	3	2	3	2	4	4	6	5	3	3		2		1	1	1			2		47
2	2	1		1	1			2	4	5	3	5	7	2	2	13	8	3	5	4	6		1	2	1			1		79
3								3	5	1	3	4	9	5	2	9	7	3	3	2	4			1			1			62
4								2	2	2	1	2	5	1	5	3	1		1	5	1			1					1	33
5				1				2	1	1	1	5	1	1	1	1	1	2						1						19
6	1							2	1	1			1	1								1								8
7														2			1													3
8												1			1															2
9									1																					1
10																														—
11			1																											1
Total number of cases	3	1	2	2	1	1	7	16	16	12	15	27	18	19	36	25	15	16	18	12	5	2	6	3	1	1	2	3	1	286

#, total number of anastomoses per placenta.

TABLE 9.2. Number of anastomoses compared to sex of twin pairs—Survey '91 Review.

Number of anastomoses per placenta	1	2	3	4	5	6	7	8	9	10	11
Survivor group (274 pairs)											
Female twins	23	52	32	12	11	5		2			
Male twins	21	34	40	21	10	5	4			1	1
Autopsy group (45 pairs)											
Female twins	3	3	3	3	2	1					
Male twins	6	10	4	5	2	2	1				

◀ ————————————————————————

FIGURE 9.3. There are four main patterns of intertwin vascular anastomoses as represented graphically (a) and in a drawing of a specific case (b). In the graph, the smaller main vertical vessels labeled A represent the surface chorionic arteries, and the larger main vertical vessels labeled V represent the chorionic veins. The circular zones joining the branches of the arteries and veins represent the villus capillary network connecting the respective artery and vein branches. The figure depicts the normal relationship at the top (normal) and then the types of anastomoses possible. There are superficial arterial (A-A) and venous (V-V) anastomoses, and parenchymal arteriovenous (A-V) connections in either direction through the villus tissue. In compound anastomoses, one or more vessels are involved in several connections in both directions simultaneously. The solid arrows indicate the usual direction of blood flow, and the dotted arrows the potential additional directions of blood flow. In (b) there are two superficial anastomoses, one arterial and one venous. When air was injected at the three sites noted on side B, it can be seen from the arrows that air went in both directions. From the top arterial anastomosis, there was an arteriovenous connection back to twin B. From the central injection, air connected through subchorionic cotyledons to veins draining to A and B. The air injected into the artery from B must have entered at least two short subchorionic horizontal branches to two separate cotyledons. From the bottom artery injection, air connected to the venous connection, back to each twin. These three sites represent examples of compound anastomoses with the potential for flow in both directions.

TABLE 9.3. Distribution of vascular anastomoses in monochorionic placentas—Survey '91 Review.

		Arterial	Venous	Parenchymal	Compound	Total
% (number) of placentas with one or more	(S)	81.4 (241)	22.6 (67)	63.2 (187)	16.6 (149)	* (296)
of each type of anastomosis	(A)	45.2 (19)	23.8 (10)	59.5 (25)	19.0 (8)	* (42)
% (number) of each type anatomosis in	(S)	36.0 (279)	9.4 (73)	47.5 (368)	7.0 (54)	100 (774)
total number of anastomoses	(A)	26.9 (25)	12.9 (12)	49.5 (46)	10.8 (10)	100 (93)

*These percentages add up to more than 100% as many placentas had more than one type of anastomosis.
S, survivor group; A, autopsy group.

as can be seen in Table 9.4. Only two placentas had three arterial shunts each, but 42 placentas had three or more parenchymal anastomoses per placenta. These variations may have significance for potential complications of these anastomoses. As evidenced by the data in Table 9.4, the distance between the cord insertions does not seem to have any particular association with the type of anastomoses that form, as the distribution basically parallels the total number of anastomoses.

Finally, the *patterns of combinations* of the four types of anastomoses were examined and the distribution is presented in Table 9.5. The percentages agree with the reported distribution[23] in some respects, but there were more arterial plus parenchymal combinations, and fewer parenchymal alone in the Survey '91 cases. The patterns of distribution were assessed by the sex of the infants and the results are presented in Table 9.6. The differences are not striking, but female sets had parenchymal-only anastomoses and the arterial plus venous combination more often than male sets; male sets had more venous only and arterial plus parenchymal combinations. The significance, if any, of this observation remains to be determined.

Autopsy Group

It has already been noted in this volume that there are differences in the patterns of placentation in the survivor group as compared with the autopsy group in the Survey '91 Review. In order to continue this comparative analysis, placenta data from monochorionic twins in the autopsy group were reviewed

TABLE 9.4. Types of intertwin anastomosis related to distance between cord insertion sites for Survey '91 Review, survivor group.

Type	#	Distance between cord insertion sites (cm)																													Total cases
		1	2	3	4	5	6	7	8	9	10	11	12	13	14	15	16	17	18	19	20	21	22	23	24	25	26	27	28	33	
AA	1	6	1	1	2		1	2	10	9	11	10	14	9	10	22	18	9	10	13	7	2	2	5	2	1			2	1	180
	2				2				3	1	1	1	2	4	1	1	2	1		1	1	1									22
	3														2																2
VV	1	3	1					3	3	5	4	3	5	3	2	8	4	1	2		1		1	1							50
	2			1								1		2	1		1														6
P	1	3	1		1			3	2	5		4	8	3	7	12	7	5	4	6	2		1	1	1				1		77
	2				2				5	2	3	2	4	6	2	5	6	1	2		4			1			1				46
	3	1							1	1	2	2	6	2		3				5	2										25
	4			1					1	1				2	2			1	1	1			1	1							12
	5							1	1																						2
	6														2			1													3
C	1	2		1				1	1	3	2	2	4	4	2	4	2	1	2	2	2			1					1	1	38
	2			1				1	1						2																5
Total number of cases		15	2	4	5	2	1	14	25	28	23	27	46	32	29	60	39	18	23	28	19	2	5	10	3	1		1	4	2	468

*, number of each type of anastomosis per placenta; AA, artery to artery (arterial); VV, vein to vein (venous); P, artery to vein (parenchymal); C, compound.

TABLE 9.5. Distribution of combinations of anastomotic types in monochorionic placentas—Survey '91 Review.

	Survivor group (310 cases) %	Autopsy group (44 cases) %	Chronic twin transfusion (19 autopsy cases) %
Arterial + parenchymal	37.7	25.0	15.8
Arterial only	20.0	11.4	10.5
Arterial + venous + parenchymal	8.4	6.8	5.3
Parencyhmal only	8.4	22.7	36.8
Arterial + venous	6.8	9.1	—
Parenchymal + compound	4.2	6.8	10.5
Arterial + compound	3.5	—	—
Venous only	2.3	4.5	—
Compound only	2.2	2.2	—
Arterial + parenchymal + compound	1.9	2.2	5.3
Venous + parenchymal + compound	1.2	4.5	—
Venous + parenchymal	1.0	2.2	5.3
Arterial + venous + compound	0.6	—	—
Arterial + venous + parenchymal + compound	0.6	2.2	—
Venous + compound	0.6	—	—

for the same relationships as have been discussed above for the survivor group. In the autopsy group, the cases span 30 years, with fewer details available in the earlier cases. Of the 107 monochorionic twin sets with one or both twins autopsied, placentas were not available for assessment by the autopsist in 5.6%, could not be assessed adequately because of fragmentation/formalin fixation/sclerosis in 14.9%, or were examined, but with no comment made about the fetal vascularization in 11.3%. A statement that "no anastomoses were found" was made in 14%, often after injection. Anastomoses were said to be "present," without other details, in 14%, and varying degrees of detail were provided in

TABLE 9.6. Patterns of anastomosis by sex of twin pairs—Survey '91 Review survivor group.

	Female twins	Male twins
Arterial + parenchymal*	54	68
Parenchymal only	25	18
Arterial only	26	23
Arterial + venous	11	5
Arterial + venous + parenchymal	14	13
Venous only	1	5
Venous + parenchymal	4	5
"Present" but no details	3	4
None identified	15	18
Total	153	159

*For this table, parenchymal includes compound anastomoses.

40.2%, so that 54.2% were documented to contain intertwin anastomoses. As might be expected, the greatest detail is available in the more recent cases, although fragmented/formalin fixed specimens continue to be a problem, and identification of the umbilical cords in the case room is still not provided in many cases.

There were fewer cases in the autopsy group than in the survivor group with sufficient data for similar comparisons. In 42 twin sets, the number and type of anastomoses could be correlated with the distance separating the cord insertions. As can be seen in Table 9.7, there is no obvious difference in the distribution patterns between the autopsy group and the survivor group as shown in Tables 9.1 and 9.4. While the number of cases is considerably smaller, the excess of numbers of anastomotic channels in male twin sets over female twin sets was not seen in the autopsy group (see Table 9.2). There were twice as many male pairs as female pairs with adequate vascular data, but the average number of anastomoses per placenta was the same—3.1 in female sets and 2.9 in male sets—compared with 2.7 and 3.1, respectively, in the survivor group. The overall ratio of male to female twin sets in the monochorionic autopsy series was 1.2 : 1. The number of cases was too small to relate the type of anastomoses to the sex of the pairs. The distribution of the type of anastomoses (see Tables 9.3 and 9.5) represents a greater proportion of parenchymal anastomoses in the autopsy group compared to the

TABLE 9.7. Number and pattern of intertwin anastomoses related to cord insertion distance from Survey '91 Review autopsy group.

(a) Numbers of anastomoses and distance between cord insertion sites

| # | Distance between cord insertion sites (cm) | | | | | | | | | | | | | | | | | | | | | | | | | | | | | Total cases |
	1	2	3	4	5	6	7	8	9	10	11	12	13	14	15	16	17	18	19	20	21	22	23	24	25	26	27	28	30	
0					2	1						1	1				3													8
1				1						1			1												1				1	5
2				1	1	1			1				2		3			1		1										11
3					1					1							1						1		1					5
4										1	1	2			1	1														6
5	1												1		1					1			1							5
6																1														1
7													1																	1
Total number of cases	1			2	2	3	1		1	3	1	6	6		5	2	5	1		2			2		2				1	42

\#, Total number of anastomoses per placenta.

(b) Types of anastomosis and distance between insertion sites

| Type | # | Distance between cord insertion sites (cm) | | | | | | | | | | | | | | | | | | | | | | | | | | | | | Total cases |
		1	2	3	4	5	6	7	8	9	10	11	12	13	14	15	16	17	18	19	20	21	22	23	24	25	26	27	28	30	
AA	1	1				2	1			1	2		1	1	1							2				1					13
	2										1	1			2	1		1													6
VV	1										1			1	1	2	1		1											1	8
	2													1				1													2
P	1	1				1	1			1	1				1	1	1	1								1					10
	2										1	1	3		1	1				2			1			1					11
	3						1								1																2
	4														1								1								2
C	1	1							1				1		2		1			1											7
	2												1				1														2
Total number of cases		3				3	3		1	2	6	2	8	3	11	2	4	3		4			2	2		3				1	63

\#, number of each type of anastomosis per placenta; AA, artery to artery (arterial); VV, vein to vein (venous); P, artery to vein (parenchymal); C, compound.

survivor group, and this relates to the much greater occurrence of syndromes due to hemodynamic imbalance across these anastomoses, as is discussed in the following sections.

Survey '91 Review—Summary

Before commenting on the documentation of intertwin vascular anastomoses, the observations from the Survey '91 Review are summarized as follows:

1. The number and pattern of intertwin vascular anastomoses does not seem to be unusually related to the distance between the umbilical cord insertion sites, with the peak of the normal distribution curve at 12, 15, and 16 cm.

2. More placentas have arterial anastomoses, but overall there are more parenchymal shunts, with arterial plus parenchymal shunts the commonest combination.

3. The pattern of compound anastomoses is defined—where several flow patterns are possible based on a more complex connection of surface and parenchymal vessels in one area.

4. There may be a difference in the number and possibly the type of anastomotic channels, based

on the sex of the twins, but this needs to be verified and, if true, explained.

5. The patterns of anastomoses in the autopsied twins did not differ in any distinct way from those in the survivor twins, except for a greater proportion of parenchymal anastomoses, related in turn to the hemodynamic consequences that brought the twins to autopsy.

Documentation of Anastomoses

The mechanics of demonstrating intertwin vascular anastomoses are discussed in Chapter 3. The value of a visual record, by means of a drawing and/or photograph, is noted. As more information becomes available about fetal blood flow in monochorionic twin sets, it is expected that more detailed information will be needed about the actual vascular anatomy, so that valid correlations can be made that will be useful in cases where hemodynamic studies are not undertaken. It is true that predicting hemodynamics from static anatomic data is conjectural, but if the anatomic data are inadequate, attempts at clinicopathologic correlation will be even more tenuous, if not impossible. The following recommendations are basic observations of the fetal vasculature in monochorionic twin placentas, and are worth collecting in all cases, but are essential in any case of less than optimal outcome for the twins. These situations would include, but not necessarily be limited to, discordant growth, anomalies, fetal or perinatal death, and fetal or perinatal neurologic or visceral morbidity suggestive of vascular problems.

1. Ensure that each umbilical cord stump is accurately identified as to twin of origin and record how that has been indicated. If there is no identification, or the assignment is equivocal, record how the descriptive order has been decided for the observations that follow. In other words, which cord is twin A's and how have you decided that?

2. Record the insertion sites of the umbilical cords relative to the nearest margin of the placenta and to each other in centimeters. For example: "Cord A inserts at its placental margin, 16 cm from the insertion site of cord B, which has a velamentous insertion 3 cm from the nearest placental margin."

3. Note the line of "attachment" of the diamniotic septum between the twins relative to the vascular equator. For example, "The base of the septum is parallel to the vascular equator but 2 cm toward cord A," or "The base of the septum is perpendicular to the vascular equator."

4. Record the relative area of the chorionic surface that the vessels from each cord occupy. For example: "Vessels from cord A are distributed over two-thirds of the surface, and vessels from cord B over one-third."

5. Record the pattern of the vascular equator between the two circulations. For example: "The two circulations are separated by an apparently avascular zone of 3 cm width that spans the chorionic surface between them," or "The circulations approach each other at several points across the vascular equator," or "The two circulations overlap extensively," or whatever variation describes the situation.

6. Record the vascular anastomoses as demonstrated by the techniques noted in Chapter 3. This can be done by verbal descriptions, adequately labeled photographs, accurate drawings, shorthand tables, or any combination depending on the dictates of the case. The observations to be noted are the following:

    (a) Which cord the vessels come from.

    (b) Type of vessel—artery or vein.

    (c) Type of anastomosis—arterial, venous, parenchymal, or compound.

    (d) Location of the anastomosis—central or peripheral. This observation may be important to hemodynamic interpretations as discussed below.

    (e) Size of anastomosing vessels—the length of the vessels involved and the diameter at the penetration point of parenchymal shunts, and the relative diameters of the vessels involved in surface shunts. Surface shunts may exist between asymmetric vessels, such as a short branch from a major artery and an artery with a long winding course, and this may have functional significance.

    (f) Pattern of vessels involved in the anastomosis—this would refer to whether the vessel is a primary, secondary, tertiary, or terminal branch from one of the main chorionic vessels, and what the angle of the branch is. It is probable that these two observations are of hemodynamic significance, although the exact extent is not yet known.

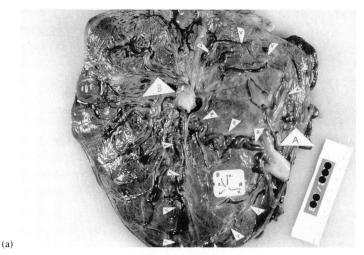

(a)

FIGURE 9.4. In this photograph of a labeled injected placenta (a), the cords are identified, and surface arterial (a,a,a) and venous (v,v,v) anastomoses and a compound anastomosis (labeled tag) are clearly located. Closer views of specific areas can be taken (b) to augment the overview picture. (The labeled tag is above and to the right of the vessels depicted.)

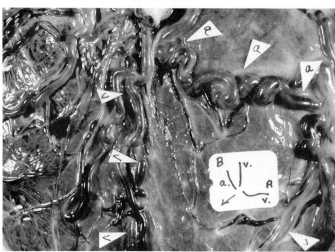

(b)

It can be seen that a well-labeled and clear photograph of the chorionic surface as in Fig. 9.4 can help considerably, and may be the only way to document and sort out a complex case.

Hemodynamic Patterns and Factors Affecting Flow

The correlation of vascular anatomy with functional blood flow in intertwin vascular anastomoses is still at the conjectural stage. Based on the observed anatomy, theoretical patterns of direction and volumes of flow can be suggested, but we still do not know all the factors that may influence fetal flow dynamics, nor the extent of their effects. Most of

our assessments to date have been based on indirect evidence of the consequences of imbalanced flow, but direct evidence from Doppler studies is beginning to be reported. It is likely that fetal blood flow through intertwin vascular anastomoses is dynamically variable, and that the net result of combinations of types of anastomoses could well be quite unpredictable.

Type of Anastomosis

The first factor influencing the hemodynamics is the type of anastomosis, and the factors of vessel anatomy have been mentioned above. Flow in an artery would be away from the twin and flow in a vein would be toward the twin. The flow in arterial or venous surface anastomoses would depend on the relative dimensions of the vessels and this, in turn, would depend on whether the involved vessels were large or small, long or short, straight or convoluted, central or peripheral in relation to the cord insertion, and at what angle they branched off the source vessel. Although the relaxed size of the surface vessels may bear little relation to their diameter in vivo, a potential direction and volume of flow may be suggested based on the midpoint diameters of the vessels involved.[13] It is probable that the flow in these surface vessels repeatedly changes direction, depending on some of the factors to be mentioned, and the activity of flow in these vessels is attested to by the fact that they are so rarely thrombosed, unless one twin has died. Depending on the vascular anatomy, and as suggested by the dotted arrows in Fig. 9.3a, what may appear to be simply a surface anastomosis could become a parenchymal anastomosis, if the flow of blood was such that another branch or a penetrating vessel was reached by the blood from the other twin. Thus, an arterial or venous anastomosis could have a fluctuating parenchymal component as well. It is generally accepted that the flow in a parenchymal anastomosis (Fig. 9.3a) is unidirectional, from the arterial to the venous vessel. However, the volume of that flow could be altered by the volume of flow through connected, ipsilateral, arteriovenous parenchymal channels. The potential flow patterns in compound anastomoses would be combinations and permutations of these suggested variations.

Blood Flow Patterns

When attempting to postulate hemodynamic events based on anatomy, it is helpful to consider some established observations about blood flow in the fetus and blood flow in general. One-half of the fetal cardiac output (55%) goes directly to the placenta through the aorta and umbilical arteries, and most of the venous return from the placenta goes through the liver before entering the inferior vena cava,[28] influencing the relative intravascular pressures. According to Poiseuille's law, the rate of flow of a nonpulsatile homogeneous fluid through a rigid tube varies inversely with the length of the tube and the viscosity of the fluid, and varies directly with the fourth power of the radius.[29] Blood flow is pulsatile, of a nonhomogeneous fluid, and the tubes are not rigid, but the major resistance

factor to flow is still the caliber of the vessel, and the drop in pressure is greater for a given distance of vessel in smaller arteries. In low flow situations, the external pressure on a vessel may become greater than the internal pressures, and flow may cease— the critical closing pressure.[29] Blood flow can be affected by local metabolic signals to contractile elements in endothelium and by local metabolic effects on the muscle of immediately proximal muscular vessels.[30] Hypoxia can be a stimulant to increased flow, and in embryonic or fetal tissue will promote the generation of new blood vessels.[31] Once flow begins in a vessel, if the flow continues, the vessel adapts and thus tends to sustain that flow (Green SI, 1991, personal communication). In order for the flow from large-caliber vessels to be distributed through even smaller branches of increased resistance, the number and caliber of the branches has to bear a set physical proportion to the parent vessel, and the angles of branching are also important.[32] These observations have been made in systems of far easier access than the human fetus and placenta, but they are presented here as potentially analogous considerations to be kept in mind when assessing intertwin hemodynamics. It is considerations such as these that prompt the suggestion that vessel diameter, length, location, and type are all important observations to be made in twin placentas.

This description of the theoretical possibilities for blood flow based on vascular anatomy suggests a potential for fluctuating hemodynamics. This is a reasonable concept and is reinforced by clinical reports of gradual fluctuations in the observed manifestations of hemodynamic imbalance, including measures of fetal growth and volumes of amniotic fluid. These are presented in the next section, along with evidence that, in some cases, major dramatic reversals of flow may take place as well.

Nonvascular Factors Affecting Flow

The observations of fluctuating consequences of imbalanced hemodynamics leads to the question of what factors affect blood flow beyond the anatomy of the vessels. The theoretical factors include fetal blood pressures and cardiac output, fetal heart rates, fetal movements, amniotic fluid pressures, and cord compression. It seems reasonable to think that if the respective fetal blood pressures and cardiac outputs are different, then fetal blood flow may vary across anastomoses, especially large ones near the umbilical cord insertions. Such differences might be encountered in twins discordantly grown for other reasons (see Chapter 6), or in heart failure of one twin. Also, fetal heart rates would be expected to affect pressure and flow. Fetal rate accelerations in twins have been noted to be concordant 50% of the time in nonstress tests, independent of gestational age, growth discordancy, or the type of placenta,[33] and they did not reflect the existence of a "dominant twin."[34] Further, concordant sleep/awake patterns have been noted 88% of the time.[35] Whether these observations would be the same where a vascular imbalance is present is not yet known, but this would seem to be worth pursuing. Cord compression is theoretically a potential source of gradual and/or sudden alterations in umbilical blood flow that may alter the hemodynamic status quo. Finally, the pressure within the amniotic cavity may have an effect on flow through surface vessels if the critical closing pressure is reached, particularly in smaller vessels.

Investigation

As noted throughout this discussion of the hemodynamics of intertwin vascular anastomoses, correlating vascular anatomy with potential blood flow patterns is still conjecture at best, although some reasonable analogies based on accepted observations are possible. The various techniques used to diagnose the presence of imbalanced flow now include Doppler studies of umbilical cord and fetal vessel flow, and refinements of these techniques. Careful clinicopathologic correlation of the findings of flow studies with chorionic vessel anatomy may help document flow patterns. However, for the most part, we are still limited to identifying the consequences of unbalanced flow, and thus assessing, indirectly, the importance of intertwin anastomoses.

Clinically Significant Patterns of Intertwin Vascular Anastomoses

In order to understand the importance of these intertwin vascular anastomoses, it will help to review the patterns of imbalanced flow that can

occur, the natural history of imbalanced flow, how it is diagnosed, what it means for the fetuses, and how it might be ameliorated. In addition, there is special concern for the consequences in the surviving twin, when the co-twin dies in utero and they share circulations.

Balanced Shunts

The potential flow patterns across intertwin vascular anastomoses could be hemodynamically balanced or imbalanced, and balanced shunts could be anticipated in several situations. Artery-to-artery or vein-to-vein anastomoses could allow shunting if there was a pressure differential across them and blood would theoretically cease flowing through them once pressure was equilibrated. The large number of patent surface anastomoses that are demonstrable in delivered placentas suggests that there is always some flow back and forth that keeps these anastomotic vessels from thrombosing and becoming obliterated. As noted above, this may reflect transient fluctuations in each twin's blood pressure, cardiac output, or other changes due to unknown fluctuations in intrauterine fetal hemodynamics.

The other potentially balanced shunting situation is when a parenchymal shunt is associated with an arterial, venous, or reverse parenchymal shunt. It is thought that a solitary parenchymal shunt could not equilibrate, but it could be compensated for by other anastomoses. Depending on the volume of the shared third circulation villus tissue, there may be an inequality of function of the villus parenchyma serving each twin, and this may have secondary effects on growth. Reportedly up to one-fifth of the placenta volume can be shared,[2] but there are fewer complications in those situations where the parenchymal anastomosis is associated with arterial or venous shunts.[3]

Nonhemodynamic consequences of these balanced shunts may include significant intertwin exchanges of blood components. It has been suggested that intermingling of blood cells of monozygotic twins during gestation may be more critical for graft tolerance than genetic unity, so that intertwin tissue grafts may be more readily tolerated between monochorionic than dichorionic monozygotic twins.[20] Blood chimeras in dizygotic twins are more problematic due to the rarity of unequivocally demonstrated anastomoses in dichorionic placentas. It is conceivable that small anastomoses were present across a septal zone devoid of chorion,[16] and that they regressed and the regional defect in the septum was not appreciated when the placenta was examined. Finally, as will be seen in the discussion that follows, these vascular anastomoses have been used to explain some of the consequences to the surviving twin of intrauterine fetal death of its co-twin, even if the hemodynamics were balanced to that point.

Imbalanced Shunts

The hemodynamically imbalanced anastomotic circulation creates a net transfer of blood from one twin to the other and has three main patterns. The pattern seen with the chorangiopagus asymmetric parasitic twin (acardius) is described in Chapter 10. The twin-to-twin transfusion syndromes (TTS) seen with initially symmetric twins are more common, and they occur gradually (chronic) or rapidly (acute), occasionally in combination. The reported percentage of placentas with demonstrable vascular anastomoses that are associated with clinically recognizable TTS varies. In one study it was stated that one third of monochorionic twin pairs may show some features of TTS.[10] In a series of 132 live-born twin pairs, 42 had monochorionic placentas, and 76% of these had vascular anastomoses.[21] Thirty-four percent of placentas with anastomoses were associated with clinical features of TTS in the twins and, of these, 18% had an acute syndrome and 82% a chronic syndrome. The same study noted that one-third of stillborn pairs had vascular anastomoses, with a diagnosis of TTS made because of differential plethora and pallor of the twins without other cause. A somewhat lower frequency was reported with 5.5% clinically apparent cases of TTS among 55 sets of twins whose placentas had anastomoses.[22] Although TTS has been reported in a dichorionic twin set,[17] and there is a reference to unlike-sex dizygotic twin pairs with TTS, but with no placenta description,[36] TTS is generally considered only possible in monochorionic placentas with vascular anastomoses.

In the Survey '91 Review, of 373 survivor twin sets with anastomoses identified, 4.6% were said to have clinical evidence of twin transfusion syndromes—one case acute, two cases fluctuating chronic, and the remainder low-grade chronic. This probably represents an underestimate as clinical data was not always available. There were a number of other sets of monochorionic twins with weight discordance of up to 64%, but there were additional placental factors that were thought to be more significant than any vascular anastomoses identified, or that the vascular anastomoses identified simply augmented the growth discordancy (see Chapter 6). Of the 107 cases of monochorionic twins in the autopsy group of the Survey '91 Review, a twin transfusion syndrome was diagnosed in 44.9% of the sets. In 22.9% of these, the placenta could not be examined for the vascular details, so the nature of the underlying shunts could not be determined. In this group, all were chronic transfusions, and one was complicated terminally by an acute transfusion. In the remaining twin sets with transfusion syndromes, 70.3% had a chronic syndrome, 8.1% had an acute syndrome, and 21.6% had a chronic syndrome with a terminal acute transfusion. The total reported occurrence of twin transfusion syndromes in all the 537 monochorionic twin sets in the Survey '91 Review was therefore 12%, or 12.6% of those twin sets with reported placental anastomoses. One or both twins died in 73.8% of affected twin sets. The conclusion would seem to be that, while clinically significant hemodynamic imbalance is not a problem in the majority of monochorionic twins, when it occurs it has a grim prognosis. It is the high mortality and morbidity of twin transfusion syndromes that has led to interest in characterizing and possibly treating the disorders.

Acute Twin-to-Twin Transfusion Syndromes

Simple Acute

The purely acute TTS is the simplest, but least common, of the hemodynamic imbalances across intertwin anastomoses. It has been suggested that the first reported case of an acute twin transfusion was between Jacob and Esau,[37] with Esau described as much redder and more vigorous. The possibility of acute exsanguination of an undelivered twin out the cord of the first delivered twin was reported in the 1600s.[1] Related cases have been described over the years, and currently there are four key characteristics that define the acute TTS,

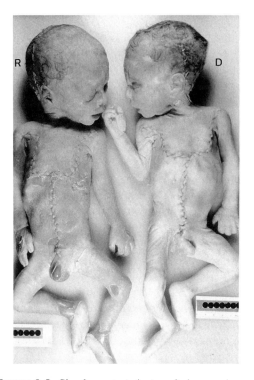

FIGURE 9.5. Simple acute twin transfusion syndrome. Note the nearly equal development of the twins but relative plethora of the recipient (R) compared to the donor (D). There were a number of superficial and parenchymal anastomoses. (Reprinted with permission from Wigglesworth and Singer, *Textbook of Fetal and Perinatal Pathology,* Chapter 8, Blackwell Scientific Publications, 1991:245.)

listed in the order they are usually encountered[3,6,12,38] (Fig. 9.5; Tables 9.8 and 9.9). Classically, there have been no abnormalities during gestation and the condition has been diagnosed at birth. The affected twins have little or no growth differential, but one is plethoric (the recipient) and one is pale (the donor), so the birth weights may differ with the plethoric twin being heavier because of congestion. The placenta is monochorionic with intertwin anastomoses of at least an arterial or venous type. Cord hemoglobin/hematocrit levels are equal at birth, but if the twins survive, fluid shifts unmask the anemia in the donor twin and polycythemia in the recipient twin, with reticulocytosis becoming evident in the donor.

The basis for the acute TTS is thought to be a rapid shift of a large volume of blood from one twin across surface vascular anastomoses and into the circulation of the other twin, creating the differential congestion. The implication of concordant growth is that flow across these anastomoses had been balanced until that event. This acute shift could be initiated if one twin went into shock in utero, as for example due to an asphyxial insult from cord compression. Alternatively, if the presence of twins is not known at delivery and the umbilical cord of the delivered twin is not clamped, transanastomotic exsanguination could occur. What is puzzling is the apparent clinical rarity of this syndrome compared to the demonstrable frequency of arterial and venous anastomoses in monochorionic placentas.[15]

In the Survey '91 Review autopsy group, 5% of cases diagnosed as twin transfusion syndrome would fit the criteria for simple acute, as in Table 9.8a, with a case example as follows. This twin pregnancy was normal to 26 weeks, when there was spontaneous premature rupture of the membranes and onset of uterine contractions. Tocolytic therapy was ineffective and labor continued with developing signs of ascending infection. The twins were freshly stillborn and the autopsy data are presented in Table 9.9a. The twins were equally well grown for age by length and the differential body and visceral weights were attributed to the considerable congestion in the recipient. In the monochorionic placenta, the cords were 12 cm apart and there was an artery-to-artery anastomosis of 1 to 2 mm diameter and a vein-to-vein anastomosis joining a vein 2 mm in diameter to one 4 mm in diameter. The findings were interpreted as representing concordant intrapartum death with acute twin transfusion, although the cause of the acute imbalance was not determined.

Other Patterns of Acute Transfusion

The simple acute pattern of twin transfusion does not appear to be recognized in early pregnancy and most reported cases have been in the third trimester. Because this imbalance is uncommon and so acute, and there appears to be no way to predict its occurrence, there has been much less published interest in this pattern than in the chronic syndrome. However, it is now recognized that acute transfusion can occur as a complication in some cases of chronic transfusion when invasive interventions are undertaken,[39] and in fact may be as frequent in

TABLE 9.8. General fetal findings in patterns of twin-to-twin transfusion syndromes.

Syndrome pattern	Transfusion status of twin	Observation				
		Body color	Linear growth	Birth weight	Hemoglobin/ hematocrit	Visceral size/weight appearance
(a) Simple acute	Donor	Pale	Equal/normal	Equal or	Equal at birth	Normal/pale
	Recipient (R)	Plethoric		R heavier		Normal/congested
(b) Acute-on-growth	Donor	Pale	Normal	Normal	Normal or low	Normal/pale
retardation	Recipient	Very plethoric	Small	Light	Usually SB*	Small/congested
(other causes)						
(c) Simple chronic	Donor	Pale	Delayed	Light	Low	Small/pale
	Recipient	Plethoric	Excessive	Heavy	High	Heavy/congested[1]
(d) Acute-on-chronic	Donor/recipient[2]	Plethoric	Delayed	Light	Usually SB	Small/congested
	Recipient/donor	Pale	Excessive	Heavy	Variable	Heavy/pale
(e) Fluctuating chronic	"Donor"[3]	Variable	Variable	Variable	Variable	Heart size may still
	"Recipient"	Variable	Variable	Variable	Variable	be discordant
(f) Acute-on-chronic	Donor/recipient	Plethoric	Delayed	Light	SB	Small/congested
feticide	Recipient/donor	Pale	Excessive	Heavy	SB	Heavy/pale

[1]The discordance of heart size is the most striking difference (see text).
[2]Chronic donor becomes acute recipient and vice versa.
[3]Status may change several times.
SB, stillborn.

these circumstances as it is as an isolated phenomenon. It should be noted, however, that not all pale members of a twin pair are necessarily donor twins of an acute TTS. Fetomaternal hemorrhage of one monochorionic twin has been described[40] and was reported once in the Survey '91 autopsy group.

In addition to the classic picture of acute twin transfusion, and the possibility that acute transfusion may complicate invasive interventions in chronic twin transfusion (Table 9.8f), two additional patterns of findings were identified in the Survey '91 Review autopsy group that suggested

acute transfusion—chronic twin transfusion with naturally occurring terminal acute transfusion (Table 9.8d), and acute transfusion between twins discordantly grown for reasons other than chronic transfusion (Table 9.8b). Further discussion of the acute-on-chronic pattern is presented in the review of chronic transfusion.

An example of an acute transfusion superimposed on growth retardation is the case of male twins who were diagnosed at 24 weeks with 2 weeks' discordant growth but equal volumes of amniotic fluid. Spontaneous fetal death occurred

TABLE 9.9. Illustrative case examples of patterns of twin transfusion syndromes.

Syndrome pattern	Twin status	Observation								
		Color	Edema	BW	CH	Brain	Heart	Liver	Kidneys	Lungs
(a) Simple acute	D	–	–	−6.5	+2.1	−4.1	−21.9	−3.8	+4.6	−19.8
	R	Congested	Slight	+21.8	+3.5	+8.3	−4.1	+53.8	+27.9	+17.2
(b) Acute-on-growth	D	–	–	+5.8	+9.4	+7.5	−17.8	−14.8	−30.2	m
retardation	R	Plethoric	–	−18.2	m	−4.2	−58.9	−57.4	−29.0	−36.4
(other causes)										
(c) Simple chronic	D	Pale	–	−25.4	−4.8	−10.1	−43.8	−20.1	−1.8	−62.9
	R	Mild congestion	–	+12.9	+2.4	−3.8	+94.7	+16.7	+90.7	−9.1
(d) Acute-on-chronic	D→R	Hyperemic	–	−29.7	−10.7	−23.0	−71.9	m	−35.2	−62.9
	R→D	Generalized palor	–	−22.8	−4.8	−24.3	+7.0	+6.5	m	−41.7
(e) Fluctuating chronic	D→R	Hyperemic	–	−10.4	+9.5	+20.8	−6.8	+11.0	+10.4	+7.3
	R→D	Pale	–	+9.6	+6.5	+11.7	+92.0	+66.5	+12.8	+23.9
(f) Acute-on-chronic	D→R	Plethoric	–	+7.8	+11.1	−6.3	−29.8	−27.0	−59.2	−46.2
after intervention	R→D	Pale	–	+53.2	+22.2	+6.5	+103.5	+56.3	+31.5	+4.5

All measurements are recorded as % above or below the mean expected for gestational age, using data of Naeye and Letts.[41]

D, donor; R, recipient; BW, birth weight; CH, crown–heel length; m, equivalent to mean for age.

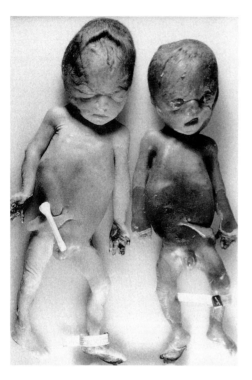

FIGURE 9.6. Acute transfusion complicating discordant fetal growth that was due to causes other than chronic transfusion. The smaller twin was growth retarded with a much smaller chorionic volume (one-fifth) and an 11-cm velamentous insertion of the cord, and appeared to have died first, although the exact cause of death was not determined. There were two anastomoses that allowed the larger twin to lose blood into the vessels of the dying and then dead co-twin, leading to his death as well. That is why the small twin is plethoric and the larger twin pale.

ble fluctuation across the arterial shunt. With this pattern of anastomoses and a growth-impaired twin, it might be postulated that if there had been a net imbalance on a chronic basis that it actually would have benefited the smaller twin and that the degree of growth impairment observed would be less than expected from the placental findings alone. Both twins had excess aspirated amniotic debris, greater in the smaller twin, and there were myocardial contraction bands in the larger twin. The interpretation was that the smaller twin was undergrown because of discordant chorion volume and abnormal cord insertion and that he died first, although the final cause of death was not determined. The loss of blood pressure in the dying and then dead twin would allow the survivor to shunt enough blood across both anastomoses to cause hypovolemic shock and death. A time frame for this process is not known, but in this case was less than a week. There were similar cases in which the plethoric smaller twin was stillborn, but the co-twin survived, related to the gestational age and/or degree of transfusion possible.

This acute-on–growth retardation pattern of acute transfusion should be suspected when a small twin is plethoric and the pale co-twin is normally grown. Careful analysis of the placental findings may suggest an acute-on–growth retardation pattern as the explanation and basis for further investigation. At least 8% of the autopsy sets with evidence of twin transfusion had this pattern and others were suggestive but with insufficient data to be definitive.

and the twins were delivered at 25 to 26 weeks' gestation. The autopsy statistics are presented in Table 9.9b and the twins in Fig. 9.6. Both twins had mild tissue autolysis, slightly more marked in the smaller twin, who was therefore thought to have died first. The monochorionic diamniotic placenta was asymmetrically partitioned with only one-fifth to one-quarter occupied by vessels from the smaller twin, who also had an 11-cm velamentous cord insertion on the placenta and a narrowed abdominal cord insertion. There were two intertwin vascular anastomoses, both described as "small," an arterial shunt and a parenchymal anastomosis from the larger to the smaller twin. The flow pattern across these two connections was conjectured to be unidirectional across the parenchymal shunt, with possi-

Chronic Twin-to-Twin Transfusion Syndromes

Mechanism

The chronic twin transfusion syndrome is commoner than the acute and is attributed to the results of long-standing hemodynamic imbalance across placental *vascular anastomoses* in monochorionic placentas. The imbalance results from a combination of vascular connections and flow patterns that leads to an imperfectly compensated flow in one direction and thus a slow net transfusion from one twin to the other.[7,20,23] Parenchymal anastomoses through common villus territories that are not associated with superficial anastomoses are particularly liable to be imbalanced.[3] These shunts do not have to be large and the actual amount of blood being lost by the donor need not be great.[2] While this asymmetry can be slight hemodynamically, it can be sufficient to cause fetal death in midpregnancy[21,42] and may explain some cases of fetus papyraceous (see Chapter 5).

While a net imbalance in the volume of blood and blood cells across the anatomic vascular shunts is considered an essential element of the chronic transfusion, there may be alterations of other *components of the transfused blood* that can augment the syndrome. It has been suggested that the transfusion also leads to differences in serum protein concentrations, which may be even more important to the full manifestation of the syndrome than the blood cell or hemodynamic imbalance. The hyperproteinemic transfusee or recipient, and the hypoproteinemic transfusor or donor, would suffer secondary effects related to fluid shifts on the basis of this altered osmolality. These shifts could be reflected in the nonshared placental tissues, altering morphology and function, and further contributing to the syndrome.[7] In other words, the protein imbalance due to the slow net transfusion could be augmented by impaired protein transport across the altered villus tissue of the donor.[40,43] The protein imbalance reported includes albumen, immunoglobulin G, transferrin and α_1-antitrypsin.[44] In addition, atriopeptin, an atrial-derived diuretic/natriuretic/vasoactive agent, has been reported to be in much higher concentrations in the recipient twin.[45] It has been postulated to contribute to the syndrome by being released in the recipient twin because of volume overload, then affecting renal function and systemic vessels, leading to hydramnios and hydrops.

Whatever the details of the mechanism of chronic TTS, the spectrum of clinical and pathological manifestations is broad. More severe examples can be identified by as early as 10 weeks of development embryopathologically,[20] and by 14 weeks ultrasonographically.[46] The intrauterine and perinatal mortality of TTS is high, up to 70% in well-defined cases,[20] although some authors consider that the complications of prematurity associated with the syndrome are the greater risk.[47] The manifestations and mechanisms of the syndrome are discussed in the order in which they are encountered—obstetric, perinatal, and pathologic. The emphasis is on untreated chronic transfusion first, followed by a discussion of variations, the types of intervention, and their effects, including the combination of acute on chronic transfusion.

Manifestations During Gestation

There has been increasing interest in those observations that can be made during gestation that will lead to a diagnosis of twin transfusion syndrome and perhaps provide an idea of prognosis, and a way to identify those cases that might be treatable.[48] A number of investigative techniques are used and although the reported observations vary somewhat, it is important for the pathologist to have an idea of the studies that are being done in order to provide appropriate pathologic correlations. The investigations include ultrasonic assessment of the fetus, placenta, and amniotic fluid, Doppler studies of fetal blood flow, cordocentesis fetal blood samples for hemoglobin levels and other studies, and studies of fetal cardiac function. These are discussed in turn.

Ultrasound

Often the first clinical manifestation of the chronic twin transfusion syndrome is a uterus that is large for dates, even for twins. This can occur any time from early second to late third trimester and is due to excessive amounts of amniotic fluid in the recipient's sac.[49] The accompanying donor twin has little or no fluid in its sac and has been characterized as a "stuck twin," because of inhibited fetal movement due to constraint.[50] It seems that this differential in volumes of amniotic fluid may be one of the first signs, preceding identifiable effects on fetal growth. A related observation has been that the urinary bladder is enlarged with a rounded contour in the twin in the hydramniotic sac, but may not be identifiable at all in the "stuck twin."[49,51] The pattern of discordant fetal growth that goes along with the differential fluid volume seems to vary. Sometimes the "stuck twin" is small for age with an appropriately grown co-twin; sometimes the smaller twin is normal for age, but the other is large for dates; sometimes they are on opposite sides of the mean for dates; and occasionally there appears to be no significant difference in size. The range of discordance at the time of diagnosis has been 0 to 5 weeks[52] and usually persists and increases unless the syndrome fluctuates (see below). The growth differential is most marked in trunk and abdomen measurements, is less in limb measurements, and the biparietal diameter appears to be the most variable, spared in some,[53] but affected in others.[51] With time, the twin in the hydramniotic sac may become edematous, beginning with pericardial and peritoneal effusions.[51,54] The "stuck twin" has been reported to become hydropic, although less frequently,[50,55] most often in association with a hydropic recipient co-twin,[52] but occasionally after fetal death of the co-twin,[56,57] and in these cases the amount of fluid around this twin may increase.[20] As the fetal hydrops in twin transfusion is partly on the basis of cardiac volume overload and heart failure, it is worth noting that cardiac enlargement has been reported in a recipient twin, whose donor twin's heart did not seem to fill completely in diastole,[49] and dilatation of the right atrium, inferior vena cava, and liver were described in a hydropic recipient twin.[54]

There have been several reports of ultrasound observations of placental features in chronic twin transfusion. In one interesting description, a normal placental pattern was seen at 22 weeks, although there was 3 weeks' discordant fetal growth.[54] Four weeks later, the parenchyma of the placenta of the larger twin was said to have maturational changes with calcification of cotyledon margins. By 28 weeks, when the larger twin was in cardiac failure, the placenta was said to have grade III calcification with central transonic areas. Unfortunately, there was no report of the gross or microscopic appearance of the placenta that might be correlated with these observations. Another report of asymmetric placental calcifications did not specify which twin's portion was affected or provide correlative histopathology.[50] A larger/thicker umbilical cord in the recipient twin has been mentioned.[54,58]

There are two additional considerations related to these ultrasound findings in twin transfusion syndrome. First, differential diagnosis of discordant fetal growth and fluid volumes must be considered.[50,59] It seems that the combination of a small "stuck twin" and larger hydramniotic twin in the second trimester, with no definable structural anomalies in either twin, is strong evidence for

chronic twin transfusion. Ultrasound findings of a single placenta with no chorion in the septum between the twins is further support for the diagnosis. Asymmetric growth retardation is well recognized in monochorionic twins (see Chapter 6), but does not usually present as a "stuck twin." Once the chronic twin transfusion syndrome is suspected on the basis of these ultrasound findings, other investigations may be done to characterize the syndrome. The second consideration is the value of these observations related to prognosis. The studies vary somewhat, but if twin transfusion is evident on the basis of discordant fluid volumes and/or fetal size at less than 24 to 26 weeks' gestation, it has been reported to be uniformly fatal,[60-62] and this mortality was irrespective of degree of weight discordance, hydrops, or hydramnios.[59] A contrasting report suggested that there was greater mortality with fetal hydrops and that the age at delivery was more important than the age at diagnosis.[63]

Doppler Studies

Twin transfusion syndromes are the result of abnormal patterns of blood flow and a number of studies have attempted to characterize this during gestation, but with somewhat mixed results.[52,57,64-67] Absent or reversed diastolic flow has been correlated with fetal or perinatal death, but could not differentiate donor from recipient and seemed unrelated to the volume of amniotic fluid.[52] Also, some twins had normal Doppler results but died. Intertwin differences of greater than 0.5 in the pulsatility index have been considered diagnostic of twin transfusion when observed in discordantly grown twins.[64] When hydrops developed in one twin, the difference became smaller. In another case, the pulsatility index in the smaller twin "cycled," and was thought to be reflecting shifts from forward through absent to reverse flow and back again through the one artery-to-artery anastomosis that was identified on the delivered placenta.[65] However, it is not clear from this report that the growth discordance in this set of twins was actually due to a chronic transfusion. Umbilical artery systolic-diastolic (SD) ratios were noted to be equal in twins discordantly grown because of chronic twin transfusion, compared with discordant twins due to placental or other lesions.[66] A contrasting report noted an elevated SD ratio in two-thirds of donor twins, but only one of six recipient twins.[67] An interesting sequence was reported in one twin pair, where the recipient twin had a normal SD ratio and the donor twin had diastolic reverse flow.[56] After the fetal death of the recipient, the donor became hydropic. As the hydrops resolved, the SD ratio was high and then normal. This sequence may reflect an acute reversal of flow after the death of the recipient (see below). Additional assessments of flow in the inferior vena cava,[68] combinations of blood flow and echocardiographic studies of cardiac function,[69] and umbilical vein flow and tricuspid valve competence[52] are reported.

Fetal Blood Studies

The external methods of assessment described above have been supplemented by studies on fetal blood.[56,70,71] Cordocentesis at 20 weeks of a recipient twin found hematocrit three times the norm, but the donor twin could not be sampled.[70] In contrast, another report noted little difference in donor/recipient cord hemoglobin/hematocrit at 21 to 23 weeks, but a difference by a factor of 2 at 36 weeks, with the donor below the norm and recipient above.[56] In this same report, both twins were relatively polycythemic in one case and in another case the donor twin was polycythemic in association with a velamentous cord insertion. It was suggested that if the smaller twin was growth retarded for reasons other than chronic twin transfusion, they could be polycythemic on that basis and this discrepancy might be a way to differentiate the small anemic donor of twin transfusion and other causes of growth retardation in twins. Hyperviscosity of fetal blood has been found to be a better predictor of survival than gestational age, with recipient gradients of less than or equal to 5.0 associated with survival at an average of 28 weeks.[71] Unequivocal prenatal evidence of intertwin vascular anastomoses has been demonstrated in two cases using adult O Rh− red cells.[56] These were injected into the umbilical vein of the donor twins and were identified in the recipients' umbilical vein blood at a rate of 7% of the recipient's sample in 16 minutes in one case, and 14.5% in 25 minutes in the other. Unfortunately, the placental vascular anatomy in these two cases was not specified. Acid-base and blood gas studies have been done on cord blood and acidemia was noted in

both recipients and donors, and other recipients were hypoxemic.[56] Studies of serum proteins and other blood components have been referred to above.[40,44,45]

Nonstressed antenatal cardiotocography has been assessed in relation to twin transfusion.[72] Although it did not identify twin transfusion specifically, it indicated if fetal distress was occurring as a result of it, reflecting significant chronic transfusion.

Pattern Variations

There are two variations of the chronic pattern of obstetric clinical signs of twin transfusion syndrome that are suggested by some of the reported cases noted above,[52,54,57] but not specifically discussed as such—fluctuating and reversed (Table 9.8d,e). The *reversed pattern* consists of evidence of chronic twin transfusion with rapid reversal of some of the findings, often associated with death of one of the twins. This can occur spontaneously or following intervention and is discussed with treatment of twin transfusion in subsequent paragraphs. Two examples of *spontaneously fluctuating signs* are presented in Figs. 9.7 and 9.8. These cases illustrate some of the anatomic complexities that can make clinicopathological correlations somewhat challenging, and reaffirm the need for pathologists to consult with clinical colleagues regarding the results of studies during pregnancy. Sorting out which twin was which before and after birth can be difficult, depending on the descriptive style of the ultrasonographer and whether delivery was vaginal or operative.

In the first case of fluctuating signs (Fig. 9.7), one twin was discordantly small for dates at 20 weeks with oligohydramnios, but began to grow and by 24 to 26 weeks was normal for age with normal fluid. Then, growth slowed, so that by 31 weeks she was below the expected size and by delivery at 35 weeks was still below the expected size 20% less than her normally grown co-twin. The placenta was monochorionic with a number of intertwin vascular anastomoses. Three of these anastomotic sites were compound, with the potential for flow in both directions. The umbilical cords were inserted 22 cm apart and the chorionic surface was vascularized equally, but there were several additional findings that might have influenced the pattern of flow in the compound sites. The cord of

FIGURE 9.7.

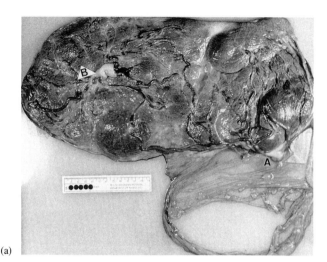

(a)

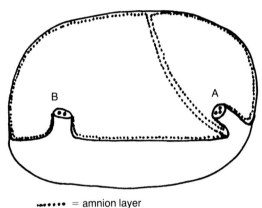

ᴍ•••• = amnion layer

(b)   ᴤᴤᴤᴤ = diamniotic septum

the smaller twin (A) had a marginal insertion, and the cord of the larger twin (B) had only one umbilical artery. The pattern of attachment of the diamniotic septum was such that the smaller twin's sac did not contain any chorionic surface. The septum arose at the placental margin, where cord A inserted and followed the margin of the disk for 15 cm on one side and 10 cm on the other side, then arched up the chorion laeve to complete a somewhat dome-shaped sac with the septum the base and the chorion laeve the dome. Thus, the intra-amniotic pressure in side B was the only one that could affect fetal surface vessels from both twins. Twin A's placental parenchyma was ischemic with accelerated villus maturity, focal villus congestion, and intravillus hemorrhage, and in side B there was mildly increased intervillus fibrin and focal villus edema. The suggestion was that the pattern of blood flow across the compound anastomoses varied in

order to account for the changes in fluid and growth rate, but the hemodynamic details and the relative influence of the cord and membrane findings are unknown. The placental histology was interpreted as consistent with chronic twin transfusion from A to B. The role of the marginal cord insertion in the latterly slowed growth remains undetermined.

In the second case of fluctuating clinical signs (Fig. 9.8), fetal growth was assessed by ultrasound measurements of femur length, biparietal diameter, trunk girth, and head circumference. Discordant growth and fluid was identified at 10 to 11 weeks and became more pronounced until 24 weeks, when there was a spontaneous catch-up growth of the smaller twin for 1 to 2 weeks, followed by a slower growth rate, but now in parallel with the growth rate of the co-twin. These changes were most evident in the femur length and trunk girth (Fig. 9.8a). At the time of birth at 32.5 weeks, the smaller twin B was

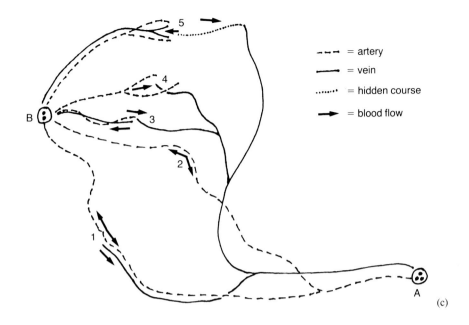

(c)

FIGURE 9.7. Spontaneously fluctuating clinical signs of chronic twin transfusion. The twins were discordantly grown at 20 weeks, twin A was smaller with oligohydramnios. At 24 to 26 weeks, she was normally grown for age with normal fluid. By delivery at 35 weeks, her birth weight was 20% less than her normal co-twin, 1,980 g versus 2,420 g. Although the placental chorionic surface was equally vascularized (a), the smaller twin A had a marginally inserted cord and an odd membrane relationship with all her surface vessels within the chorionic sac of her co-twin (b). Of the five anastomotic sites identified, three were compound with the potential for blood flow in several directions (c). At site 1 anastomosis, the arterial blood from B could be part of a parenchymal shunt as well as the arterial shunt. Site 2 is a simple arterial anastomosis. At site 3, the arterial blood from B could go into one or both of two nearby venous channels, to A or back to B. At site 4 is a parenchymal anastomosis from B to A. At site 5, the arterial blood from B returned to cord B but also connected through an undetermined subchorionic vessel to a vein of A at some distance, a rather unusual pattern. Note that not all surface vessels are represented in these drawings, which are from drawings originally created at the time of the injection. What actual role the single artery cord from twin B and the other gross features noted had on the flow patterns remains conjectural.

38% discordant by weight, with twin A slightly heavier than expected (A = 1,850 g, B = 1,155 g). Complicating the picture was a hemoglobin of 126 g/L in the larger twin and 142 g/L in the smaller twin, with the suggestion of an acute reversal of the twin transfusion in the 3 days before delivery. The smaller twin B had a 6-cm velamentous cord insertion, 15 cm from cord A, and the vessels ramified over only one-fifth of the chorionic surface. Cord A was held tightly to the separating membranes by a fold of amnion, creating the possibility of kinking at the top of this fold. The maturation of the villus tissue of twin B was irregular with increased perivillus fibrin, and there was generalized villus immaturity in twin A's portion. Six anastomoses were demonstrated and two were compound—the rela-

tive sizes and possible flow patterns are presented in Fig. 9.8b. In this case, it is hard to assess the relative contribution of twin transfusion and chorionic abnormality (velamentous cord and smaller volume) to the growth changes in the smaller twin B. It may be that baseline growth potential was influenced by the placental anatomy, but that this was modified in a fluctuating fashion by the anastomoses. The factors influencing the flow patterns in the compound anastomoses are not known.

Manifestations During Gestation—Summary

The intragestational manifestations of chronic twin transfusion syndrome are variable in pattern, degree, and time of identification. Diagnosis of

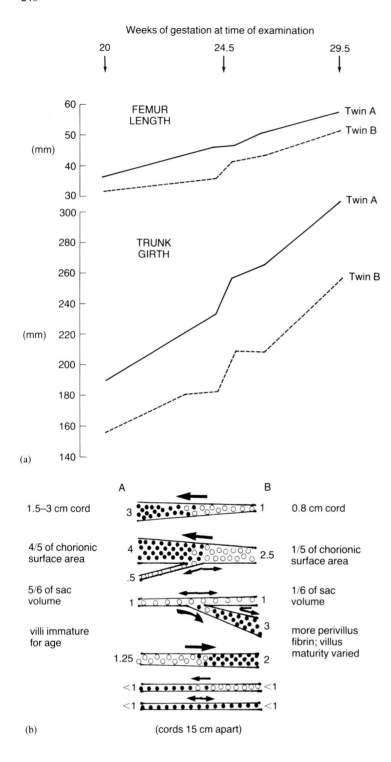

(a)

(b)

A   B

1.5–3 cm cord   0.8 cm cord

4/5 of chorionic   1/5 of chorionic
surface area   surface area

5/6 of sac   1/6 of sac
volume   volume

villi immature   more perivillus
for age   fibrin; villus
                       maturity varied

(cords 15 cm apart)

FIGURE 9.8. Fluctuating chronic twin transfusion. In (a) are represented the observed femur lengths and trunk diameters at ultrasound examinations at successive times during the gestation prior to delivery at 32.5 weeks. The variation in growth patterns can be seen with a catch-up phase toward the end of the second trimester. In (b) is a representation of the anastomoses identified in the placenta with the relative sizes and probable and possible directions of blood flow, in an attempt to try to visualize the net result. The solid circles represent venous blood and open circles arterial blood. The confounding placental form variables are also noted that may have affected fetal growth directly as well as by influencing flow through the anastomoses.

chronic transfusion is suggested by discordant fetal growth and fluid volumes, particularly a "stuck twin" in the second trimester, and a number of other assessments are possible. The findings may progress, fluctuate, or reverse in an as yet unpredictable fashion, but earlier and more pronounced abnormalities seem to equate with uniformly fatal outcome. Guidelines for surveillance of such pregnancies have not been established, but it has been recommended that extensive sonographic monitoring of suspected monochorionic twins be started "as early as possible and repeated at intervals dictated by the clinical situation."[48] The pathologist who is examining the placenta and infants from cases of chronic twin transfusion needs to be aware of the results of any assessment used during pregnancy.

Neonatal Manifestations

Although the mortality rate is high, some twins survive and a number of neonatal observations have been reported.[4–6,20,26,38,73] In the classic and uncomplicated case of chronic twin transfusion, the neonatal appearance reflects the findings in utero—the donor twin is small for age with varying degrees of the oligohydramnios phenotype, and is pale and anemic; the recipient twin is large for age, plethoric, possibly hydropic, and polycythemic. As with the prenatal observations, diagnosis of chronic twin transfusion in the newborn requires a combination of observations and elimination of other diagnoses. It is not sufficient to diagnose twin transfusion on the basis of weight discordance or hematocrit differences alone, even if the placenta is monochorionic.[74] Discordant growth and discordant hematology can have other implications as noted in this and other chapters, and these must be ruled out.

The degree of *growth discordance* varies from none to 1,000 g or more[4,5,20] and a birth weight difference of greater than 20% has been suggested as a diagnostic feature.[38] However, discordant birth weight of this degree can be seen with dichorionic as well as monochorionic twins.[75] In the Survey '91 Review, growth discordance of greater than 20% among the survivor twins was twice as common in dichorionic as monochorionic twin sets (see Table 6.3). In the autopsy series of the Survey '91 Review, dichorionic twins still accounted for 20% to 55% of the greater than 20% growth discordant sets.

A *hemoglobin difference* of greater than 50 g/L has been used as a diagnostic feature,[6] although in extreme cases it may be as much as 190 g/L.[4,5,20] A study using venous blood obtained in the first day of life found intertwin hemoglobin differences of greater than 50 g/L in just as many dichorionic as monochorionic twins.[75] It has been suggested, however, that only cord blood samples collected at the time of delivery would reflect the in utero state, and that there are rapid changes in fluid compartments after birth that could lead to less relevant results.[76] A test for fetal cells in the maternal circulation is essential in all cases of neonatal anemia to rule out fetomaternal hemorrhage, which can be unilateral in twins.[40] Serum ferritin levels at birth and at 1 month of age, as a measure of tissue iron stores, have been reported in twin transfusion with low and rising levels in the donor, and high and falling levels in the recipient.[77]

There are several other observations that have been made of naturally surviving twins in the newborn period. *Discordant bone densities* that resolved over time were noted in a set of twins that were diagnosed as twin transfusion syndrome on the basis of discordant weight/color/hemoglobin/white cell count, although the placenta was not described.[78] The larger polycythemic twin was osteopenic and the smaller anemic twin was osteosclerotic. Bone length (ulna) and body length were the same by 3 months of age (corrected) and the bone densities were approaching the norm for age. There were related changes in plasma calcium, phosphate, and alkaline phosphatase. The postulate was that the anemic twin had fewer macrophages for activation and transformation to osteoclasts, with the reverse situation in the plethoric twin, and that the problem resolved as normal osteoclast populations were established postnatally. *Discordant heart size* is one of the key autopsy criteria for the diagnosis of chronic twin transfusion (see below), and this discrepancy should be readily identifiable in the neonate; but does not seem to be used as a diagnostic clue in reported cases. Increased pulmonary vasculature has been reported in surviving newborn recipient twins, and while initially thought due to congenital heart disease, was eventually attributed to hypervolemia.[79] It was not stated when this finding resolved, and no placenta details were provided. Whether some of the other pathologic findings can be translated into clinical observations in the newborn remains to be determined.

It was noted in Chapter 4, that one of the predisposing factors to preterm delivery of twins was excess uterine distention, as with hydramnios. Because hydramnios is so common in chronic twin transfusion, premature delivery occurs in over half the cases with chronic twin transfusion of any consequence.[4,50] Thus, the neonatal problem of twin survivors include all the complications of prematurity.[63] In addition, the *recipient twin* may suffer from complications of the plethora and hemoconcentration.[80] These are cardiac failure, vascular thrombosis, and hyperbilirubinemia, with or without kernicterus, due to hemolysis. The *donor twin* may be at risk for ischemic/anoxic lesions due to the anemia. However, the risk to the donor seems to be less than to the recipient for consequences of abnormal blood volume and composition.[21,47] Cutaneous hematopoiesis has been identified in donor twins consisting of normoblasts and some myeloid precursors in the dermis and subcutaneous fat.[47] This is an interesting observation in light of the fact that neutropenia in anemic donor twins has been attributed to diminished neutrophil production, based on neutrophil kinetic studies.[81]

Pathology

The pathologic spectrum in chronic twin transfusion is a combination of placental and fetal findings as demonstrated in Fig. 9.9. The following discussion reviews the placental findings and then the fetal pathology in simple chronic twin transfusion. Chronic transfusion compounded by other processes is discussed, followed by a review of therapeutic measures and their consequences. Finally, the consequences of fetal death of one twin related to intertwin vascular anastomoses is discussed.

Patterns of Mortality

Before reviewing the pathology of fatal chronic twin transfusion, it may be instructive to examine the patterns of mortality—which twin dies, and when. The relative rates of mortality of donor and recipient, the proportion of concordant death, the relative timing of donor and recipient demise, and the gestational age and sex of affected twin sets have been assessed from the Survey '91 Review autopsy series of chronic twin transfusion (nonintervention cases), and cases extracted from the

literature.[3,4,6,21,46,48,52,57,63,66,82–90] As can be seen from Table 9.10 concordant death is more common than death of only one twin, and fetal death is more common than postnatal death. In Table 9.11 are the patterns of donor and recipient death and it can be seen that donors die more frequently than recipients prenatally, but that postnatal death rates appear to be equal. When death is concordant, the donor dies before the recipient twice as often as the reverse, and when there is only one death, the donor dies twice as often as the recipient. When the donor died first and was stillborn, the recipient died 3 days to 2½ years later. When both donor and recipient were live-born but the donor died first, the interval was 30 mins to 3.5 months, 58% within 24 hours. When the recipient died first in utero, the live-born donor survived 5 days to 8 weeks. When both were live-born but the recipient died first, the interval to the donor's death was 3 hours to 48 hours, 50% within 12 hours. These differences may be related to gestational age at delivery. As might be expected, concordant stillbirth tends to be more common earlier in gestation (Table 9.12), likely related to the severity of the process. Concordant postnatal death is also more frequent in the early second half of gestation, more probably on the basis of complications of prematurity. When stillbirth was combined with postnatal death, the delivery times are scattered across the gestational timetable.

Placenta

The placental findings in untreated chronic twin transfusion syndrome include general observations of twin placentas as described in Chapter 3, details of the fetal vasculature as described above, and the morphology of the villus tissue. In 20% of Survey '91 Review autopsy series cases of chronic twin transfusion, both donor and recipient twins had cord *anomalies* in equal numbers, consisting equally of marginal and velamentous insertions, and one each of single-artery cords. Thirteen percent of donor twins, but only 2.6% of recipient twins, had either the smaller proportion of the chorionic volume or fewer than the normal number of surface vessels. Eight percent of donor twins had both an abnormally inserted umbilical cord and smaller chorionic volume. The importance of these observations is that when there is discordant/abnormal chorionic development, in addition to intertwin vascular anas-

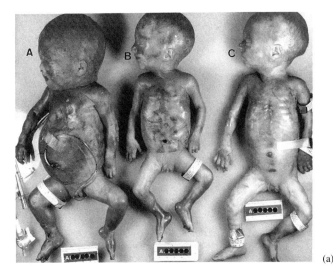

(a)

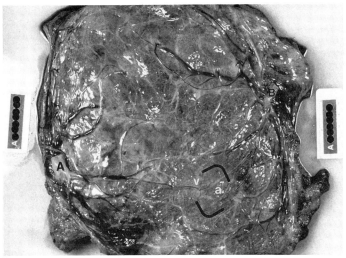

(b)

FIGURE 9.9. An example of the classic features of the straightforward chronic twin-to-twin transfusion syndrome. The presence of triplets provided an unusual opportunity for a normal comparison within the same gestation. These triplets were delivered by section at 26 weeks after 4 weeks of repeated amniocenteses because of hydramnios. Triplets A and B were monochorionic diamniotic with intertwin anastomoses and twin-to-twin transfusion syndrome. Triplet C was a dizygotic (by blood group) normal triplet for gestational age, used here as a standard for the other two. In the picture of the triplets (a), note the plethoric, edematous, and largest triplet A (1,011 g), the recipient of the twin-to-twin transfusion syndrome; the smallest triplet B (580 g), the donor of the twin-to-twin transfusion syndrome; and the normally grown triplet C (840 g). In the placenta of the twin-to-twin transfusion syndrome pair (b), the disk is 660 g and the cords are 18 cm apart. The surface is symmetrically vascularized with equal numbers of chorionic vessels. An arteriovenous shunt is located in the bracketed area with the artery (a) of triplet B to the vein (v) of triplet A.

tomoses, both factors must be considered in any discussion of the effect of the hemodynamics of the anastomoses on fetal growth or pathology. In other words, is the smaller twin small because of placental developmental factors, or because he/she was the donor of a twin transfusion syndrome, or does one situation compound the other, as noted in some cases of acute-on–growth retardation transfusion described in the previous discussion of acute transfusion? An additional feature on the chorionic sur-

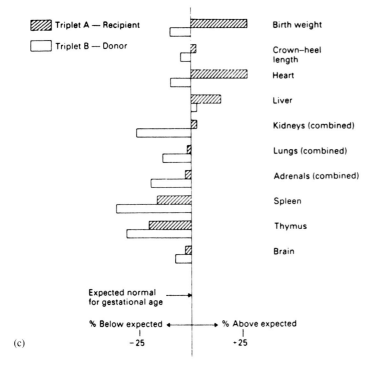

Triplet A — Recipient
Triplet B — Donor

Birth weight
Crown–heel length
Heart
Liver
Kidneys (combined)
Lungs (combined)
Adrenals (combined)
Spleen
Thymus
Brain

Expected normal for gestational age

% Below expected ← → % Above expected
−25   +25

(c)

FIGURE 9.9. *Continued.* In the graph of comparative growth and organ weights of the twin transfusion pair (c), note particularly the disparity of birth weight and heart weight. Even when the viscera weighed less than the expected in both twins, the donor's organs weighed less than those of the recipient. Note the relative sizes of the hearts of all the triplets (d). Triplet C's heart is the expected size for age. Triplet A's heart (the recipient) is twice the expected weight, and triplet B's heart (the donor) is less than the expected weight by 27%.

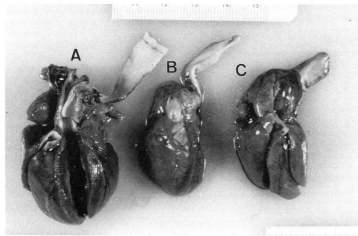

(d)

face of placentas from cases of chronic transfusion may be the presence of focal degenerative lesions of the amnion, possibly with amnion nodosum, in the sac of the donor twin.[4,20]

It has been suggested in the previous discussion, that we need to record more details than we have in the past about the quantitative *vascular anatomy* of the shared vessels, in order to analyze the outcomes more routinely. It is unlikely that most service pathologists would be in a position to provide

analyses of the complexity displayed by Schatz (as reproduced in ref. 1), but using the suggested techniques described in Chapter 3 and above, more useful information can be provided on a regular basis than is currently available.

The pattern of anastomoses in the literature cases was insufficiently detailed for analysis, so the Survey '91 Review was the basis for a review of vascular anastomoses in twin transfusion compared to monochorionic placentas in general. Of the un-

FIGURE 9.9. *Continued.* In the three low-power photographs of the placental histology of the triplets (e), note the well-vascularized and normally cellular villi of the normal triplet (N), the sparser and poorly vascularized villi of the donor (D), and the bulkier edematous villi of the recipient (R).

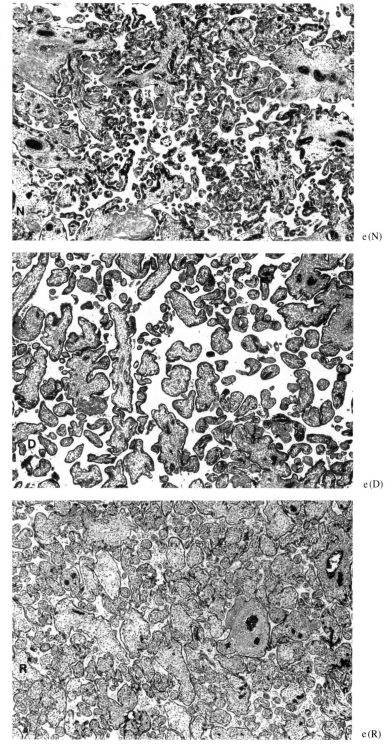

e (N)

e (D)

e (R)

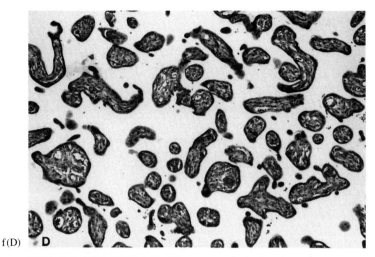

f(D)

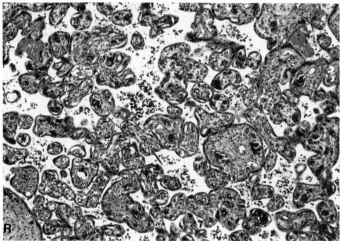

f(R)

FIGURE 9.9. *Continued.* In (f) is another example of placental histology at 24 weeks' gestation in a different case of twin-to-twin transfusion syndrome to demonstrate the degree to which donor (D) and recipient (R) villus territories may differ. This photograph was taken in the midzone of the placenta at the same magnification in each case. The donor tissue has a distinctly hypotrophic and ischemic appearance. (Reprinted with permission from Wigglesworth and Singer, *Textbook of Fetal and Perinatal Pathology,* Chapter 8, Blackwell Scientific Publications, 1991:248–249.)

treated cases of chronic twin transfusion, there were adequate placental data to assess in 19. The cord insertions ranged from 1 cm to 25 cm apart. Although the numbers are relatively small, it can be seen from Table 9.5 that the pattern of anastomoses is different in autopsy cases with chronic twin transfusion. The 36.8% of cases with only parenchymal anastomoses consists of only unidirectional arteriovenous anastomoses from donor to recipient in 21% and only bidirectional arteriovenous anastomoses between donor and recipient in another 15.8%. Compared to the frequency of parenchymal

TABLE 9.10. Deaths related to chronic twin transfusion syndrome—concordance patterns.

	Concordant death			Death of only one twin			
	Literature	Survey '91	Total*	Literature	Survey '91	Total*	Totals*
Fetal death	28	12	40	13	5	18	58
Postnatal death	18	11	29	6	5	11	40
Fetal/postnatal	7	5	12	–	–	–	12
Male pairs	4	16	20	4	5	9	29
Female pairs	7	17	24	4	3	7	31

*Total presented as total number twin sets in death time category.

TABLE 9.11. Deaths related to chronic twin transfusion syndrome—donor/recipient patterns.

	Fetal death			Postnatal death			
	Literature	Survey '91	Total	Literature	Survey '91	Total	Totals
All donors	40	19	59	24	15	39	98
All recipients	33	15	48	22	17	39	87
Concordant deaths							
Donor first	3	5	8	5	7	12	20
Recipient first	2	4	6	3	1	4	10
Single twin deaths							
Donor only	10	4	14	4	1	5	19
Recipient only	3	1	4	1	4	5	9

TABLE 9.12. Gestational age of twin deaths due to chronic twin transfusion syndrome.*

	Gestational age (weeks)†									
	20–21	22–23	24–25	26–27	28–29	30–31	32–33	34–35	36–37	38+
**Both stillborn	4	6	2	3	2	1	4	1	1	2
**Both postnatal deaths	1	7	9	5	5	1	1	–	1	–
**Stillbirth + postnatal death	–	–	2	1	1	1	2	1	–	3
Only one death										
Stillbirth	–	–	1	1	3	1	1	2	2	4
Postnatal	–	–	–	1	2	2	–	–	2	2
Total number of infant deaths	10	26	27	20	21	9	15	6	8	14

*Literature and Survey '91 cases combined.
†Gestational age = age at delivery whether stillborn or postnatal death.
**Number of sets.

anastomoses in the general survivor and autopsy case placentas as noted in Table 9.3, arteriovenous anastomoses were reported in 78.9% of autopsied chronic twin transfusion cases, and represented 66.6% of all the anastomoses identified in those cases.

These observations are consistent with earlier reports[7] and are not surprising because an unbalanced blood flow is the pathophysiologic basis of chronic twin transfusion, and flow in parenchymal anastomoses is probably unidirectional and may vary less widely than in surface vessel shunts. It becomes an interesting question as to how to explain findings consistent with chronic twin transfusion in the infants, where only a surface arterial anastomosis is identified. These infrequent cases may be ones in which there is an undetected penetrating vessel arising from the inferior surface on the recipient's side of the arterial anastomosis, so that an undetected arteriovenous shunt may be present as well. Such cases point out the detail that may be needed in order to assess what appear to be incon-

sistent findings at first review. In those cases with bidirectional parenchymal anastomoses, or parenchymal with surface anastomoses, we can only assume that the net flow across these combinations was sufficiently imbalanced to cause the syndrome. It may be that differences in the anatomy of the cord insertions become important in these cases.[91]

The same analysis was done of the vascular patterns described in 11 cases of survivor group twin placentas reported to be associated with signs of chronic twin transfusion. The only discernible difference between the cases that survived and those that died was that, although parenchymal anastomoses represented 64.3% of all the anastomoses identified, and 81.8% of these placentas had parenchymal anastomoses, in two-thirds of the placentas there were surface arterial, venous, and/or compound, and therefore potentially balancing anastomoses as well. These may have been the reason the syndrome was manifest later or less severely in the group that survived.

The appearance of the decidual surface of the placenta may reflect differences in the villus tissue and mirror the respective twin's appearance.

The *donor portions* of the placenta have been described as bulky and pale with large pleomorphic and edematous villi.[7] The mechanism of the villus edema was not clear as fetal edema was not usually associated with these edematous villi, so some local placental process was suggested. This edema enlarged the villus surface area to twice that of the recipient, possibly reducing the intervillus space and affecting maternal perfusion.[73] In spite of this, vasculosyncytial membranes were few, thick, and small as compared to the villi of the co-twin, and the syncytiotrophoblast was still fairly thick with few knots, but a large number of sprouts, creating a relatively immature appearance.[91] The cytotrophoblast was normal and the loose stromal tissues contained frequent Hofbauer cells with granular or vacuolated cytoplasm. The villus capillaries were interpreted as being long and thin because they had the same surface area as those in the recipient but were half the caliber. This suggested that even if the donor twin was anemic with the probability of a hyperdynamic circulation, the villus capillary flow was poor due to the increased resistance. This would contribute to poor transport and result in an infant who appeared to be suffering from intrauterine malnutrition.[4] There was also intracapillary erythroblastosis and there was more intervillus fibrin than in the recipient. In some cases the donor placenta has been reported to have an atrophied or ischemic appearance compared to that of the co-twin,[20] although it is not clear whether this represents a later stage of the above process or a different pattern of placental response.

The *recipient's placental portion* has been described as enlarged because of congestion, but has also been reported to be smaller than the donor's.[92] The villi are more uniformly of normal size and appearance but the capillaries are usually markedly dilated and congested, creating many large, thin, vasculosyncytial membranes. This appearance may mean facilitated fetomaternal exchange in the recipient and hence explain the greater growth rate.[92]

The histology of the *shared cotyledons* has been reported as well.[7] In cases without a clinical transfusion syndrome, but with common villus territories, the villi were normal. In shared areas in chronic transfusion syndrome cases where the donor's artery supplied the territory, the villi were normal. In the shared areas where the recipient's artery was the supply, the villi looked like the rest of the donor territory.

Mineralization of villus basement membranes was described in some of the Survey '91 autopsy cases of chronic twin transfusion, and was seen in both donor and recipient villus territories, but not always concordantly. This is a finding of unknown significance that remains to be explained as it is also seen with fetal hydrops and fetal death in singletons, as well as in a variety of genital, renal, and hematologic conditions.[82,93]

Fetal Findings

The pathologic features of twins affected by chronic twin transfusion consist of gross and microscopic alterations in *growth* and development related to nutrient and oxygenation imbalance and pressure/volume adaptations. The linear growth of the infants may be more or less affected and discordant, but body weights can be strikingly different. Classically, the recipient twin is larger than expected for age and the donor smaller, occasionally disproportionately so. The organ weights are often discordant in the same pattern, although brain weight may be spared. In some cases, some organ weights may be below the expected weight in both twins, but the donor organs are still smaller than the recipient's.

The reduced organ weights in the donor were attributed by Naeye[4,5] to reduced cytoplasmic mass in a manner analogous to the changes seen with chronic malnutrition. The liver, spleen, thymus, and fetal adrenal cortex were more affected than the brain, pancreas, kidney, or permanent adrenal cortex. The suggested cause of these exaggerated malnourished appearances in the donor was the loss of plasma nutrients to the recipient partners. He also postulated that placental oxygen transport and transplacental exchange of other nutrients may be abnormal in all twin gestations, and that this may contribute to the syndrome. Transport defects could be due to maternal uterine blood flow that is inadequate for the demands of the twin conception and/or could be related to placental villus changes associated with the transfusion state as described above.[7,92]

Some of the classic features of simple chronic twin transfusion syndrome are presented for com-

FIGURE 9.10. Simple chronic twin transfusion (see Table 9.9c). Note the marked discrepancy in the size of the heart and lungs of the donor (D) and recipient (R) twins in (a). The donor died before the recipient and was autopsied separately, so his viscera were formalin fixed at the time of the second autopsy. The discordant birth weight and viscera weights, especially the heart, are represented graphically in (b) as a percentage of the mean for age (dotted line).

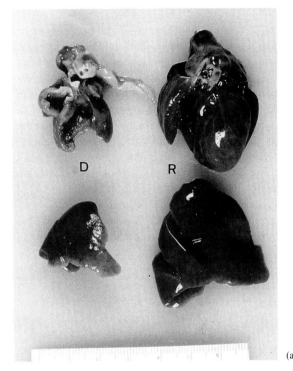

(a)

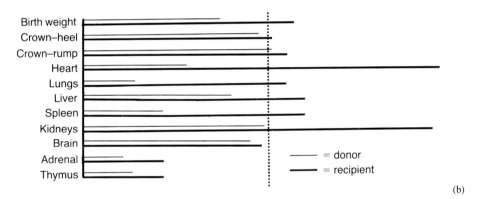

(b)

parison in Table 9.8c and in an illustrative case as follows. A twin gestation was complicated by hydramnios at 20 weeks and a total of 4,450 cc of fluid was withdrawn in three amniocenteses for symptomatic therapy of the mother. Although tocolysis helped suppress uterine contractions, they eventually led to delivery at 23 weeks. Both male twins died within 5 hours of birth. The autopsy data are presented in Table 9.9c and presented graphically with a picture of the heart and lungs in Fig. 9.10. The umbilical cord insertions were 25 cm apart on the symmetrically vascularized monochorionic placenta and the recipient had a marginally inserted cord. There were two arteriovenous anastomoses from the smaller to the larger twin, one of 2-mm-diameter vessels and the other with a 1-mm-diameter artery connected to a 2-mm- diameter vein. There was also one superficial arterial shunt 1 mm in diameter. The pattern of growth discordance and placental findings were considered compatible with simple chronic twin transfusion. As in other cases noted in the Survey '91 Review, the difference in weight of the hearts approached a factor of four, a degree of discordance not seen in any other pattern of intertwin weight/growth discordance with otherwise normally developed twins.

As noted in the case example above, some of the most striking differences that have been observed between donor and recipient are in the *cardiovascular system*. In Naeye's[4,5] review, the heart of the donor twin was much smaller than normal due to decreased number and mass of cardiac fibers, while the heart of the recipient was hyperplastic and on occasion weighed twice that of the donor. This was interpreted as a myocardial response to increased cardiac workload due to the increased blood viscosity and hypervolemic hypertension. This discrepancy can be evident at as early as 10 weeks of gestation[20] and may be the first identifiable features of chronic intertwin hemodynamic imbalance.[94] As a corollary, the muscle mass of the pulmonary and systemic arteries was increased in the recipient as an adaptation to the long-standing hypertension, with opposite changes in the donor.[4,5,57] Elastic arteries can be affected as well with intimal thickening of the aorta by multiple layers of smooth-muscle cells parallel to the long axis of the aorta reported in recipient twins.[95] Discordant calcification of the elastic fibers of the pulmonary trunk has been seen in recipients when there is an unusually large difference in the respective cardiac weights.[96]

The *lungs* in the donor twin are usually smaller than expected, based in part on the relative malnutrition mentioned above. In addition, there may be an element of chest compression as part of the oligohydramnios phenotype in the "stuck twin." Donor lungs have been described as less mature histologically, attributed to the relative ischemia of the donor state.[97]

As might be expected on the basis of discordant volumes of amniotic fluid in twin transfusion, there are differences in the *kidneys*. Recipient kidneys are larger than normal with congested enlarged glomeruli,[7,51] not only as a morphologic response to nutritional forces, but also to the plethora, and this leads to polyuria and hence excess amniotic fluid.

The donor kidneys are small with small glomeruli, but with additional abnormalities of the proximal convoluted tubules. These tubules have been described to contain degenerative changes with calcification,[51] or to be undeveloped with glomeruli surrounded by small undifferentiated appearing tubules.[83,97] This has been attributed to renal hypoperfusion,[83] and may be associated with other evidence of developmental lag, such as increased blastema.[97] In this context, it is of interest that a similar lesion of proximal tubules has been reported in cases of angiotensin converting enzyme inhibition fetopathy.[98] There is one report of scattered glomerular crescents in a donor twin's kidneys, attributed to chronic hypoxemia, but the tubules were said to be normal.[99]

A differential *erythropoietic response* has been observed in twins with chronic transfusion.[56] Recipient twins may have excess hepatic hematopoiesis on the basis of transfused donor erythropoietin.[1] The anemic donor twin may also have increased extramedullary hematopoiesis, but this seems more variable, and cutaneous hematopoiesis has been reported.[47]

There has been considerable attention in the literature to lesions of the *central nervous system* in twins and the possible relationship of these findings to intertwin vascular anastomoses. This is discussed in the following section on consequences of fetal death in twins.

Differential Diagnosis

It has been noted above that the diagnosis of acute or chronic twin transfusion syndrome, as an explanation for discordant twin growth, color, other observations, or fetal death, can be complicated if other processes are present as well. The problem of other causes of fetal growth retardation has already been mentioned. The case of an hydropia growth retarded twin pair has been reported that was initially thought to be due to chronic twin transfusion, but was identified as due to human parvovirus B19 infection.[100] Three examples of other problem cases from the Survey '91 Review are presented briefly.

Case one—differential diagnosis with discordant endocardial fibroelastosis (EFE). Twins were diagnosed at 11 weeks and progressive discordant growth and fluid volumes noted. Hydramnios led to preterm labor at 27 weeks. At birth, the hydropic larger twin was 3.5% longer and 23% heavier than expected, with cord hematocrit of 31% and cardiomegaly on x-ray. She died at age 10½ hrs and at autopsy her heart was twice the expected weight with biventricular EFE and visceral findings of congestive heart failure. The co-twin was 6.8% shorter and 21.3% lighter than expected, with a "normal" cord hematocrit. She lived 18 days and died with severe bronchopulmonary dysplasia. The heart was slightly large for the infant at the time of autopsy, as it was normal weight for age while the twin was still small, but had no sign of EFE.

The monochorionic placenta was asymmetrically portioned with 40% to the larger and 60% to the smaller twin. The cords were 12 cm apart and there were two parenchymal shunts from the smaller to the larger twin, each less than 1 mm in diameter, a 1-mm venous shunt, and an arterial shunt of arteries 4 mm in diameter on the large twin's side and less than 1 mm on the smaller twin's side.

There is certainly evidence for chronic twin transfusion, but how much did heart failure from EFE contribute to the fluid differences? EFE has not been reported in twin transfusion recipients so it seems an independent factor.

Case two—differential diagnosis with vessel calcification and hydrops. Twins with discordant growth and differential fluid volumes with hydrops of the larger twin were identified by ultrasound at 17 weeks, and at 23 weeks both sacs had excess fluid. The hydropic twin died in utero and the pregnancy was delivered 7 to 10 days later at 29 weeks. The length of the stillborn twin was 3.5% above the expected mean (at death), while the survivor was 7.3% less than expected. The weight of the survivor was 7.8% less than the mean and the macerated stillborn twin was at the mean. The survivor's heart weight was 16.6% above the expected and the stillborn's heart 9.6% below the mean. The survivor's cord hematocrit was 31%. The stillborn twin had residual hydrops and idiopathic arterial calcification of the aorta and major branches as well as pulmonary arteries, with myocardial fibrosis and focal calcification. The surviving co-twin died in less than 24 hours with hyaline membrane disease and barotrauma. There was no calcification of any systemic or pulmonary vessel. He had increased hematopoiesis in the liver and adrenal with mild anasarca and general congestion. An unexpected finding was a hypoperfusion injury of the brain, consisting of periventricular infarction and gliosis consistent with the timing of the co-twin's fetal death. There was also acute periventricular hemorrhage, but no vessel pathology.

The monochorionic placenta was only slightly asymmetric with the larger side to the stillborn twin. The umbilical cords were 14 cm apart and the liveborn twin had a marginally inserted single artery cord. There were a number of anastomoses: 1 cm diameter venous shunt, 2-mm-diameter arterial shunt, another arterial shunt with

a 4- to 5-mm-diameter vessel on the live-born twin's side and a 1- to 2-mm-diameter vessel on the stillborn twin's side, and a compound anastomosis consisting of a 4-mm artery to a 2-mm artery (live-born to stillborn), with a branch that joined a 1- to 2-mm- vein from the stillborn twin, which vein was also connected to a separate 1- to 2-mm-artery from the live-born twin. The overall impression therefore would be that any chronic imbalance would have been from the live-born to the stillborn twin, making the hydrops in the stillborn twin on the basis of being a recipient twin, and pulmonary vessel calcification has been reported in recipient twins.[96] However, idiopathic arterial calcification is also associated with hydrops, although the mechanism is not known.[101]

In this case, then, it is difficult to decide which process is more important in the twin who died in utero. The stillborn twin may have had two problems and fetal death may have been due to cardiac failure on the basis of both these entities. It is suggested that, at the time of his death, there was a period of shock in the surviving twin because of altered hemodynamics across the anastomoses, leading to the hypoperfusional lesions in the brain identified at autopsy. He may have recovered, but then deteriorated into impending heart failure by the time of birth. The significance of the single-artery marginal cord to his overall picture is not known.

Case three—differential diagnosis with fetomaternal hemorrhage (FMH). In this case, twins were diagnosed at 31 weeks and unilateral hydramnios was noted. Absent fetal movements at 37 weeks led to hospital admission. A slow fetal heart rate was identified with a scalp electrode, but both twins were stillborn at emergency section. The larger twin appeared to have died first on the basis of degree of maceration and she was pale. She was 12% longer and 23% heavier than expected with a heart that was twice the expected weight. The co-twin was 3.4% longer than expected and 7.5% less in weight, with a heart weight equivalent to the mean expected. The cords were 10 cm apart on the monochorionic placenta, and the smaller twin had vessels over one-quarter of the chorionic surface with a marginally inserted cord. There were three anastomoses, two arterial shunts of 1 mm each, and a parenchymal shunt from a 2.5-mm artery from the smaller to a 4-mm vein from the larger twin. The appearances were compatible with the chronic twin transfusion syndrome, except that the larger supposed recipient was very pale.

The explanation was suggested by the placenta, where there was a 6 × 4 cm infarcted chorangioma in the recipient twin's portion, and 5.2% fetal cells (estimate 126 ml) in the maternal circulation. The sequence in this case was therefore interpreted as severe fetomaternal hemorrhage from the recipient twin related to the chorangioma,[102] with shock and death, followed by shock and death in the donor twin on the basis of acutely altered hemodynamics. Both twins were well grown, and one suspects that without the FMH both might have been live-born.

These three cases are uncommon events, but have been presented as examples of cases where chronic twin transfusion is not the only factor contributing to the clinical and pathologic findings. The pathologist needs to be aware that intertwin vascular anastomoses may not be the only source of twin discordance, and that other processes may augment or compound the classic chronic twin transfusion findings.

Acute-on-Chronic Transfusion

It was mentioned in the section on acute transfusion that the simple acute transfusion was rare, and that acute transfusion as a complication of a chronic transfusion might be more common. In fact, 45% of the autopsy cases of chronic transfusion identified in the Survey '91 Review were interpreted as acute-on-chronic just prior to fetal death. As noted in Table 9.8d, the key features of these sets of twins has been growth discordance that was compatible with the chronic transfusion, but a reversal of the plethora/pallor so that the larger twin was pale and the smaller twin plethoric. The possibility of reversal or acute change in the chronic hemodynamics was suggested by the details in some reports in the literature, although the discussions did not dwell on that aspect of the cases.[52,54,57,84] The concept of acute on chronic was reported in detail in a case of apparently monoamniotic twins,[103] and used to explain the brain damage noted in some survivors after fetal death of one monochorionic twin.[39,104] These cases imply that some acute event has occurred to upset the previously stable, albeit imbalanced, flow, and that surface anastomoses are present to allow a large volume to shift rapidly.

An example of the acute-on-chronic pattern as outlined in Table 9.8d is presented as follows. This twin pregnancy was diagnosed at 8 weeks with normal fetal growth at 13 weeks. At 17 weeks, there was a slight discrepancy in size and by 19 weeks 4 days, there was a smaller twin with oligohydramnios and a larger twin with polyhydramnios. Premature labor was associated with ascending infection after premature rupture of the membranes, and both twins were stillborn at 23 weeks. The autopsy data are presented in Table 9.9d. The evidence for

chronic twin transfusion was the growth discordance, most particularly of the heart (Fig. 9.11a). The organ weights of the smaller twin were not as low as expected for their size, because of intense congestion. The evidence for acute-on-chronic transfusion was the marked reversal of color with severe pallor of the larger twin and marked congestion of the smaller twin (Fig. 9.11b). (The test for fetal cells in the maternal circulation was negative.) Unfortunately, in this case the placenta was retained and required manual removal, so it was in fragments and the pattern of intertwin anastomoses could not be detailed. This is an example of the difficulty that is sometimes encountered when attempting to provide a complete analysis of all components of a case. The precipitating factor was not determined, although it was thought temporally related to the rupture of membranes.

One final example of the variability of chronic twin transfusion that may change patterns clinically and present confusing features at autopsy is as follows. Twins were diagnosed at 14 to 15 weeks, and by 22 weeks discordant fluid and 3 weeks' discordant growth were seen with ultrasound. At 25 weeks, the Doppler ratio was 2.9 in the larger twin and 7.7 in the smaller twin. At 26 weeks, there was more fluid around the smaller twin, and by 27 weeks there had been growth arrest of the larger twin, catch up growth of the smaller twin, with decreased fluid in both sacs. The vascular resistance in the larger twin was 2.3, but was $5 + n$ in the smaller twin with no end diastolic flow. Fetal distress, consisting of sequential and progressive variable decelerations, was followed by fetal death, and the twins were stillborn the following day at 28 weeks. The autopsy data are presented in Table 9.9e. As can be seen from Fig. 9.12a, the twins are relatively evenly grown, as noted clinically, except for the noteworthy difference in the diameters of the umbilical cords—the more plethoric twin A, who seems to have died first on the basis of degree of maceration, has a much thinner cord, 0.8 cm compared with 1.3 cm for twin B. The additional pathologic evidence of chronic twin transfusion was the organ weight discordance, although the degree of discordance was lessened by the intense congestion of the hyperemic twin's smaller organs. The most striking difference was the heart weight with a nearly 100% difference between the twins (Fig. 9.12b). The evidence for acute transfusion was the

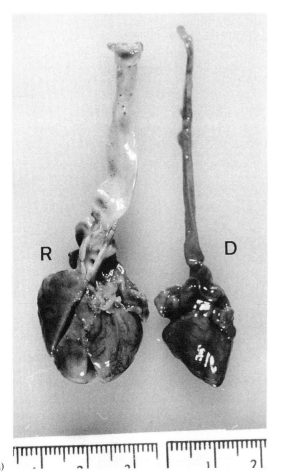

(a)

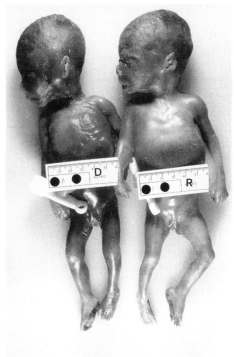

(b)

FIGURE 9.11. Acute-on-chronic twin transfusion (see Table 9.9d). The discordant heart sizes as seen in (a) are evidence for the underlying chronic transfusion, while the discordant reversed plethora of the smaller donor twin (b) is evidence for the terminal acute reversal of the shunt. D, chronic donor; R, chronic recipient.

differential color, particularly of the intensely congested, though smaller, liver in twin A.

The umbilical cords were 12 cm apart on the monochorionic placenta and their circulations overlapped extensively, so that a true vascular equator was not definable (Fig. 9.12c). There were a number of intertwin anastomoses compatible with the interpretation of reversing chronic transfusion with a terminal acute transfusion, as suggested clinically.

Externally, these twins looked like a simple acute transfusion, except for the discordant umbilical cord sizes. Internally, the evidence for a preceding chronic imbalance were the discordant heart sizes, with parallel discordant circumferences of the descending aorta, 50% greater in twin B. The chronic imbalance was altered at 25 to 26 weeks, but the precipitating factor was uncertain. The basis and timing of the apparent acute transfusion was also undetermined. It could not be said whether something led to the acute transfusion with death of the previous donor/now recipient, followed by death of the previous recipient/now donor, or whether the previous donor died for undetermined reasons and then acted as a no-pressure drain for blood from the previous recipient, who then died. One suggested mechanism was that the original donor's small heart could not cope with the altered hemodynamics.

These examples of variations of chronic and acute transfusion serve to remind us that not every case is logically straightforward, and that a number of contributing forces need to be kept in mind when interpreting clinical and pathologic findings. When

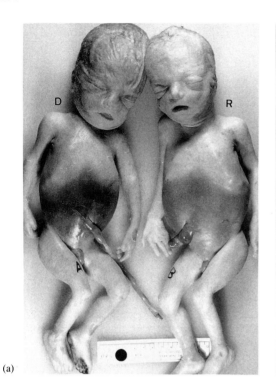

(a)

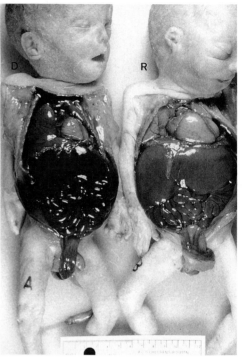

(b)

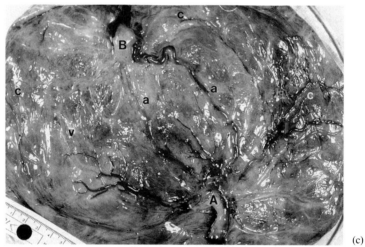

(c)

FIGURE 9.12. Reversing chronic transfusion with terminal acute transfusion. D, original donor; R, original recipient of chronic transfusion. The twins seem to be the same size (a), but the differing umbilical cord diameters reflect a chronic transfusion, as do the strikingly discordant heart sizes (b). The original donor (twin A) is plethoric at the time of autopsy, reflecting the terminal acute transfusion. The chorionic circulations were overlapping (c) with a number of intertwin anastomoses: two arterial (a) and one venous (v) surface shunts, and three regions of compound anastomoses (c) with the potential for flow in either direction.

there are variations identified, particularly the acute-on-chronic, it is important first to try to identify what might have led to the sudden change, and second, to determine the consequences for each twin. This is true, not only for the spontaneous cases, but may explain undesired outcomes in cases where therapeutic interventions have been tried.

Intervention Procedures

Because of the dismal outcome of twin transfusion diagnosed in midtrimester, there have been a number of procedures used to try to obtain at least one normal living infant, and have included, in order of increasing vigor, bed rest, maternal medication, decompression amniocentesis, fetal therapy, selective feticide, anastomotic interruption, and surgical removal of one twin. Bed rest and tocolysis do not appear to offer any noteworthy benefit and while indomethacin can be effective in reducing fetal urine output and hence the amounts of amniotic fluid, long-term use is not encouraged.[61,63,105] Digoxin, given to a mother at 26 weeks and for the rest of the pregnancy, led to resolution of fetal hydrops and the twins were less discordant at birth at 34 weeks than they had been at 22 weeks, with a 10% difference in hematocrit—both survived.[106] One parenchymal anastomosis was mentioned in this case.

Decompression Amniocentesis

Aggressive therapeutic/decompression amniocentesis has been variably successful in cases of chronic twin transfusion. One of the most successful series consisted of 17 cases that ranged from 16 to 28 weeks' gestation at diagnosis, required 1 to 10 amniocenteses (mean = 4) for 225 to 5,000 ml fluid (mean 1,683 ml).[107] Pregnancy was prolonged 31 to 139 days (mean 80 days) with 60% resolution of hydrops and 79% perinatal survival. Unfortunately, there was no information about the patterns of intertwin anastomoses in any of these cases. A contrasting report of serial amniocentesis in 13 patients did not find any significant difference in gestational age at diagnosis, interval between diagnosis and delivery, or survival rate comparing cases with and without amniocentesis, but no correlative placental findings were reported.[63] The absence of placental findings in the majority of the articles on the effects of decompression amniocentesis makes it very difficult to assess the significance of the reported success or failure of the procedure.

The explanation for the successful cases following amniocentesis is not clear. One suggestion was that decompression permitted better circulation in the "stuck twin," leading to normalizing of amniotic fluid volumes.[107] Another proposal was that repeated amniocentesis affects fetal urine output, but the mechanism was not determined and vascular anatomy was not described.[108] Other explanations for beneficial effects of repeated amniocentesis include a reduction in the risk of polyhydramnios-mediated premature delivery, or a maturational reduction in the significance of intertwin anastomoses with increasing fetoplacental blood volume in later pregnancy.[109] It has been noted that fetal anemia/polycythemia persists when amniocentesis is the only treatment,[108,110] but the significance of this finding to the outcome is not yet understood.

The timing of the procedure may be important. Therapeutic amniocentesis was reported to be most effective if done before there was severe maternal abdominal distention or signs of labor, although no correlative placental findings were provided.[111] When amniocentesis becomes essential for maternal symptomatic relief, it may mean irreversible pathology, as there were no surviving infants in one reported series.[46] Although it has been noted that reaccumulation of fluid does not follow a discernible pattern, and that the intervals between amniocentesis vary markedly, both from case to case and within individual cases, this has not been correlated with placental findings.[112]

The procedural complications reported include rupture of amnion and abruptio placenta, as well as preterm labor and intra-amniotic infection.[112] Surviving "stuck twins" have been reported to have evidence of antenatal brain damage, but this was not correlated with placental findings.[112] Other reports of periventricular leukomalacia in hydramniotic twins and renal damage in "stuck twins" after serial amniocentesis are also not correlated with details of intertwin vascular anatomy on the placenta.[113]

It can be seen from the preceding paragraphs that aggressive amniocentesis of the hydramniotic sac has been associated with varying success, but has not been correlated with placental findings. The significance of alterations in intra-amniotic pressure may depend on the vascular pattern present

FIGURE 9.13. Amniocentesis for hydramnios due to chronic twin transfusion syndrome. Although repeated amniocenteses were used for 800 to 1,400 ml of fluid each time between 24 and 27 weeks, the donor twin died at 27 weeks. No further amniocenteses were needed and the well survivor was born spontaneously at 33 weeks. This stillborn twin was growth retarded for the age at death with no anomalies. One-third of the monochorionic placenta was sclerosed. Only three anastomoses could be demonstrated 6 weeks after fetal death, probably because they had been kept patent by the survivor.

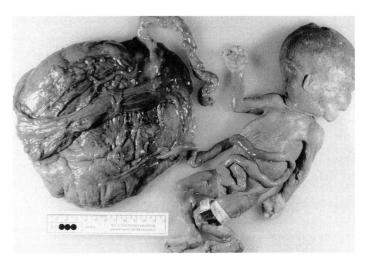

within the hydramniotic sac. It may be, therefore, that the variations reported can be explained by variations in the anatomy (and thus potential hemodynamics) of the intertwin vascular anastomoses. Amniocentesis was used in two cases in the Survey '91 Review.

Case 1—Twins were identified by ultrasound at 7.5 weeks and discordant size and fluid suggestive of twin transfusion was seen at 13 weeks. The larger twin in the hydramniotic sac was growing normally, while the smaller twin was progressively restricted and eventually 4 weeks behind in size by 24 weeks. Weekly decompression amniocentesis for 800 to 1,400 ml fluid were performed between 24 and 27 weeks. Intermittent severe bradycardia of the smaller twin was noted at 26 weeks and he died 1 week later. No further amniocenteses were required, although hydramnios without fetal hydrops persisted around the survivor. Spontaneous delivery occurred at 33 weeks with a healthy 2,050-g live-born male twin and a macerated co-twin (Fig. 9.13). The linear measurements of the stillborn twin were indicative of growth retardation at the time of death at 27 weeks— crown–heel length was 14.2% less than the mean for that age. The monochorionic placental portion of the stillborn twin was one-third the total volume and involuted. The umbilical cords inserted 8.5 cm apart and three anastomotic sites were described—arterial with the original donor's vessel 1 mm and the recipient's vessel 3 mm; arterial with equal 1-mm vessels; parenchymal with a 2-mm artery from the original recipient to a 1- mm vein of the original donor. Unfortunately, many of the original donor's chorionic vessels were sclerosed and the possibility of other anastomoses could not be ruled out. One suspects that there were other parenchymal anastomoses

from the stillborn to the live- born twin, but that they sclerosed after the death of the donor. The three connections that could be demonstrated were likely kept patent by virtue of originating from the survivor. It is probable that blood in all three returned to the survivor through unidentified penetrating vessels as the placental parenchyma of the donor was sclerosed. Part of the original shared villus territory may have been recruited to the survivor's circulation. The mechanism of fetal death is difficult to determine 6 weeks after the event, but one possibility is that the reduction in intra-amniotic pressure after amniocentesis altered blood flow in the anastomotic surface vessels, so that the donor gradually went into shock and died. It is not known why the recipient did not bleed back across the anastomoses and suffer a similar fate.

Case 2—This twin pregnancy was marked by suddenly increased uterine size at 18 weeks with fetal and fluid discordance compatible with twin transfusion, including mild hydrops of the larger twin in the hydramniotic sac. Amniocentesis of 1,800 cc at 18 weeks and another 1,000 cc at 21 weeks was followed by normalization of fluid levels and fetal growth until 34 weeks, when oligohydramnios with mature ultrasound placenta pattern was seen. Section delivery was performed for abnormal fetal position and twin boys, 2,350 g and 2,200 g were live-born and did well. The placenta was monochorionic diamniotic with 15 cm between the cords (Fig. 9.14). There were three parenchymal anastomoses from the smaller to the larger twin, and a venous anastomosis that was part of a compound parenchymal anastomosis from the larger to the smaller twin. One might suspect that it was this latter zone that was the basis for fluctuation, and that removal of the amniotic fluid permitted a balancing flow in this region.

It is interesting to speculate on the importance of

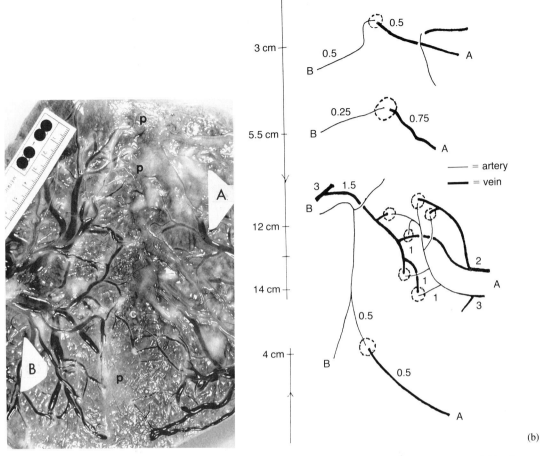

FIGURE 9.14. In this case of therapeutic amniocentesis for hydramnios due to chronic twin transfusion syndrome, both twins did well. Twin B was the original donor with a number of arteriovenous parenchymal anastomoses from B to A [p in (a) and top two and bottom circles in (b)]. The central compound anastomosis in region marked c in (a), with a venous shunt and multiple parenchymal shunts as drawn in (b), may have represented the variable that responded to the pressure changes after amniocentesis, allowing shunting from A to B. (Drawing made at time of injection studies. Scale on left is distance of anastomoses from nearest margin of placenta. Diameters of vessels are in millimeters.)

the diamniotic separating membrane in cases of chronic twin transfusion syndrome. It was noted in Chapter 8 that monoamniotic twins are rarely affected by chronic twin transfusion. Also, decompression of the hydramniotic sac has had a beneficial effect on some aspects of the syndrome in many cases. These observations suggest that there is some differentiating feature between the two sacs of a diamniotic monochorionic twin placenta that is important to the perpetuation and progression of the syndrome. What this might be is not clear, as theoretically the pressure should be equal across a pliable membrane like the diamniotic septum (Green SI, 1992, personal communication). Although monoamniotic twins are at risk for entanglements, is there a possibility that creation of a window through the septum between the twins would help stabilize a chronic transfusion state? If this has been tried, it does not appear to have been reported.

Fetal Therapy

Direct fetal therapy has been reported, both inadvertent and intentional. During one of serial amniocenteses in two cases of twin transfusion, a surface chorionic vessel of the recipient twin was punctured and intra-amniotic hemorrhage occurred.[114] Although the twins continued to be growth discordant, volumes of amniotic fluid normalized and living and normally developing twins were born, 4 weeks in one case and 10 weeks in the other case, after the hemorrhage.[115] Also, reference has been made to partial exchange transfusions for anemia or polycythemia with some suggestion of an effect on fetal hydrops.[110]

Selective Feticide

Selective feticide of the donor twin has been reported using a variety of techniques but with limited success, although selective feticide in discordantly anomalous or diseased dichorionic twins has been reported for a number of conditions and has been successful.[39] The difference is that in monochorionic twins threatened by twin transfusion syndrome, the intertwin vascular anastomoses that have caused the problem are also the source of potential damaging or lethal complications of any feticide procedure. Anything injected into the circulation of the selected twin has the potential to reach the co-twin, and, depending on the vascular anatomy, death of one twin could lead to shock in the co-twin, followed by death, or recovery but with damage. The successes and problems with selective feticide using intracardiac fluid injections are exemplified by the following cases.

Case one—Successful feticide of a donor twin at 25 weeks using pericardial tamponade with normal saline led to resolution of uterine irritability and hydramnios with normal fetal growth of the survivor until delivery at 37 weeks.[116] The surviving twin has continued to develop normally with no signs of cerebral or other damage. The papyraceous twin had a single artery 6 mm velamentously inserted cord and its placental portion was completely sclerosed, so it was not possible to document anastomotic vessels (Fig. 9.15).

Case two—Intracardiac intraventricular saline used to achieve asystole, followed by potassium chloride, was successful in one reported case after pericardial saline tamponade failed, but no placental findings were noted.[70] In a similar Survey '91 case, intracardiac potassium chloride was used after an unsuccessful injection of saline, and this was followed by death of the injected twin and then death of the co-twin at 24 weeks.[39] At autopsy, there were bidirectional parenchymal anastomoses in an asymmetrically vascularized monochorionic placenta

(donor had one-third area). The appearances and measurements of the twins were interpreted as an acute reversal of the imbalance after death of the original donor (Fig. 9.16; Tables 9.8f and 9.9f).

Case three—In this case, the only intervention at 25 weeks was penetration of the chest of the smaller twin by the needle as the procedure had to be stopped for maternal reasons and bradycardia of both twins.[39] Decompression amniocenteses were used thereafter for symptomatic relief of the mother, and section delivery took place 4 weeks later. Both twins were live-born, but the recipient twin had severe hypoxic ischemic brain damage corresponding to the interval from the attempted feticide, and she died at 3 days of age. The donor twin had caught up in length, had a normal hemoglobin and, after a stormy neonatal course, has done well. Three unidirectional parenchymal shunts from the smaller to the larger twin were confirmed between the 19 cm distant cords on the monochorionic placenta, and two more parenchymal shunts in the same direction were obstructed by arteriolar thrombosis. There was an additional venous anastomosis. The interpretation was that the initial bradycardia meant that both twins were in shock, with relatively more severe hypotension in the plethoric recipient, resulting in the cerebral lesion. Thrombosis of two of the five parenchymal shunts may have contributed to a lesser drain on the donor twin, balanced by the venous anastomosis, and she responded with increased growth.

Mechanical obstruction of one twin's circulation has also been attempted, again with varying success. Thrombogenic coils have been used to try to stimulate thrombosis in the heart without risking transfusion of a noxious substance or fluid volume to the co-twin,[117] and were tried in one case in the Survey '91 Review autopsy series.[118] Twins were diagnosed at 8 weeks and a "stuck twin" with 3 weeks' discordant growth compared to the larger hydramniotic twin with early hydrops was seen at 19 weeks 3 days. The hydrops evolved from ascites and pericardial effusion to skin edema in 3 days. At 20 weeks, five thrombogenic coils were inserted into the donor's heart with ultrasound guidance over 2 hours, with no detectable effect on this twin's circulation by Doppler study. Spontaneous delivery occurred later the same day and both twins were live-born, but died within minutes. The appearance and autopsy measurements of the twins were consistent with simple chronic twin transfusion (Fig. 9.17), especially the heart weights of -8.7% in the donor and $+130\%$ in the recipient compared to the mean expected for age. The coils in the donor were located in the right atrium, right ventricle,

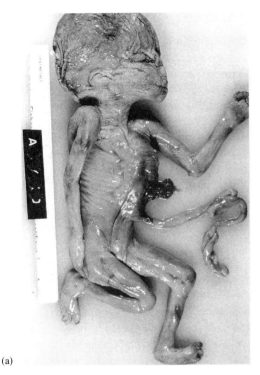

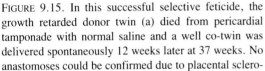

(a)

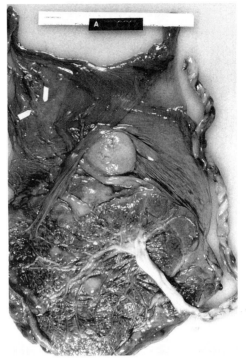

(b)

FIGURE 9.15. In this successful selective feticide, the growth retarded donor twin (a) died from pericardial tamponade with normal saline and a well co-twin was delivered spontaneously 12 weeks later at 37 weeks. No anastomoses could be confirmed due to placental sclero-sis (b). The terminated twin had a velamentous cord insertion (between white arrows), and its portion of the placenta was sclerosed. (Reprinted with permission from ref. 39.)

pericardial cavity, and two in the lower lobe of the right lung, without apparent thrombotic effect. Unfortunately, the placenta was received in multiple fragments, so the underlying vascular anatomy could not be assessed.

Hemostatic sealant [TISSEEL (Immuno [Canada, Ltd.])] has been used in an attempt to obstruct the cardiac circulation of the donor twin in another case from the Survey '91 Review autopsy series. In this case, twin transfusion was diagnosed at 18 weeks with an appropriately grown hydramniotic twin and a 2-week smaller "stuck twin," and the mother was in early labor. At 19 weeks, TISSEEL was injected into the heart of the donor twin with cardiac arrest. The co-twin's heart beat was normal at the end of the procedure, but contractility was decreasing 3 hours after the procedure, and fetal death of the second twin was documented 8 hours later. Delivery was induced by amniocentesis. The appearances and measurements of the twins were indicative of an acute-on-chronic transfusion pat-tern (Fig. 9.18a). The sealant filled the donor's heart, systemic and pulmonary arterial circulations, and pericardium; it was interstitial in the diaphragm (Fig. 9.18b), and extended into one umbilical artery. In the monochorionic placenta, the cords were 10 cm apart, and the donor cord inserted at one margin. The surface vascularity was asymmetric with 40% to the donor and 60% to the recipient. The circulations were partially overlapping and anastomotic sites were numerous, often compound, and involved vessels of very small caliber (Fig. 9.18c,d). Injection studies were hampered by fragmentation of the parenchyma, but bidirectional parenchymal and surface arterial anastomoses were demonstrated (Fig. 9.18d). In this case, the interpretation was that, after the death of the donor twin, the original recipient twin exsanguinated back across to the original donor, leading to death and the reverse congestion/pallor noted at autopsy.

A number of considerations important to decision-making for selective feticide have been dis-

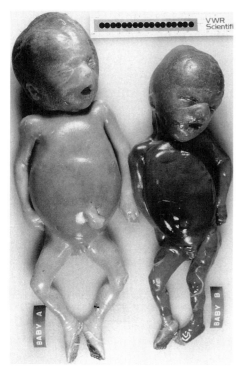

FIGURE 9.16. In this case of acute reversal of chronic twin transfusion complicating selective feticide of the donor, the smaller original donor became a receptacle for blood from the original recipient, who also died. Bidirectional parenchymal anastomoses were found in the asymmetrically vascularized monochorionic placenta. The original donor had one-third of the area. (Reprinted with permission from ref. 39.)

cussed in a report of several of the above cases.[39] The key concerns are the certainty of the diagnosis, the selection of the twin to be terminated, the method, the timing, and the potential consequences for the co-twin and mother. There is also considerable ethical discussion that needs to take place in each case on a case by case basis, with fully informed involvement of the parents and use of expert opinion in all aspects of each case. This is not a procedure to be undertaken lightly and requires full pathologic evaluation of the placenta, the terminated twin, and the co-twin if necessary. Both successful and unsuccessful procedures need careful clinicopathological correlation in order to determine whether these techniques are reasonable options and under what circumstances.

Interruption of Anastomoses

The source of the problem in twin transfusion is the intertwin vascular anastomosis, so it is reasonable to consider ways to intervene at that level. It is a somewhat daunting prospect, however, based on the problems encountered trying to identify anastomoses in the delivered placenta in the laboratory. Even when shunts are identified, it is only conjecture as to which were the most important. It seems a considerable challenge to be able to identify and interfere with significant anastomoses in utero. Vessels between the lobes of the normally bilobed rhesus placenta were successfully occluded by fetoscopically delivered laser energy,[119] and this led to trials in human twin transfusion.[120] In three cases of chronic twin transfusion, vessels that could be traced from the recipient's cord insertion were photocoagulated if they were seen to join with a donor vessel, or passed beneath the septum. There was stabilization or resolution of the syndrome in all cases and four of the six infants survived, compared to the 100% mortality expected. Placental evidence of the success of the procedure was presented. This is the most direct and specific treatment possible, but it is limited by the placental position in the uterus, by the line of the septum in relation to the chorionic vessels, and possibly by the availability of a sufficiently interested, skilled, and experienced physician. What is particularly interesting about the in utero view of this procedure is the remarkable prominence of even small vessels when seen through the fetoscope (De Lia JE, 1992, personal communication). The difference from the appearance of the delivered placenta on the pathology bench is striking, and reaffirms that we have much to learn about the hemodynamics of intertwin anastomoses.

Removal of Fetus

An extension of the selective feticide approach to management of chronic twin transfusion is surgical removal of one twin.[121] The donor twin was removed at 21 to 22 weeks and was said to be normal, although no autopsy findings were presented. The surviving co-twin was delivered by section at 28 weeks because of spontaneous labor and was appropriate by weight, but no other data were given. He

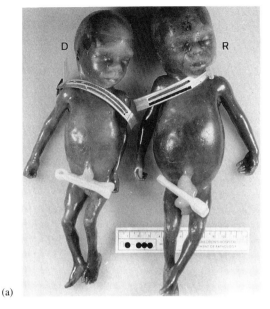

(a)

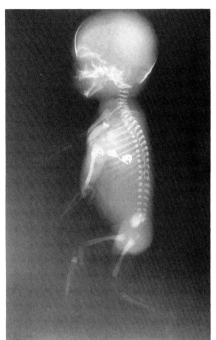

(b)

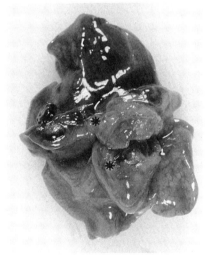

(c)

FIGURE 9.17. Selective feticide was attempted in these twins using thrombogenic coils in the donor, but was unsuccessful. The twins were discordant in size and color, compatible with chronic twin transfusion (a). The smaller donor (D) is paler than the larger recipient (R). The intrathoracic coils can be seen in the x-ray of the donor (b), and in the thoracic tissues at autopsy (c—two coils can be seen in this view of the heart just beside the *).

had aortic stenosis and died related to cardiac surgery, but no autopsy data were reported. The placental anatomy was not described. The occurrence of the valve lesion in this case is noteworthy as this has been seen previously in a surviving monochorionic twin with fetus papyraceous.[122]

Consequences of Fetal Death of One Twin

The unpredictable variability of the anatomy and consequences of intertwin vascular anastomoses have been presented in some detail in this chapter to

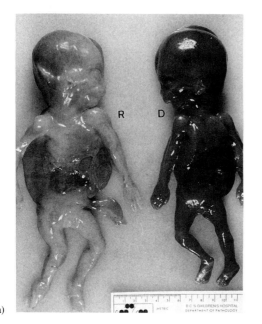

(a)

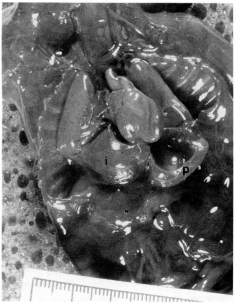

(b)

(c)

FIGURE 9.18. Selective feticide was achieved with injection of fibrin sealant in the donor twin, but the co-twin died shortly after. The twins presented an acute-on-chronic appearance, because the smaller original chronic donor (D) twin was plethoric and the larger original chronic recipient (R) was pale (a). In (b), the sealant was found in the donor's heart chambers, systemic and pulmonary circulations, formed a pericardial cast around the heart (p), and was interstitial in the diaphragm (i). The circulations were overlapping in the asymmetrically vascularized placenta (c). (The white line marks the approximate vascular equator between the two chorionic circulations.)

FIGURE 9.18. *Continued*. There were numerous anastomoses, often compound, involving vessels of very small caliber (d). (The drawings are taken from the originals made at the time of injection studies.)

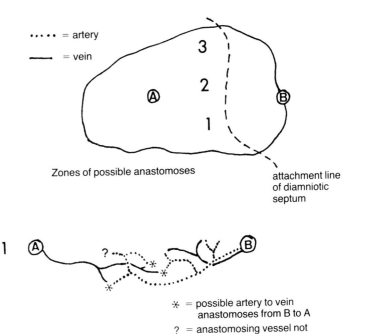

Zones of possible anastomoses

attachment line of diamniotic septum

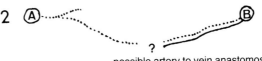

* = possible artery to vein anastomoses from B to A

? = anastomosing vessel not found

possible artery to vein anastomosis from A to B

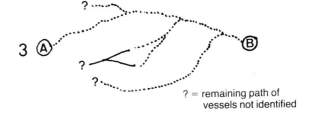

? = remaining path of vessels not identified   (d)

demonstrate the importance of clinicopathological consultation and correlation to the interpretation of clinical events and pathologic findings. This has become particularly critical in those cases of fetal death of one twin with visceral damage in the co-twin, where neurologic deficit in the survivor is the basis for a dispute or challenge concerning medical care and compensation. It is suggested that detailed written and graphic documentation is essential for all placentas of twin sets where there has been fetal death of one twin and there is evidence, or even concern, that the surviving co-twin has, or is at

risk for, problems. Only if there is solid evidence of appropriate placental findings, can a vascular basis for prenatal or perinatal morbidity be confirmed, and even then, there may be compounding variables, such as other discordant placental findings, or discordant fetal and/or perinatal insults.

One of the first suggestions that the death of one monochorionic twin could adversely affect the survivor, based on complications of intertwin vascular anastomoses, came from a set of monoamniotic twins described by Benirschke[3] in 1961. This twin pair consisted of a macerated fetus and a live-born infant who died at 62 hours of age with complete renal cortical necrosis, cardiac hypertrophy, infarct of the spleen, and severe symmetric necrosis in the brain. There were extensive vascular anastomoses between the two circulations around the insertion sites of the adjacent umbilical cords, and massive fibrin deposits in the cortical stem vessels of the brain and vessels in the kidney in the live-born twin. These findings suggested that thromboplastin-rich macerating blood from the dead twin crossed to the live twin, initiating a coagulopathy and leading to the consequences reported. However, the umbilical cords were also intimately entwined, so anoxic/ischemic lesions or coagulopathy on the basis of cord compression alone could not be excluded.

Patterns of Lesions and Placental Findings

In the years following Benirschke's case, there have been a number of other reported twins where lesions in the survivor of a macerated co-twin have been attributed to transchorionic coagulopathy. The defects described have included additional examples of renal cortical and cerebral necrosis,[85,123] brain damage including hydrancephaly, porencephaly, and multicystic encephalomalacia,[124,125] intestinal atresia,[86] congenital skin defects,[126] and foot necrosis.[127] Unfortunately, monozygosity was proven in only a few instances, and even fewer reports referred to the placenta as monochorionic or described any vascular communications. The lack of such corroborating evidence leads to uncertainty about the explanations proposed in many of these reports. Discussions of more recent cases are suggesting that there are probably a number of potential mechanisms for these apparently hypoxic/ischemic/vascular lesions in twins—mechanisms that are related to intertwin vascular anastomoses but in different ways—and that there may be cases that look similar but are due to other processes. The following discussion reviews examples of discordant visceral damage in twins and the potential mechanisms involved.

When twins are connected by placental vascular anastomoses, death of one twin can be reasonably expected to have some effect on the co-twin, although the nature and extent of that effect depends on the anatomic and functional pattern of the anas-tomoses, and on the stage of gestation at which it occurs. It has already been noted in this chapter that the death of one twin in midgestation can have either beneficial or lethal consequences for the co-twin. Spontaneous death of the donor twin[57] and selective feticide of the donor twin[116] have led to resolution of hydrops/hydramnios and resulted in live birth of the survivor. In contrast, both spontaneous and iatrogenic death, again usually of the donor twin, has been followed by apparent exsanguination of the survivor across the anastomoses with subsequent death (see case reported in previous section).

It seems that vasculogenic lesions in the survivor can be related to the period of gestation in which the insult occurs, analogous to lesions seen in singletons. It has been suggested that death of one twin in early pregnancy presents little risk to the survivor,[87,128] but there are also contrasting reports of ventriculomegaly/porencephaly, with bowel atresias in surviving twins after fetal death at 13 to 18 weeks' gestation.[129] In the second trimester, visceral infarcts in developing tissues may be resorbed with resultant absence of structures/tissues or atresias, and in the third trimester the infarcts persist as healing necrosis, with the degree of scarring and calcification dependent on the interval to diagnosis.[86,130]

The importance of the particular anatomic pattern of the anastomoses in cases of morbidity in the survivor is evident from recent studies that have included such data. Antenatal multifocal necrosis of cerebral white matter has been strongly associated with the presence of a vein-to-vein anastomosis as one of multiple intertwin anastomoses, together with additional arterial and parenchymal shunts—six of eight infants in four twin pairs, both donors and recipients, were affected.[131] An important additional observation was that cerebral white matter necrosis did not have to be preceded by fetal death.[131,132,133] A similar although less dramatic trend was noted when the incidence of fetal abnormalities in the surviving co-twin was assessed in all cases of intertwin anastomoses—19% of all twin sets with arterial and venous, or arterial and parenchymal combinations had abnormalities, 10% of all sets with venous ± parenchymal combinations, and 11% of all sets with only parenchymal shunts, compared to 3% of sets with arterial anastomoses only.[128]

FIGURE 9.19. Brain damage in a recipient twin resulting from an episode of shock following unsuccessful attempt at feticide of the donor twin 4 weeks prior to delivery. In these coronal sections can be seen hydrocephalus, intraventricular hemorrhage, and severe periventricular leukomalacia. This twin died at 3 days of age, while the donor survived and did well. (Reprinted with permission from ref. 39.)

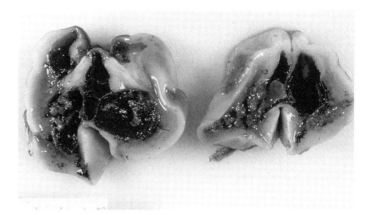

Central Nervous System

The patterns of brain pathology that have been described in monochorionic twins include hypoxic/ischemic lesions of white matter, hemorrhagic lesions in parenchyma or ventricles, and malformations.[134] The hypoxic/ischemic lesions include ischemic infarcts, most often in middle cerebral artery territory, leukomalacia, microcephaly, and hydranencephaly. Hemorrhagic lesions may be complicated by posthemorrhagic hydrocephalus. Neural tube defects have been associated with fetal death, but the association with vascular anastomoses is not clear.[88,134] Optic nerve hypoplasia has been reported in association with prenatal vascular encephalopathy in twins, but without placental findings.[135] The commonest lesions are the hypoxic/ischemic pattern and usually it is the recipient who is affected in association with a macerated donor co-twin, although donor twins have been damaged as well. While thromboembolic phenomena may account for some findings, episodes of hypotension may affect both donor and recipient twins.[133,134] Unstable circulatory volumes across anastomoses have been suggested as a cause for germinal matrix hemorrhage in the recipient and periventricular leukomalacia in the associated donor.[136]

Hypotension, with or without an associated coagulopathy, can explain hypoxic/ischemic lesions in singletons as well as twins, and hypotension can have a number of causes. All the processes that can cause fetal and perinatal brain damage in singletons[137] can apply just as well to twins,[138] and twins that share vascular anastomoses have an additional potential source of acute circulatory imbalance.

That acute circulatory imbalance may occur after the death of one twin,[104] or be associated with transient alterations of fetal heart rate/blood pressure[39] (Fig. 9.19). A source of hypotensive, hypoxic/ischemic lesions unique to monoamniotic twins is cord compression due to entanglement, either with the other twin or the other cord. This mechanism may be as important as transchorionic coagulopathy in cases of damaged monoamniotic twins with macerated co-twins.[3,123] Prenatal disruption of the diamniotic septum has been reported, creating secondarily monoamniotic twin pairs, with similar complications.[139,140] These cases have led to the suggestion that when amniocenteses are performed in twin gestations, the septum should be avoided whenever possible.[140]

Other Reported Visceral Damage

Bilateral *renal cortical necrosis* has been reported in surviving monochorionic twins after fetal death,[3,85,123] and the concepts of pathogenesis referred to in relation to cerebral damage apply to the kidneys as well. Renal cortical necrosis in a monozygotic twin with macerated co-twin with encephalocele, was associated with fetal anemia due to fetomaternal transfusion, but the placenta was not examined and the basis of monozygosity was not stated.[89] Corticomedullary and cortical renal infarcts with scarring and calcification, and focal infarction of basal ganglia and white matter, occurred prenatally in one of monochorionic twins who were both live-born.[90] The affected twin was growth retarded, with a velamentous cord insertion into only one-third of the chorionic volume. No surface anastomoses were seen with injection, but parenchymal anastomoses were not mentioned. Whether the hypoxic/ischemic lesions in the smaller twin were related to the abnormal cord/placental development or an undetected shunt was not ascertained.

Aplasia cutis of trunk and limbs has been associated with twinning, particularly with a fetus papyraceous, suggesting that this pattern was distinct from defects in the vertex of the scalp and might be related to complications of intertwin vascular anastomoses.[126] Trunk and scalp defects,[141] and scalp and knee defects[142] have been reported in monochorionic twins with fetus papyraceous, and unilateral scalp defect in symmetric live-born monoamniotic twins,[143] so the relationship of skin lesion pattern and fetal death to vascular anastomosis is not clear-cut. In one case of trunk skin defects with fetus papyraceous, the fetal death was attributed to toxoplasmosis, but no placental findings were reported and zygosity was not determined.[144] The lack of details of placental findings in these and other examples of discordant lesions in twins makes it difficult to be definitive about possible connections between the lesions and intertwin vascular communications, particularly if the placentation has not even been confirmed to be monochorionic.

Other than discordant heart size, pulmonary hypertension, and possible arterial calcifications, few *cardiovascular* lesions have been reported with twin transfusion. An unusual example of apparently acquired stenosis of a normally formed aortic valve with normal ascending aorta, endocardial sclerosis in a dilated left ventricle, and dilatation of the left atrium with fibrosed nonpatent foramen ovale, was associated with a fetus papyraceous and monochorionic placenta with anastomoses.[122] The lesions were attributed to altered hemodynamics following fetal death, although mechanistic details were not suggested.

Possible Mechanisms of Fetal Damage

The two pathogenetic concepts for discordant fetal lesions associated with death of one twin in utero—transchorionic coagulopathy and hemodynamic imbalance—warrant further comment.

Transchorionic Coagulopathy

There are two questions to consider regarding transchorionic coagulopathy—what evidence is there that it exists, and how might it take place. There is no doubt that intravascular thrombi, consistent with thrombotic phenomena, have been seen in surviving twins with visceral damage. However, it remains to be determined whether the stimulus arose from thromboplastins or actual thromboemboli from the dying or deceased twin, or arose within the affected twin itself. In two twin sets with fetal death, one with porencephaly in the survivor, fetal blood samples from the surviving twin had normal coagulation profiles, but the interval since fetal death was not stated, nor were placental details provided.[145] In one case of monochorionic twin transfusion with fetal death of the recipient, the donor developed renal cortical necrosis and porencephaly with ventriculomegaly.[146] The interval from fetal death to the onset of these findings was not clear from the report, but the survivor was described as having consumptive thrombocytopenia at cesarean birth at 28 weeks. No details of placental vascularity were given. Other reports suggesting absence of any coagulopathy in surviving twins are difficult to assess, because the pattern of placentation and intervals from fetal death to assessment of coagulation are not clear.[147,148] One might suspect that if coagulopathy in the survivor was induced by material from the dead twin, that there might be a temporal relationship, limited by details of the shared fetal circulation, so that the results of any coagulation studies must be related to the time of fetal death. If, in fact, the visceral lesions in the survivors were due to a coagulopathy, whether exogenous or endogenous, one might suspect that hematologic evidence of such a disturbance might have subsided by the time the lesions were well developed.

There are some additional problems to consider when assessing the relationship of intrauterine death of an infant and complicating coagulopathy. When a fetus of a multiple pregnancy dies and is delivered, but the placenta is retained, neither the mother nor the surviving twin apparently suffer any consequences (see Chapter 4). When the fetus is retained, coagulopathies in both the mother and the co-twin have been reported or suspected, but in no cases have both the mother and the co-twin been affected. Most reports suggest that maternal coagulopathy is not a problem in cases of fetal death of one twin with retention of the dead fetus.[149,150] In a case where a dead twin was cited as the cause of a coagulopathy in the mother,[151] there was no evidence of it in the co-twin, even though vascular shunts on the placenta were demonstrated. Alternatively, although a dead twin has been reported to be associated with disseminated intravascular coagulopathy in the mother, there do not appear to be any examples of maternal coagulopathy in any of the reports of abnormalities in a surviving twin that are attributed to transchorionic coagulopathy. Is the coagulopathy in the mother different from coagulopathy in the co-twin? In one report, the maternal coagulopathy did not recur after the second successfully treated episode, suggesting that the inciting factor may no longer be in the circulation, might be somehow altered, that possibly the maternal response was altered, or that the two conditions might not even be related.[151] Even in the accepted cases of maternal coagulopathy with retained dead single fetus, the exact source of the stimulus to the coagulopathy has not been clarified.[152] Presumably, the dead fetus is contained within its gestational sac, its placental vessels eventually sclerose because of cessation of fetal blood flow, and maternal intervillus blood continues to nourish and maintain the trophoblast covering the villi. A breach in the placental barrier must occur, or there must be some unknown change in the intervillus space to stimulate a coagulopathy. It has been suggested that a retained dead fetus can provoke immunologic injury of the placenta, but the details and mechanism remain to be determined.[153]

The other aspect of transchorionic coagulopathy to consider is the mechanism of transfer of the thrombogenic material or thromboemboli. The few reports of autopsy findings in the dead twin have not mentioned intravascular thrombi that could be a source of emboli, but coagulopathy can be difficult to identify histologically.[154] The phrase in the literature has been that this transfer is "from the dead twin," implying that it is a sequel to fetal death, yet it is difficult to imagine the movement of blood from a dead twin with no propelling force. There are three possible situations that could be invoked. If the doomed twin is dying in shock and has a coagulopathy as part of that process, there may still be enough cross-circulation to allow an effect on the other twin before the dying twin succumbs. Alternatively, after the demise of one twin, there may be alterations in blood flow patterns through shared villus territory. Depending on the

vascular anatomy, a cotyledon that was mainly or totally perfused by the now dead twin, may become perfused by the survivor. There may be endothelial damage from temporary hypoperfusion during the changeover, and this might be a source of thrombogenic stimuli. Finally, if the circulation of the dying twin is erratic for a period of time, mural thrombi might form in the larger chorionic vessels, and, depending on the vascular anatomy and flow patterns before and after fetal death, thrombi or thrombogenic materials could conceivably reach the survivor's circulation.

There were two examples in the Survey '91 Review autopsy series that are pertinent here. In Fig. 8.9 of monoamniotic twins, where one died as a result of cord compression (the cord was around the neck of the co-twin), the surviving twin appeared to have recruited almost the entire placenta, so that no involuted placental tissues could be defined, although fetal death had occurred 6 to 7 weeks before delivery. The cords were 3 cm apart and injection of arteries or veins from the surviving twin's cord led to immediate filling of vessels originally from the dead twin's cord—arterial and venous anastomoses were numerous and up to 1 cm diameter. There were two parenchymal anastomoses from the dead to the surviving twin, with vessels 3 to 5 mm in diameter. No sclerotic villi were seen in multiple parenchymal sections. The surviving co-twin was entirely normal. In Fig. 9.20 is another clear example of recruitment by the surviving twin of vessels that were originally from the dead twin. In this case, fetal death occurred 18 weeks before term delivery, perhaps related to the 9 cm velamentous insertion and one loop of cord around the ankle. The possibility of twin transfusion was not mentioned in the notes prior to fetal death. At the time of examination of the placenta after delivery, the surviving twin appeared to have recruited the entire arterial circulation from the dead twin, through a preexisting artery-to-artery anastomosis, through which blood crossed the first branch point of the single cord artery at the velamentous insertion to connect to the remaining branches from the umbilical artery. There were venous branches from the dead twin that were also recruited to a branch point, by virtue of the parenchymal connections now perfused by the survivor. There was no reported clinical suspicion of visceral damage in the 4.4-kg surviving twin.

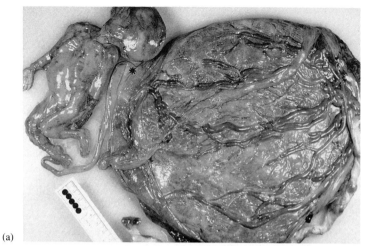

(a)

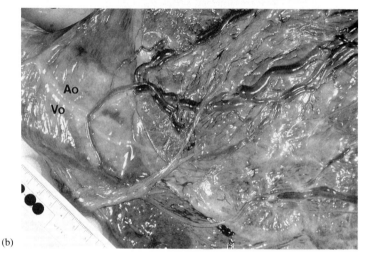

(b)

FIGURE 9.20. Recruitment of vessels after fetal death. Note the velamentous insertion of the cord from the dead twin (*) and that there does not seem to be evidence of involuted placental tissue corresponding to the dead twin (a). In a closer view of the cord from the dead twin (b), a few sclerosed vessels are seen in the membranes [Ao and Vo—the intramembranous branches from the velamentous insertion of the two vessel cord from twin B, and the venous branches Vo · 1 and Vo · 2 in the diagram (c)]. The majority of the vessels are quite patent, having been taken over by the surviving twin, with flow paths as shown in (c). The original anastomoses that allowed this takeover were an arterial shunt (number 3), from which twin B's own parenchymal shunt was taken over (A2 → V2); a parenchymal shunt from B to A at number 1, taken over by way of the arterial shunt and twin B's artery branches A1 and A2; and two more of twin B's own parenchymal shunts at number 2 and number 4, which served to recruit V1 and V2 of twin B's circulation. There was only a microscopic rim of sclerosed villus tissue at the margin of the placenta that could be considered from twin B. (Drawing made at time of injection studies.)

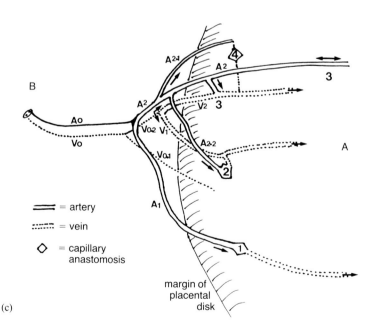

(c)

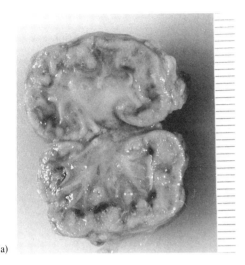

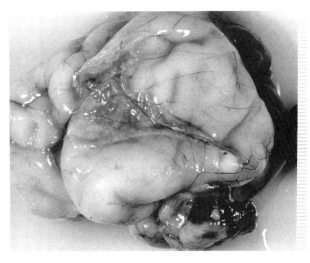

(a)   (b)

FIGURE 9.21. Fetal blood flow problems causing visceral damage. These organs were from the original recipient survivor of a chronic twin transfusion. The donor died in utero 1 week before delivery, attributed to a cord anomaly and it was postulated that the original recipient lost enough blood acutely back across vascular anastomoses into the dead twin, so that she sustained hypoxic/ischemic lesions of the kidneys (a) and brain (b), in addition to other visceral damage. She died at 7 days of age.

Although there did not appear to be problems with transchorionic coagulopathy in these two cases, they are presented as an example of a possible mechanism for such a process, in other words the recruitment of vessels and villus tissue from the dying/dead twin by the surviving twin.

Fetal Perfusion

The other main postulated mechanism of fetal death with visceral damage in the co-twin, is acute or subacute changes in fetal perfusion that either cause the death of the one twin with secondary hypotension in the survivor, or affect both twins concurrently, but with differential severity. The evidence that this occurs is indirect and based mainly on those cases of acute-on-chronic transfusion, where the previous donor is plethoric and the previous recipient is pale[97] (see cases described above). An example of fluctuating flow contributing to brain damage in the recipient was one of the cases of attempted intervention described above.[39]

In the Survey '91 Review, there was one twin set with discordant visceral damage and fetal death. Monochorionic female twins were delivered spontaneously at 31 weeks, about 1 week after one fetal death. There had been no reported problems. The surviving twin died at 7 days of age with renal cortical necrosis, cavitating and gliotic periventricular infarcts with descending degeneration (Fig. 9.21), other foci of gliotic cerebral infarcts, and splenic infarction, all considered compatible with the interval from fetal death. The surviving twin was appropriately grown at birth (+2.8% above the mean for crown–heel length), but was anemic and pale. The macerated twin was congested and slightly smaller (3.5% below the mean for crown–heel length). Evidence for chronic twin transfusion was the discordant heart size—the dead twin/donor heart was −40% compared to the mean, and this was greater than the degree of weight reduction of other viscera attributable to autolysis, and the recipient's/survivor's heart was +19.6% compared to the mean. The fetal death was attributed to a velamentous insertion of the cord, with transient acute hemorrhage of the surviving twin into the donor twin, with recovery but with visceral damage. Unfortunately, the placental circulations were not detailed, so this explanation remains hypothetical.

Doppler studies of umbilical artery flow in twin transfusion have been discussed above and no consistent pattern is reported yet. Resolution of abnormal patterns of flow following fetal death has been described,[52] but so has no detectable change in umbilical flow in the 24 hours following fetal death with at least one arterial anastomosis.[65]

Prevention

As with any investigation of pathophysiology, the ultimate goal of determining why, how, and when something goes wrong is to establish if a specific treatment approach is warranted. As might be expected from the preceding discussion, it is difficult to arrive at dogmatic recommendations based on information in the literature.[155] Also, the basic process is sufficiently unpredictable that no uniform policy has been proposed.[134] Expectant monitoring has been suggested as the basis for further management.[48] Early delivery of the survivor has not prevented lesions attributable to coagulopathy,[156] as the damage has probably already occurred, but prevention of mortality or morbidity in the viable potential survivor may be achieved by intervention before the anticipated fetal death.[104] This approach still has the risks based on prematurity depending on the gestational age at delivery.

Conclusion

Intertwin vascular anastomoses develop in monochorionic placentas and can be arterial, venous, parenchymal, or compound, in any number, pattern, and direction of combinations. Currently, the blood flow patterns in utero are only conjecture and probably potentially dynamically variable, depending on factors of intrafetal physiology, umbilical cord circulation, fetal movements, amniotic fluid pressures, and perhaps other forces as well. The clinical importance of these connections is when net blood flow is imbalanced, either acutely or chronically, or both. The results range from fetal death of one or both twins, through degrees of discordant morbidity, to minimal differences in well-grown twins. The earlier severe imbalances, with near-uniform mortality, have led to a number of techniques aimed at interrupting the imbalance in order to achieve survival of at least one twin. There is also considerable medical and medicolegal attention being paid to the occurrence and mechanism of discordant morbidity following fetal death of one twin.

There remains a great deal to be learned about the anatomy, physiology, and pathophysiology of in-

tertwin vascular anastomoses, and the pathologist has a critical role to play. In order for useful clinicopathological correlations to take place in these cases, placenta examinations must be thorough, precise and adequately documented, including details of fetal vessel patterns and anastomoses in particular. Clinical and autopsy findings need to be correlated carefully with the placental details on a case by case basis, particularly when there has been an unexpected adverse outcome. As can be seen from this chapter, any discussion of events with intertwin vascular anastomoses remains hypothetical without adequate pathologic examination.

References

1. Strong SJ, Corney G. *The Placenta in Twin Pregnancy*. London: Pergamon Press; 1967:1–13.
2. Kloosterman GJ. The "Third Circulation" in identical twins. *Ned Tijdschr Verlosk Gynaecol.* 1963;63:395–412.
3. Benirschke K. Twin placenta in perinatal mortality. *NY State J Med.* 1961;61:1499–1508.
4. Naeye RL. Human intrauterine parabiotic syndrome and its complications. *N Engl J Med.* 1963;268:804–809.
5. Naeye RL. Organ abnormalities in a human parabiotic syndrome. *Am J Pathol.* 1965;46:829–842.
6. Rausen AR, Seki M, Strauss L. Twin transfusion syndrome. *J Pediatr.* 1965;66:613–628.
7. Aherne W, Strong SJ, Corney G. The structure of the placenta in the twin transfusion syndrome. *Biol Neonate.* 1968;12:121–135.
8. Benirschke K, Kaufmann P. *Pathology of the Human Placenta.* 2nd ed. New York: Springer-Verlag; 1990:662.
9. Benirschke K, Kaufmann P. *Pathology of the Human Placenta.* 2nd ed. New York: Springer-Verlag; 1990:205–207.
10. Boyd JD, Hamilton WJ. *The Human Placenta.* Cambridge: W Heffer; 1970:222–227.
11. Arts NFT. Investigations on the vascular system of the placenta. I and II. *Am J Obstet Gynecol.* 1961;82:147–158,159–166.
12. Benirschke K, Driscoll SG. *The Pathology of the Human Placenta.* New York: Springer-Verlag; 1967:91–179.
13. Shanklin DR, Perrin EVDK. Multiple gestation. In: Perrin EVDK, ed. *Pathology of the Placenta.* Vol 5. *Contemporary Issues in Surgical Pathology,* Roth LM, ed. New York: Churchill Livingstone; 1984:165–182.
14. Bhargava I, Chakravarty A. Vascular anastomoses

in twin placentae and their recognition. *Acta Anat.* 1975;93:471–480.

15. Cameron AH. The Birmingham twin survey. *R Soc Med Proc.* 1968;61:229–234.

16. Nylander PPS, Osunkoya BO. Unusual monochorionic placentation with heterosexual twins. *Obstet Gynecol.* 1970;36:621–625.

17. Lage JM, Vanmarter LJ, Mikhail E. Vascular anastomoses in fused, dichorionic twin placentas resulting in twin transfusion syndrome. *Placenta.* 1989;10:55–59.

18. Benirschke K. Origin and clinical significance of twinning. *Clin Obstet Gynecol.* 1972;15:220–235.

19. Altschuler G. Medical implications of basic concepts in gemellology. In: Iffy L, Kaminetzky HA, eds. *Principles and Practice of Obstetrics and Perinatology.* New York: John Wiley; 1981:1171–1181.

20. Benirschke K, Kim CK. Multiple pregnancy. *N Engl J Med.* 1973;288:1276–1284,1329–1336.

21. Galea P, Scott JM, Goel KM. Feto-fetal transfusion syndrome. *Arch Dis Child.* 1982;57:781–794.

22. Robertson EG, Neer KJ. Placental injection studies in twin gestation. *Am J Obstet Gynecol.* 1983;147:170–174.

23. Leroy F. Major fetal hazzards in multiple pregnancy. *Acta Genet Med Gemellol.* 1976;25:299–306.

24. Boyd, JD, Hamilton WJ. (1970) *The Human Placenta.* Cambridge: W. Heffer; 1970:61–75.

25. Arts NFTh, Lohman AHM. The vascular anatomy of monochorionic diamniotic twin placentas and the transfusion syndrome. *Eur J Obstet Gynecol.* 1971;3:85–93.

26. Sekiya S, Hafez ESE. Physiomorphology of twin transfusion syndrome; a study of 86 twin gestations. *Obstet Gynecol.* 1977;50:288–292.

27. Bleisch VR. Placental circulation of human twins. Constant arterial anastomoses in monochorionic placentas. *Am J Obstet Gynecol.* 1965;91:862–869.

28. Berne RM, Levy MN. Cardiovascular Physiology. 5th ed. St. Louis: CV Mosby; 1986:231–233.

29. Smith JJ, Kampine JP. *Circulatory Physiology—The Essentials.* 3rd ed. Baltimore: Williams & Wilkins; 1990:16–30.

30. Smith JJ, Kampine JP. *Circulatory Physiology—The Essentials.* 3rd ed. St. Louis: CV Mosby; 1986:133.

31. Smith JJ, Kampine JP. *Circulatory Physiology—The Essentials.* 3rd ed. St. Louis: CV Mosby; 1986:159.

32. La Barbera M. Inner currents. How fluid dynamics channels natural selection. *The Sciences.* 1991; 31:30–37.

33. Sherer DM, Nawrocki MN, Peco NE, Metlay LA, Woods JR. The occurrence of simultaneous fetal heart rate accelerations in twins during nonstress testing. *Obstet Gynecol.* 1990;76:817–821.

34. Sherer DM, Nawrocki MN, Abramowicz JS, Peco NE, Metlay L, Woods JR. Is there a "Dominant Twin" in utero? (Abstract). *Am J Obstet Gynecol.* 1991;164:421

35. Gallagher MW, Johnson TRB. Fetal heart rate accelerations, fetal movement and fetal behavior patterns in twin gestations (Abstract). *Am J Obstet Gynecol.* 1992;166:416.

36. Van Allen MI. Fetal vascular disruptions: mechanisms and some resulting birth defects. *Pediatr Ann.* 1981;10:219–233.

37. King James Bible. *Genesis.* 25:21–26.

38. Tan KL, Tan R, Tan SH, Tan AM. The twin transfusion syndrome, clinical observations in 35 affected pairs. *Clin Pediatr.* 1979;18:111–114.

39. Baldwin VJ, Wittmann BK. Pathology of intragestational intervention in twin to twin transfusion syndrome. *Pediatr Pathol.* 1990;10:79–93.

40. Bryan EM. IgG deficiency in association with placental edema. *Early Hum Dev.* 1977;1/2:133–143.

41. Naeye RL, Letts HW. Body measurements of fetal and neonatal twins. *Arch Pathol.* 1964;77:393–396.

42. Benirschke K, Des Roches Harper V. The acardiac anomaly. *Teratology.* 1977;15:311–316.

43. Corney G. Twin placentation and some effects on twins of known zygosity. In: Nance WE, ed. Twin Research: Biology and Epidemiology. *Prog Clin Biol Res.* 1978;24B:9–16.

44. Bryan E, Slavin B. Serum IgG levels in feto-fetal transfusion syndrome. *Arch Dis Child.* 1974;49:908–910.

45. Nageotte MP, Hurwitz SR, Kaupke CJ, Vaziri ND, Pandian MR. Atriopeptin in the twin transfusion syndrome. *Obstet Gynecol.* 1989;73:867–870.

46. Bebbington MW, Wittmann BK. Fetal transfusion syndrome: antenatal factors predicting outcome. *Am J Obstet Gynecol.* 1989;160:913–915.

47. Schwartz JL, Manisculco WM, Lane AT, Currao WJ. Twin transfusion syndrome causing cutaneous erythropoiesis. *Pediatrics.* 1984;74:527–529.

48. Blickstein I. The twin-twin transfusion syndrome. *Obstet Gynecol.* 1990;76:714–722.

49. Elejalde BR, de Elejalde MM, Wagner AM, Lebel RR. Diagnosis of twin transfusion syndrome at 18 weeks of gestation. *J Clin Ultrasound.* 1983;11:442–446.

50. Patten RM, Mack LA, Harvey D, Cyr DR, Pretorius DH. Disparity of amniotic fluid volume and fetal size: problem of the stuck twin—US Studies. *Radiology* 1989;172:153–157.

51. Achiron R, Rosen N, Zakut H. Pathophysiologic

mechanism of hydramnios development in twin transfusion syndrome. *J Reprod Med.* 1987; 32:305–308.

52. Pretorius DH, Manchester D, Barkin S, Parker S, Nelson TR. Doppler ultrasound of twin transfusion syndrome. *J Ultrasound Med.* 1988;7:117–124.

53. Brown DL, Benson CB, Driscoll SG, Doubilet PM. Twin-twin transfusion syndrome: sonographic findings. *Radiology* 1989;170:61–63.

54. Brennan JN, Diwan RV, Rosen MG, Bellon EM. Fetofetal transfusion syndrome: prenatal ultrasonographic diagnosis. *Radiology* 1982;143:535–536.

55. Lubinsky M, Rapoport P. Transient fetal hydrops and "prune belly" in one identical female twin. *N Engl J Med.* 1983;308:256–257.

56. Fisk NM, Borrell A, Hubinont C, Tannirandorn Y, Nicolini U, Rodeck CH. Fetofetal transfusion syndrome: do the neonatal criteria apply in utero? *Arch Dis Child.* 1990;65:657–661.

57. Kirshon B, Moise KJ, Mari G, Rothchild J, Wasserstrum N. In utero resolution of hydrops fetalis following the death of one twin in twin-twin transfusion. *Am J Perinatol.* 1990;7:107–109.

58. Okane M, Okamoto H, Hamada H, Mesaki N, Kubo T, Iwasaki H. Significance of twin to twin transfusion syndrome in the prognosis of twin pregnancies and its prenatal diagnosis by ultrasonography. *Nippon Sanka Fujinka Gakkai Zasshi.* 1990;42:599–604.

59. Wittmann BK, Baldwin VJ, Nichol B. Antenatal diagnosis of twin transfusion syndrome by ultrasound. *Obstet Gynecol.* 1981;58:123–127.

60. Moore TR, Garrett V, Benirschke K. Prognostic factors for survival in the twin transfusion syndrome (Abstract). *Am J Obstet Gynecol.* 1991; 164:289.

61. Castanez J, Cetrulo C, D'Alton M. Twin to twin transfusion (Abstract). *Am J Obstet Gynecol.* 1992;166:357.

62. Chescheir NC, Seeds JW. Polyhydramnios and oligohydramnios in twin gestations. *Obstet Gynecol.* 1988;71:882–884.

63. Gonsoulin W, Moise KJ, Kirshon B, Cotton DB, Wheeler SM, Carpenter RJ. Outcome of twin-twin transfusion diagnosed before 28 weeks of gestation. *Obstet Gynecol.* 1990;75:214–216.

64. Yamada A, Kasugai M, Ohno Y, Ishizuka T, Mizutani S, Tomoda Y. Antenatal diagnosis of twin-twin transfusion syndrome by Doppler ultrasound. *Obstet Gynecol.* 1991;78:1058–1061.

65. Erskine RLA, Ritchie JWK, Murnaghan GA. Antenatal diagnosis of placental anastomosis in a twin pregnancy using Doppler ultrasound. *Br J Obstet Gynecol.* 1986;93:955–959.

66. Giles WB, Trudinger BJ, Cook CM, Connelly AJ.

Doppler umbilical artery studies in the twin-twin transfusion syndrome. *Obstet Gynecol.* 1990;76: 1097–1099.

67. Gaziano EP, Knox E, Bendel RP, Calvin S, Brandt D. Is pulsed Doppler velocimetry useful in the management of multiple-gestation pregnancies? *Am J Obstet Gynecol.* 1991;164:1426–1433.

68. Kanzaki T, Chiba Y. Evaluation of the preload condition of the fetus by inferior vena caval blood flow pattern. *Fetal Diagn Ther.* 1990;5:168–174.

69. Chiba Y, Kobayashi H, Kunzaki T, Murakami M. Quantitative analysis of cardiac function in nonimmunological hydrops fetalis. *Fetal Diagn Ther.* 1990;5:175–188.

70. Weiner CP. Diagnosis and treatment of twin to twin transfusion in the mid second trimester of pregnancy. *Fetal Ther.* 1987;2:71–74.

71. Ludomirski A, Weiner S, Craparo F, Bhutani U. Twin to twin transfusion syndrome: role of Doppler flow and fetal hyperviscosity in predicting outcome (Abstract). *Am J Obstet Gynecol.* 1991;164:243.

72. Goldberg HJ, Oats JN, Ratten V, Beischer NA. Timely diagnosis by cardiotocography of critical fetal reserve due to fetofetal transfusion syndrome. *Aust NZ J Obstet Gynaecol.* 1986;26:182–184.

73. Abraham JM. Intrauterine fetofetal transfusion syndrome. *Clin Pediatr.* 1967;6:405–410.

74. Shah DM, Chaffin D. Perinatal outcome in very preterm births with twin-twin transfusion syndrome. *Am J Obstet Gynecol.* 1989;161:1111–1113.

75. Danskin FH, Neilson JP. Twin to twin transfusion syndrome: what are appropriate diagnostic criteria? *Am J Obstet Gynecol.* 1989;161:365–369.

76. Giles W, Trudinger B, Wilcox G. Discrepancies in hemoglobin levels (Letter). *Am J Obstet Gynecol.* 1989;163:1713.

77. Caglar MK, Kolle LAA. Determination of serum ferritin in the evaluation of iron depletion and iron overload in chronic twin-to-twin transfusion syndrome. *J Perinat Med.* 1989;17:357–359.

78. Bishop NJ, King FJ, Ward P, Rennie JM, Dixon AK. Paradoxical bone mineralization in the twin to twin transfusion syndrome. *Arch Dis Child.* 1990;65:705–706.

79. Ashley WE, Sanders I. Twin to twin transfusion: cause of increased pulmonary vasculature in the newborn. *AJR.* 1981;137:617–618.

80. Oh W. Neonatal polycythemia and hyperviscosity. *Pediatr Clin North Am.* 1986;33:523–532.

81. Koenig JM, Hunter DD, Christensen RD. Neutropenia in donor (anemic) twins involved in the twin-to-twin transfusion syndrome. *J Perinatol.* 1991;11:355–358.

82. Baldwin VJ. Placenta. In: Dimmick JD, Kalousek

DK, eds. *Developmental Pathology of the Embryo and Fetus*. Philadelphia: JB Lippincott; 1992:271–319.

83. Genest DR, Lage JM. Absence of normal-appearing proximal tubules in the fetal and neonatal kidney: prevalence and significance. *Hum Pathol*. 1991;22:147–153.

84. Betts DA. Twin transfusion syndrome: a case report. *J Am Assoc Nurse Anaesth*. 1982;50:378–381.

85. Moore CM, McAdams AJ, Sutherland J. Intrauterine disseminated intravascular coagulation: a syndrome of multiple pregnancy with a dead twin fetus. *J Pediatr*. 1969;74:523–528.

86. Hoyme HE, Higginbottom MC, Jones KL. Vascular etiology of disruptive structural defects in monozygotic twins. *Pediatrics*. 1981;67:288–291.

87. Yoshida K, Soma H. Outcome of the surviving cotwin of a fetus papyraceous or of a dead fetus. *Acta Genet Med Gemellol*. 1986;35:91–98.

88. Luebke HJ, Reiser CA, Pauli RM. Fetal disruptions: assessment of frequency, heterogeneity, and embryologic mechanism in a population referred to a community-based stillbirth assessment program. *Am J Med Genet*. 1990;36:56–72.

89. Reisman LE, Pathak A. Bilateral renal cortical necrosis in the newborn. *Am J Dis Child*. 1966;111:541–543.

90. Dimmick JE, Hardwick DF, Ho-Yuen B. A case of renal necrosis and fibrosis in the immediate newborn period. *Am J Dis Child*. 1971;122:345–347.

91. Fries MH, Goldstein RB, Kilpatrick SJ, Golbus MS, Callen PW, Filly RA. The role of velamentous cord insertion in the etiology of twin-twin transfusion syndrome. *Obstet Gynecol*. 1993;81:569–574.

92. Sala MA, Matheus M. Placental characteristics in twin transfusion syndrome. *Arch Gynecol Obstet*. 1989;246:51–56.

93. Krohn K, Ljungqvist A, Robertson B. Trophoblastic and subtrophoblastic mineral salt deposition in hydramnios. *Acta Pathol Microbiol Scand*. 1967;69:514–520.

94. Barr M, Pridjian G. Growth effects in twins: clinical implications (Abstract). *Teratology*. 1991;43:424.

95. Nicosia RF, Krouse TB, Mobini J. Congenital aortic intimal thickening: its occurrence in a case of twin-twin transfusion syndrome. *Arch Pathol Lab Med*. 1981;105:247–249.

96. Popek EJ, Strain JD, Neumann A, Wilson H. In utero development of pulmonary artery calcification in monochorionic twin (Abstract). *Mod Pathol*. 1990;3:7P. (Poster presentation, Society for Pediatric Pathology, Boston, March 1990.)

97. Hawkins EP, Page LM, Langston C. Twin-twin transfusion: effects on organ maturation (Abstract). *Mod Pathol*. 1989;2:3P. (Poster presentation, Society for Pediatric Pathology, San Francisco, March 1989.)

98. Barr M Jr, Cohen MM Jr. ACE inhibitor fetopathy and hypocalvaria: the kidney-skull connection. *Teratology*. 1991;44:485–495.

99. Altemani AM, Vassalo J, Billis A. Congenital focal glomerular lesions in only one monozygotic twin related to a probable twin transfusion syndrome. *Histopathology*. 1986;10:991–994.

100. Weiner CP, Naides SJ. Fetal survival after human parvovirus B19 infection: spectrum of intrauterine response in a twin gestation. *Am J Perinatol*. 1992;9(1):66–68.

101. Darnell Jones DE, Pritchard KI, Gioannini CA, Moore DT, Bradford WP. Hydrops fetalis associated with idiopathic arterial calcification. *Obstet Gynecol*. 1972;39:435–440.

102. Santamaria M, Benirschke K, Carpenter PM, Baldwin VJ, Pritchard JA. Transplacental hemorrhage associated with placental neoplasms. *Pediatr Pathol*. 1987;7:601–615.

103. Bendon RW, Siddiqi T. Clinical pathology conference: acute twin-to-twin in utero transfusion. *Pediatr Pathol*. 1989;9:591–598.

104. Fusi L, McParland P, Fisk N, Nicolini U, Wigglesworth J. Acute twin-twin transfusion: a possible mechanism for brain-damaged survivors after intrauterine death of a monochorionic twin. *Obstet Gynecol*. 1991;78:517–520.

105. Rosen DJD, Fejgin MD, Rabinowitz R, Regev RH, Beyth Y. Indomethacin therapy and fetal urine production in twins with polyhydramnios. *J Perinat Med*. 1991;19:173–176.

106. De Lia JE, Emery MG, Sheafor SA, Jennison TA. Twin transfusion syndrome: successful in utero treatment with digoxin. *Int J Gynecol Obstet*. 1985;23:197–201.

107. Elliott JP, Urig MA, Clewell WH. Aggressive therapeutic amniocentesis for treatment of twin-twin transfusion syndrome. *Obstet Gynecol*. 1991;77:537–540.

108. Rosen DJD, Rabinowitz R, Beyth Y, Fejgin MD, Nicolaides KH. Fetal urine production in normal twins and in twins with acute polyhydramnios. *Fetal Diagn Ther*. 1990;5:57–60.

109. Saunders WH, Snijders RJM, Nicolaides KH. Therapeutic amniocentesis in twin-twin transfusion syndrome appearing in the second trimester of pregnancy. *Am J Obstet Gynecol*. 1992;166:820–824.

110. Weiner C, Ludomirsky A. Diagnosis and treatment of twin to twin transfusion syndrome. (TTTS) (Abstract). *Am J Obstet Gynecol*. 1992;166:284.

111. Urig MA, Newell WH, Elliott JP. Twin-twin transfusion syndrome. *Am J Obstet Gynecol*. 1990; 163:1522–1526.

112. Mahony BS, Petty CN, Nyberg DA, Luthy DA, Hickok DE, Hirsch JH. The "stuck twin" phenomenon: ultrasonographic findings, pregnancy outcome, and management with serial amniocenteses. *Am J Obstet Gynecol*. 1990;163:1513–1522.

113. Feingold M, Cetrulo CL, Newton ER, Weiss J, Shakr C, Shmoys S. Serial amniocenteses in the treatment of twin to twin transfusion complicated with acute polyhydramnios. *Acta Genet Med Gemellol*. 1986;35:107–113.

114. Schneider KTM, Vetter K, Huch R, Huch A. Acute polyhydramnios complicating twin pregnancies. *Acta Genet Med Gemellol*. 1985;34:179–184.

115. Vetter K, Schneider KTM. Iatrogenous remission of twin transfusion syndrome (Letter). *Am J Obstet Gynecol*. 1988;158:221.

116. Wittmann BK, Farquharson DF, Thomas WDS, Baldwin VJ, Wadsworth LD. The role of feticide in the management of severe twin transfusion syndrome. *Am J Obstet Gynecol*. 1986;155:1023–1026.

117. Burke MS, Heyborne K, Bruno A, Porreco RP. Selective feticide in the second trimester: percutaneous ultrasound guided intracardiac placement of a thrombogenic coil (Abstract). *Am J Obstet Gynecol*. 1991;164:337.

118. Bebbington MW, Wilson RD, Machan L, Wittmann BK Selective feticide in fetal transfusion syndrome using ultrasound guided insertion of thrombogenic coils. (In press. Submitted to *Obstet Gynecol*.)

119. De Lia JE, Cukierski MA, Lundergan DK, Kochenour NK. Neodymium:yttrium-aluminum-garnet laser occlusion of rhesus placental vasculature via fetoscopy. *Am J Obstet Gynecol*. 1989;160:485–489.

120. De Lia JE, Cruikshank DP, Keye WR Jr. Fetoscopic neodymium:yag laser occlusion of placental vessels in severe twin-twin transfusion syndrome. *Obstet Gynecol*. 1990;75:1046–1053.

121. Urig MA, Simpson GF, Elliott JP, Clewell WH. Twin-twin transfusion syndrome: the surgical removal of one twin as a treatment option. *Fetal Ther*. 1988;3:185–188.

122. Kaplan C. (1984) Isolated aortic stenosis with fetus papyraceous: a new vascular disruptive anomaly. In: Ryder OA, Byrd ML, eds. *One Medicine*. Heidelberg: Springer-Verlag; 1984:77–83.

123. Bulla M, von Lilien T, Goecke H, Roth B, Ortmann M, Heising J. Renal and cerebral necrosis in survivor after in utero death of co-twin. *Arch Gynecol*. 1987;240:119–124.

124. Yoshioka H, Kadomoto Y, Mino M, Morikawa Y, Kasubuchi Y, Kusunoki T. Multicystic encephalomalacia in liveborn twin with a stillborn macerated co-twin. *J Pediatr*. 1979;95:798–800.

125. Jung JH, Graham JM, Schultz N, Smith DW. Congenital hydranencephaly/porencephaly due to vascular disruption in monozygotic twins. *Pediatrics*. 1984;73:467–469.

126. Mannino FL, Jones KL, Benirschke K. Congenital skin defects and fetus papyraceous. *J Pediatr*. 1977;91:559–564.

127. Margono F, Feinkind L, Minkoff HL. Foot necrosis in a surviving fetus associated with twin-twin transfusion syndrome and monochorionic placenta. *Obstet Gynecol*. 1992;79:867–869.

128. Yoshida K, Matayoshi K. A study on prognosis of surviving cotwin. *Acta Genet Med Gemellol*. 1990;39:383–387.

129. Anderson RL, Golbus MS, Curry CJR, Callen PW, Hastrup WH. Central nervous system damage and other anomalies in surviving fetus following second trimester antenatal death of cotwin. *Prenat Diagn*. 1990;10:513–518.

130. Jones KL, Benirschke K. The developmental pathogenesis of structural defects: the contribution of monozygotic twins. *Semin Perinatol*. 1983;7: 239–243.

131. Bejar R, Vigliocco G, Gramajo H, Solona C, Benirschke K, Berry C, Coen R, Resnik R. Antenatal origin of neurologic damage in newborn infants. II Multiple gestations. *Am J Obstet Gynecol*. 1990;162:1230–1236.

132. Eglowstein M, D'Alton M. Single intrauterine demise in twin pregnancy (Abstract). *Am J Obstet Gynecol*. 1992;166:369.

133. Grafe MR. Antenatal cerebral necrosis in monochorionic twins. *Pediatr Pathol*. 1993;13:15–19.

134. Larroche JCl, Droull P, Delezoide AL, Narcy F, Nessmann C. Brain damage in monozygous twins. *Biol Neonate*. 1990;57:261–278.

135. Burke JP, O'Keefe M, Bowell R. Optic nerve hypoplasia, encephalopathy, and neurodevelopmental handicap. *Br J Ophthalmol*. 1991;75:236–239.

136. Hurst RW, Abbitt PL. Fetal intracranial hemorrhage and periventricular leukomalacia: complication of twin-twin transfusion. *AJNR*. 1989;10:562–563.

137. Norman MG. Perinatal brain damage. *Perspect Pediatr Pathol*. 1978;4:41–92.

138. Norman MG. Mechanisms of brain damage in twins. *Can J Neurol Sci*. 1982;9:339–344.

139. D'Alton ME, Newton ER, Cetrulo CL. Intrauterine fetal demise in multiple gestation. *Acta Genet Med Gemellol*. 1984;33:43–49.

140. Gilbert WM, Davis SE, Kaplan C, Pretorius D, Merritt TA, Benirschke K. Morbidity associated with prenatal disruption of the dividing membrane in twin gestations. *Obstet Gynecol*. 1991;78:623–630.

141. Cruikshank SH, Granados JL. Increased amniotic acetyl cholinesterase activity with a fetus papyraceous and aplasia cutis congenita. *Obstet Gynecol*. 1988;71:997–999.

142. Wagner DS, Klein RL, Robinson HB, Novak RW. Placental emboli from a fetus papyraceous. *J Pediatr Surg*. 1990;25:538–542.

143. Yagupsky P, Reuveni H, Karplus M, Moses S. Aplasia cutis congenita in one of monozygotic twins. *Pediatr Dermatol*. 1986;3:403–405.

144. McCrossin DB, Roberton NRC. Congenital skin defects, twins and toxoplasmosis. *J R Soc Med*. 1989;82:108–109.

145. Cox WL, Forestier F, Capella-Pavlovsky M, Daffos F. Fetal blood sampling in twin pregnancies. *Fetal Ther*. 1987;2:101–108.

146. Patten RM, Mack LA, Nyberg DA, Filly RA. Twin embolization syndrome: prenatal sonographic detection and significance. *Radiology*. 1989;173:685–689.

147. Carlson NJ, Towers CV. Multiple gestation complicated by the death of one fetus. *Obstet Gynecol*. 1989;73:685–689.

148. Cattanach SA, Wedel M, White S, Young M. Single intrauterine fetal death in a suspected monozygotic twin pregnancy. *Aust NZ J Obstet Gynecol*. 1990;30:137–140.

149. Lumme R, Saarikoski S. Antepartal fetal death of one twin. *Int J Gynecol Obstet*. 1987;25:331–336.

150. Cherouny PH, Hoskins IA, Johnson TRB, Niebyl JR. Multiple pregnancy with late death of one fetus. *Obstet Gynecol*. 1989;74:318–320.

151. Romero R, Duffy TP, Berkowitz RL, Chang E, Hobbins JC. Prolongation of a preterm pregnancy complicated by death of a single twin in utero and disseminated intravascular coagulation. *N Engl J Med*. 1984;310:772–774.

152. Pritchard JA. Hematological problems associated with delivery, placental abruption, retained dead fetus and amniotic fluid embolism. *Clin Hematol*. 1973;2:563–586.

153. Ikarashi T, Takeuchi S, Ohnishi Y. Immunocytochemical study of a placenta of a twin pregnancy with retained dead fetus. *Asia-Oceana J Obstet Gynaecol*. 1987;13:227–234.

154. Conover PT, Abramowsky C, Beyer-Patterson P. Immunohistochemical diagnosis of disseminated intravascular coagulation in newborns. *Pediatr Pathol*. 1990;10:707–716.

155. Landy HJ, Weingold AB. Management of a multiple gestation complicated by an antepartum fetal demise. *Obstet Gynecol Surv*. 1989;44:171–176.

156. Puckett JD. Fetal death of second twin in second trimester. *Am J Obstet Gynecol*. 1988;159:740–741.

10
Anomalies of Monozygotic Duplication

Although monozygotic twins are often called "identical," implying symmetrically distinct duplication, much of the literature on abnormalities of monozygotic twinning describes the remarkable variety of asymmetric or incomplete duplications that are encountered. These include the so-called acardius-acephalus group, parasitic partial duplication, fetus in fetu, and the varieties of conjoined twins. Some of the most bizarre human anomalies occur in this group of conceptions and they have been the stuff of "freak shows" and museums for centuries. Public curiosity continues, and tabloid and national newspaper and magazine media regularly publish accounts of these unfortunate infants.[1-3] These abnormalities are rare but they deserve close attention and documentation for the lessons in development they may provide, and the pathologist has a particular opportunity to study the anatomy and consider the pathoembryology of these fetuses and infants. An equally important role for the pathologist is to identify these often grotesque abnormalities as probably sporadic developmental "mistakes of nature" due to as yet unknown causes. Such an interpretation may help alleviate the emotional suffering of the parents and equip them to deal more effectively with family and friends. Also, it has been the author's experience that these parents benefit greatly by discussing autopsy findings directly with the pathologist, and such discussions are encouraged in these cases particularly.

Possible Mechanisms

The patterns of normal and aberrant monozygotic duplication can be summarized as in Figure 10.1, but the mechanisms of formation of asymmetric or incomplete twins, and the basis for the spectrum of the observed patterns of anomalous duplication are not understood completely. The concept that single-egg twinning is an abnormality itself is discussed in Chapter 2. It is suggested in that discussion that the female zygote may be more susceptible to this abnormal process as evidenced by increasing rates of female twin pairs with increasing proximity of the twins, including conjoined twins, so it is curious that this association does not seem to hold with some forms of asymmetric twinning.

From animal studies, it has been suggested that if the developing embryos are sufficiently separate, whether as a result of fission or codominant axes, dichorionic or monochorionic symmetric individuals develop.[4] Also, if the two axes are sufficiently close together that they overlap and develop an area common to both, or if a portion of the axis undergoes fission and parts of equal size develop, the parts formed are as strongly inclined to be normal as are single individuals. Both these situations would tend to lead to symmetric outcomes, separate and conjoined, respectively.

Alternatively, if one developing embryo has an advantage over the other, the one suffering the disadvantage will be reduced in size and may be very abnormal in form. This disparity could arise from some of the variations referred to in Figure 7.1, such as unequal twinning, or discordant postzygotic nondisjunction, mutation, or mitotic crossing over. Then, the abnormal embryo can survive only if it is able to parasitize the more normal co-twin, either by anastomoses of chorionic circulations (chorangiopagus parasiticus, also known as acardia/acephalus), or by actually attaching to the co-twin externally (ectoparasite or heteroparasite) or internally (endoparasite or fetus in

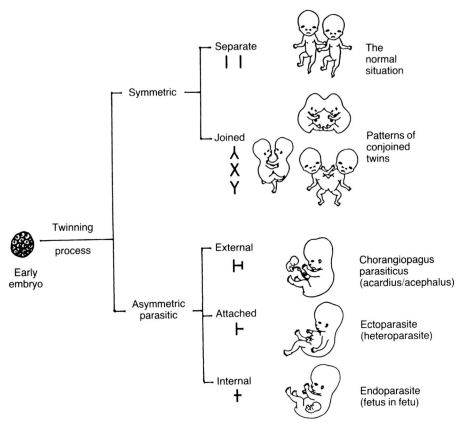

FIGURE 10.1. In this scheme are represented the main patterns of fetal outcome from monozygotic twinning. Symmetric twins may be separate, as in the normal situation, or variably joined as in the varieties of conjoined twins. Asymmetric twinning may create an aberrant fetus that survives only because it can parasitize the more normal twin, through umbilical cord or chorionic anastomoses, body surface, or visceral connections. The symbols are a simple way to represent the patterns. The differentiation of some asymmetric twins from teratomas is discussed in the text.

fetu). This parasitism would allow the abnormal member of a twin pair to survive in spite of being afflicted with pronounced disturbances in structure, even if it has been reduced to a poorly differentiated mass of tissue more closely resembling a tumor than a twin. Occasionally, it may be difficult to differentiate between abnormalities that result from twinning and those caused by primary neoplasia or by abnormal development of an isolated portion of the body.[5,6]

The following discussion describes the patterns of asymmetric duplication including the controversy of twin versus teratoma, expands particularly on the chorangiopagus parasiticus pattern, and reviews symmetric duplication of conjoined twins. Localized duplication of body parts is probably not

a true twinning abnormality, but is considered where appropriate.

Asymmetric Duplication

The boundaries between the three patterns of asymmetric parasitic twins are far from distinct, and the group itself is sometimes not readily differentiated from some of the cases described as conjoined twins or from some of the more complex teratomas. For example, the most frequent site of external parasitic twin attachment is ventral, either thoracic or epigastric, and this attachment is similar to the commonest position of conjoined twins, i.e., thoracopagus and xiphopagus, and is related to the omphalomesenteric conjunction of the chorangiopagus parasiticus twins. Also, intracranial, retroperitoneal, and sacrococcygeal masses with fetal tissues have been variously described as twins or teratomas, and a parasitic twin may be included within the abdomen of its co-twin, anastomosed to a branch of the omphalomesenteric circulation, so the differential diagnosis between an asymmetric twin and a teratoma can be difficult in some of these cases as well.

Twins versus Teratomas

The controversy over what is a twin and what is a tumor arises most often with fetoform structures found within a mass contained within a normal individual, but the *criteria* for differentiating teratomas from abnormal twins are difficult to derive from the literature. It has been suggested in spite of morphologic overlap, that teratomas and abnormal included twins do not represent a continuum,[5,7] even though they have been reported to occur together within the same mass.[8,9] In contrast, it has been argued that many examples of endoparasitic twins are actually remarkably complex, well-differentiated, highly organized teratomas.[10] The controversy might be settled by differentiation of the underlying pathoembryology, but this does not seem to be understood completely, partly because of the remarkable variation in the reported location and vascular supply of the masses, and the gross and microscopic appearances of the contents. There does not appear to be any problem making a diagnosis of teratoma for a broadly attached midline mass in the cranial vault, retroperitoneum, or sacrococcygeal area, which is solid and cystic with a mixture of cell types from all three embryonic layers.[11] These cells are more or less differentiated and arranged in more or less organoid fashion, with related structures from several embryonic layers, and component tissues can vary in developmental maturity in different areas of the mass. Malignant foci occur and metastatic disease is a concern in the management of these cases. These tumors are said to arise from a pluripotent primordial group of cells that escaped the primary organizer in early embryonic life, failed to participate in the normal architecture of the body in the area where they arose, and therefore underwent their own independent differentiation, although contiguous tissues within the

tumor can exert an inductive effect on one another. The commonest of these teratomas in infants is in the sacrococcygeal area and the majority occur in females.

Interpretation becomes more difficult when the fetal tissues in these masses become more recognizable with grossly definable body parts. These fetoform masses seem to present in two main patterns— body segments, usually limb-like, embedded within the solid tissue mass, or a rudimentary to remarkably well-developed "fetus" suspended in a "sac" by a "pedicle". In the first case, the presence of more or less complete limbs within an otherwise typical teratomatous mass is generally considered to represent focally well-differentiated teratoma. Some examples of the second pattern have been referred to as teratomas with homunculi, and the recognizable parts have been head-like structures and/or limbs in the majority, with parts of the spine or pelvis in a few, and genital-like structures in a few, but little or no visceral tissue.[12] These have been pedunculated structures attached to the inside of benign cystic teratomas of the ovary. It has been suggested that they are parthenogenetic in origin, and are encountered after the first decade of life. Although these structures are remarkably fetoform, they are incomplete and are not generally considered to represent endoparasitic twins. However, many descriptions of cases that are called endoparasitic twins are remarkably similar,[13] and the distinguishing criteria are far from clear in some cases.[11]

Even more complicated is the case of a congenital intracerebral mass with five fetoform masses— three of them each consisting of four extremities attached to a central mass, and two of them with limbs, spine, and trunk, but different amounts of cranial structures.[14] These "fetuses" were embedded within the tumor mass without apparent fetal membranes. The two better-developed ones had umbilical cords, but no placental tissue was identified microscopically and the exact vascular supply was not apparent. If the criteria for a twin include an oriented, longitudinal, partly symmetrical structure with a definable trunk and vertebral column,[5,7] then at least two of these "fetuses" were twins. If the criteria include a definable set of histologically normal fetal membranes,[10] then these represented fetoform differentiation in a teratoma.

The question of how differentiated a teratoma can be considers not only the fetoform mass within the "tumor," but the sac that contains the "fetus." The better-differentiated fetoform masses are usually described as being contained within a sac, and connected to the wall of the sac by a vascular pedicle that is interpreted as analogous to an umbilical cord. The histology of these structures is not usually presented in the case reports, but in one instance was described in detail.[10] The finding of nerves, vasa vasora, and other unusual components suggested that the "amnion" and "umbilical cord" were in fact teratomatous tissues, not twin-derived membranes or body stalk. The implication is more than academic. In some cases, operative removal of the sac has been technically difficult and it has been left in situ.[15] If these lesions are truly teratomas, removal of the sac might be warranted in spite of the difficulties. Another approach might be to question whether a "fetus" has to have a normal body stalk or fetal membranes in order to be considered an abnormal twin. Perhaps the histologic appearance of these structures is different because the twin is developing where it is, rather than within its own chorionic sac. Histologically confirmed chorionic tissue has been reported in at least one case, although the exact anatomic relationship was not clear.[13] Chorionic gonadotrophin levels do not appear to have been assessed in cases of internal fetoform masses. Further definition of the origin and nature of the sac and pedicle will require careful histologic evaluation of these cases in the future.

Another aspect of the characterization of these anomalies is the nature (amount and type) of internal structures that can be identified. These are usually minimal to nonexistent in reported cases, with microscopically identifiable intestine being the main structure, along with varying amounts of fat, vessels, nerves, and other mesodermal derivatives.[16] The histologic appearances have been likened to the haphazard differentiation seen in a typical teratoma. Conversely, the absence of definable viscera is reminiscent of a less well differentiated external chorangiopagus parasiticus twin, especially when the internal parasitic "fetus" consists mainly of rudimentary axial trunk and limbs. The resemblance of some examples of "included" or fetus-in-fetu twins to chorangiopagus twins is discussed in the following section on endoparasitic twins.

Some of the difficulty separating twins and teratomas may revolve around the definition of the words used. In most English dictionaries, the word "twin" has two connotations—being born at the same time and/or being one of two separate but closely related things, or persons or things that are very much alike in appearance, shape, and structure. Etymologically, it may be stretching the definition to include infants from interval delivery, or any conjoined infants other than thoracopagi as twins, but medical usage has broadened the term to include these patterns. Whether it is broad enough to include the asymmetric internal and attached fetoform masses might be worth reconsidering. The term "teratoma" was first used by Virchow in 1863 to refer to a malformed or monstrous tumor, and a familial relationship of twinning and teratomas was reported in 1941, suggesting common genetic features,[17] as yet unspecified. Teratomas and twinning is described in Chapter 8, but the significance of cases such as a protruding teratoma of the hard palate in the female of unlike-sex twins remains undetermined.[18]

If teratomas are to be differentiated from "included" twins, there needs to be an explanation for the *origin* of the aberrant twin that is distinct from the teratoma. This may be difficult as the line between a tumor that arises from pluripotential embryonic cells and a twin that does the same relates to fundamental questions of cell differentiation. The potential for malignancy in one or more components of true teratomas seems to be the main intrinsic biologic difference beyond the commonality of disordered development. Malignancy does not appear to have been reported in an internal or externally attached fetoform mass, even those rare cases that have lasted the lifetime of the individual.[19] Developmentally, the rather regular location of the internal pedunculated/sacular fetoform masses—midline retroperitoneal in the majority—suggests that if there is an abnormal twin developing along with the more normal twin, if it happens to be located near the yolk sac, then perhaps its developing vascular body stalk becomes connected to omphalomesenteric vessels of its co-twin, and the sac around it forms from delaminating amnion. Then, because of the aberrant location, this pedicle and sac become invested with vessels and nerves and lymphoid tissue from the host fetus.[10,16] It has been argued as evidence against the "twin," that the developmental timetable is not the same as for the host twin.[10] However, these internal fetuses are developmentally abnormal, and parallel growth would be unexpected.

Finally, these abnormal and incomplete duplications may yet be identified as due to regional developmental programming aberrations on the basis of anomalies of homeobox function, as has been observed in insects, birds, amphibians, and mammals.[6,20–22] This concept may not end the controversy relating to aberrant-included twin/duplication versus teratoma, but it may explain some of the ectoparasitic/attached twins/duplications where differentiation from true teratomas is less of a problem. Whether homeobox anomalies can explain minimally separate symmetric conjoined twins is not clear, but it would seem that the chorangiopagus parasiticus twin is an unrelated and separate entity.

The other situation that sometimes raises the question of differentiating a teratoma from an anomalous twin is the presence of *fetoform masses attached to the placenta*. Masses designated as teratomas have been described attached to the umbilical cord,[23] present within the placental membranes,[24] or arising from the chorionic surface of the placenta with[25] or without[26] their own vascular stalk. Fox and Butler-Manuel[24] explained the various locations of teratomas of the placenta as due to aberrantly migrated germ cells. They suggested that these could pass through the loose tissues at the base of the mesentery of the evaginated gut in the umbilical cord and, theoretically, could migrate even further in the loose tissues of the chorionic plate. Their criteria for differentiating a teratoma from an amorphous fetus was the presence in the amorphous fetus of an axial skeleton and an umbilical cord, however rudimentary. The intramembranous mass in their case would thus qualify as a teratoma. One of the other reported cases exemplifies the problem of differential diagnosis because the small skin-covered mass had only fragments of mature and recognizable tissues but was attached to the surface of the placenta by a vascular stalk distinct from the cord insertion of the twin, and was thus a vascular parasite of the twin.[25] The twin was anomalous and lacked a right arm and leg, kidney, and umbilical artery, with a right parietal bony defect as well. The five cord lesions described as teratomas are consistent with Fox's criteria.[23] They ranged in size from 1 to 2 cm in diameter to the size of a "child's head." They were variably solid or cystic. All had skin and intestinal epithelium. Some

had muscle, nerves, cartilage, bone, and neural tissues. Two of the associated infants survived, one was stillborn and one died as a neonatal death, but whether the cord lesion contributed was not discussed.

A recent extensive review of over 100 reported cases of amorphous or variably fetoform masses failed to support the value of presence or absence of an umbilical cord and/or skeletal organization to differentiate a fetus amorphus from a teratoma.[27] Stephens et al.[27] found that the presence or absence of an umbilical cord did not relate at all to the developmental state of the specimen. They considered that the extent of skeletal development might be a more valid criterion, but note that the degree of internal organization in these cases presented an anatomical continuum that made differential naming meaningless.

Reports of *cytogenetic studies* of asymmetric parasitic twins seem to have been limited to the chorangiopagus parasiticus twin, but there is an interesting exception. Cytogenetic analysis of a spherical mass of tissue without organoid differentiation, but with its own separate cord attachment to the placental surface, provided a $47,XY+C$ karyotype.[28] The karyotypes of the healthy male co-twin and the parents were normal. This suggests that chromosome analysis may be worthwhile on all suspected asymmetric twins, in order to identify the role of heterokaryotic twinning as a cause.

In the Survey '91 Review, there was one possible teratoma of the placenta (Fig. 10.2). This was an ovoid skin-covered mass on a vascular pedicle. It contained microscopically identifiable parts of mature gastrointestinal tract structures and respiratory epithelium but had no complete organs and no axial structure.

In *summary*, the differentiation of a teratoma from an amorphous fetus, whether internal or external, if in fact they are different, remains to be determined. These cases are sufficiently rare that as much should be learned from each one as possible. If an internal fetoform mass is identified, blood tests for chorionic products could be done before surgery. The site of attachment and anatomic relationships should be established as clearly as possible during the operation. The material removed should be subject to detailed gross and microscopic examination with photographs/drawings as appropriate. Parallel cytogenetic and DNA analysis on the "fe-

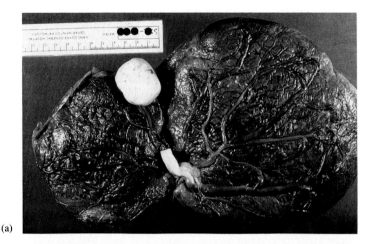

(a)

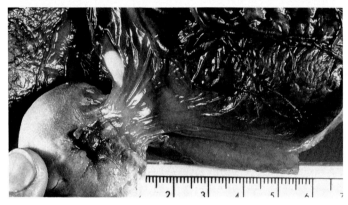

(b)

FIGURE 10.2. This ovoid skin-covered mass (a) was attached to the placental surface by a vascular pedicle (b), which contained one artery and one vein. The irregular opening on the underside of the mass (b) led into a zone of respiratory tissues with an adjacent segment of small bowel, and nearby portions of bone and cartilage. The majority of the mass was edematous and fatty areolar tissues beneath the keratinizing stratified squamous non–hair-bearing epithelium. It was not settled whether this was a twinning abnormality (note yolk sac nearby) because it had a vascular stalk, or a teratoma because it had no axial organization.

tus" and the host is more valuable than of the "fetus" alone. If a number of cases can be analyzed to this extent, and then collated, we may not be much further ahead but our uncertainty will be at a more sophisticated level, and we may be able to progress from there.

Endoparasite

In spite of the preceding discussion of the problems differentiating teratomas from included twins, the concept of fetus in fetu or endoparasitic twin is nearly two centuries old (attributed to Meckel[16]), and for that reason alone warrants further consideration. The reported cases have a superficial similarity but with differing details, and a few unusual findings are reported. The following summary is from a selection of 16 reported cases spanning 40 years, to try to characterize this anomaly and provide an idea of the spectrum of findings.[8–10,13–16,29–37]

These internal masses were found equally often in males and females, were variably symptomatic although occasionally incidental findings, and were identified within the first year of life in the majority. The affected host twins were not recorded to have any other anomalies or problems, and the majority survived operative removal of the mass without difficulty. In those few cases where it was mentioned, there was no family history of twins or teratomas.

The masses were located in the upper retroperitoneum in 75% of the cases, intracranially in 12.5%,[14,33] and intrascrotal/testis related in 12.5%.[32,36] The reported size ranged from 5 cm in diameter to 17 × 14 cm, the largest mass weighed 1.8 kg,[13] and another 1-kg mass represented 18% of the infant's weight.[8]

All but the intracranial masses were within a capsule of some form. This capsule was sometimes described as thick and fibrous, sometimes thin and membranous. The wall was occasionally described as containing nerves, vessels or lymphoid aggregates, and if the capsule was lined by squamous epithelium, skin derivatives as well, especially hair and sebaceous glands. Other lining layers were described as endothelium[31] or amnion,[35] but histology was not always provided. Chorionic villus-like tissue was reported in only one case.[13] The connection of this capsule to the circulation of the host was not always clear. Sometimes an area of thickening of the capsule was associated with one or more vessels that seemed to arise there and pass to major vessels of the host as a "pedicle" of sorts. The host vessel most often mentioned was the superior mesenteric artery, but in the majority of cases the vascular supply was not noted. The sac created by this capsule usually contained fluid, from a few to several hundred milliliters, and usually it was described as yellowish and turbid, occasionally with vernix fragments.

The reported connection of the fetoform mass within the capsule varied, while the connection of the "fetus" in those cases with teratomatous tissues or within the cranium was not defined. The ventral portion of the "fetus" was described as adherent to the inner capsule wall,[35] or a cord-like structure was noted going from the aberrant twin's "abdomen" to the capsule wall,[32] sometimes to the area of thickening from which arose the capsular vessels.[29] This structure was not usually described histologically, although one report noted that it did not look like umbilical cord microscopically because it contained nerve trunks and the artery had a well-developed internal elastic membrane.[10]

The fetoform masses were usually single, occasionally two were found,[9,29,37] and five were reported in one case.[14] The complexity of form ranged from a rudimentary nodular axis with limb-like protuberances and no viscera, to relatively well-differentiated outer forms resembling chorangiopagus parasiticus (CAPP) twins. Like the usual CAPP twins (see discussion below), lower extremities were better formed than upper limbs, the size of the "trunk" varied, genitalia were not always evident, and the differentiation of a true "head" was rare. Instead, a hair-bearing domed upper pole with varying face-like clefts or protuberances was seen, with an anencephaly-like x-ray appearance. In the better-differentiated "fetuses," the body cavity often contained varying amounts of intestine. Kidney, adrenals, and gonads were mentioned occasionally,

but other viscera were rare and cardiac structures absent. Lungs were reported to be well developed in the intraventricular intracerebral "fetus," an unexpected observation as the description was of a four-limbed mass with no heart, kidney, or gonad, but with small and large intestine.[33] Lung tissue is not usually reported even in the developed CAPP twins, so its presence in this case is puzzling. Another unusual case had a bifid fetoform mass: the small amorphous mass was composed of tissues from the upper body, and the larger mass consisted of the lower half of the body with features analogous to the CAPP twins.[34]

This resemblance of the endoparasitic "twin" to the external chorangiopagus twin suggests some homology of pathoembryology in these two patterns of asymmetric twinning. However, the issue becomes confused with reports of cases such as that of an asymmetric twin resembling a CAPP twin attached to the intestinal tract of the host twin in an omphalopagus pattern.[38] We have much to learn about these remarkable anomalies. Unfortunately, there were no examples of endoparasitic asymmetric twins in the Survey '91 Review.

Ectoparasite

The terminology and characterization of external duplication abnormalities is not well defined, because these lesions are the least common of the asymmetric anomalies. It is not even clear that these lesions are truly disorders of the twinning process, because the gross appearances often resemble the anomalies created experimentally by transplanting morphogenetic fields in amphibians,[6] suggesting a very localized postzygotic phenomenon. This category of defects does not usually include limited duplication anomalies such as the relatively common polydactyly. Although digital duplication does follow certain patterns of form and is often part of a more widespread syndromic developmental disorder, it is probably due to a regional ectodermal/mesodermal growth factor/inductive interaction rather than a disordered twinning process (Kalousek DK, 1992, personal communication).

The entities usually considered in the category of ectoparasitic twins are those body segments that are externally attached to the body of a relatively normal appearing fetus or infant. The reported sites of attachment are the inferior pelvic (lumbosacral/

perineal) and the epigastric (xiphoid to omphalus) regions. These are sometimes termed heteropagus conjoined twins, but this may create confusion with the other forms of conjoined twins that are symmetric, and are sometimes termed diplopagus. The host twin is sometimes termed the autosite, while the parasitic "twin" may be labeled based on its location, such as epigastrius, or its form, such as dipygus for caudal duplications. The host twins tend to have other developmental abnormalities, in contrast to the otherwise normal hosts of endoparasitic "twins". This observation may argue for a more generally disturbed developmental program in the case of the ectoparasitic anomaly, rather than a twinning disturbance. Alternatively, the adherent portions may influence regional development adversely as a secondary phenomenon.

The *inferior pelvic* location for duplication anomalies raises the question of differentiation from sacrococcygeal teratomas. Cases such as a mature presacral sacrococcygeal teratoma associated with a well-developed lower limb in flexion with four well-developed toes[39] are analogous to the internal lesions described in the preceding section. The explanation of fetal structures as well defined and complete as a limb contained within a classical teratoma remains to be determined.

The more usual extra tissues in the pelvic area consist of caudal duplications with variably well-developed legs and pelvic structures, usually located between the legs of the host.[40-43] Anal and external genital structures may be duplicated, as may internal rectal, genital, and urinary viscera and ducts. There is a similarity among the reported cases that suggests they represent a specific entity, possibly related to axis development and limb bud organization, but what the underlying influence is remains to be determined. The additional host twin anomalies have been of two types—regional ones associated with distortions from the accessory fetal tissues, and more distal anomalies of uncertain cause. The distant lesions have included an omphalocele and multiple hemivertebrae,[38] omphalocele with situs inversus and tetralogy of Fallot,[41] and omphalocele alone.[42,43] It is not clear why omphaloceles seem to be part of the complex except as a further manifestation of disturbed midline structures. The regional lesions are abnormalities of internal genitalia, anorectal, and lower urinary tract anomalies in conjunction with structures

associated with the parasitic portions. The extra rudimentary pelvis is usually interposed between the pubic rami of the host. The accessory limbs are incomplete, sometimes sensate but usually nonmobile, while the main limbs seem to function normally once the pelvis can be realigned. In the four reports cited, there were two males and two females affected.

There was an atypical lumbosacral duplication reported that consisted of a hypoplastic limb with a four-digit foot, an anus with a blind pouch, and two well-formed fetal breasts.[44] This unusual collection of structures had no associated viscera, and was readily separated from the underlying tissues. The female host had no other apparent problems, and it remains unexplained.

The *epigastric* ectoparasitic duplications are puzzling because, even here, the duplicated tissues are most commonly the pelvis and legs, with varying amounts of additional tissues and viscera.[45-47] One wonders if this pattern reflects aberrant morphogenetic fields, and affects lower limb fields because they are more susceptible to variation than upper limbs. It has been observed that these appended limbs have no motor innervation and little or no muscle, perhaps reflecting development beyond the influence of neuroectodermal derivatives.[45] The anterior body wall location of these parasitic portions may be higher (thoracoparasiticus) or lower (gastroparasiticus).[45] The parasitic portion may be quite superficial with minimal visceral structures[45,47] or part of a much greater distortion of underlying structures with associated duplication anomalies of intestines and heart,[45] conjunction of liver, and duplication of lower urinary tract.[46] The higher adherences may be accompanied by an omphalocele in the host, but not always,[47] and other anomalies such as facial asymmetry have been noted.[47]

One puzzling case was that of a well-grown female with discontinuous facial and epigastric duplications.[48] She had a soft tubular noncystic structure covered by skin connecting the midline forehead to the midchin which resembled nares histologically. The tongue, lower lip, and mandible were duplicated. The upper epigastric mass consisted of skin-covered irregular skeletal structures with breast tissue. In the adjacent omphalocele of the autosite host was a well-developed kidney and small and large bowel with appendix, all attached to the upper mass by a soft-tissue stalk. The host twin had tetralogy of Fallot. The authors postulated that a single factor affected all these areas at 3 weeks of development, but were not able to suggest what that might have been. Interestingly, bifid great toes have been noted in the parasitic limbs.[45]

Ventral ectoparasitic "twins" consisting of head and upper body parts are dramatic but rare.[3,49] The head may be remarkably well developed, although craniofacial microsomia attributed to reduced blood supply has been described in considerable detail.[49] The explanation for an ectopic head remains to be determined. A case of occipital encephalocele, which contained a remarkably well-developed cerebrum, was excised from a male infant who appeared to have no neurologic deficit as a result.[50] Whether this represents a regional duplication analogous to polydactyly, or is part of the parasitic duplications described here remains to be determined.

It is interesting to note that, of the five cases of ventral duplication anomalies, four were males. The significance of this distribution compared to equal involvement of the sexes in the sacral duplications and endoparasitic "twins" is not known.

This category of ventral or epigastric duplication anomalies begins to merge with the patterns of conjoined symmetric twins who are joined at the thorax and/or epigastrium, in an unusual case of much more complex asymmetric twinning.[51] In this case, one twin was considerably smaller than the other and the bony fusion included not only the sternum but the pelvis as well, with one set of external genitalia. The smaller twin had craniofacial anomalies and more serious cardiac anomalies. The lower gastrointestinal tracts were shared and there were two bladders, each receiving ureters from each twin. This case appears to resemble conjoined twins more than an ectoparasitic anomaly, but it is asymmetric with a pattern of fusion not usually encountered in ventral symmetric conjoined twins. It is unclear where this pattern fits in the spectrum, but is mentioned here for consideration.

There is another spectrum to consider—the varieties of craniofacial duplications.[52,53] These anomalies range from simple nasal duplication to two complete faces on a single head (diprosopus), to two separate and complete heads, and the latter phenomenon merges with some cases of symmetric conjoined twins. Although this appears to be a continuum, it has been suggested that facial dupli-

cations are different from twinning anomalies, and are due to regional duplications such as forking of the notochord, duplications of portions of the anterior neural tube, or duplications of mesodermal growth centers around the stomatodeum.[52] A female to male ratio of 2 : 1 has been noted in these cases.

In the Survey '91 Review, there was one example of an ectoparasitic anomaly portrayed in Fig. 10.3.

Chorangiopagus Parasiticus Twins

Chorangiopagus parasiticus (CAPP) twinning represents the commonest form of asymmetric twinning, occurring in up to 1% of monozygotic monochorionic twin pairs or 1 in 35,000 births.[54] This anomaly was first described in the 16th century[55] and the aberrations of the human form that it presents led to descriptions of imaginary races of beings in unexplored lands and outer space.[56] In 1850, Hempel noted the chorionic vascular anastomoses between the anomalous and normal twin, and the resulting reversal of circulation in the parasitic twin.[56] A number of examples have been described in detail over the years, and cases have been detected by ultrasound at as early as 12 weeks of gestation.[57]

The reported form of CAPP twins constitutes a gradient of malformations and reduction anomalies of virtually all tissues, and ranges from a fetus weighing several thousand grams who has a partially developed head, a deformed face, trunk and arms, and partial internal viscera, to an amorphous mass that might be confused with a teratoma.[7,24,27,58] Two CAPP twin fetuses with a normal triplet[59] and conjoined CAPP fetuses with a normal fetus in a triplet gestation[53] have been described, as has a CAPP fetus conjoined to a normal twin through the gastrointestinal tract analogous to the endoparasitic asymmetric twin.[38] The general pattern of reduction malformation is modified by infinite variations and this is reflected in the terminology, although attempts have been made to use terminology that suggests the pathophysiology instead.

Terminology

The classification of the asymmetric abnormality of monozygotic twinning referred to as "external" in Fig. 10.1 has gone through several phases. Al-

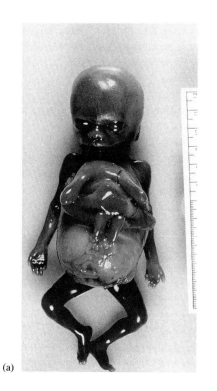

(a)

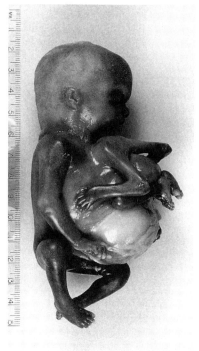

(b)

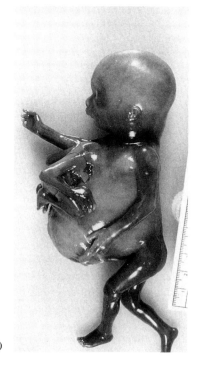

(c)

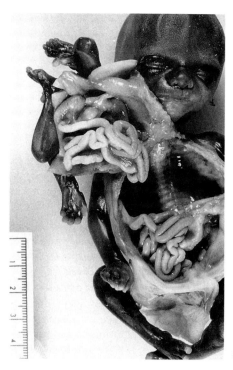

(d)

TABLE 10.1. Classification and distribution of chorangiopagus parasiticus (CAPP) twins.

Expanded classification with distribution*	Percent	Simplified classification†
Acardius holosomus 14.7%		
Holocranius	12.5	→ Acardius anceps
Hemicranius	2.3	
Acardius hemisomus 68%		
Acephalus	10.2	
Holocranius	3.4	
Hemicranius	6.8	→ Acardius acephalus
Acranius	35.2	
Athorax	6.8	
Arrhachis	3.4	
Acormus		
Incompletus	1.1	→ Acardius acormus
Completus	1.1	
Acardius amorphus 17%		
Externus	8.0 →	Acardius myelocephalus
Totalis	9.1 →	Acardius amorphus

*Ogatu terminology quoted by Sato et al.[61] with percentages from Sato's data.
† Terminology of Simonds and Gowen,[60] 1925.

though there are basic similarities, no two examples of this anomaly are identical, so the purely descriptive nosology based on external appearance has become quite complex and perhaps more confusing than helpful. This is particularly so when classifications are modified, stating features of radiographic and dissection findings. Up to 12 different classes of the anomaly have been described, some of which have several names that are dissimilar.[60,61] As can be seen from Table 10.1, the term "acardius" is common to all types, and has been used to refer to the group as a whole. However, a number of these abnormal twins actually have rudimentary and occasionally functioning hearts. Accordingly, alternative terminology based on the apparent vascular pathophysiology was suggested[62] and the term "twin reversed arterial perfusion" (TRAP) sequence was proposed.[63,64]

One of the key features of the vascular pathophysiology of this anomaly is that the asymmetric twin survives only by parasitizing the more normally developed co-twin by way of circulatory conjunction of umbilical or chorionic plate vessels. Therefore, the anomaly can be considered to be a form of conjoined twin in which the conjunction is of the chorionic circulation, hence chorangiopagus parasiticus, a term used by Schwalbe in 1906–1907.[65] This term represents the most uniform aspect of these cases because the term indicates where these twins are joined, without implications as to the shape of the abnormal twin or the presence or absence of other contributing abnormalities such as chromosomal errors. Even the acronym, CAPP, is to an extent descriptive of the gross form. Therefore, CAPP or chorangiopagus parasiticus is recommended as the simplest and most inclusive term for this anomaly and is used in this volume.

Pathogenesis

The scientific study of CAPP twins began in the early 1700s, but they were considered the result of

◄ ─────────────────────────

FIGURE 10.3. This ectoparasitic anomaly was identified by ultrasound examination at 17 weeks' gestation by dates and delivery was induced at 18 weeks. Linear growth of the host was appropriate for 16 weeks and he had a small mandible and large omphalocele caudal to the sternoepigastric attachment of the parasitic portion (a—anterior, b—right lateral, c—left lateral views). The parasite consisted of four quite well-developed limbs: the upper limbs had shoulders, and the lower limbs had popliteal pterygia and an abnormal rump. There was no natal cleft or anus, but male external genitalia with an abnormal phallic structure were present. Radiographically, there were limb bones, clavicles, and pelvic remnants, but no spinal structures. The viscera in the omphalocele of the host autosite belonged to the parasite (d). The lungs were three times the size of the host lungs and histologically resembled type III cystic adenomatoid malformation. There was no heart. Both the gastrointestinal and respiratory tracts ended cranially in 1-cm cystic structures in the anterior mediastinum of the host. The intestine also ended blindly inferiorly in the pelvic area of the parasite, but contained normal neural plexi. There were two histologically normal but mildly hydronephrotic kidneys with mild hydroureter, a small bladder, and patent urethra. Two normal adrenal glands were present, but no pancreas or spleen. There were no nerve trunks in the limbs microscopically. The testes were different sizes and the smaller one was missing germ cells. The squarish liver was conjoined with the host liver with two separate biliary systems. The host had bilateral diaphragmatic defects, with small and irregularly lobed lungs. Other than the shared liver, the abdominal viscera of the host were normal.

"maternal impression" such as by the guillotine, until about 1775.[66] Then, it was suggested that they were determined at conception and related to some vascular problem.[66] This was actually demonstrated in 1836 with injection studies,[66] and the possibility of altered circulation suggested shortly after.[56] The bizarre forms of this anomaly led to the concept that it was primarily a developmental abnormality, while the unusual vascular anastomosis suggested to others that it was the result of destructive effects of altered circulation. The current concept of pathogenesis suggests that both mechanisms are important.

There have been a number of *primary developmental defects* identified in the anomalous twin of the CAPP pair. These have been major aberrations and were considered sufficient to explain the problem, with the anomalous twin being able to survive only because it could parasitize the normal co-twin. It has been suggested that failure of cardiac development was the primary abnormality,[5,67] or that absence of one umbilical artery was the key defect.[68] However, not all examples of this anomaly are truly acardiac, and many have normal three-vessel cords. Careful cytogenetic analyses of anomalous CAPP twins that failed to identify any abnormality were interpreted to indicate that chromosomal errors were not a factor.[69,70] In contrast, discordant karyotypes have been identified in other examples of CAPP twin sets, suggesting that they might be important in some cases. In some CAPP twin sets, only the anomalous twin was karyotypically abnormal: 45,X with 46,XX co-twin[71]; 47,XY,+21 with 46,XY co-twin[72]; 46,X,i(Xp) with 46,XX co-twin[73]; 45,XX,t (4;21)del(4p) with 46,XX co-twin.[74] In other sets, both twins were cytogenetically abnormal: concordant 47,XXY[75]; 94,XXXXYY with 47,XXY co-twin.[75] In one reported set, the co-twin had trisomy 18, but cytogenetics could not be assessed in the CAPP twin because of formalin fixation.[76] This case was unusual because the anomalous twin had more cranial vault and less lower limb structure than commonly seen in examples of this size, and no vascular anastomoses were described, although some must have been present as no heart was found.

A particularly important case, not only for concepts of CAPP twinning but for twinning mechanisms in general, was that of Bieber et al.[77] who described a CAPP twin pair that was the result of fertilization of an ovum and its first polar body. The normal twin was a normal 46,XY infant, the CAPP twin was 70,XXX,+15 predominantly, and the HLA typing of fibroblasts revealed that the triploidy was meiotic in origin with three distinct haplotypes including two from the mother. They concluded that part of the CAPP anomaly was due to the reduced cytoplasmic mass of the polar body as well as to the chromosomal error, and suggested that while abnormalities of vascular connections and perfusion might determine the form of the CAPP fetus, they might not be the primary cause in some cases. In their case the triploidy was clearly present long before the differentiation of the vasculature. It was their conclusion that a CAPP fetus may be the result of a variety of asymmetric twinning mechanisms that all result in a blighted conceptus that survives because of the vascular anastomosis with the co-twin.

The pattern of chorionic vascular anastomoses between the CAPP twin and the co-twin is part of the definition of this anomaly, and the aberrant hemodynamics that result have led to the *secondary destructive vascular theory*. These anastomoses differ from those described in Chapter 9 because only umbilical cord or chorionic surface vessels are involved, and the anomalous twin has no placental parenchymal circulation of its own. Thus, with only artery-to-artery and vein-to-vein connections providing the path for circulation to the anomalous twin, the circulation must be the reverse of normal—blood returning to the fetus through the umbilical artery and leaving via the umbilical vein.[78] This aspect of the anomaly is termed twin reversed arterial perfusion (TRAP).[63,64] Careful dissection of limb muscles in nine cases of TRAP sequence infants identified a number of primary abnormalities in muscularization.[64] This suggested that if vascular causes were important they had to act before limb development was complete, in order to affect early developmental events that could lead to muscle rearrangements. These observations did not rule out additional degenerative changes after the structures were formed.

Both the direction of blood flow and the volume and quality of the blood seem to be important. Because the anomalous perfused twin is receiving blood directly from the umbilical or chorionic arteries of the pump twin, it is being perfused with deoxygenated "used" blood that has already gone around one twin's system.[79] It is this hypoxic blood flowing in an abnormal direction that is thought responsible for the resorption and reduction of previously formed tissues,[7,78] with the caudal end of the embryo usually slightly better perfused and therefore more complete.[70] This concept is supported in part by studies in experimental embryology that indicate a role for pattern of blood flow in the development of the heart.[80] Also, even in cases where there is a "heart" of some form, the normal vascular anatomy of the body cavity is usually replaced by a primitive, apparently haphazard, vascular plexus.[73]

So many of these abnormal twins had only one umbilical artery[68] or an incomplete or hypoplastic second artery in the cord,[81] that the anomalous body stalk development was suggested as a prerequisite for the syndrome.[68] However, enough cases with truly three- vessel cords have been described[61,74] to suggest that the aberrant anastomoses are more important than the number of vessels in the cord. However, that concept does not rule out a role for the two-vessel cord as a threshold factor in the anomaly in these cases.

If part of the pathophysiology of this anomaly is related to abnormal flow patterns of hypoxic blood, one might expect additional evidence in the form of vessel thrombi. This has been mentioned only rarely. A small mural thrombus was noted in the umbilical vein of a functionally two-vessel cord.[69] In another case, the presence of heavily calcified mural thrombi in both vessels of the two vessel cord of the CAPP twin suggested an additional vascular factor—thrombotic or thromboembolic occlusion of the thoracic and upper abdominal vessels with later resorption of tissue in the affected areas.[73] However, there were no thrombi seen in the internal vascular plexus of the anomalous twin in this case.

The primary developmental theory and the secondary vascular destructive theory can be unified as follows. As described by van Allen et al.,[74] there are two key requirements for a CAPP twin pair. First, there must be close proximity of the developing vessels of the two embryos on a common placenta, so that direct vascular anastomoses can occur at the 18- to 21-day stage when the vascular network of the placenta connects with the umbilical-allantoic vessels of the embryo. Second, there must be discordant development of the embryos that allows the normal or pump twin to assume the

circulation of the abnormal or perfused twin. The source of this discordant abnormality, developmental delay, or structural asymmetry could be any one of a number of problems such as the heterokaryotic chromosomal anomalies, triploid polar body twinning, or two vessel body stalk as mentioned above, or unequal monozygotic twinning as discussed in Chapter 7.

The aberrant vascular connections and altered blood flow patterns then have consequences for both twins. In the perfused twin, the abnormal flow pattern leads to altered cardiovascular development, which may in turn influence primary tissue development in other organs. Perfusion with hypoxic blood leads to degenerative changes in the tissues that do form. In this situation, the pump twin is also receiving an increased load of deoxygenated "used" blood because the flow from the CAPP twin returns directly to the co-twin without going through the placenta. This may contribute to prenatal growth developmental deficiency. Because the pump twin has to circulate its blood through the extra mass of the anomalous twin, cardiomegaly and high output failure can occur.

What remains to be explained is the remarkable variety of forms that this twinning anomaly presents. What determines the size, completeness, and degree of organization of the CAPP twin? It may depend in part on the specific embryonic anomaly, which will determine the level of development at the time the vascular connections form.[82] The timing of the onset of flow through the anastomoses, and the volume of flow, are additional potential sources of variation of both further development and degree of degenerative/regressive changes. Further, superimposed thrombi could add additional ischemic insult. Also pertinent in this context is the report of an amorphous fetus termed a "pseudoamorphus".[83] The external form of this 564-g term male fetus fits easily into the spectrum seen with CAPP twin pairs, except it was a singleton. In addition, it did have a heart with a common atrium, and a truncus arteriosus arising from a muscular bulbus. Also, most viscera were represented and centrally well developed around a normal diaphragm, but becoming more abnormal cephalad and caudad, in keeping with the aberrant external form with related anomalies of musculoskeletal system. Brain and spinal cord were considered normal. The malformation was interpreted as a result of an early disturbance in the segmentation of the sclerotomes and myotomes, and in the formation of the heart, with possible secondary circulatory effects. Another reported case was somewhat similar in that the typical CAPP twin had a primitive single ventricle heart and was said to be part of a dichorionic diamniotic twin pair with no vascular anastomoses.[84] However, the umbilical cords were described as inserting at a "common site" and the photograph of the microscopic appearance of the septum between the twins contains amnion only, so the true nature of this case is uncertain. All reported cases to date have been in monochorionic twin pairs.

There are some interesting aspects to the *incidence* of this anomaly that may have significance for its pathophysiology. The sex ratio varies in the reported series, from equal[60,85] to nearly 4 : 1 female predominance,[74] but females are in excess in most reports. This may be a reflection of the general trend of increased female twin sets as proximity of the embryos increases (see Chapter 2). CAPP twin pairs seem to occur as part of a triplet set more often than would be expected by the relative rates of twins and triplets. In one series, 3.5% were part of triplets,[61] 21.5% of another series occurred in triplets,[74] and in a review of 340 cases, CAPP fetuses were part of a monozygotic pair occurring within triplets three times as often as among monozygotic pairs alone.[85] This is an intriguing observation that needs further study to determine its implications. It was suggested in Chapter 3 that the pattern of membranes and placentation was related to the timing of the twinning process, so it is interesting that monoamniotic placentations seem unusually common with CAPP twin pairs,[85] up to 40% of cases.[74] If this observation implies a process occurring in an embryo after creation of the amnion, then the potential span of occurrence of the CAPP anomaly would seem to be long indeed, from the time of the first meiotic division in cases of polar body twinning[77] to about 8 days, when the amnion delaminates.[86] The coincidence of apparent CAPP twinning with deformations due to amniotic bands also raises questions of timing of the findings.[82,87]

There are *animal models* of this anomaly that provide additional observations and questions. A number of examples have been observed in ruminants, mainly cattle, but also goats and sheep.[60,69,88] In cattle, there can be circulatory fusion of chorionic vessels within an unlike-sex pair, resulting in a sterile female or freemartin, and CAPP twins have been reported in that circumstance. This would tend to argue against a twinning process anomaly and favor a primary developmental defect augmented by the circulatory dynamics, in those cases at least. It appears that the anomaly is limited to animals that can have placental vascular fusion. In the armadillo, where monozygotic multiples of 4 to 15 occur regularly, and the placentas are monochorionic, vascular anastomoses have not been seen, nor have CAPP type anomalies been reported.[88]

There do not seem to be any common factors in the maternal obstetric or general health history, in family history, or environmental exposures that might be considered contributory.

Whatever the underlying mechanisms and pathophysiology, the recurrence risk does not appear to be increased in subsequent pregnancies as a recurrence does not seem to have been reported, even in those families with recurrent monozygotic twinning. Thus, the pathologist has an important contribution to make in these cases—to identify these often nightmarish "monsters" as monozygotic twinning anomalies, so that appropriate counseling can be provided to the understandably upset families.

Morphology

This twinning anomaly was reportedly first described in 1533[64] and over 400 cases have been reported since. The descriptions of these cases in the literature represent seemingly limitless variations on the theme of reduction malformations involving every organ system. While no two cases are identical, there are recurrent similarities. The commonest pattern of the better-developed anomalous twin is a variably edematous fetoform mass with relatively well-developed legs, variable perineal structures, a trunk with normally situated umbilical cord, and replacement of the upper half of the body by a rounded dome that may have rudimentary upper limbs and barely discernible indications of facial structures. Radiographically, the legs and pelvis may be reasonably complete, but there may be vertebral and rib anomalies, and often little or no upper limb or cranial structures, as the spine ends cranially in a knot of bone. Brain development may be minimal or absent but spinal cord is usually present. There is usually a single body cavity with some portions of abdominal viscera, but usually few if any thoracic structures. The interstitial and subcutaneous tissues may be quite edematous, and even cystic in the "neck" region. The commonest pattern of the more amorphous anomalous twin is an ovoid mass of varying size with deformed limb rudiments, usually no perineal development, and often insertion of the cord near a hair-bearing flap of skin. In these, there are rudiments of an axial skeleton radiographically, and a small body cavity with few visceral remnants. The subcutaneous zone is thick with edematous mesenchymal tissues. In all patterns, this parasitic perfused twin has no placental villus vascular connections of its own, and its cord vessels are conjoined with those of the supporting or parasitized pump twin on the surface of the placenta or somewhere along the cord in direct artery-to-artery and vein-to-vein anastomoses.

The morphology of the CAPP twin pair includes consideration of the anomalous or perfused twin, the sustaining or pump twin, and the placental findings. The following discussion summarizes selected literature reviews. In one review, the *CAPP fetus* weighed 906 g on average (range 16–6,260 g), while the co-twin weighed 1,345 g on average (range 60–3,200 g).[61] However, in 15 individual sets with enough data, the CAPP twin weighed more than the pump twin twice as often as the pump twin was the heavier of the pair, and this was not related to the sex of the pair.[55,61,62,68-73,81,82,89,90] The heavier twin was 1.1 to 4.5 times the weight of the lighter twin, and the degree of difference was not related to which twin was heavier except in those cases with marked hydrops of the anomalous twin. The size of the fetus does not seem to be related to the completeness of development, as some of the heaviest CAPP twins have been quite rudimentary.[74] While these pregnancies tend to end prematurely—average gestational age at delivery was 30 weeks (range 18–44 weeks)[61]—small and large CAPP twins have been noted at most gestational ages.

The range of abnormalities of the anomalous twin is remarkable. They are often quite edematous, with subcutaneous tissue edema that is generalized or more prominent in the upper half. This is attributed to tissue hypoxia as a result of perfusion with "used" blood.[74] The pattern of reduction malformations defies simple categorization, as exemplified by the

findings in three series totaling 120 cases as summarized in Table 10.2. The histologic assessment has generally reflected the gross appearances, with more variation reported in the kidneys. The kidney is one of the organs more commonly present in these cases, and histologic abnormalities have included cystic changes,[89] hypoplasia with fewer glomerular generations than normal[69] and fewer tubules widely separated by fibrous tissue with abnormal glomeruli,[72] tubular disorganization,[71] and agenesis of proximal renal tubules in a hypoplastic unilateral kidney, attributed to renal hypoperfusion.[92]

It seems reasonable to suspect that the pattern of malformations and reductions will depend on the nature of the primary defect, if any, and the pattern and timing of vascular anastomoses. Correlations of this type will require not only morphologic evaluation of the affected twin, including cytogenetics, but also details of the pump twin, again with cytogenetics, and precise placental findings. There may be those who will argue that such detail is not needed for accurate diagnosis of a nonrecurrent twinning anomaly, and this is true. However, there are lessons to be learned from these cases about embryonic development, and for that reason alone they should be documented as carefully as possible to provide sufficient data for correlative analysis.

Perinatal mortality of the *pump twin* is high— 40% are stillborn and an additional 12.5% die in the neonatal period[61] of cardiovascular overload[74] and complications of prematurity.[61] If delivery can be delayed beyond 37 weeks, survival reaches 79%.[61] Although it was once suggested that there was no vascular consequence to the normal co-twin,[93] the evidence of cardiovascular overload in affected cases consists of cardiac enlargement with right ventricular hypertrophy and relative pulmonary stenosis, hepatosplenomegaly with ascites, and subcutaneous hydrops in severe cases.[74] The basis for the hydrops is not only high output failure, but also hypoproteinemia due to hepatic decompensation.[74,94] A further manifestation of the circulatory overload in one case was diffuse visceral arterial medial calcification and interruption of elastic fibers.[95] There was calcification of one large placental artery and striking calcification of trophoblastic basement membranes. The associated CAPP twin had a single-artery cord inserting into its co-twin's cord, but no vascular calcification was seen in the

TABLE 10.2. Patterns of malformation in CAPP fetuses.

Percent of cases with findings noted	Tissues/organs present and other features		
	van Allen et al.[74] (14 cases)	Sato et al.[61] (88 cases)	Lachman et al.[91] (18 cases)
100%	Growth abnormality		Skin
	Diaphragmatic defect		Hair
	Syndactyly/oligodactyl of hands		Vertebrae
	Esophageal atresia		Long bones
	Short intestine		Intestines
	Incomplete rotation of gut		
	Ascites		
	Myxedematous thickening of skin		
75–100%	Anophthalmia or microphthalmia	Legs and vertebrae	Gonads
	Talipes equinovarus	Hair	Meninges
	Absent lungs	Identifiable gonad	
	Absent spleen		
	Absent or hypoplastic pancreas		
	Absent or hypoplastic gonads		
50–75%	Cranial vault and brain absent	Adrenals	Kidneys
	Radial aplasia	Renal tissue	Adrenals
	Syndactyly/oligodactyly of feet	Skull and cerebrum	Cerebrum
	Reduced thorax	Diffuse edema	Thyroid
	Unfolded heart tube		Thymus
	Interrupted intestine		
	Omphalocele		
	Absent liver		
	Bilateral renal agenesis		
	Hypoplastic or lobulated kidneys		
	Absent adrenals		
25–50%	Cranial vault present, open or intact	Cysts of subcutaneous	Lung
	Facial features absent or present with defects	tissues	Liver
	such as cleft lip and/or palate	Arms	Pituitary
	Arms and/or legs rudimentary or absent	Pancreas	Pancreas
	Thorax absent	Thyroid	Lymph nodes
	Anus imperforate		Single umbilical artery
	Liver small or gallbladder absent		
	No heart tissue but a primitive vascular plexus		
	Two vessel cord		
0–25%	Partial cranial vault	Pulmonary tissue	Spleen
	Necrotic brain	Cardiac tissue	
	Holoprosencephaly	Splenic tissue	
	Rudimentary facial features	Hepatic tissue	
	Absent lower limbs		
	Necrotic or rudimentary lungs		
	Simple midline hepatic lobe		
	Folded heart with common chamber		
	Gastroschisis or cloacal exstrophy		

cord or body. Pulmonary artery calcification alone has been reported in pump twins, and was thought to be related to the greater size of the CAPP twin being perfused, compared to cases without vessel calcification.[96] Although this suggested sequence of cardiac failure in the pump twin based on the size and thus the cardiac load of the anomalous twin seems reasonable, it becomes difficult to explain the absence of signs of cardiac failure in a normally grown surviving pump twin at 32 weeks whose parasitic twin was almost as long and 4.5 times heavier.[90] Because the pump twin receives doubly "used" blood back from the perfused twin, embolic phenomena have been looked for, but none were found.[74] Other than the signs of cardiac failure, the pump twins are remarkably free of abnormalities. They tend to be mildly growth impaired and up to 10% have been reported to have malformations, often of a similar type as in the CAPP twin that they nourish.[97]

As indicated by the name of this anomaly, the details of the *placental vascular connections* are one of the keys to the diagnosis and should be recorded carefully. CAPP twins are often considered to be characterized by two-vessel cords as part of the defect,[68] but three-vessel cords have been reported in 25%[61] to 57%[74] of anomalous twins, and sometimes both twins have two-vessel cords.[71] Unfortunately, the patterns of vascular anastomoses are not clear in many reported cases, but in one series of 50 cases with adequate data, there was a direct connection of the umbilical cord of the CAPP twin to the cord of the pump twin in 14%,[61] and these have been described occurring within the separating membranes.[62] When the anastomosis is beyond the cord insertions on the placental surface, it usually consists of one large caliber artery-to-artery and vein-to-vein anastamosis each, sometimes up to 1 cm in diameter,[94] often joining vessels between nearby cord insertion sites on the chorionic surface or at the margin.[61,69,70,82]

There are other placental features to note as well. All cases to date are in monochorionic placentas, but both diamniotic and monoamniotic sets are described. When the CAPP twin has no kidneys or has an obstructed or nonfunctional renal system, amnion nodosum is found in its sac when the placenta is diamniotic.[70,89] Most reports describe the villus histology as normal, while other authors describe maturation dissociation or retardation, which they suggest may be analogous to maturation defects in placentas with fetuses with sacrococcygeal teratomas.[82]

There were 13 CAPP twin pairs in the *Survey '91 Review cases*. The range of morphology is presented in Figs. 10.4 to 10.13, and the available details are summarized in Table 10.3, but some of the findings warrant further comment. In contrast to the reported series, 77% of the cases were male twins. This remains unexplained. Unlike many of the reported cases, the external form of the Survey '91 CAPP twins was generally quite recognizable when compared to the magnitude of the visceral defects. The amount of true edema of the CAPP twin varied, and the nuchal loculations extended down the entire dorsum in one case (case 1, Table 10.3). The degree of brain development was predictable based on skull size, but in both cases where

brain development had occurred, there were major secondary destructive lesion residues (cases 2 and 9, Table 10.3). The facial features were always rudimentary or absent. Even when upper or lower limbs were reasonably well defined, there were digital reduction anomalies, as though the most distal structures were the most deprived. Definable external genitalia were seen in both male and female CAPP twins and the degree of development seemed to parallel that of the legs and pelvis, but anal development was not always equal to genital definition. The majority of the umbilical cords of the CAPP twins had only two vessels, but in two-thirds of these there was an additional artery remnant that was hypoplastic and sometimes thrombosed, occasionally identified only in microscopic sections of the anterior abdominal wall. Radiographically, the skull was the most frequently reduced structure, followed by arm bones, shoulder components, and leg bones. The pelvis and axial spine, including the ribs, were less often affected.

The internal viscera findings were similar to the reported cases. The spinal cord was often present in spite of the absence of any definable brain. Just under one third of the cases in this series had simple tubular hearts, some with superimposed thrombosis. The peripheral major vessels described were usually a major dorsal artery and vein with erratic branches, sometimes traceable to the viscera. In other cases, the viscera appeared to be supplied from an ill-defined plexiform circulation embedded in mesenchymal connective tissues that filled the nonvisceral space in the body cavity. These vessels were noted to contain thrombi in one case (case 2, Table 10.3). The upper region of the body cavity sometimes contained blind ending tracheoesophageal structures as though foregut growth was arrested before branching took place, but the tissues that were present matured normally histologically. The presence of a rudimentary defined face did not indicate that foregut development would be found (case 4, Table 10.3). A normal diaphragm was reported in about a third of the cases with no apparent relation to the degree of development of the viscera present above or below. The stomach was never described and the bowel present was always a varying length of ileum, a cecum with appendix, and varying length of colon, usually malrotated. When there was no anus, the colon ended blindly. The ganglion development in the

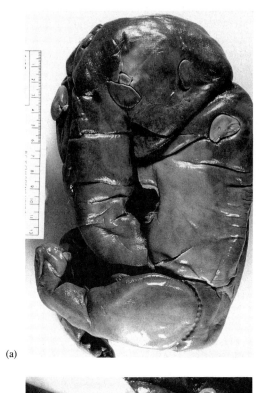

(a)

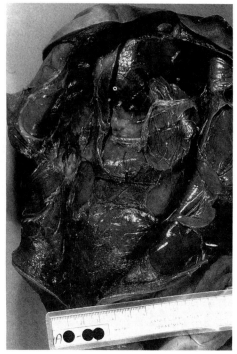

(b)

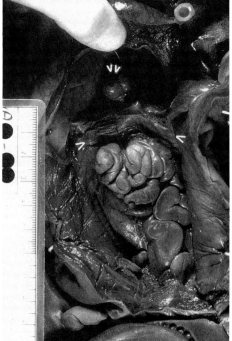

(c)

FIGURE 10.4. CAPP twin with thrombosed tubular heart. This was the second largest CAPP twin in the Survey '91 Review (case 1, Table 10.3). There were well-developed legs and recognizable genitalia (hypospadius, testes in abdomen), with flipper-like rudiments of upper limbs, absence of definable shoulders or neck, and rudimentary tags and clefts of facial structures with bilateral cleft lip (a). Most of the dorsal region was thickened with multi-loculated thin-walled fluid-filled cysts (b). The body cavity was divided by an intact diaphragm (between arrows) with a heart (double arrow), esophagus, trachea and lung tissue above, and intestine, testes, adrenals, kidney, and bladder below (c).

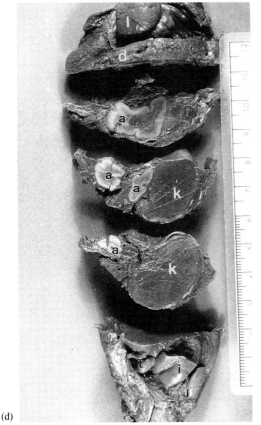

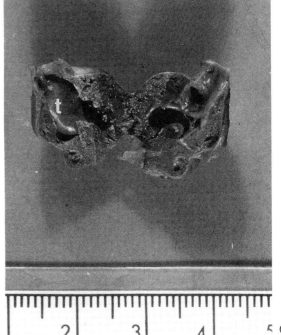

FIGURE 10.4. *Continued*. In serial sections through the visceral block (d) can be seen a nodule of lung (l) and diaphragm (d), a portion of adrenal (a), portions of two adrenals (a,a) and the one kidney (k), portions of one adrenal (a) and the one kidney (k), and intestine (i) and testes (t). The hemisected heart in (e) was a simple tubular structure with organized thrombus (t) in the largest chamber. [(a) and (e): Reprinted with permission from Baldwin, VJ, *Developmental Pathology of the Embryo and Fetus*, JB Lippincott, 1992:336.]

bowel varied but no pattern emerged related to other findings. Liver and pancreas were usually absent, although pancreas was found microscopically in nearly one-quarter of the cases. The paired viscera of adrenals, kidneys, and gonads were both present more often than only one, and were all found in the majority. Histologic abnormalities of renal development were the most frequent microscopic abnormality reported, and were similar to the literature cases. Unfortunately, the reports reviewed did not contain enough information to correlate internal gonadal development with development of external genitalia. Thymic tissue was identified in two cases, but spleen in only one.

The descriptions of the associated placental components unfortunately were incomplete. Two main patterns of anastomoses were observed—conjunction of the cords above the insertion of the pump twin's cord onto the placenta, and an extension of one artery and one vein from the pump twin's chorionic surface vessels to become the umbilical cord of the CAPP twin. Two distinct cord insertion sites on the placental surface, with chorionic vascular anastomoses between, was described once. Amnion nodosum on the CAPP twin's side and mural thrombi in some chorionic surface vessels were mentioned in some cases, but no other consistent findings were noted.

The pump twin findings were similar to the literature cases. The two survivors were associated with the most rudimentary CAPP twins (cases 8 and 13, Table 10.3), although one of these was quite

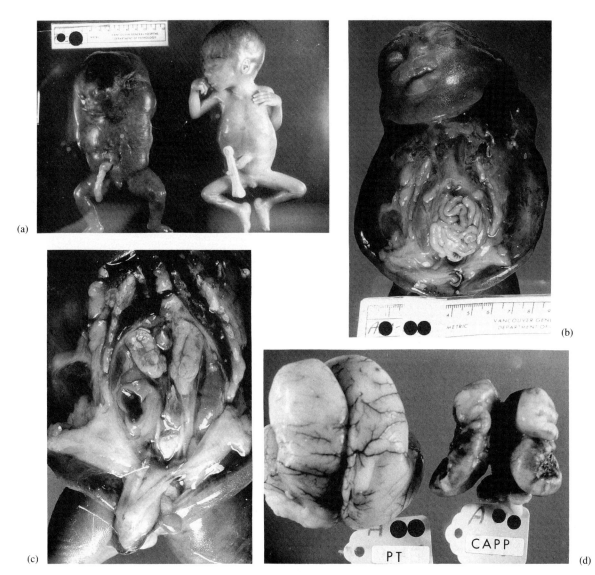

FIGURE 10.5. One of the more completely developed CAPP twins in the Survey '91 Review (case 2, Table 10.3). Note the near equivalent size of the twin pair (a), the CAPP twin is edematous and the pump twin is growth retarded. The neck of the CAPP twin is obscured by edema, but the face and cranium are quite recognizable (a,b). In the face the ears are represented by skin tags only (and had no canals), eyelids are fused (and only a left eye globe was present), left nostril and choanae are patent, lips and mouth are normal. Internally, the thorax is small (b,c) with only a blind tracheoesophageal structure above the diaphragm, and doubly blind ended intestine with Meckel's diverticulum and microscopic pancreas, complete urinary tract, hypoplastic ovaries without other internal genitalia, and both adrenals below the diaphragm. The connective tissues in both parts of the body cavity were angiomatous and many of the vessels were thrombosed. The brain of the CAPP twin is small (CAPP) compared to the pump twin (PT) (d) with both reduction anomalies and gliosis and calcification seen microscopically.

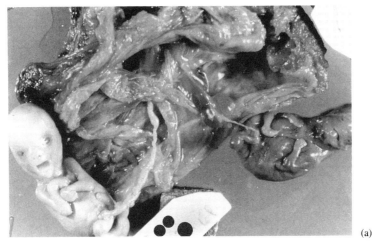

(a)

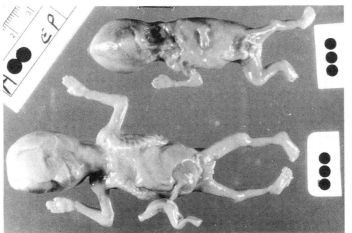

(b)

FIGURE 10.6. Embryofetal examples of CAPP twin pairs. (a) This twin pair was at least 11 weeks gestational age by size; no history was provided. They are macerated, but one can still see the relatively well-defined head (unfortunately partially beyond the edge of the photograph), neck and upper limbs in the CAPP twin, although most internal viscera were missing (case 3, Table 10.3). Difficult to see in this photograph but present were pterygia binding the upper arms to the trunk, syndactyly in the left hand, and lobster claw deformity of the left foot. (b) These twins were delivered at 20 weeks by dates, but were only 10 to 11 weeks in size (case 4, Table 10.3). Note the relatively normal external form of the smaller CAPP twin, who was missing most of his internal viscera. The left arm and hand are small, there is syndactyly in the right hand and left foot.

large. In the seven cases where it was assessed, cardiomegaly was noted in six, ranging from slight to nearly three times the expected heart weight for age, and was reported in cases from 21 to 29 weeks. Additional signs of cardiac failure were less frequently noted and hydrops was not reported in any case. Growth failure, excessive hepatic hematopoiesis, and pulmonary hypoplasia were mentioned in a few cases. In only one pump twin were structural anomalies noted, reduction lesions of

kidney and adrenal, and a Meckel's diverticulum (case 11, Table 10.3).

No cytogenetic abnormality was found in the cases suitable for analysis.

In summary, other than the contrary predominance of male twins, these cases of CAPP twinning from the Survey '91 Review are consistent with the reported descriptions of this anomaly. The distinctive aspect of the abnormal circulation was particularly striking in the two cases with better cranial and

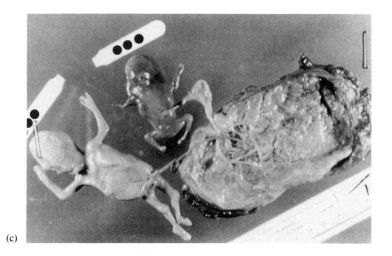

(c)

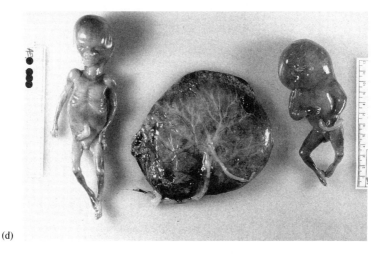

(d)

FIGURE 10.6. *Continued.* (c) The gestational dating of this pair was not known, but growth was equivalent to 9.5 to 12 weeks developmental age (case 5, Table 10.3). Although unfortunately poorly focused, the external features of the smaller twin are relatively well developed in spite of the fact that most internal viscera were absent. The arms were webbed and there were only two toes on each foot and four fingers on the left hand. The posterior palate was cleft. (d) The gestational age at delivery in this case is not known, but the pump twin was 16 to 17 weeks gestational age size (case 6, Table 10.3). Note the well-developed limbs, but reduced head and face in the smaller CAPP twin. Note immediately adjacent insertion of the umbilical cords on the placenta.

brain development. The presence of thrombi in the "heart," internal vascular plexus, and chorionic vessels in some cases likely reflects the abnormal circulation as well, and may have further augmented the findings. The thoroughness of the analyses of these cases varies depending on the interest of the investigator, but it can be seen from the above review and the literature cases, that the more details there are, the more relevant any pathophysiologic hypotheses can be.

Clinical Aspects

There are three areas of clinical concern with CAPP twinning—antenatal findings, neonatal features in live-born pump twins, and therapeutic measures applied during pregnancy.

The *obstetric aspects* include antenatal diagnostic features, maternal complications, and problems of labor and delivery. The mother is often in her first pregnancy,[59] and large for dates with only one

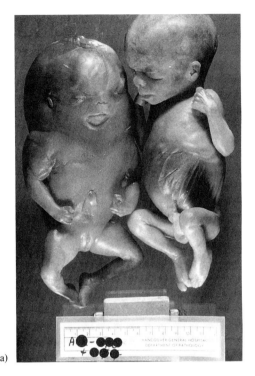

(a)

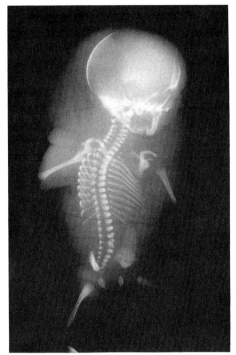

(b)

FIGURE 10.7. CAPP twin pair with remarkable visceral defects in externally quite well-developed anomalous twin (case 7, Table 10.3). The smaller twin is slightly shorter than the pump twin, but heavier because of pronounced nuchal edema (a). The head is small with reduction of facial features, and there are reduction/syndactyly anomalies of the hands and feet, although the arms and legs are normal. The unusually well-developed calvarium is seen in the radiograph (b), although the distal limbs are masked. Internally (c) the intestines are easily seen but few other viscera were present. Sternum and 12th ribs were absent.

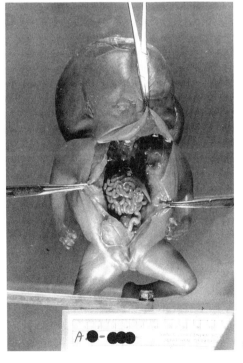

(c)

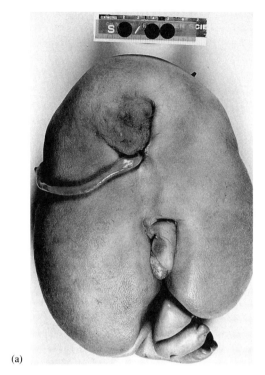

(a)

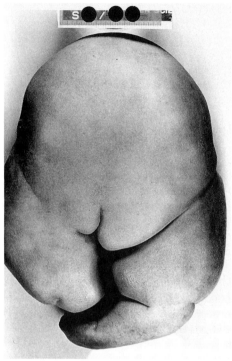

(b)

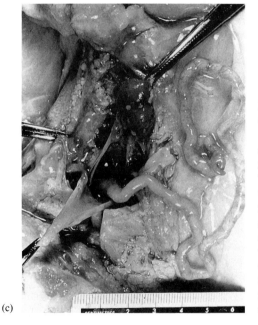

(c)

FIGURE 10.8. This was one of the most rudimentary CAPP twins, but the largest by weight (case 8, Table 10.3) of the Survey '91 Review cases, and it has been described more briefly before.[57] Note the basic formlessness of the large ovoid mass with malformed lower "limbs," redundant penile structure, and a two-vessel umbilical cord emerging from below a hair-bearing skin flap anteriorly (a), and a short natal cleft (with patent anus) posteriorly (b). Internally, there is a tiny body cavity (c), with cranially blind terminal ileum, cecum with appendix, and colon, and crossed fused renal ectopia on the left, as the most visible structures. There were two ureters. The prostate and right seminal vesicle were found. The thick edematous subcutaneous tissues are also evident.

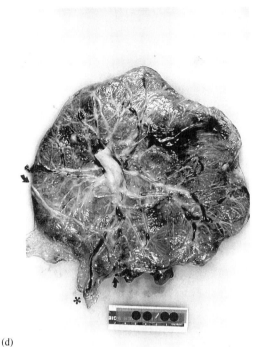
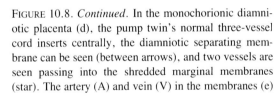

(d)

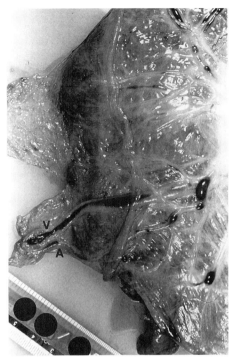

(e)

FIGURE 10.8. *Continued*. In the monochorionic diamni-otic placenta (d), the pump twin's normal three-vessel cord inserts centrally, the diamniotic separating mem-brane can be seen (between arrows), and two vessels are seen passing into the shredded marginal membranes (star). The artery (A) and vein (V) in the membranes (e) are considered the vascular supply to the CAPP twin, although the specimen is torn. The CAPP twin had a two-vessel cord, but at the body wall a second hypoplastic umbilical artery was found with luminal thrombosis. [(a): Reprinted from *Medical Ultrasound* 8:105–107, 1984, with permission from John Wiley and Sons.]

detectable fetal heartbeat.[98] Polyhydramnios is re-ported in up to 87% of cases,[61] and is readily identified with ultrasound examination, along with the anomalous fetus that has no moving heart in a second sac, and fetal death of one twin may be diagnosed.[59,99] However, follow-up ultrasound ex-aminations reveal growth of the noncardiac fetus along with its co-twin, and this, plus the pattern of anomalies, suggests the diagnosis of a CAPP twin pair. Continued monitoring of the pump twin is usually undertaken to look for signs of heart failure, such as developing hydrops, so that elective deliv-ery can be timely.[100] Diagnostic features may be present from 12 to 16 weeks,[57] and occasionally the actual anastomotic vessel can be seen ultrasono-graphically.[82] In the cases with better developed cardiac structures, fetal echocardiography may identify the distinct independent abnormal function and can be used to monitor cardiac function in the pump twin.[84] Pulsed Doppler velocimetric studies have provided in vivo confirmation of the reversed flow in the umbilical cord of the CAPP twin.[101,102] The S/D ratios in the pump twin reflect the vascular resistance of the placenta and the perfused acardiac twin, while the S/D ratio in the CAPP twin repre-sents its systemic resistance.[103] Amniotic alpha-fetoprotein has been reported increased to 5 to 10 multiples of the mean in cases with rather small and relatively amorphic CAPP twins, creating problems of diagnosis and management in those cases.[104,105]

It has been noted above that preterm delivery is a feature of these cases and one of the limiting factors for survival of the pump twin. The risk of preterm delivery has been related to the weight of the CAPP twin.[106] The closer the weight of the CAPP twin was to the weight of the pump twin, the greater the frequency of hydramnios and congestive heart fail-ure in the pump twin, and the greater risk of preterm delivery with perinatal mortality. Thus, elective delivery of the twins becomes a difficult decision,

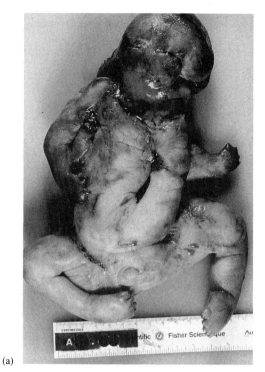

(a)

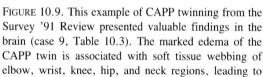

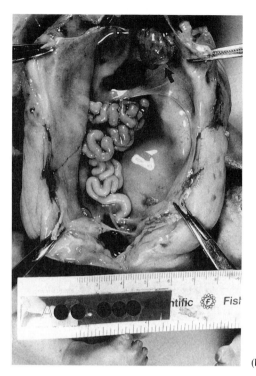

(b)

FIGURE 10.9. This example of CAPP twinning from the Survey '91 Review presented valuable findings in the brain (case 9, Table 10.3). The marked edema of the CAPP twin is associated with soft tissue webbing of elbow, wrist, knee, hip, and neck regions, leading to distorted positioning (a). Marked digital reductions in hands and feet are evident as well as small clefts representing the "face." The edematous subcutaneous tissues can be seen in (b) along with intestine, kidneys, and a "thoracic" mass near the "neck" that is the heart (arrow).

balancing adequate maturation with onset of cardiac decompensation.

There have been a couple of additional interesting findings in *live-born pump twins*. Severe hypoproteinemia has been noted, possibly on the basis of hepatic decompensation due to hypoxia, acidosis, and/or elevated venous pressure.[94] Hypoproteinemia thus may both result from, and contribute to, cardiac failure. Rather striking anemia in the pump twin has been reported with hemoglobin levels of 85 g/L at 28 weeks and 86 g/L at 31 weeks.[84,99] No cause was suggested and no test for fetomaternal bleeding was reported, so this finding remains to be confirmed and explained.

Because of the increased perinatal mortality of the usually normally formed pump twin, efforts have been directed toward ameliorating the circulatory failure, or reducing the cardiovascular load. *Therapy* with maternal digitalization was successful in leading to resolution of hydrops in the pump twin, with unremarkable perinatal outcome at 34 weeks, even though the CAPP twin was the same size and thus represented a major circulatory load.[107] Indomethacin has been used to reduce the volume of amniotic fluid and reduce the risk of preterm labor.[108] In that case, there was never hydrops of the pump twin who did well after birth at 34 weeks. The CAPP twin was less than half its size. Monitoring of the fetal ductus and neonatal renal function is indicated if indomethacin is used.[109] As the anomalous twin will not survive, selective interruption of the CAPP twin cord has been suggested.[110] A thrombogenic coil has been successfully placed in the umbilical artery of the CAPP twin, with elective delivery of a vigorous co-twin at 39 weeks.[111] By blocking the artery, and thereby reducing venous return, the risk of thromboemboli from the CAPP twin was reduced. The most invasive approach has been hysterotomy with selective delivery of the anomalous twin.[112–114] The procedure has been done at 19 to 26 weeks, with 6/7 surviving pump twins 4 to 16 weeks later at

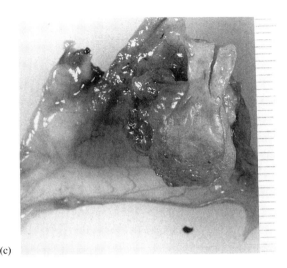

(c)

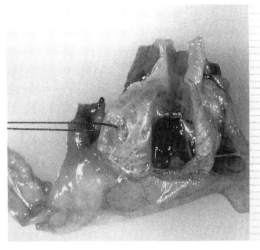

(d)

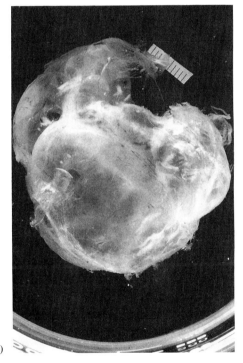

(e)

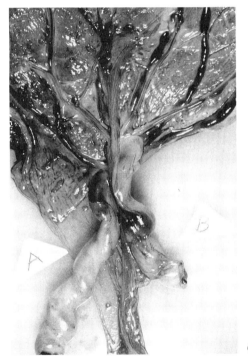

(f)

FIGURE 10.9. *Continued.* The "heart" has a pericardial sac (c), and consisted of a single ventricular mass with two atria and a single arterial trunk (d). There is a thrombus in the ventricle but no thrombi in other vessels. The brain of the CAPP twin has been reduced to a cerebral fibroglial cyst (e) attached to a lobulated glial mass representing brain stem, cerebellum, and spinal cord. The absence of ocular tissues, the presence of damaged cerebellum, and the presence of the pineal suggested a destructive process beginning at about 26 days' gestation and lasting over a period of time, worse in the anterior circulation (carotid supply) than the posterior (basilar). The two-vessel CAPP twin cord (A) inserts into the pump twin's cord (B) with direct artery-to-artery and vein-to-vein anastomoses just above the cord insertion at the placental margin (f).

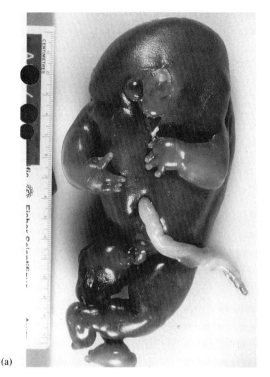

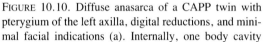

(a)

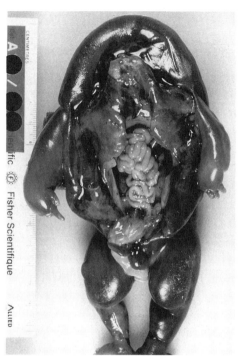

(b)

FIGURE 10.10. Diffuse anasarca of a CAPP twin with pterygium of the left axilla, digital reductions, and minimal facial indications (a). Internally, one body cavity with intestines is easily visible (b). The bony nubbin at the top of the spine is evident (case 10, Table 10.3).

27 to 38 weeks' gestation. The one fetal loss was in the 26-week case and due to placental abruption 2 hours after the procedure.[113]

Selective obstruction of the umbilical cord of the CAPP twin was attempted in one of the Survey '91 cases (case 11, Table 10.3; Fig. 10.13), and the problems and findings exemplify the value of clinical-pathological correlation. The CAPP twinning abnormality was identified by ultrasound examination in late first trimester during investigation of vaginal bleeding in this third pregnancy of a well 35 year old woman. Medical, family, and other obstetric history was noncontributory. The abnormal twin had a definable heart with a heart rate of 130 beats per minute, but with oligohydramnios, so that the umbilical cord could not be discerned adequately for Doppler studies. The normally grown pump twin was missing one kidney and had increased amniotic fluid. The gestation was monitored and management options reviewed. After extensive discussions with the family, and hospital Ethics and Pregnancy Termination Committees, selective termination of the CAPP twin with injected fibrin

sealant was chosen. At about 20 weeks' gestation, fibrin polymer [TISSEEL, Immuno (Canada, Ltd.)] was injected into the larger of the two visible vessels in the umbilical cord of the abnormal twin, with discernible arrest of pulsation in the cord. However, this arrest was transient and cardiac activity was detected several hours later in the abnormal twin. A second attempt a week later, with fibrin polymer injected into the thorax of the abnormal twin was unsuccessful. On the third attempt the next day, the second injection of 4 cc of polymer into a pulsating vessel in the cord of the abnormal twin led to flow arrest in the cord, but was followed almost immediately by bradycardia in the pump twin. This did not improve and fetal death of the pump twin was documented 2 hours later. Delivery was induced 4 days later. The postmortem findings are presented in Fig. 10.13.

Theoretically, the use of fibrin polymer to block the cord circulation of the abnormal twin should have worked well. However, the vascular anatomy of the cords of both the abnormal twin and the pump twin, as well as additional pathologic findings in the

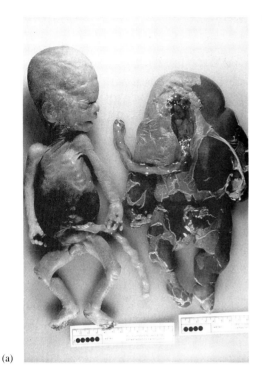

(a)

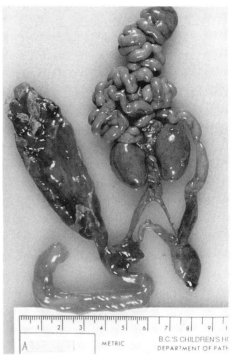

(b)

FIGURE 10.11. The edematous CAPP twin of this pair (case 12, Table 10.3) has an unusual anterior soft-tissue defect above the umbilical cord (a). The nature of this lesion was not determined. The CAPP twin is quite macerated, but the absence of definable head and neck is evident. The internal viscera of the CAPP twin (b) consist of bowel, adrenals (with cytomegaly in the fetal cortex), normal kidneys, and testes. (The large ovoid mass is the skin defect and subjacent tissues removed en bloc for histology.) In the placenta (c), the cords anastomose just before the placental margin, with multiple mural thrombi in the CAPP twin's umbilical vein (B) and venous branches of the placental surface.

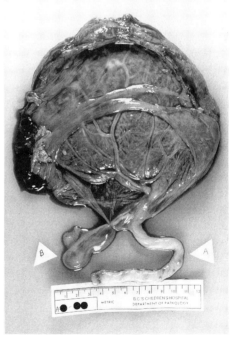

(c)

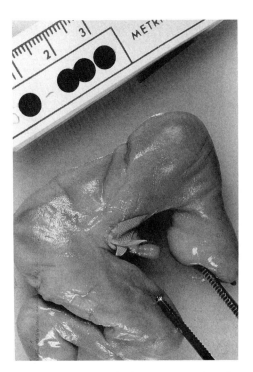

FIGURE 10.12. This was the least remnant classed as a CAPP twin in the Survey '91 Review. Only 15-weeks-size lower limbs with digital reductions were found and unfortunately the vascular connection was not described, although a tiny cord can be seen above the penile structure and isolated by a triangle of cloth for the photograph (case 13, Table 10.3).

placenta, none of which could have been anticipated, confounded the outcome. Based on the clinical events and the pathologic findings, the following sequence was postulated. The first injection of polymer was into the larger of the umbilical arteries in the three vessel portion of the cord closer to the CAPP fetus. The effect was transient because the flow continued from the arterial segment in the more distal two-vessel portion of the cord, through the branching anastomosis into the smaller second artery and into the CAPP twin. The second injection into the region of the heart did not reach the intracardiac space and simply spread through the body cavity. The final successful intravascular injection was into the single umbilical artery of the CAPP twin in the cord segment closer to the placenta. The volume of material injected led to its distribution into the majority of the chorionic arterial tree through the arterial anastomosis, and this included some retrograde flow into the larger of the

two arteries in the cord of the pump twin. This sudden obstruction of the larger of the two arteries led to bradycardia. The smaller artery could not sustain the cardiac output and sluggish venous return led to thrombosis, causing death of the pump twin. The hemorrhagic endovasculopathy lesion was evidence of problems with chorionic flow prior to the procedure and would have further compromised the circulatory reserve of the pump twin.

CAPP—Summary

The CAPP or choriangiopagus parasiticus twinning anomaly is the consequence of a combination of two main conditions. The first is any one of a variety of developmental abnormalities in one twin, with survival of that twin because it becomes attached to, and directly supplied by, the circulation of its co-twin. The second is that the anatomy of the vascular anastomosis leads to reversed flow of hypoxic blood into the anomalous twin with secondary degenerative effects on its body form. The morphologic appearances are broadly varied and so far not related to primary defect, fetal sex, or timing or pattern of abnormal flow. The anomaly is lethal in the affected twin, while the co-twin is at risk for fetal or perinatal death from cardiac failure and prematurity. Some therapeutic approaches have been successful.

The role of the pathologist in these cases is twofold. On the one hand, accurate diagnosis of this often bizarre twin as a twinning anomaly with no increased risk of recurrence is essential for the appropriate comfort and counseling of the family. On the other hand, careful recording of the anomalies in the CAPP twin, findings in the pump twin, and details of placentation, supplemented with additional studies, such as cytogenetics of both twins, provides valuable information for eventual unraveling of the embryonic developmental puzzles presented by this anomaly.

Symmetric Duplication—Conjoined Twins

The anomaly of incomplete twinning that is probably best known to the general public consists of conjoined twins, twins of approximately equal size that are incompletely separated but retain a degree

FIGURE 10.13. Attempted selective termination of a CAPP twin with injection of fibrin polymer into the umbilical cord of the abnormal twin A (see text for details of procedure). At postmortem examination, the parasitic twin A was edematous and macerated, had no identifiable head or upper limbs, and the lower limbs were malformed with webbing of the left leg at the knee and digital reductions (a). There was a lumbosacral neural tube defect consisting of a meningomyelocele, an unusual anomaly in CAPP twins. Lower limbs and pelvis were seen by x-ray with a central vertebral column and irregular distorted ribs, but no bony structures above the upper ribs (b). The central body cavity of the abnormal twin contained a small tubular heart, a right adrenal and kidney, right testicle, urinary bladder, and two blind segments of bowel with blind rectum. Much of the intestine was encased in fibrin polymer. The pump twin B was appropriately grown, externally developmentally normal, with edema and maceration (a). Internally, there was cardiomegaly, and agenesis of right kidney and ureter with a small right adrenal. Bony skeleton was normal (b). The placenta, with membranes still attached is shown in (c), with the cord of twin B angled down to show the thrombosed vein and distended artery to better advantage. Findings are clarified in (d), taken from the drawing made at the time of dissection.

The umbilical cord from the abnormal twin appeared to contain only two vessels and it inserted onto the placental surface near the margin (c,d). The artery anastomosed to the arterial chorionic circulation of twin B, just as it reached the placental surface [solid arrow in (c) and a-a arrow in (d)]. The vein anastomosed with the umbilical vein of twin B at the cord insertion of twin B [obscured in (c),v-v arrow in (d)].

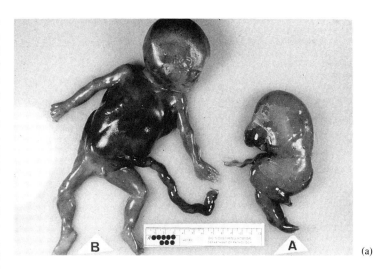

(a)

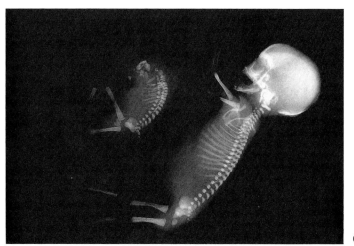

(b)

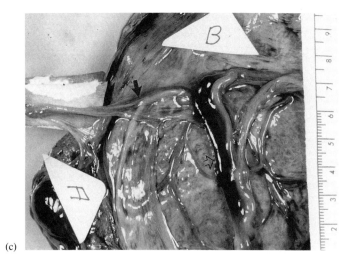

(c)

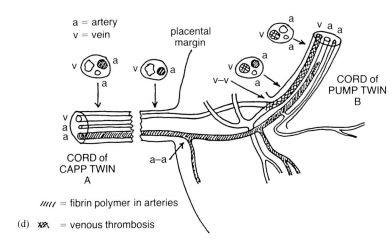

a = artery
v = vein

placental
margin

CORD of
CAPP TWIN
A

CORD of
PUMP TWIN
B

a–a

///// = fibrin polymer in arteries

(d) ✕✕ = venous thrombosis

FIGURE 10.13. *Continued.* The chorionic surface veins on the placenta were engorged and the arteries were firm and white. In the three vessel umbilical cord of twin B, the vein was distended and hemorrhagic for 9 cm upward from the insertion [open arrow in (c) and cross-hatch in (d)]. Microscopically, the umbilical cord of the CAPP twin had a larger and smaller umbilical artery in the portion attached to the fetus, but only one umbilical artery in the portion attached to the placenta (d). The umbilical vein was empty, the larger of the two arteries was distended with fibrin polymer throughout its length [diagonal hatching in (d)], and the smaller artery was empty. Although the entire cord specimen received was serially blocked, the site of anastomosis of the two arteries was not found. The interpretation was that the CAPP twin cord contained an abnormally long Hyrtl anastomosis, the origin of which was damaged when the fetus was delivered and the cord cut. Polymer was also found in the internal course of the umbilical artery and in several major internal arteries. In the cord of twin B, one artery was smaller than the other microscopically, only half the size in some sections (d). In the first 9 cm of the cord from the placental surface, the larger artery was occluded by fibrin polymer and the vein contained thrombus. In multiple sections of the chorionic vessels of the placental surface, fibrin polymer was identified in the chorionic arteries as they fanned out from the insertion of cord B, small fragments of polymer were found in some of the penetrating branches of these arteries and the chorionic veins were distended and some contained thrombus fragments. In the subchorionic villus tissue, there was extensive hemorrhagic endovasculopathy, which was most pronounced nearest the cord insertion.

of overall symmetry no matter what the pattern of conjunction. Incomplete twinning is recognized in plants and animals[115] and double-headed turtles and snakes are well represented in the lay press.[116,117] Perhaps one of the oldest representations of this anomaly in humans is a neolithic double-headed twin goddess from Turkey, dated about 6500 B.C.[118] Biographical reviews of some of the famous conjoined twins throughout history are fascinating and delightful reading, and should be consulted for

TABLE 10.3. CAPP twin pairs from Survey '91 Review.

			CAPP twin																																		
			General form											Skeletal elements										Internal viscera													
Case figure	Sex GA	Weight CAPP pump	E	LL	G	A	T	UL	H/F	N	H	F	UC	Sk	F	Sp	Rb	Sh	Pg	UL	LL	H/F	B/Sc	Ht	Lu	TE	Th	D	L	S	P	Ad	K	Gd	ICC	IG
1 / 10.4	M 32	1220 / 2000	Tr/G	PN/PN	PN/PA	O/O	PN/PN	R/O	O/PA	O/O	R/PA	R/PA	O/2+	O/PN	O/PA	PN/PN	PN/PN	R/PA	PN/PA	O/O	PA/PN	O/PA	O/NC · PA/PN	PA/O	M/O	PA/PA	NC/NC	PN/PN	O/O	O/O	O/M	2/PN	1/PN	2/PN	PA/PA	NC/O
2 / 10.5	F 25–27	336 / 340	G/Nu	PN	PA	O/NC	PN	O	O/PA · PA/PA	O/PA	PA/PA	PA/PA	NC	PN/PA	PA	(no radiograph reported)						PA/PN · NC	O/O	O/O	PA/NC	NC/PA	PN/PN	O/PA	O/O	M/NC	2/PN · NC	2/PN · NC	2/PA	PA/PA	O/PN
3 / 10.6a	F 11?	3 / 5	O	PN	PN	NC	PN	PA	PA/PA	PA	PA	PA	NC	PA	PA	(no radiograph reported)						PA/NC · NC	O	O	NC	PA	PN	PA	O	NC	PN	NC	PA	PA	PN
4 / 10.6b	M 20	9 / 16	O	PN	PN	PN	PN	PA	PA/PA	PN	PN	PN	3			(no radiograph reported)						PA/NC · NC	O	PA	O	O	NC	PA	O	O	2	IR	2	PA	NC
5 / 10.6c	M 14?	9 / 22	O	PA	NC	NC	PN	PA	PA/PA	O	PA	R	2	PA		(no radiograph reported)						PA/NC · NC	PA	NC	O	O	NC	PA	O	O	IL	IL	NC	PA	NC
6 / 10.6d	M 16–17?	NC / 110	O	PN	NC	NC	NC	PN	NC/NC	PA	PA	R	2			(no radiograph reported)						PA/PN*	O	O	R	NC	NC	O	PN	O	2/PA*	2/PN	O	PA	O
7 / 10.7	F 22	465 / 440	Nu/Tr	PN	PN	PN	PN	PN	PA/PA	O	PA	R	2	PA	PA	PN	PN	PN	PN	PN	PN	PA/PN	O	O	R	M	PN	O	PN	O	1/*	2/PN*	1/M	PA	O
8 / 10.8	M 36	1770 / 2820	G	PA	PA	PN	PA	O	O/PA	O	O	O	2+	O	O	O	O	O	PA	O	PA	O	O	O	O	O	O	O	O	O	O	2/PN	2/PN*	2/1	PA/*	PA
9 / 10.9	M 32	620 / 1400	G	PA	PA	PN	PN	PA	PA/PA	O	PA	R	2+	PA	PA	PN	PA	*	PN	O	PA	R/PA	PA/PN	PA	O	PA	NC	O	O	O	M	2/PA*	2/PA*	2/PN	PA	PA
10 / 10.10	M 21	300 / 290	Tr/Nu	PN	PN	PN	PN	PN	PA/PA	O	R	R	2+	R	O	PN	PN	PN	PN	PN	PN	R/PA	O/PN	O	O	O	NC	O	O	O	M	2/PN*	2/PN*	2/PN	PA	NC
11 / 10.13	M 29	125 / 335	G	PA	O	O	PA	O	O/R	O	O	O	2+	R	O	PA	PA	O	PA	O	PA	O/O	O/PN	PA	O	O	NC	O	O	O	O	1R/PN	1R/PN	1R/PN	PA	R
12 / 10.11	M 29	446 / 522	G/O	PN/PA	PN	NC	PA	O	PA/PA · PN	O	O	O	2+	PA	PA	PN	PA	PA	PA	PN	PN	PA/O · PN	O/NC · PN	O	O	O	O	O	O	O	O	2/PN*	2/PN	2/PN	PA	NC
13 / 10.12	M 40	NC / 3070	O	O	O	O	O	O	O	O	O	O	NC	(no radiograph reported)								O	O	O	O	O	O	O	O	O	O	O	O	O	O	O

TABLE 10.3. *Continued*

Case figure	Sex	GA	Weight		Pump twin		Placenta	
			CAPP	pump	General findings	Signs cardiac overload	Anastomosis	Other findings
1 / 10.4	M	32	1220	2000	Fresh stillbirth; no abnormalities reported	NC	"A connection of the vessels between the two cords"	"One two-vessel cord had organized thrombus in one vessel"
2 / 10.5	F	25–27	336	340	IUGR; length = 20 weeks	CM—7g (2.5g); VC; HS	NC	In fragments (retained)
3	F	11?	3	5	No abnormalities reported	NC	NC separate cord insertion	NC
4 / 10.6a / 10.6b	M	20	9	16	Macerated; no abnormalities reported	NC	(No specimen received)	
5 / 10.6c	M	14?	9	22	Macerated; no abnormalities reported	NC		Fragmented, especially at cord attachment sites
6 / 10.6d	M	16-17?	NC	110	Normal 46,XY	Hepatomegaly only	Cord insertions adjacent with direct arterial and venous anastomoses	NC
7 / 10.7	F	22	465	440	Increased hematopoiesis in liver	CM—7g (3.8g); VC; HS	NC	Fragments only; amnion nodosum on side CAPP twin
8 / 10.8	M	36	1770	2820	Did well	NC	One artery and one vein from normal cord became CAPP cord	Villi immature for dates; amnion nodosum CAPP side
9 / 10.9	M	32	620	1400	IUGR—10% for age	CM—18g (9.6g)	Cords anastomosed just above marginal insertion	NC
10 / 10.10	M	21	300	290	Lungs small; centrilobular hepatic hemosiderin	CM—4g (2.4–2.9); HS	Possible cord junction above specimen as received	NC
11 / 10.13	M	29	125	335	Macerated; well grown; absent left kidney and ureter; right adrenal half size of left; Meckel's	CM—heart weight normal though macerated	Arterial and venous on surface	See detailed description in text of attempted selective termination
12 / 10.11	M	29	446	522	IUGR; marked hematopoiesis liver; adrenal cytomegaly; pulmonary hypoplasia 7.9 g (18 g)	Slight CM	Cords anastomosed just before placental margin	Amnion nodosum CAPP side
13 / 10.12	M	40	NC	3070	Normal	NC	NC	Monoamniotic

Case 1—Diagnosed antenatally; delivery spontaneous, CAPP twin first, both stillborn. Second pregnancy in 30-year-old woman; no significant history. Only the CAPP twin is in Survey records; macerated and was received formalin fixed. Death of CAPP twin possibly associated with spontaneous thrombosis of one cord vessel.

Case 2—Diagnosed antenatally with fetal death of malformed twin suggested by absence fetal heart, movement or growth 8 weeks prior to spontaneous labor. CAPP twin born first, then pump twin who died shortly after birth. Twenty-two-year-old well secundagravida. CAPP twin not macerated, contrary to prenatal diagnosis. Pump twin not edematous but sac had excess fluid. 46,XX normal karotype from CAPP twin.

Case 3—No history available, received formalin fixed.

Case 4—Well 26-year-old mother, fifth pregnancy, two normal children, two spontaneous first trimester abortions, no other details. Spontaneous delivery of these twins at 20 weeks by dates, no details provided.

Case 5—No history available, other than spontaneous abortion.

Case 6—Reportedly diagnosed antenatally in 21-year-old woman, no other information available. In this case there were two small ocular anlagen in the disorganized mesenchyme that replaced the cerebral hemispheres suggesting normal brain development to that stage with subsequent destruction. The adrenals were fused in the midline. The CAPP twin had a normal 46,XY karyotype.

Case 7—Both twins stillborn at 22 weeks. No other history provided. The kidneys were histologically more immature than expected with tubules surrounded by primitive mesenchyme and too widely spaced in some areas. Occasional tubules had dystrophic calcification. Adrenal was ectopically placed above the diaphragm. Cultures for cytogenetics failed to grow from either twin.

Case 8—This case has been reported previously.[57] The mother was a well, 32-year-old primigravida and the abnormal twin condition was seen with ultrasound at 12 weeks. It was diagnosed as a CAPP twin pair at 23 weeks after monitoring growth of the mass with absence of definable heart. The normal twin was monitored by ultrasound examination every 2 weeks, and labor and delivery induced at 36 weeks because of onset of oligohydramnios in its sac. The kidneys were histologically appropriately mature for age but had only two-thirds the normal number of glomeruli. The bowel was aganglionic.

Case 9—CAPP twinning diagnosed by ultrasound at 16 weeks. The pump twin grew normally but began developing venous dilatation, increased chest circumference, and placental hydrops. Spontaneous rupture of membranes occurred at 32 weeks with section delivery. The CAPP twin was freshly stillborn. The second born pump twin was normal at birth with a hematocrit of 52. He died at 5 days of age from complications of aortic thrombosis consequent to umbilical artery catheterization. The heart size was considered too greatly increased to be all postnatal enlargement. The mother was 41 years of age with one living child, three spontaneous abortions, one elective termination, but no details are available. The CAPP twin had a normal male karyotype, the clavicles were absent, the adrenals were fused posteriorly, the kidneys were hypoplastic and "disorganized". The microscopic pancreas was dysplastic.

Case 10—Spontaneous stillbirth at 21 weeks to a well, 19-year-old primigravida. No other history. The pump twin delivered first.

Case 11—This was a case of attempted selective termination and is described in more detail in the text.

Case 12—A twinning anomaly was identified at 18 weeks with ultrasound examination and CAPP twins identified at 22 weeks. The pump twin was not growing, so mother was admitted to hospital for bed rest. Doppler studies indicated increasing resistance in the pump twin's cord with eventual loss of diastolic flow and then reversed flow. Conservative management was elected by the family. Fetal death occurred at 29 weeks and labor and delivery were induced. The pump twin delivered as a double footing breach, followed by the vertex presenting CAPP twin.

Case 13—This partial twin was an incidental finding on the placenta of an apparently otherwise normal infant.

F, female; M, male; GA, gestational age in weeks at delivery; ?, minimum GA based on fetal size where GA by dates not known; Weight, autopsy weight (grams); if liveborn, is birthweight; PN, present and normal; O, absent; PA, present but with reduction anomalies; R, rudimentary; NC, not commented on; M, microscopically identified; *, see comment for more details; 1,2, one or both of paired viscera; L, left; R, right if stated; Ht, heart; Lu, lungs; TE, trachea/esophagus; Th, thymus; D, diaphragm; L, liver; S, spleen; P, pancreas; Ad, adrenal; K, kidney (whenever kidney present, corresponding lower duct system always present, including bladder and urethra); Gd, gonads; ICC, ileum/cecum/colon (stomach and upper small bowel never identified; intestine found almost always consisted of varying lengths ileum with cecum and appendix, and varying lengths of colon; if anus absent, bowel segment ended blindly below as well as above; IG, internal genitalia (seminal vesicles and prostate in male; tubes, uterus, cervix in female); E, subcutaneous edema: Nu, pronounced in "neck" region, Tr, mainly torso, G, generalized; LL, lower limbs; G, genitalia; A, anus; T, trunk; UL, upper limb; H/F, hands/feet; N, neck; H, head; Fa, face; UC, umbilical cord: 2, 2 vessels, 3, 3 vessels, 2+ , 2 vessels with hypoplastic 2nd artery; Sk, skull; SP, spine; Rb, ribs; Sh, shoulder girdle; Pg, pelvic girdle; B/Sc, brain/spinal cord; CM, cardiomegaly, observed (expected) weights; VC, visceral congestion; HS, congested hepatosplenomegally; IUGR, growth retardation; Placenta, all monochorionic diamniotic unless stated.

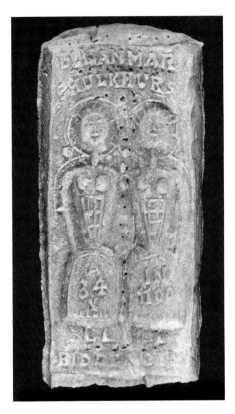

FIGURE 10.14. The Biddenden maids were the earliest known English double terata, and were probably pyopagus twins. "Cakes" (flour and water) were imprinted with their image and were passed out to the poor once a year, using funds from their bequest of land to the local church when they died in 1134. Their shoulders are always shown close together, but that probably simply represents the fact that they walked with their arms around each other.

an appreciation of the psychosocial impact of this anomaly of reproduction[119–121] These cases include the Biddenden maids of 1100 (Fig. 10.14), the original "Siamese twins" of the 1800s (Chang and Eng Bunker from Siam), a tantalizing description of the only known pregnancy and delivery in one member of a set of pyopagus twins, and the first autopsy of conjoined twins in the new world, done to determine the spiritual unity or duality of the pair.

The unity or duality of conjoined twins is one of the major considerations that this physical phenomenon presents. Social and religious debate has focused on this aspect, particularly in those cases where surgical separation is considered possible but only if one is sacrificed for the survival of the other.[122] There does not seem to be agreement as to whether such twins are simply one person with a parasitic growth or two persons whose lives must be considered. The degree of duplication is probably important but because the anomaly represents a continuum, definitive criteria for distinct personhood may be hard to establish. Two reasonably complete individuals that are joined are no problem—but what of the case with separate heads but a single body and set of limbs? Some may consider that there is more to an individual than a head.[120] If separation is considered, further conflicts arise regarding simply an inviolable right to life, as opposed to a more complex discussion of quality of life. Each case, therefore, seems to be considered in its own setting as there appear to be no generally agreed guidelines among Jewish or Christian religious leaders.[123] Even the pathologist may be faced with the mundane decision as to whether to assign one autopsy number or two to a set of conjoined twins. However, there seems to be general agreement from a psychosocial point of view that if separation is contemplated, the sooner it is done the better, preferably within the first 6 months of life.[123] Decisions as to separation must be made promptly, and detailed investigation of the infants is required soon after birth. Thus, the purely medical and surgical considerations regarding the possibility and actual process of separation represent another major aspect of conjoined twins.

The surgical separation of conjoined twins has been reported since 1689, when a set of twins joined at the umbilicus were divided successfully with a ligature.[124,125] The success of separation procedures depends on three considerations: the actual anatomy of the conjunction and degree to which vital organs are shared, the degree to which that anatomy can be defined prior to surgery, and the skill and experience of the necessarily large team of physicians and support staff required. Prior to the availability of ultrasound, these twins were rarely diagnosed before some complication of labor was encountered.[126] Current technology allows ultrasonic diagnosis as early as 8.5 weeks gestational age,[127] and remarkably detailed structural information can be obtained with magnetic resonance imaging.[128] Additional studies such as fetal echocardiograms may be helpful.[129] The more detailed the antenatal information available, the more appropriate the counseling and obstetric management can be,[130] and the more specific the advance planning can be for neonatal assessment and surgical separation, should that be possible.[124,131,132] Remarkably complex procedures are being performed, particularly in cases of conjunctions of the lower half of the bodies, but the long-term outcomes remain to be determined.

One of the important contributions to successful management of conjoined twins has been provided by careful clinicopathologic correlations by interested pathologists, typified by the Birth Defects Original Article Series report on conjoined twins.[133] Because examples of this phenomenon are rare in any one individual's experience, the pathologist is particularly enjoined to provide a thorough description of each case that he or she encounters. In this way, as much information will be available as possible to those who must make a decision for separation. Also, accumulated data from detailed pathologic analyses may eventually provide enough clues so that mechanisms of conjoined twinning can be clarified.

Etiology and Pathogenesis

Theoretically, the incidence of conjoined twins would be related to the incidence of monozygotic twinning, reflecting those factors that influence single-egg twinning. However, the reported statistics are difficult to compare as they usually give the incidence of conjoined twins among all deliveries. The reported incidence ranges from 1 : 192,000 births in southern Africa,[134] through 1 : 33,000 to 1 : 165,000 in North America,[135–138] 1 : 100,000 in Japan,[139] 1 : 75,000 in Sweden,[140] 1 : 68,000 in Hungary,[141] 1 : 58,000 in Singapore[142] and 1 : 6,454 in Taipei.[143] These variations seem to reflect the relative proportion of monozygotic twins in these populations, except for the relatively low incidence in Japan, which remains unexplained. Conjoined twins have been reported with an unexpectedly high frequency in triplets. Nine cases of conjoined twins as part of a triplet set have been described.[144] Two-thirds were thoracopagus twins and the normal triplet was of the same sex in all but one case, although zygosity was not stated. Conjoined CAPP twins have been described in a monochorionic triplet pregnancy.[54] Up to 6% of conjoined twins may be part of a triplet set,[97] and they have been reported with quadruplets,[126] although it

is not clear what these occurrences signify regarding etiology or pathogenesis.

The incidence of conjoined twins as related to maternal factors, family history, and sex ratio has been studied. Conjoined twinning does not appear to be related to factors of maternal age or gravidity, but the relationship to a family history of twins is less certain. More than 1,000 descendants of Chang and Eng Bunker have been traced with only one set of twins identified.[145] In contrast, a family history of monozygotic twins was identified in a group of Arab conjoined twins,[146] and a strong history of twinning, including another conjoined twin, was identified in the family of a mother with a dicephalus dipus tribrachius twin set.[147] It is possible that the sex ratio of conjoined twins is important because there is striking female preponderance of up to 90% to 95% of the reported cases,[5,148] although females usually represent around 70% in many series.[134,137–139,141] This excess of females may be related to the pathogenesis of the anomaly analogous to the discussion of the mechanisms of monozygotic twinning and its relation to delay factors and the female zygote (see Chapters 2 and 7). In this context, it is interesting to note the report of a female set of thoracoabdominally united twins in an abdominal pregnancy.[149]

Possible teratogenic factors have been considered for conjoined twins. A variety of agents and manipulations have been identified in animal experiments as contributing to conjoined twinning.[150] In man, periconceptual use of oral contraceptives, clomiphene ovulation induction, and therapy with oral griseofulvin have been reported in a few cases, but the significance of these associations is not determined.[141,151]

Just as the contributing etiologic factors remains to be determined, the actual pathogenetic mechanisms have yet to be clarified. While it was originally thought that these monsters arose as a result of fusion of homologous developed parts,[152] current explanations focus on events much earlier in embryogenesis, and consider either incomplete fission of the developing embryo, or the development of codominant axes with apposition of parts of the axes that leads to conjunction of a few or many cells.

Whether the incomplete fission theory or codominant axis theory is invoked, the abnormal influences that lead to conjoined twins are considered to be present in the microclimate around the fertilized ovum.[153] The process begins around days 13 to 15 postfertilization when the primitive streak and axiation commence.[150] The result is an overlap of contiguous embryonic areas or formative fields that may be subject thereby to conflicting organizing centers that normally induce and align body regions and organ systems.[6,7,150,154,155] The orientation of these contiguously developing axes to one another, and the location and extent of the overlap of their fields of influence, determine the site and extent of sharing or conjunction of the resulting tissues.[156,157] In addition to the effects of too closely located organizers, organs developing in unaccustomed proximity may exert an immobilizing effect on each other, contributing to further malformations other than being fused.[158,159]

Whatever theory of pathogenesis is proposed, it must take into account the fairly regular forms of the spectrum of conjoined twins, and some apparent limits to those forms. For example, it has been observed that only like parts are joined, that junction of limbs alone does not seem to occur, and that the axes of conjunction are more often symmetric than not, with the exception of some cases of cranial conjunction. This may be because conjunction is more likely to occur if specific growing sites of the embryos are too closely apposed—cranial or caudal neuropores, pharyngeal or cloacal membranes, edges of the enfolding embryonic disks, or cardiac anlagen.[157] Also, while one is reluctant to refer to unusual cases described in the lay press that have not been corroborated by a scientific report, there is a tantalizing story of thoracopagus twins with what may have been a third endoparasitic fetus between them, the only possible triplet conjunction noted in the review for this volume.[160]

Patterns and Classification

The patterns of conjoined twins actually observed exemplify many of the theoretical possibilities that the mechanisms described above could imply. If the twins are more separate than fused, they are usually joined anteriorly, posteriorly, cranially, or caudally. If they are more fused than separate, they are usually joined laterally.[5] The degrees of conjunction in any of these alignments can be considered as part of a continuum from the single individual to the separate pair of twin individuals, and whole systems of conjoined twins are possible.[153] An analysis

---

Terata katadidyma—single in the lower body and double above; a pair of twins joined by some portion of the lower body.

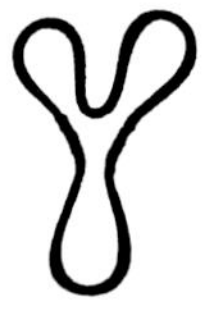

Diprosopus: 2 faces side by side with 1 head and 1 body.

Dicephalus: 2 heads and necks side by side with one body.

Ischiopagus: joined by the inferior margins of the coccyx and sacrum, the two completely separate spinal columns lying in the same axis, side by side.

Pyopagus: joined by the lateral and posterior surfaces of the coccyx and sacrum which are single; the rest of the two bodies being normally duplicated. These twins are almost back to back.

Terata anadidyma—single in the upper portion of the body and double below, or a pair of twins joined by some region of the upper part of the body.

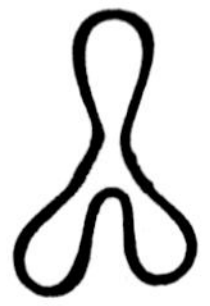

Dipygus: 1 head, thorax, and abdomen with 2 pelves with or without two sets of external genitalia and up to 4 legs, variably oriented.

Syncephalus: joined by the face. The faces are turned laterally and the twins may be separate except for this or further joined by the thorax, but are separate from the umbilicus down, bodies facing each other.

Craniopagus: joined at some homologous portion of the cranial vault, being separate at all other points; axes of the twins variably related.

Terata anakatadidyma—Twins joined by the midportion of the body and being separate and double above and below the region possessed in common.

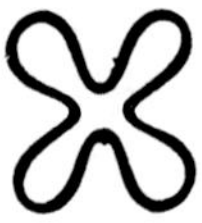

Thoracopagus: part of the thoracic wall and contained viscera is common to both twins, face to face.

Omphalopagus: these twins are joined from the umbilicus to the zyphoid, face to face.

Rachipagus: twins united at the vertebral column at any point above the sacrum, back to back.

FIGURE 10.15. Guttmacher's classification of conjoined twins.[152]

TABLE 10.4. Frequencies of different patterns of conjoined twins.[138]

Katadidyma (6.2)	Dicephalus	3.7
	Pyopagus	2.5
	Ischiopagus	–
Anadidyma (8.7)	Syncephalus	2.5
	Craniopagus	6.2
Anakatadidyma (59.3)	Thoracopagus	18.5
	Omphalopagus	9.9
	Xiphopagus	2.5
	Thoraco-omphalopagus	28.4
Other (25.9)	Parasitic	9.9
	Combination	12.3
	Not stated	3.7

The numbers refer to percentages of each type.

of visceral situs using cross sectional drawings of skull, thorax, and pelvis in major types of conjoined twins identified two interesting patterns.[161] A face-to-face conjunction created what was termed "line" or "axial" symmetry, the conjoining portion was shared by both twins, and no abnormality of situs was noted. A side-by-side union created "midsagittal plane" symmetry with the possibility of a dominant twin, and abnormal situs of one twin was always associated. Other types of twins lay between these two patterns. These observations suggest a relationship to differing influences on embryonic development, depending on the orientation of the

colliding developing embryonic plates or visceral anlagen to each other.[157,161]

Because of the variety of conjunctions possible, the classification of these twins is complicated and tends to be descriptive of the site and extent of the union, sometimes including details of head and extremity numbers and orientation. The resulting names can be intimidating and may not contribute to the fundamental understanding of the mode of origin. Also, there does not seem to be agreement on whether to emphasize the zone that is conjoined or to describe the portions that are duplicated. Basically, the conjunction can be of upper body portions, of lower body components or middle zone regions, as indicated by the symbols in Fig. 10.15. The classification used by Guttmacher and Nichols[152] is etymologically accurate and straightforward, and it is useful as a broad scheme of categorization into which most cases could be placed, with further descriptive modifiers as needed (Fig. 10.15).

A few additional terms are used with some frequency as synonyms in the literature. Syncephalus twins are also called janiceps or cephalothoracopagus twins, depending on the degree of fusion.[155] The diprosopus twins have been termed lateral cephalothoracopagus anomalies.[162] Spencer[157] has suggested the term "parapagus" (side

TABLE 10.5. Selected references concerning conjoined twins.

Topic	Author(s)	Year	Reference #
General reviews	Bergsma, Blattner, Nichols, Rudolph	1967	133
	Tan, Goon, Salmon, Wee	1971	142
	Potter, Craig	1975	5
	Edmunds, Layde	1982	138
	Zake	1984	165
	Little, Bryan	1988	166
Specific types			
Thoracopagus and thoraco-omphalopagus	Nichols, Blattner, Rudolph (42 cases)	1967	125
Xipghopagus and omphalopagus	Harper, Kenigsberg, Sia, Horn, et al. (36 cases)	1980	163
Cephalothoracopagus (syncephalus)	Herring, Rowlatt (11 cases)	1981	155
	Delprado, Baird (7 cases)	1984	167
	Baron, Shermeta, Ismail, Ben-Ami, et al. (11 cases)	1990	168
Craniopagus	Winston, Rockoff, Milliken, Strand, et al. (31 cases)	1987	169
	Bucholz, Yoon, Shively (21 cases)	1987	170
Dicephalus	Konstantinova	1976	171
	Ursell, Wigger	1983	164
	Siebert, Machin, Sperber	1989	172
Diprosopus	Barr	1982	52
	Chervenak, Pinto, Heller, Norooz (31 cases)	1985	53
Pyopagus and ischiopagus	Gupta	1966	173
	Albert, Drummond, O'Neill, Watts (17 cases)	1992	174

fixed) could replace the terms "diprosopus" and "dicephalus" used to describe the anterolateral conjunctions of the face and head. Omphalopagus conjunctions are also referred to as xiphopagus twins.[163] Unfortunately, the laterally joined duplications have defied simplification and have been described in some of the most complex terms, with combinations of words used to specify the number of heads, arms, and legs in each case, e.g., dicephalus tribrachius dipus.[164]

When the frequencies of the different patterns of conjunction are analyzed (Table 10.4), centrally conjoined twins are considerably more common than all of the others combined. Since somite development begins centrally and spreads caudally and cranially, the extremities of the embryo may be able to complete separate duplication later than the central portions, possibly after the influences leading to central conjunction, such as fusion of cardiac anlagen or the edge of the infolding embryonic disks, have exerted their effect. This may account for the preponderance of thoracopagus twins.

Pathology

The pathologic findings of conjoined twins include analysis of patterns of malformation, causes of death, and placentation. While the autopsy examination of a set of conjoined twins may seem an intimidating prospect to the inexperienced, help is available. One of the most extensive photographic catalogues is provided by Potter and Craig[5] and the references given in Table 10.5 can be consulted for further details of the specific types. At the time of writing this text, Spencer is preparing what will be the most extensive review of human conjoined twins, probably more than a thousand cases from early embryonic examples onward (Spencer R, 1993, personal communication). When it is available, her review will be the definitive reference. A detailed presentation of each of these types is beyond the scope of this book so an overview description of the more common patterns is presented in the next sections, with several general comments first. The illustrations have been chosen to display how these cases can be documented on a busy service by a variety of pathologists with differing interests in these cases. The review of the examples in the Survey '91 caseload has reinforced the value of simple line drawings and readily staged photodocumentation as supplements to even excellent word descriptions.

Placenta, Anomalies, and Mortality

The placentas are always monochorionic monoamniotic, and there may be a single cord from the surface of the placenta, which may divide before inserting into the twins, or two cords that originate separately and fuse closer to the infant(s). In one interesting case, a bilaminar web of amnion contained the separate portions of the distally united cord segments and tethered these cord segments to the placental surface as well.[175] The twins were joined from the lower sternum to the umbilicus, with a single cord containing six vessels, four arteries and two veins. This observation may have significance for the timing of the abnormal twinning process, if one considers the discussion of amniogenesis in monochorionic placentas as presented in Chapter 8. Another report of a case of partially septated amniotic cavity with abdomino-omphalopagus feti was referred to but could not be located for details.[176] The number of cord vessels ranges from one artery and one vein to four arteries and two veins. No specific parenchymal lesions have been reported.

The malformations and anomalies found in conjoined twins can be considered in two basic groups termed secondary and primary.[38] There are those malformations of the conjoined organs, most probably secondary to the aberrant twinning process, and often with profound effects on their normal pattern of symmetry or asymmetry.[158] The nonconjoined organs may be primarily malformed or have disturbed symmetry as well, unrelated to the anomalous twinning, although it may be difficult to determine how widespread the abnormal developmental influences can be.[158] Both types of malformation may be concordant or discordant, with discordance of major malformations reported as high as 20%.[141] The patterns observed likely reflect both the original orientation of the respective embryonic cell masses and organizers, as well as superimposed effects of vascular development.

The cardiovascular conjunction of conjoined twins is usually the limiting factor to survival or a consideration for separation. Analysis of the degree of fusion and altered symmetry of the shared hearts can be a daunting prospect clinically,[177,178] and pathologically,[158,179] but a suggested classification of five degrees of conjunction is helpful.[180] First, there may be no significant fusion, even in cephalothoracopagus twins. Second, large vessels may be fused and common in dicephalus or cephalothoracopagus twins. Third, atrial fusion with varying patterns of symmetry can be seen in dicephalus and thoracopagus twins. Fourth, atrioventricular fusion is the severest degree of conjunction in thoracopagus twins. Fifth, the presence of only one heart in one of conjoined twins was seen in a dicephalus pair.

It is no surprise that conjoined twins have a high mortality rate.[138] Nearly 40% are stillborn and a further one third die within 24 hours of birth. The cases that die soon after birth are usually extensively joined with serious abnormalities of internal organs, which are often fused. The mechanism of death in these cases is often related to a severely abnormal conjoined heart or to the pulmonary hypoplasia that accompanies the distortion of fused thoracic cages. In contrast, there have been sets of minimally conjoined twins whose cause of death is not easily explained. These twins often lived for some time, but when one died as a result of natural causes, the other apparently well twin died very soon after, within minutes or hours. The best known example of this phenomenon was Chang and Eng Bunker.[121] It has been suggested that the death of one twin leads to a lethal disseminated intravascular coagulopathy in the other but this has not been verified. We may never know the answer because current management of such twins usually means surgical separation at the earliest possible opportunity.

Thoracopagus Twins

The commonest pattern of conjoined twins is face to face fusion of the thorax and variable portions of the abdomen—thoracopagus—and there is an extensive literature available concerning the anatomy of such twins with particular reference to the possibility of surgical separation.[131–133,159,178,180] Although thoracopagus twins are basically symmetrical, there is often a degree of disparity of size and hardiness and this enters into considerations regarding separation.[125]

One of the most critical factors to survival or separation of thoracopagus twins is the degree of cardiac fusion. Although cardiac fusion is present in 75% of cases,[159] the degree of fusion cannot be predicted by the degree of thoracic fusion.[158] A common pericardium is observed in 90% of cases and atrial fusion is almost always present if any cardiac fusion exists at all. The conjoined heart is in the frontal plane although the bodies are in the lateral plane. There are several approaches to the anatomic classification of the conjoined hearts,[125,159,178,179,180] depending on the number of chambers or what is fused and how much, and these references are recommended to those who wish to provide the best descriptions of these challenging organs. The other limiting factor in the survival of these infants is that there is often a lethal degree of pulmonary hypoplasia due to loss of thoracic volume secondary to the conjunction, even though pleural spaces are usually separate.

Less life threatening but still important to considerations of separation, are the degrees of fusion of other viscera and the presence of other anomalies. Many of the anomalies in these twins seem to be manifestations of alterations in body symmetry.[158] The normally asymmetrical structures (heart and great vessels, lungs, liver, spleen, and gastrointestinal tract) are rendered more symmetric. The normally symmetrical structures (brain, upper respiratory tract, urogenital system, and skeleton) are less severely affected or not affected at all. The degree of fusion of other viscera varies. The liver is shared in all cases but the intestinal tract is shared in only about half of the cases. There may be an omphalocele at the site of the conjoined umbilicus. There is an unfortunately incomplete reference to a set of thoracopagus twins as being clearly of opposite sex.[148] Monozygotic twins can be heterokaryotic (see Chapter 7), but discordant external genitalia have not been reported in any other case of conjoined twins.

In the Survey '91 Review, 7 of the 12 sets of conjoined twins were thoracopagus twins and all were female. The major features are summarized in Table 10.6 with representative illustrations in Figs. 10.16 to 10.21. Most of the more recent cases of conjoined twins have been identified early in pregnancy with elective termination before midgestation. The characteristics of the thoracopagus twins, both clinical and pathological, were in keeping with the reported cases in the literature.

TABLE 10.6. Conjoined twins from the Survey '91 Review.

Case figure	Age sex weight	Shared structures	Situs anomalies other viscera	Other anomalies	Placental findings
			(a) Thoracopagus conjunction		
1 —	8 wks (36) F 3800 g	Sternal notch to umbilicus 3-vessel umbilical cord; vessels branched after fetal insertion Cardiac—heart in frontal plane when infants in lateral plane; pericardium; right atria; left ventricles Liver—parenchyma fused with interconnected venous drainage to each inferior vena cava; biliary systems distinct but small with normal drainage Diaphragm—peritoneal fold separated the respective cavities	Mirror-image cleft lips and alveolar ridge R pulmonary isomerism DA; L pulmonary isomerism DB Asplenia DA Malrotated stomach DB	VSD (C) ASD (C) AVC—DA; TA—DB; PA—DA	(Discarded in case room without examination)
2 10.16	SB (34) F 2470 g	From clavicles to umbilicus with a 4 cm omphalocele 4 vessels in cord—2 arteries (R in A; L in B), 2 veins All 4 clavicles met at the "manubrium" on the umbilical (anterior) side Cardiac—pericardium; common ventricles; (see Fig. 10.16h) Diaphragm—peritoneal cavities communicate around liver Liver—T-shaped, larger portion in A; increased connective tissue around central veins throughout; separate biliary systems	R pulmonary isomerism DA Asplenia DA Mirror-image aorta on right in A	"Dermatoglyphics less similar than generally found in nonconjoined monozygotic twins" Pleuropericardial window DB Fused adrenals DA Celiac axis and superior mesenteric artery arise as one vessel	(Discarded without examination)

				Unavailable for examination
3 10.17	23 days (33) F 4090 g	3rd costochondral region to umbilicus (4 cm omphalocele); asymmetrically with a higher zone in A joined to lower zone in B Umbilical cord with 5 vessels, 3 from A, 2 from B (right umbilical artery only) Cardiac—pericardium; atria; atrioventricular valves; and left ventricle of A to right ventricle of B (see Fig. 10.17e) Diaphragm; peritoneal cavity Liver curved over abdominal viscera in anteroposterior plane Duodenum (2nd part of A to 3rd part of B) and small bowel to bifurcation 4 cm proximal to Meckel's diverticulum in B	L pulmonary isomerism DB	Idiopathic nephromegaly (twice normal; histologically normal) (C) Absent gallbladder DB Pulmonary hypoplasia (C) Small dysplastic ovaries DB
4 10.18	45 min (40) F 5300 g	Manubrium to umbilicus with 7 × 4 cm omphalocele Umbilical cord with 5 vessels—4 arteries, 1 vein. Cardiac—pericardium; 3/4 of heart located on twin B's side of coronal plane between twins; cardiac sharing—see Fig. 10.18b Pleural cavities Diaphragm; peritoneal cavity Intestine from 2nd part duodenums with conjoined region receiving bile from separate biliary systems through one ampulla of vater, for 25 cm, then enter 6 cm diameter sac in omphalocele from which 2 small bowel tubes emerge to continue independently Liver—"fused extensively at porta hepatis resulting in saddle-shaped organ hung over the joined duodenum as a mussel shell"; twin A's portion smaller with atresia of umbilical vein	Malrotation cecum DA L pulmonary isomerism DA	Thoracolumbar scoliosis with convexity to right in A, and lesser curvature to left in B	35-cm umbilical cord with 5 vessels, inserts in membranes 1.5 cm from margin; placenta trimmed weight = 740 g; no other findings

TABLE 10.6. *Continued*

Case figure	Age sex weight	Shared structures	Situs anomalies other viscera	Other anomalies	Placental findings
5 10.19	ET (14) F 196 g	From base of neck to umbilicus Umbilical cord with 5 vessels—3 arteries, 2 veins Common larynx with separate glottises; common esophagus, stomach and small bowel to terminal ileum Single diaphragm, common liver, one gallbladder, single pancreas, one spleen Pericardium with union of atria, ventricles and great vessles of heart (see Fig. 10.19b)	NR	NR	The 5-vessel cord bifurcated just above insertion to a 2-vessel cord and a 3-vessel cord
6 10.20	ET (17) F 238 g	Manubrium sterni to just above umbilical cord Single 6-vessel cord—4 arteries, 2 veins Pericardium and heart (no details provided) Liver—saddle shaped with one gallbladder	NR	NR	Cord split into two 3-vessel cords 3 cm above placental surface
7 10.21	ET (13) F 44 g	Manubrium sterni to just above umbilical cord Single 6-vessel cord—4 arteries, 2 veins Pericardium and heart (no details provided) Liver	NR	NR	Cord single to placental insertion

(b) Omphalopagus conjunction

Case figure	Age sex weight	Shared structures	Situs anomalies other viscera	Other anomalies	Placental findings
1 10.22	ET (14) F 48 g	Xiphisternal cartilage Outer surface pericardial sacs below xiphisternum Liver—symmetric fusion of identical halves, each with gallbladder and umbilical vein; peritoneal cavities separate Single 6-vessel umbilical cord—4 arteries, 2 veins	Thoracoabdominal situs inversus DA Bilateral superior vena cavae DB	Hypoplastic right heart DA Hypoplastic left lung (C)	The 15-cm-long 6-vessel cord divided into two 3-vessel cords 1 cm above the placenta and vessels for each supplied about one-half the chorionic surface; focal anastomoses mentioned but not described

		(c) Cephalothoracopagus		
1 10.23	2 hrs (33–34) F 3050 g	Mandible to umbilicus with 3-vessel cord—2 arteries, 1 vein Esophagus, stomach, bowel to terminal ileum Diaphragm Liver—asymmetric with asymmetric biliary systems	Lung situs indeterminate (C) Rotational changes in situs for pharyngeal and neck structures, heart, lungs, liver	Cleft lip/palate DB	3-vessel cord; placenta normal

		(d) Dicephalus		
1 10.24	10 min (36) F 3415 g	Shoulders to pelvis and perineum side by side; inferior portion of sternums anteriorly, ribs posteriorly Cardiac—one IVC and one descending thoracic and abdominal aorta to and from heart B for all abdominal viscera, paired or fused; greater defects twin A's heart Terminal ileum to cloaca T-shaped liver with separate biliary systems Nodule of dysplastic kidney between the two normal kidneys Cloacal termination of partially hypoplastic genitourinary ducts and common rectum (see Fig. 10.24c) and double vulva	All four lungs two lobes only, bronchial pattern not reported Pelvic viscera aligned front to back instead of side to side as in rest of body	Bifid uvula (C) TV atresia, PA stenosis, VSD, transposed aorta DA Thymus A 1/6 size of thymus B	2-vessel cord, SUA on left; placenta not received
2 10.25	63 mins (35) M 4350 g	Side by side with spines separate to pelvis, with absence medial transverse processes of lumbar spines, union of ribs and one clavicular structure posteriorly; two arms, two legs Cardiac fusion with greater defects in right-sided heart (see Fig. 10.25f) Infradiaphragmatic structures single and normal; single intestine from duodenum at level duplicate pancreatic ducts to ileum	NR	Bilateral diaphragmatic hernias with liver and both stomachs in thorax Pulmonary hypoplasia, severe	Normal 21-cm 3-vessel cord and normal placenta

TABLE 10.6. *Continued*

Case figure	Age sex weight	Shared structures	Situs anomalies other viscera	Other anomalies	Placental findings
				(e) Diprosopus	
1 10.26	ET (16.5) M 107 g	Medially fused symmetrically double bases of skulls and all vertebrae. Single pharynx and remaining intestinal tract below double tongue	Both lungs 2 lobes, no comment re bronchi	Absent cranial vault. Total spinal dysrhaphism. Ectopic pancreas at bifurcation of trachea. Mosaic 46,XY; 47XYY. 11 pairs ribs	Normal for age with 3-vessel cord

Case (a)1—Diagnosed prior to labor, criteria not stated; classical section delivery, both breech. Symmetric linear measurements and head circumference. Electrocardiogram pattern was of a single cardiac electrical field, although synchronous and asynchronous pulses recorded in chart. Blood pressures in arms/legs differed by 2–6 mm systolic. Respirations independent, occasionally synchronous, rates approximately equal. Independent intestinal function and pain response. Death due to congestive heart failure, respirations ceased 20 seconds apart.

Case (a)2—Diagnosed during labor, delivered vaginally. Single-heart sounds during labor, with bradycardia and heart beat detected after birth, but no respiratory efforts after birth, no resusitation. Paternal family history of twinning, zygosity unknown. Twin B 3 cm shorter crown–heel length.

Case (a)3—Twins diagnosed before delivery by section at 33 weeks for fetal distress, not known whether conjunction identified before delivery. Sharing of liver and part of intestine suggested clinically. Twins maintained until cardiovascular studies complete, with assisted ventilation for respiratory distress, first twin A, then twin B, as needed. Electrocardiagram had two different complexes patterns, but mutual interference made interpretation difficult. The cardiac lesion was assessed to preclude separation, even with sacrifice of one twin, so they were not resuscitated from an episode of respiratory deterioration with cardiac arrest.

Case (a)4—Not known when twins diagnosed, but ultrasound examination in early labor revealed A cephalic and B breech. Emergency section delivery occurred 10 hours after artificial rupture of membranes at term because of failure of progress and fetal distress. They were not resuscitated because of apparent degree of conjunction.

Case (a)5—This pregnancy was conceived while mother was lactating from previous normal pregnancy, so ultrasound examination was done to determine dating and conjoined twins diagnosed. Prostaglandin termination elected. Twins equal size.

Case (a)6—These conjoined twins were identified by ultrasound examination at 17 weeks and detailed ultrasound studies indicated that separation was not possible, so elective termination of the pregnancy with prostaglandin was chosen. The twins were equal size, but only 14 weeks developmental age when delivered at 18 weeks.

Case (a)7—These twins were identified by ultrasound at 13 weeks gestational age and elective termination chosen. They were equally grown.

Case (b)1—The conjoined twins were identified by ultrasound at 14 weeks to have conjoined liver and possibly other midgut structures, elective termination with prostaglandin chosen.

Case (c)1—Conjoined twins were diagnosed by ultrasound examination done because the mother was large for dates. The degree of conjunction was such that operative delivery for maternal reasons was chosen, as she had polyhydramnios with increasing discomfort. Although live-born, there was no resuscitation.

Case (d)1—These twins were diagnosed after operative delivery. Twins had been identified earlier and it was stated that "first baby presenting as a vertex and second in a breech presentation" (!). Twin B slightly larger.

Case (d)2—Ultrasound examination done because the uterus was large for dates identified the twinning abnormality and section delivery performed electively. He (they) were not resuscitated. As the body parts were more joined than separate, this case was assigned only one accession number. There was said to be a strong family history of twinning on both sides, but no zygosity details provided.

Case (e)1—Routine ultrasound identified an anomalous fetus with cranial defect and the pregnancy was terminated.

*Age at death if liveborn (gestational age at birth in weeks). F, female; M, male; C, concordant; D, discordant, twin A or B; R, right; L, left; NR, none recorded; SB, stillborn; ET, elective termination; Weight, birthweight if known, otherwise autopsy weight; ASD, atrial septal defect; AVC, atrioventricular septal defect with single artrioventricular valve; VSD, ventricular septal defect; PA, pulmonary valve atresia; PH, pulmonary artery hypoplasia; TA, tricuspid atresia; TAPVR, total anomalous pulmonary venous return [infradiaphragmatic in case (a)2A].

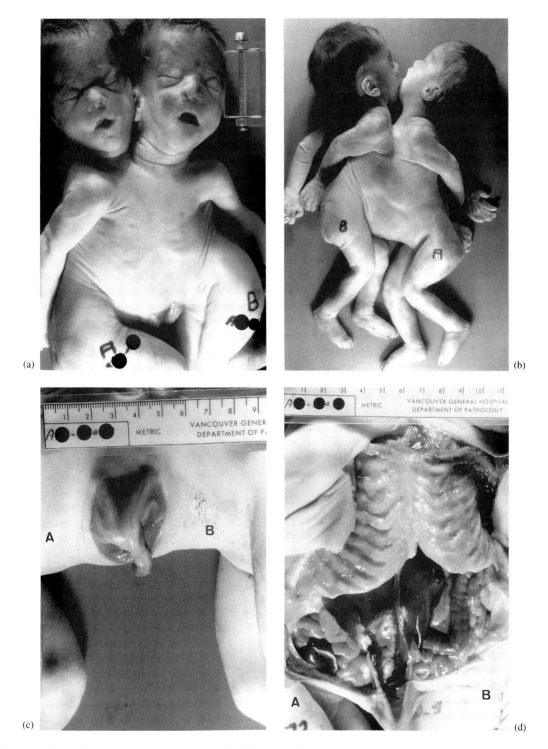

(a)

(b)

(c)

(d)

FIGURE 10.16. Thoracopagus twins [case (a)2, Table 10.6]. These twins are typical of thoracopagus twins and are shown in some detail to provide an example of how they can be documented. Although the twins are basically face to face, they are not completely parallel, so that the conjoined area has its own posterior (a) and anterior (b) orientation, based in part on the location of the umbilicus (a,c), and the clavicular attachments to the conjoined hemi sternae (d—anterior view, e—view of inside posterior chest wall).

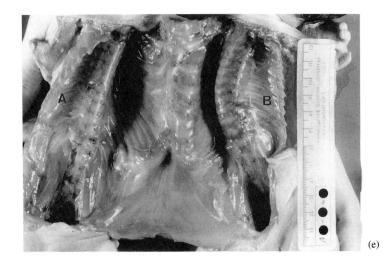

(e)

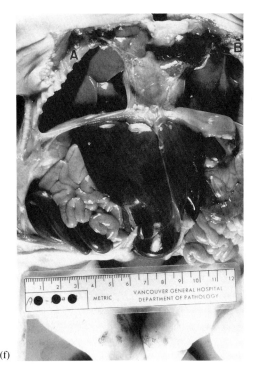

(f)

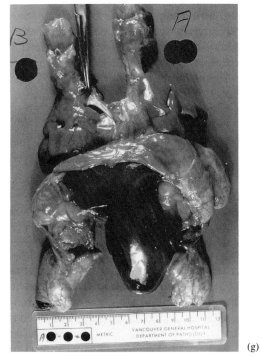

(g)

FIGURE 10.16. *Continued.* Note the spinal curvatures in (e). Note the greater prominence of the heart and the T-shaped liver in the anterior view of the viscera (f), compared to the posterior aspect (g).

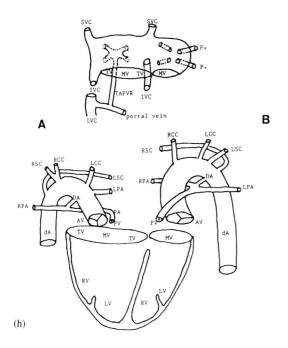

(h)

FIGURE 10.16. *Continued*. The drawings (h), made at the time of dissection, clarify the anatomy of the conjoined hearts. Systemic venous return from each twin is to a common atrium, and passes through a partially shared atrioventricular valve into a common ventricle, which is irregularly septated. The ventricular outflow consists of bilaterally hypoplastic pulmonary arteries, with aberrant right pulmonary artery in A, and reasonably normal sized aortas which are mirror images. SVC, superior vena cava; IVC, inferior vena cava; Pv, pulmonary vein; TV, tricuspid valve; MV, mitral valve; PV, pulmonary valve; AV, aortic valve; RV, right ventricle; LV, left ventricle; DA, ductus arteriosus; LPA, left pulmonary artery; RPA, right pulmonary artery; dA, descending aorta; RCC, right common carotid; LCC, left common carotid; LSC, left subclavian; RSC, right subclavian; TAPVR, total anomalous pulmonary venous return.

Other Patterns

There are four other patterns of conjoined twins that occur sufficiently frequently that they might be encountered in a pediatric pathology practice affiliated with a busy obstetric unit: omphalopagus twins, cephalothoracopagus twins, lateral conjunctions, and varieties of craniofacial duplication. These are defined briefly.

The most readily separable conjoined twins are the *omphalopagus* twins, since their union may involve only skin and portions of liver (as in Chang and Eng Bunker), occasionally including portions of the sternum.[125] A review of 36 cases of what were termed xiphopagus twins found the following distribution of conjoined tissue: liver in 81% of cases, cartilage in 56%, diaphragm in 17%, genitourinary tract in 3%, and skin alone in 6%.[163] In 53% of the cases, both twins survived. Twenty-five percent had concordant cardiac malformations and 33% had concordant gastrointestinal anomalies. Ventral conjunction at concordant gastroschises with discordant cloacal defect has been reported, and there were two separate three-vessel umbilical cords, situated to the left of the gastroschisis in each twin.[181] The cords fused before inserting into the placenta. Although the degree of conjunction of omphalopagus twins can be quite limited, such as partial fusion of a short segment of mid-ileum through a common umbilical hernia, there still can be severe abnormalities in the conjoined system and in other systems, such as amyoplasia and arthrogryposis multiplex.[182] Whether the additional intestinal and musculoskeletal anomalies reflected the abnormal influences that led to the conjunction, or were a result of disturbed vascular flow due to the conjunction, or both, was not determined. Because this pattern of twinning involves relatively malleable structures, these twins may rotate and tend to lie head to toe, presenting a potentially confusing false negative finding during initial clinical evaluation antenatally.

There is a particularly fascinating report of what appeared to be the twin transfusion syndrome in male twins who shared small intestine with bilateral discordant degrees of colonic atresia, and had conjoined bladders at the urachus level.[183] The briefly live-born twin was pale and wasted and his attached stillborn co-twin was large, plethoric, and hydropic (1,490 g vs 2,700 g, crown–heel length 34 cm vs 37.5 cm). Unfortunately, no cardiac weights were recorded and the heart and great vessels were said to be normal in both twins, so one of the key diagnostic criteria for chronic twin transfusion in separate twins was not present (see Chapter 9), but it is difficult to suggest any other interpretation than differential circulations.

The one example of omphalopagus conjunction in the Survey '91 Review was identified in early pregnancy and electively delivered at 14 weeks. The findings are summarized in Table 10.6 and it is shown in Fig. 10.22.

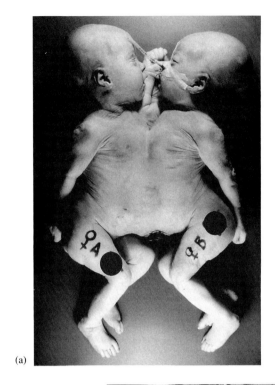

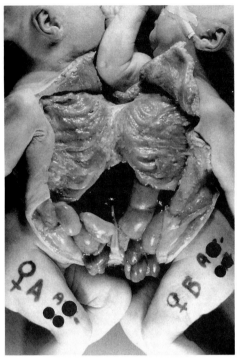

(a)   (b)

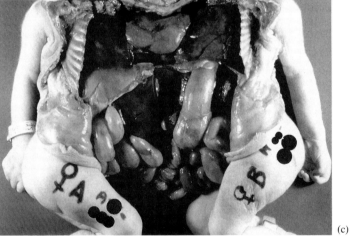

(c)

FIGURE 10.17. Thoracopagus twins [case (a)3, Table 10.6]. In this pair, the conjunction is more asymmetric with greater visceral fusion. The 35-cm circumference bridge (a,b) begins 3 cm below the sternal notch in A and 4 cm in B, and ends 8 cm from the pubic symphysis in A and 4 cm in B. Twin A's spine is relatively straight, while twin B has marked kyphosis. Twin B is 2 cm shorter in crown–heel length.

FIGURE 10.17. *Continued*. The anterior component of the central horseshoe-shaped liver can be seen (b,c) and the common diaphragm and irregular heart (d). In (e) are the drawings made of the heart and duodenal conjunction at the time of dissection. In the heart, the common atrium with rudimentary left atrium for twin A is seen with anomalous pulmonary venous return. The atrioventricular flow is through two valves consisting of two tricuspid valves together and twin B's mitral valve. There is a ventricular septal defect in A and the left ventricle of A is incompletely separated from the right ventricle of B. There is concordant transposition of the great vessels with pulmonary valve atresia in A. In B, the aortic valve was bicuspid and there was no ductus arteriosus. A coronary vessel from B supplied part of A's myocardium across the posterior side of the heart. A, aorta; PA, pulmonary artery; RA, right atrium; LA, left atrium; RIVC, right inferior vena cava; RSVC, right superior vena cava. (Remainder of key as in Fig. 10.16h.) The union of the duodenums (D) is diagramed, indicating separate pancreases (P) and stomachs (S) with bile duct (BD) to gallbladder in A but direct to liver in B.

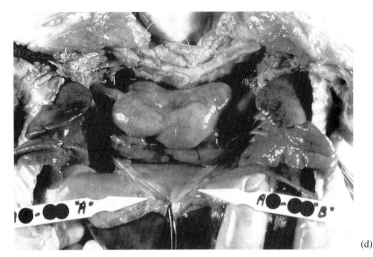

(d)

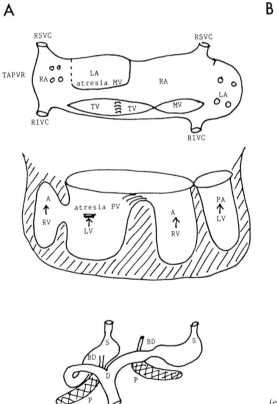

(e)

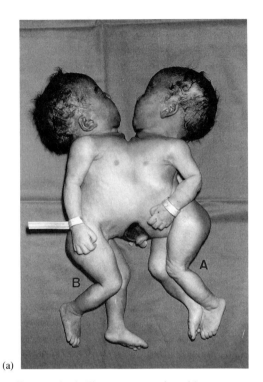

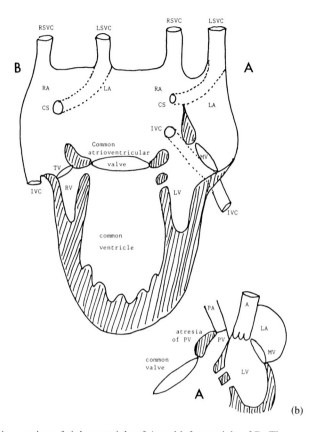

(a)

(b)

FIGURE 10.18. Thoracopagus twins with more symmetric conjunction, including conjoined heart [case (a)4, Table 10.6]. The twins are discordant in crown–heel length by 4.5 cm (A smaller)(a). In the heart, diagramed at the time of dissection (b), there is bilateral persistence of the left superior vena cava, a common atrium with hypoplasia of left auricle, a common atrioventricular valve composed of tricuspid valve from A and mitral valve from B, and union of right ventricle of A and left ventricle of B. The common ventricle communicates with the other two ventricles. The outflow from this common ventricle was to a normal aorta in B and toward a normal conus but atretic pulmonary valve in A, supplied by the ductus arteriosus. CS, coronary sinus; LSVC, left superior vena cava. (Remainder of key as in Figs. 10.16h and 10.17e.)

FIGURE 10.19. Embryofetal thoracopagus twins. This pair is joined more extensively with union of neck viscera [case (a)5, Table 10.6]. The external fusion begins in the region of the neck (a) and there is more conjunction of endodermal- derived viscera and cardiac structures as diagramed in (b). The separate pharynxes (P), separate glottises in a common larynx (L), separate tracheas and bronchi, common esophagus (E), stomach (S) and bowel are depicted. The conjoined heart has been reduced to only two atria and a single ventricle with only two asymmetric great vessels as shown. (Key: as in Figs. 10.16h and 10.17e.)

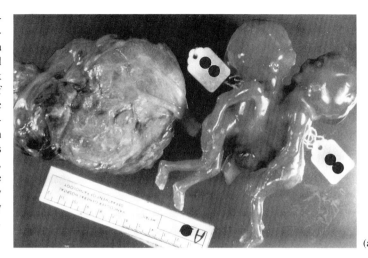

(a)

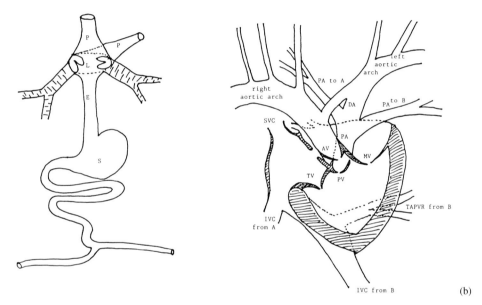

(b)

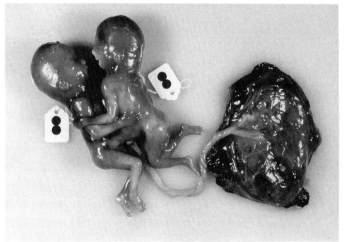

(a)

FIGURE 10.20. Embryofetal thoracopagus twins terminated electively after antenatal studies indicated separation was not possible [case (a)6, Table 10.6]. The typical manubrium to umbilicus conjunction is evident, along with forking of the six- vessel cord to two three-vessel cords just above the placenta (a), and the central common liver (b).

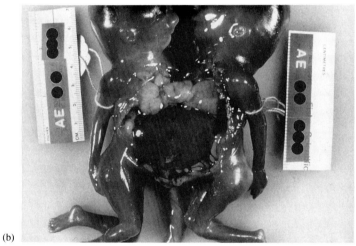

(b)

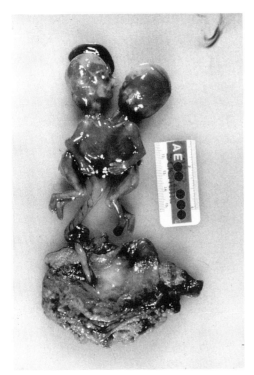

FIGURE 10.21. Embryofetal thoracopagus twins terminated at 13 weeks [case (a)7, Table 10.6]. Classical manubrium to umbilicus conjunction with shared heart and common liver, single six-vessel cord, and no other lesions reported. Fine details may be difficult to determine in small sets as macerated as these twins.

In the *cephalothoracopagus* twins, the cranial fusions may be lateral with a single distorted facial zone, or the double facial zones on either side as in the janiceps type.[155] It has been suggested that each face in the janiceps type is made up of the right side of one twin and the left side of the other,[152] but this may not be true of all cases. The degree of conjunction and deformity depends on the extent of fusion of the trunks.[162,167,168,184] The thoracic and abdominal organs are often duplicated. The heart and anterior intestinal derivatives tend to be oriented anteroposteriorly and to be shared by the twins rather than belonging to the right or left individual. The posterior organs tend to maintain a right and left orientation. There was one example of cephalothoracopagus twinning in the Survey '91 Review and it is summarized in Table 10.6 and illustrated in Fig. 10.23.

In the *lateral conjunctions* of the lower body,

sometimes referred to as rostral duplication,[164] there are varying degrees of separation of the cerebrospinal axis. This may consist of two heads only or involve separation of the bodies to the level of a single pelvis with duplication of the viscera roughly proportional to that of the cerebrospinal axis. These twins tend to be more fused than separate,[5] one may be more dominant, and abnormal situs in one twin is common.[161] The naming of this pattern of conjoined twins is often the most difficult, usually consisting of a compound of the number of heads, arms, and legs. There were two examples of this pattern of conjoined twin in the Survey '91 Review and they are summarized in Table 10.6 and illustrated in Figs. 10.24 and 10.25.

There are two aspects to consider with *craniofacial duplications*. First, they are frequently associated with neural tube defects.[155,173] This is particularly interesting in reference to discussions regarding the associated incidences of monozygotic twins, neural tube defects, and female zygotes[185] (see Chapter 7). Second, while there is a spectrum of facial duplication from isolated nasal duplication to the complete doubling of all facial structures as in the diprosopus,[53] it might be questioned whether this type of anomaly is truly a conjoined twin or merely a regional duplication for some other reason. Is there in fact a class of so-called conjoined twins who are not the result of incomplete fission or codominant axes, but who are the result of forces leading to variable duplications of localized parts, analogous to other regional duplications such as polydactyly? In an extensive review of the varieties of facial duplications, Barr[52] makes the additional point that they are to be considered separate from the median cleft face syndromes.

The one case of diprosopus in the Survey '91 Review was one of the two male sets of the 12 sets of conjoined twins. The anomaly had been identified in early pregnancy and elective termination occurred at 16 weeks. The features are summarized in Table 10.6 and it is illustrated in Fig. 10.26.

Pathology—Summary

Detailed analyses of any pattern of conjoined twins at autopsy is rarely urgent and deserves careful thought. The literature cited should be consulted prior to dissection so that the maximum information

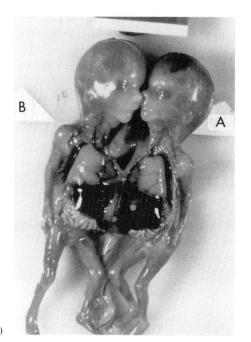

(a)

▶

FIGURE 10.22. Embryofetal omphalopagus twins terminated at 14 weeks [case (b)1, Table 10.6]. The conjoined liver is prominent and the peritoneal septum is evident (a,b), and part of the situs inversus in twin A can be seen with trilobed left lung in (b).

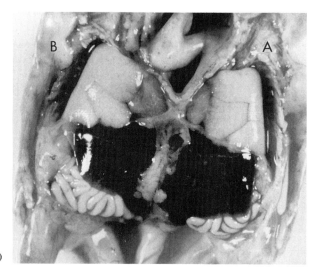

(b)

FIGURE 10.23. These cephalothoracopagus twins are fused from the mandibles to the umbilicus, with complimentary partial rotation of the coronal planes so that they are not directly facing, and this is reflected in the viscera [case (c)1, Table 10.6]. On side A/B (a), the shoulders are 7 cm apart and the nipples 4 cm, while on side B/A (b), the shoulders are 8 cm apart and the nipples 3 cm. The umbilical region is more visible on side A/B. There are differences in the pattern of viscera visible on the A/B or "anterior" (c), and B/A or "posterior" (d) sides. The heart (H) of A presents anteriorly and the heart of B posteriorly, with a common pericardial sac, but there was conjunction of the great vessels only. The lungs (Lu) of A are anterior and B's are posterior, and all are multilobed with indeterminate bronchial branching. The fused liver is horseshoe shaped (Li), asymmetrically oriented with a much larger portion posteriorly, and with separate biliary systems, also asymmetric in size. Kidneys (K) and adrenals (Ad) are visible on both sides, but the intestine is present only on the "anterior" A/B side with separate cecums (C) and attached appendices visible.

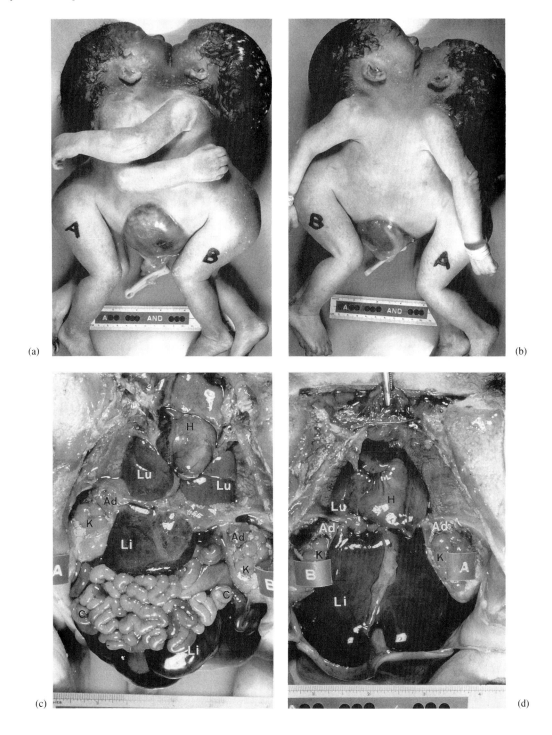

(a)

(b)

(c)

(d)

FIGURE 10.23. *Continued.* When the viscera are removed after taking off the intestines and elevating the anterior flap of liver (e), the single esophagus (E), elongate vertical stomach with duplicated fundus (S) can be seen in the "anterior" or A/B view, along with the two pancreases (P) and spleens (Sp), and small biliary tract to the smaller liver lobe (white arrow) and the larger to the larger lobe (black arrow). The intestine was common to a point 30 cm proximal to the cecum in A and 28 cm in B, branching just before a 1-cm Meckel's diverticulum in B. As can be seen from (f), the heads are slightly rotated in opposite directions, and the pharyngeal viscera were even more rotated so there are separate tongues and glottises but only one esophagus (g).

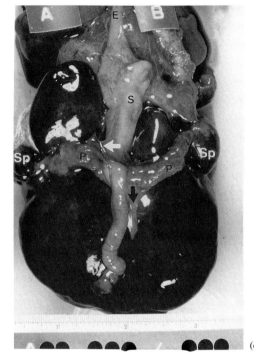

(e)

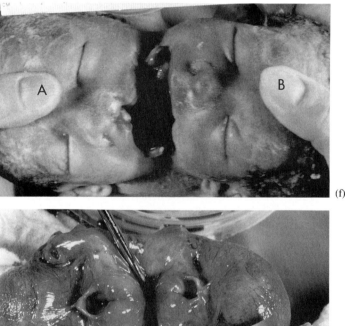

(f)

(g)

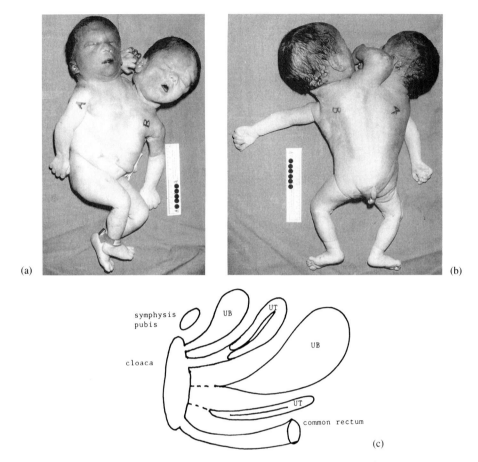

FIGURE 10.24. These were dicephalus tripus tribrachius (2 heads, 3 legs, 3 arms) twins (a,b) [case (d)1, Table 10.6]. The third arm, seen posteriorly, seems to be arising from twin B because of its orientation, but it has two well-formed hands. The level of union of the spines is not stated but there was a single pelvis with a posterior rudimentary third leg with small foot and single digit at the level of the sacrum. There was a remnant of a third kidney internally with asymmetric hypoplasia of the lower urinary tract and internal genitalia and a common rectum, all opening into a cloaca as depicted in the sagittal drawing (c). The right ureter entered a normal bladder (UB), with normal urethra; the left ureter entered a distended bladder with atretic urethra. There was a normal vagina (V), uterus (UT), tubes and ovaries behind the normal bladder; there was an atretic vagina and hypoplastic uterus with one tube and ovary behind the atretic urethra and dilated bladder.

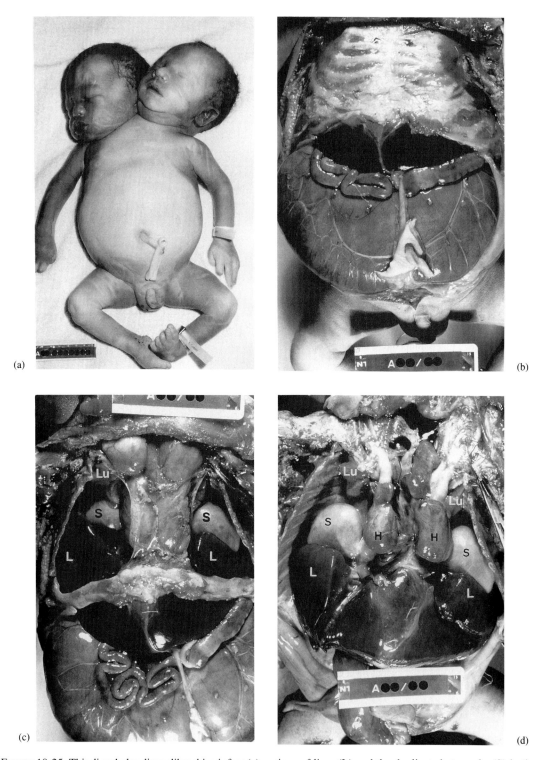

FIGURE 10.25. This dicephalus dipus dibrachius infant (a) had focal massive dilatation of the ileum (b) with no cause identified, bilateral diaphragmatic herniae (c) with por- tions of liver (L) and the duplicated stomachs (S) in the respective hemithorax (c,d) with severe pulmonary hy- poplasia (Lu) [case (d)2, Table 10.6].

FIGURE 10.25. *Continued*. The separate spines to the level of the pelvis are seen in (e). There are two hearts (H), joined at the atrial level with left atrium to right atrium, with communications through secundum septal defects and deroofed coronary sinus (f). In the right heart, there is a common atrioventricular valve, inverted and rotated ventricles with horizontal septum ("upstairs-downstairs heart"), great vessels from a right-sided type ventricle with pulmonary atresia, d-malrotation of great vessels, total anomalous pulmonary venous return to the azygous system; the left heart was essentially normal with persistent left superior vena cava to the coronary sinus. The major branches from the hearts are diagramed in (g). RH, structures connected with viscera of right-sided head; LH, structures connected with viscera of left-sided head; R, right; L, left; A, artery; V, vein; SC, subclavian; CC—common carotid; J, jugular; SVC, superior vena cava; IVC, inferior vena cava; PA, pulmonary artery; TAPVR, total anomalous pulmonary venous return; DA, ductus arteriosus; dA, descending aorta; LV, left ventricle; RV, right ventricle.

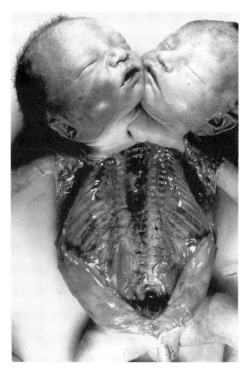

(e)

can be obtained. Radiographic studies and extensive photographic documentation supplemented by careful, accurate, and clear diagrams, done in a measured stepwise fashion, is the most useful and least stressful approach. As long as the information is available, it can be reviewed along with other cases by those with a special affinity and understanding of these problems, so that the embryologic and teratologic lessons they contain can be deciphered at last.

Concluding Comments

Just when we think we are perhaps beginning to understand these anomalies of monozygotic twinning, a twinning anomaly occurs that takes us back to basics. One such example is presented briefly in Fig. 10.27 as a reminder that we still have much to learn.

Although we do not understand why a single zygote/early embryo undergoes division sufficient to create more than one embryo/fetus, we recognize that this twinning process can go awry and lead to bizarre anomalies indeed. The key

feature of all these malformations is incomplete separation of the "twins". This ranges from twins where one is joined to the other by chorionic or umbilical cord vessels only (chorangiopagus parasiticus), to near total singularity with duplication of all or part of the head only (diprosopus). The malformation may be one of symmetry, with asymmetrically grown or abnormally developed parasitic twins able to survive because they are connected to the host twin, as with the CAPP, ectoparasitic, or endoparasitic anomalies. Alternatively, the malformation may be one of orientation, with abnormally oriented separately developing embryonic axes unable to complete their separate development in one or more regions, as with the varieties of conjoined twins. The developmental abnormalities that occur as a direct result of the aberrant twinning process are often accompanied by additional malformations as a consequence of developmental disturbances due to distorted proximities, tissue influences, and vascularizations.

These anomalies of monozygotic duplication are individually uncommon or rare, do not appear to have any increased risk of recurrence, and are often readily identifiable as twinning anomalies, so one

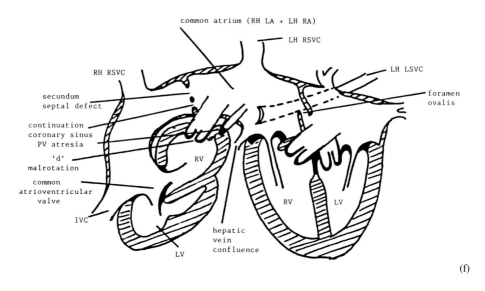

(f)

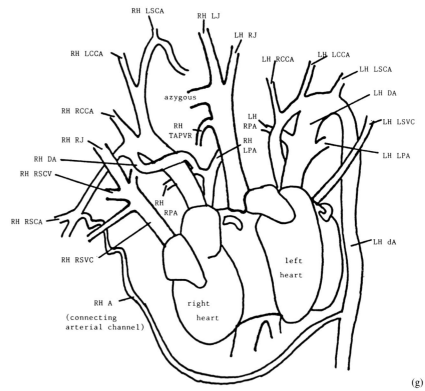

FIGURE 10.25. *Continued.*

(g)

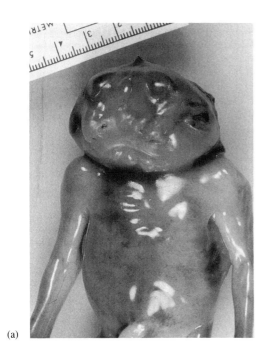
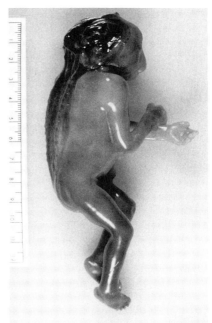

(a)   (b)

FIGURE 10.26. This twinning anomaly of diprosopus contains several interesting features [case (e)1, Table 10.6]. In addition to the duplication of the face (a), with one pair of ears and two small but distinct mandibles, there was craniospinal rachischisis in the double but medially fused craniospinal axes (b), and mosaicism for two cell lines, 46,XY and 47,XYY. The association of neural tube defects with cranially fused conjoined twins is recognized, but the significance of the mosaicism is not known.

might question the value of analyzing any of them beyond the point of diagnosis. In fact there are two avenues of investigation that can be aided by thoughtful documentation of these cases—pathobiology of embryonic development and clinically significant pathophysiology—as suggested by the following comments for each type of anomaly. First, until the pathobiology of teratomas and endoparasitic "twins" can be clarified, unequivocal diagnostic criteria will be difficult to define, and this may even have an impact on surgical procedures in some cases, as noted in the relevant discussion in the section on twins versus teratomas, above. Second, the development of knowledge of homeobox genes as orientation and field organizers in the embryo leads to the question of whether ectoparasitic "twins" are truly a twinning anomaly or due to some more regional problem. If this question can be answered, perhaps the mechanisms underlying twinning itself can be clarified. Third, the presence of a parasitic CAPP twin in the chorionic circulatory path of a normal co-twin has considerable potential clinical implications for both the co-twin and the mother. The details of the underlying pathobiology remain to be determined and the pathologist may be called upon to provide pathological correlations for clinical events, especially if antenatal therapeutic intervention is undertaken. Finally, in addition to its importance to an understanding of the underlying pathobiology, clinicopathological correlation is essential to the prenatal and postnatal investigation and management of conjoined twins, so that therapeutic decisions can be based on the most accurate information possible.

Because the diagnosis of these anomalies as aberrations of twinning can be made from relatively superficial examination in the majority of cases, and appropriate counseling can be given promptly, the detailed pathologic documentation can be done in a measured fashion. Some procedures, such as chorionic product assays in cases of suspected endoparasitic twins, and cytogenetic/DNA studies on the host and aberrant parasitic twin, as well as documentation of orientation and vascular connec-

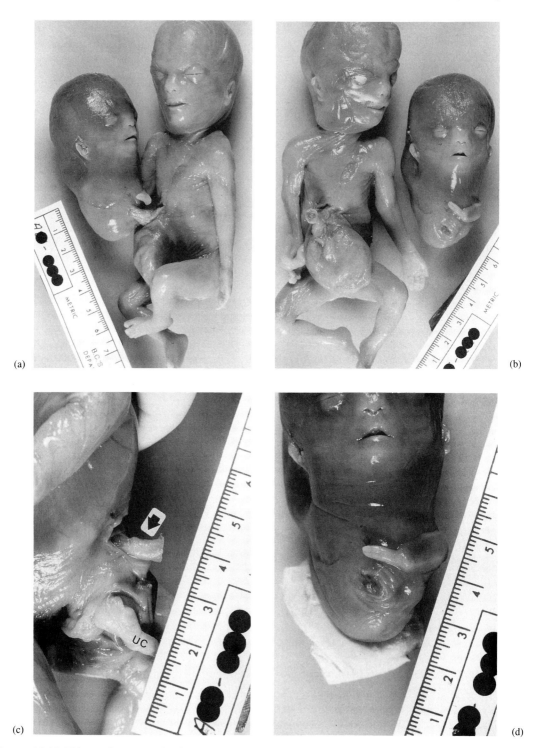

FIGURE 10.27. This case is an example of the concept that anomalies of monozygotic twinning may be infinitely varied and not always amenable to rigid classification. These asymmetric male twins were delivered electively at about 17 weeks' gestation, after being seen by xerora-diography done because of elevated maternal serum alpha-fetoprotein. The external parasitic twin has total caudal regression and is attached with a 10 × 5 mm omphalomesenteric epigastric pedicle to the co-twin (a).

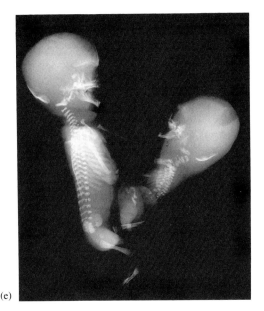

(e)

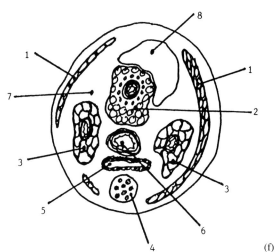

(f)

FIGURE 10.27. *Continued*. The normal twin has a large omphalocele (a,b,c) containing macerated liver, gastrointestinal tract on universal mesentery, and Meckel's diverticulum. The anomalous twin has amelia of the right arm and reduction malformation of the left arm. The respiratory tract was intact with normally lobated but hypoplastic lungs. The heart was tubular with absence of the left ventricle and truncus arteriosus. Below the intact diaphragm, most abdominal viscera were absent: interruption of the intestinal tract distal to the pancreas, bilateral renal agenesis with absence of the lower ducts, midline adrenal fusion, only one testicle found, hepatic tissue limited to epigastric band, absent pelvis and legs, but with cartilaginous extensions and musculovascular leg equivalents present in epigastric band. The external form and epigastric/omphalomesenteric band of the abnormal twin can be seen (a,b,c,d). The band joins the normal twin at the apex of the omphalocele (c—arrow), and the umbilical cord (UC) of the normal twin is also seen. The anomalous left "arm" and degree of caudal reduction are seen in (d) and in the lateral x-ray (e).

Because it was important to determine the vascular connections between the twins, the pedicle/band was serially blocked and sectioned. The appearance of the structures in the band suggested that rudiments of the caudal end of the parasitic twin were represented (f). In the representative cross section through the midportion of the band there was a cartilaginous extension (4) that might represent a spinal equivalent, but looked more like primitive notochord. Two large vessels, a venous sinus that might represent inferior vena cava (5) and a muscular artery representing aorta (6), were flanked by bundles of striated skeletal muscle with a large central artery and smaller branches, termed leg equivalents (3). Above was

a neurovascular bundle surrounded by autolyzed glandular tissue suggestive of superior mesenteric artery and pancreas (2), with quite autolyzed liver (8) above that. On either side was a band of striated skeletal muscle (1) interpreted as an extension of body wall muscle. The remaining tissues were interstitial connective tissue consisting largely of areolar tissues with occasional small vessels and small amounts of fat (7). In other blocks of this pedicle, an isolated segment of intestine with inspissated contents and peritoneal reflections contiguous with the peritoneum of the normal twin were seen. The liver tissue merged with the liver in the omphalocele. The actual vascular anatomy could not be followed completely, but the sections suggested that each twin had his own hepatic arterial supply and that hepatic venous drainage was conjoined through the joined liver.

The features of this particular case do not fit easily within the patterns of anomalous twinning described in this chapter. It is not an endoparasitic twin. It is not like the ectoparasitic twin as it is attached with a pedicle, although the region of attachment fits, and upper-body-only parasitic twins are known. It is not the chorangiopagus parasiticus twin as the fetal portion is the reverse of that anomaly and the circulation pattern is not appropriate. It is not truly a conjoined twin if the sense of that group is limited to nearly symmetric conjunctions. This may be a bridging case between ectoparasitic twinning and conjoined twinning with caudal agenesis, depending on one's point of view. (This case is described with the kind consent of Dr. Stephen Kassel, Director of Laboratories, and Dr. Cynthia Cury, Medical Geneticist, both of Valley Children's Hospital, Fresno, California, who submitted it to this author for examination and interpretation.)

tions, must be undertaken at the appropriate times during clinical investigation and management. However, the morphologic details of the resected or deceased twin(s) can be recorded in words, supplemented with drawings, photographs, and radiographs, after consideration and consultation as needed. If detailed case material is available, it can be collated and analyzed on a broader scale in cooperative studies, in order to answer the developmental questions posed by these striking anomalies.

References

1. Hollobon J. Making individuals out of siamese twins. *Globe and Mail*. 1984; Aug 7:14.
2. Hluchy P. A new chance at life for siamese twins. *MacLeans*. 1984; Aug 13:38–42.
3. O'Donovan S. Tragic tale of two-headed baby has happy ending. *National Examiner*. 1989; Feb 7:25.
4. Stockard CR. Developmental rate and structural expression: an experimental study of twins, "double monsters" and single deformities, and the interaction among embryonic organs during their origin and development. *Am J Anat*. 1921;28:115–277.
5. Potter EL, Craig JM. *Pathology of the Fetus and the Infant*. 3rd ed. Chicago: Year Book Medical Publishers; 1975:180–197,207–237.
6. De Robertis EM, Oliver G, Wright CVE. Homeobox genes and the vertebrate body plan. *Sci Am*. 1990;263:46–52.
7. Willis RA. *The Borderland of Embryology and Pathology*. 2nd ed. London: Butterworths; 1962: 135–147,442–462.
8. Du Plessis JPG, Winship WS, Kirstein JDL. Fetus in fetu and teratoma. *South Afr Med J*. 1974; 48:2119–2122.
9. Nadimpalli VR, Reyes H, Manaligod JR. Retroperitoneal teratoma with fetuses. *Teratology*. 1989; 39:233–236.
10. Heifetz SA, Alrabeeah A, Brown B StJ, Lau H. Fetus in fetu: a fetoform teratoma. *Pediatr Pathol*. 1988;8:215–226.
11. Gonzalez-Crussi F. Extragonadal teratomas. In: *Atlas of Tumor Pathology*, Second series, Fascicle 18. Washington, DC: Armed Forces Institute of Pathology, 1982.
12. Weldon-Linne CM, Rushovich AM. Benign cystic teratomas with homunculi. *Obstet Gynecol*. 1983; 61:88S-94S.
13. Lamabadusuriya SP, Atukorale AW, Soysa PE, Walpita PR. A case of fetus in fetu. *Arch Dis Child*. 1972;47:305–307.
14. Kimmel DL, Moyer EK, Peale AR, Winborne LW,

Gotwals JE. A cerebral tumor containing five human fetuses. *Anat Rec*. 1950;106:141–165.
15. Knox AJS, Webb AJ. The clinical features and treatment of fetus in fetu: two case reports and review of the literature. *J Pediatr Surg*. 1975; 10:483–489.
16. Lewis RH. Foetus in foetu and the retroperitoneal teratoma. *Arch Dis Child*. 1961;36:220–226.
17. Edmonds HW, Hawkins JW. The relationship of twins, teratomas and ovarian dermoids. *Cancer Res*. 1941;1:896–899.
18. Vohra K, Iqbal S, Dasilva M, Sahdev S, Shahar Y, Jhaveri R. Visual diagnosis casebook: epignathus. *J Perinatol*. 1989;9:448–450.
19. Newman A. *The Illustrated Treasury of Medical Curiosa*. New York: McGraw-Hill; 1988:226,294.
20. Manley JL, Levine MS. The homeo box and mammalian development. *Cell*. 1985;43:1–2.
21. Gehring WJ. The homeo box: a key to the understanding of development? *Cell*. 1985;43:3–5.
22. Gehring WJ, Hiromi Y. Homeotic genes and the homeobox. *Annu Rev Genet*. 1986;20:147–173.
23. Smith D, Majmudar B. Teratoma of umbilical cord. *Hum Pathol*. 1985;16:190–193.
24. Fox H, Butler-Manuel R. A teratoma of the placenta. *J Pathol Bact*. 1964;88:137–140.
25. Fujikura T, Wellings SR. A teratoma like mass in the placenta of a malformed infant. *Am J Obstet Gynecol*. 1964;89:824–825.
26. Nickell KA, Stocker JT. Placental teratoma: a case report. *Pediatr Pathol*. 1987;7:645–650.
27. Stephens TD, Spall R, Urfer AG, Martin R. Fetus amorphus or placental teratoma? *Teratology*. 1989; 40:1–10.
28. Kerr MG, Rashad MN. Autosomal trisomy in a discordant monozygotic twin. *Nature*. 1966; 212:726–727.
29. Gross RE, Clatworthy HW. Twin fetuses in fetu. *J Pediatr*. 1951;38:502–508.
30. Janovski NA. Fetus in fetu. *J Pediatr*. 1962; 61:100–104.
31. Boyce MJ, Lockyer JW, Wood CBS. Foetus in foetu: serologic assessment of monozygotic origin by automated analysis. *J Clin Pathol*. 1972;25: 793–798.
32. Kakizoe T, Tahara M. Fetus in fetu located in the scrotal sac of a newborn infant: a case report. *J Urol*. 1972;107:506–508.
33. Afshar F, King TT, Berry CL. Intraventricular fetus in fetu. *J Neurosurg*. 1982;56:845–849.
34. Chi JG, Lee YS, Park YS, Chang KY. Fetus-in-fetu: report of a case. *Am J Clin Pathol*. 1984; 82:115–119.
35. Yasuda Y, Mitomori T, Matsuura A, Tanimura T.

Fetus in fetu: report of a case. *Teratology*. 1985; 31:337–344.

36. Alpers CE, Harrison MR. Fetus in fetu associated with an undescended testis. *Pediatr Pathol*. 1985;4:37–46.

37. Martinez-Urrutia MJ, Pereira PL, Lassaletta L, Gracia R, Utrilla J. Abdominal mass: "fetus in fetu." *Acta Pediatr Scand*. 1990;79:121–122.

38. Ornoy A, Navot D, Menashi M, Laufer N, Chemke J. Asymmetry and discordance for congenital anomalies in conjoined twins: a report of six cases. *Teratology*. 1980;22:145–154.

39. Drut RM, Drut R, Fontana A, Grosso JJ. Mature presacral sacrococcygeal teratoma associated with a sacral "epignathus." *Pediatr Pathol*. 1992;12:99–103.

40. Rowe MI, Ravitch MM, Ranniger K. Operative correction of caudal duplication (dipygus). *Surgery*. 1968;63:840–848.

41. Simpson JS, Gibson DA, Cook GT. Surgical correction of caudal duplication (dipygus). *J Pediatr Surg*. 1973;8:935–938.

42. Spitz L, Rickwood AMK, Pilling D. Dipygus (caudal duplication). *J Pediatr Surg*. 1979;14:557–560.

43. Braun P, Addor C, Cuendet A. Surgical correction of caudal duplication. *J Pediatr Surg*. 1979;14:561–563.

44. Sathiakumar N, Ifere OAS, Salawu SAI, Mbamali EI. Heteropagus: a case report. *Ann Trop Pediatr*. 1988;8:38–41.

45. Stephens TD, Siebert JR, Graham JM Jr, Beckwith JB. Parasitic conjoined twins, two cases, and their relation to limb morphogenesis. *Teratology*. 1982; 26:115–121.

46. Yasuda Y, Ohtsuki H, Torii S, Tomoyoshi E, Clark CF. Epigastrius with oomphalocoele—report of a case. *Teratology*. 1984;30:297–309.

47. Takayanagi K. A rare case of caudal duplication. *J Pediatr Surg*. 1991;26:228–229.

48. Husain AN, Muraskas J, Lambert G, Dado D, Lynch J. Parasitic conjoined twins with oomphalo-coele and tetralogy of Fallot. *Pediatr Pathol*. 1989;9:321–328.

49. Silbermann M, Bar-Maor JA, Auslander L. Craniofacial microsomia in a parasite of a heteropagus conjoined twin: a clinical and histopathologic evaluation. *Head Neck Surg*. 1984;6:792–800.

50. Antunes JL, Sharer LR, Pellock JM. Occipital encephalocoele—a case of conjoined twinning? *Neurosurgery*. 1983;13:703–707.

51. Chen W-J, Chen K-M, Chen M-T, Liu T-K, Chu S-H, Tsai FC, Hwang F-Y. Emergency separation of omphaloischiopagus tetrapus conjoined twins in

the newborn period. *J Pediatr Surg*. 1989;24: 1221–1224.

52. Barr M Jr. Facial duplication: case, review and embryogenesis. *Teratology*. 1982;25:153–159.

53. Chervenak FA, Pinto MM, Heller CI, Norooz H. Obstetric significance of fetal craniofacial duplication. A case report. *J Reprod Med*. 1985;30:74–76.

54. Amatuzio JC, Gorlin RJ. Conjoined acardiac monsters. *Arch Pathol Lab Med*. 1981;105:253–255.

55. Napolitani FD, Schreiber I. The acardiac monster. A review of the world literature and presentation of 2 cases. *Am J Obstet Gynecol*. 1960;80:582–589.

56. Warkany J. *Congenital Malformations.*. Chicago: Year Book Medical Publishers; 1971:474.

57. Lindahl SA, Baldwin VJ, Wakeford J, Wittmann BK. Early diagnosis of an acardiac acephalus twin by ultrasound. *Med Ultrasound*. 1984;8:105–107.

58. Fox H. Pathology of the Placenta. Vol 7. *Major Problems in Pathology,* Bennington JL, ed. London: WB Saunders; 1978:73–94.

59. Sanfilippo J, Bianchine JQ, Walsh A, Badawy S. Acardius myelacephalus. Two monsters in a triplet pregnancy. *NY State J Med*. 1979;79:P245–247.

60. Simonds JP, Gowen GA. Fetus amorphus (report of a case). *Surg Gynecol Obstet*. 1925;41:171–179.

61. Sato T, Kaneko K, Konuma S, Sato I, Tamada T. Acardiac anomalies: review of 88 cases in Japan. *Asia Oceana J Obstet Gynecol*. 1984;10:45–52.

62. Auerback P, Wiglesworth FW. Congenital absence of the heart: observation of a human funiculopagus twinning with insertiofuniculi furcata, fusion, forking and interposito velamentosa. *Teratology*. 1978;17:143–150.

63. van Allen MI. Fetal vascular disruptions: mechanisms and some resulting birth defects. *Pediatr Ann*. 1981;10:219–233.

64. Stephens TD. Muscle abnormalities associated with the twin-reversed-arterial-perfusion (TRAP) sequence (acardia). *Teratology*. 1984;30:311–318.

65. Ketchum J, Motyloff L. Chorangiopagus parasiticus (Schwalbe). Report of a case of acardius acephalus and of a case of fetus amorphus. *Am J Obstet Gynecol*. 1957;73:1349–1354.

66. Price B. Primary biases in twin studies—a review of prenatal and natal difference-producing factors in monozygotic pairs. *Am J Hum Genet*. 1950; 2:293–352.

67. Severn CB, Holyoke EA. Human acardiac anomalies. *Am J Obstet Gynecol*. 1973;116:358–365.

68. Kyriazis A, Arean VM, Shanklin DR. Placental-radiographic analysis of parasitic acardiac fetus: partially common umbilical circulation. *J Reprod Med*. 1974;12:74–81.

69. Benirschke K, Des Roches Harper V. The acardiac anomaly. *Teratology*. 1977;15:311–316.

70. Kaplan C, Benirschke K. The acardiac anomaly. New case reports and current status. *Acta Genet Med Gemellol*. 1979;28:51–59.

71. Deacon JS, Machin GA, Martin JME, Nicholson S, Nwankwo DC, Wintemute R. Investigation of acephalus. *Am J Med Genet*. 1980;5:85–99.

72. Scott JM, Ferguson-Smith MA. Heterokaryotypic monozygotic twins and the acardiac monster. *J Obstet Gynecol Br Cwlth*. 1973;80:52–59.

73. Wolf HK, MacDonald J, Bradford WB, Lahman JT. Acardius anceps with evidence of intrauterine vascular occlusion: report of a case and discussion of pathogenesis. *Pediatr Pathol*. 1991;11:143–152.

74. van Allen MI, Smith DW, Shepard TH. Twin reversed arterial perfusion (TRAP) sequence: a study of 14 twin pregnancies with acardius. *Semin Perinatol*. 1983;7:285–293.

75. Moore CA, Buehler BA, McManus BM, Harmon JP, Mirkin LD, Goldstein DJ. Brief clinical report: acephalus-acardia in twins with aneuploidy. *Am J Med Genet Suppl*. 1987;3:139–143.

76. Bhatnagar KP, Sharma SC, Bisker J. The holoacardius: a correlative computerized tomographic, radiologic, and ultrasonographic investigation of a new case with review of literature. *Acta Genet Med Gemellol*. 1986;35:77–89.

77. Bieber FR, Nance WE, Morton CC, Brown JA, Redwine FO, Jordan RL, Mohanakumar T. Genetic studies of an acardiac monster: evidence of polar body twinning in man. *Science*. 1981;213:775–777.

78. Campbell M, Shepherd HD. The circulatory and anatomical abnormalities of an acardiac fetus of rare form. *Lancet*. 1905;Sept 30:941–944.

79. Leroy F. Major fetal hazzards in multiple pregnancy. *Acta Genet Med Gemellol*. 1976;25:299–306.

80. Gessner IH. Spectrum of congenital cardiac anomalies produced in chick embryos by mechanical interference with cardiogenesis. *Circ Res*. 1966;18:625–633.

81. Keith L. Holoacardius. *J Reprod Med*. 1974;12:82–85.

82. Nerlich A, Wisser J, Draeger A, Nathrath W, Remberger K. Human acardiac anomaly: a report of three cases. *Eur J Obstet Gynecol Reprod Biol*. 1990;38:79–85.

83. Svejda J. A case of foetus pseudo-amorphus. *J Pathol Bact*. 1947;59:647–655.

84. Gewolb IH, Freedman RM, Kleinman CS, Hobbins JC. Prenatal diagnosis of a human pseudo-

85. James WH. A note on the epidemiology of acardiac monsters. *Teratology*. 1978;16:211–216.

86. Benirschke K, Driscoll SG. *The Pathology of the Human Placenta*. New York: Springer-Verlag; 1967:166–168.

87. Draeger A, Nerlich A. Syndrome des bandes amniotiques associe a une malformation acardiaque observe dans une grossesse gemellaire. A propos d'un cas. *Ann Pathol*. 1988;8:317–320.

88. Benirschke K. Lessons from multiple pregnancies in mammals. In: Gedda L, Parisi P, Nance WE, eds. Twin Research 3: Twin Biology and Multiple Pregnancy. *Prog Clin Biol Res*. 1981;69A:135–139.

89. Richart R, Benirschke K. Holoacardius amorphus. Report of a case with chromosomal analysis. *Am J Obstet Gynecol*. 1963;86:329–332.

90. Imai A, Hirose R, Kawabata I, Tamaya T. Acardiac acephalic monster extremely larger than the co-twin. A case report. *Gynecol Obstet Invest*. 1991;32:62–64.

91. Lachman R, McNabb M, Furmanski M, Karp L. The acardiac monster. *Eur J Pediatr*. 1980;134:195–200.

92. Genest DR, Lage JM. Absence of normal-appearing proximal tubules in the fetal and neonatal kidney: prevalence and significance. *Hum Pathol*. 1991;22:147–153.

93. Weissberg SM. Fetus acardius. *J Reprod Med*. 1974;12:71–73.

94. Harkavy KL, Scanlon JW. Hydrops fetalis in a parabiotic acardiac twin. *Am J Dis Child*. 1978;132:638–639.

95. Royston D, Geoghegan F. Disseminated arterial calcification associated with acardius acephalus. *Arch Dis Child*. 1983;58:641–643.

96. Popek EJ, Strain JD, Neumann A, Wilson H. In utero development of pulmonary artery calcification in monochorionic twins: report of three cases (Abstract). *Mod Pathol*. 1990;3:7P. (Poster—Society for Pediatric Pathology, Boston 1990.)

97. Schinzel AAGL, Smith DW, Miller JR. Monozygotic twinning and structural defects. *J Pediatr*. 1979;95:921–930.

98. Billah KL, Shah K, Odwin C. Ultrasound diagnosis and management of acardius anencephalic twin pregnancy. *Med Ultrasound*. 1984;8:108–109.

99. Stiller RJ, Romero R, Pace S, Hobbins JC. Prenatal identification of twin reversed arterial perfusion syndrome in the first trimester. *Am J Obstet Gynecol*. 1989;160:1194–1196.

100. Gibson JY, D'Cruz CA, Patel RB, Palmer SM.

Acardiac anomaly: review of the subject with case report and emphasis on practical sonography. *J Clin Ultrasound*. 1986;14:541–545.

101. Kirkinen P, Herva R, Räsänen J, Airaksinen J, Ikaheimo M. Documentation of paradoxical umbilical blood supply of an acardiac twin in the antepartum state. *J Perinat Med*. 1989;17:63–65.

102. Benson CB, Bieber FR, Genest DR, Doubilet PM. Doppler demonstration of reversed umbilical blood flow in an acardiac twin. *J Clin Ultrasound*. 1989;17:291–295.

103. Sherer DM, Armstrong B, Shah YG, Metlay LA, Woods JR Jr. Prenatal sonographic diagnosis, Doppler velocimetric umbilical cord studies and subsequent management of an acardiac twin pregnancy. *Obstet Gynecol*. 1989;74:472–475.

104. Harger JH, Doshi N, Marchese S, Hinkle RS, Garver KL. Increased amnionic fluid alpha-fetoprotein due to a holoacardius amorphus twin. *Clin Genet*. 1981;19:257–261.

105. Read AP, Donnai D, Tracey J, Fennell SJ. Increased amniotic alphafetoprotein due to a holoacardius amorphus twin. *Clin Genet*. 1982;21:382–383.

106. Moore TR, Gale S, Benirschke K. Perinatal outcome of forty-nine pregnancies complicated by acardiac twinning. *Am J Obstet Gynecol*. 1990;163:907–912.

107. Simpson PC, Trudinger BJ, Walker A, Baird PJ. The intrauterine treatment of fetal cardiac failure in a twin pregnancy with an acardiac, acephalic monster. *Am J Obstet Gynecol*. 1983;147:842–844.

108. Ash K, Harman CR, Gritter H. TRAP sequence—successful outcome with indomethacin treatment. *Obstet Gynecol*. 1990;76:960–962.

109. Thomas B, Buderus S, Gembruch U. Is the 'safety' of indomethacin treatment of polyhydramnios in the mother to be questioned? (Abstract). *Fetal Diagn Ther*. 1991;6:174.

110. Platt LD, DeVore GR, Bieniarz A, Benner P, Rao R. Antenatal diagnosis of acephalus acardia: a proposed management scheme. *Am J Obstet Gynecol*. 1983;146:857–859.

111. Porrero RP, Barton SM, Haverkamp AD. Occlusion of umbilical artery in acardiac acephalic twin. *Lancet* 1991;337:326–327.

112. Robie GF, Payne GG, Morgan MA. Selective delivery of an acardiac acephalic twin. *N Engl J Med*. 1989;320:512–513.

113. Fries MH, Goldberg JD, Golbus MS. Treatment of acardiac-acephalus twin gestation by hysterotomy and selective delivery. *Obstet Gynecol*. 1992;79:601–604.

114. Ginsberg NA, Applebaum M, Rabin SA, Caffarelli MA, Kuuspalu M, Daskal JL, Verlinsky Y, Strom CM, Barton JJ. Term birth after midtrimester hysterotomy and selective delivery of an acardiac twin. *Am J Obstet Gynecol*. 1992;167:33–37.

115. Benirschke K. The pathophysiology of the twinning process. In: Iffy L, Kaminetzky HA, eds. *Principles and Practice of Obstetrics and Perinatology*. New York: John Wiley; 1981:1165–1170.

116. Shaw CE. Split personality. The two-headed snake. *Zoonooz*. 1954;27:4.

117. The strangest thing. *The Globe and Mail*. 1986; Sept 24:48.

118. Warkany J. *Congenital Malformations*. Chicago: Year Book Medical Publishers; 1971:6–9.

119. Gedda L. *Twinning in History and Science*. Springfield: Charles C Thomas; 1961:106–118.

120. Newman HH. *Multiple Human Births*. New York: Doubleday, Doran; 1940:60–74.

121. Guttmacher AF. Biographical notes on some famous conjoined twins. *Birth Defects*. 1967;3(1): 10–17.

122. Annas GJ. Siamese twins: killing one to save the other. *Hastings Cent Rep*. 1987;17:27–29.

123. Pepper CK. Ethical and moral considerations in the separation of conjoined twins. *Birth Defects*. 1967;3(1):128–134.

124. Votteler TP. Conjoined twins. In: Welch KJ, Randolph JG, Ravich MM, O'Neill JA, Rowe MI, eds. *Pediatric Surgery*. 4th ed. Vol 2. Chicago: Year Book Medical Publishers; 1986:771–779.

125. Nichols BL, Blattner RJ, Rudolph AJ. General clinical management of thoracopagus twins. *Birth Defects*. 1967;3(1):38–51.

126. Ripman HA. Conjoined twins as an obstetric problem. *Guy's Hosp Rep*. 1958;107:173–184.

127. Maggio M, Callan NA, Hamod KA, Sanders RC. The first trimester ultrasonographic diagnosis of conjoined twins. *Am J Obstet Gynecol*. 1985; 152:833–835.

128. Turner RJ, Hankins GDU, Weinreb JC, Ziaya PR, Davis TN, Lowe TW, Gilstrap LC. Magnetic resonance imaging and ultrasonography in the antenatal evaluation of conjoined twins. *Am J Obstet Gynecol*. 1986;155:645–649.

129. Sanders SP, Chin AJ, Parness IA, Benacerraf B, Greene MF, Epstein MF, Colan SD, Frigoletto FD. Prenatal diagnosis of congenital heart defects in thoracoabdominally conjoined twins. *N Engl J Med*. 1985;313:370–374.

130. Sakala EP. Obstetric management of conjoined twins. *Obstet Gynecol*. 1986;67:21S-25S.

131. Filler RM. Conjoined twins and their separation. *Semin Perinatol*. 1986;10:82–91.

132. O'Neill JA, Holcomb GW, Schnaufer L, Temple-

ton JM, Bishop HC, Ross AJ, Duckett JW, Norwood WI, Ziegler MM, Koop CE. Surgical experience with thirteen conjoined twins. *Ann Surg.* 1988;208:299–312.

133. Bergsma D, Blattner RJ, Nichols BL, Rudolph AJ. Conjoined twins. *Birth Defects.* 1967;3(1):1–147.

134. Viljoen DL, Nelson MM, Beighton P. The epidemiology of conjoined twinning in southern Africa. *Clin Genet.* 1983;24:15–21.

135. Rudolph AJ, Michaels JP, Nichols BL. Obstetric management of conjoined twins. *Birth Defects.* 1967;3(1):28–57.

136. Benirschke K, Kim CK. Multiple pregnancy. *N Engl J Med.* 1973;288:1276–1284,1329–1336.

137. Myrianthopoulos MC. Congenital malformations in twins: epidemiologic survey. *Birth Defects.* 1975;11(8):1–39.

138. Edmunds LD, Layde PM. Conjoined twins in the United States, 1970–1977. *Teratology.* 1982;25:301–308.

139. Imaizumi Y. Conjoined twins in Japan, 1979–1985. *Acta Genet Med Gemellol.* 1988;37:339–345.

140. Källén B, Rybo G. Conjoined twinning in Sweden. *Acta Genet Med Gemellol.* 1978;57:257–259.

141. Métneki J, Czeuzel A. Conjoined twins in Hungary, 1970–1986. *Acta Genet Med Gemellol.* 1989;38:285–299.

142. Tan KL, Goon SM, Salmon Y, Wee JH. Conjoined twins. *Acta Obstet Gynecol Scand.* 1971;50:373–380.

143. Emanuel I, Huang SW, Gutman LT, Yu FC, Linn CC. The incidence of congenital malformations in a Chinese population: The Taipei collaborative study. *Teratology.* 1972;5:159–169.

144. Tan K-L, Tock EPC, Dawood MY, Ratnam SS. Conjoined twins in a triplet pregnancy. *Am J Dis Child.* 1971;122:455–458.

145. Aird I. Conjoined twins—further observations. *Br Med J.* 1959;1:1313–1315.

146. Jaschevatzky OE, Goldman B, Kampf D, Wexler H, Grunstein S. Etiologic aspects of double monsters. *Eur J Obstet Gynecol Reprod Biol.* 1980;10:343–349.

147. Hamon A, Dinno N. Dicephalus dipus tribrachius conjoined twins in a female infant. *Birth Defects.* 1978;14(6A):213–218.

148. Milham S Jr. Symmetrical conjoined twins: an analysis of the birth records of twenty-two sets. *J Pediatr.* 1966;69:643–647.

149. Offringa PJ, Wildschut HIJ, Tutein Nolthenius-Puylaert MCBJE, Leon S, Boersma ER. Conjoined twins and abdominal pregnancy. *Int J Gynecol Obstet.* 1989;30:73–76.

150. Benirschke K, Temple WW, Bloor CM. Conjoined twins: nosology and congenital malformations. *Birth Defects.* 1978;14(6A):179–192.

151. Rosa FW. Twins, conjoined, teratogenicity. In: Buyse ML, ed. *Birth Defects Encyclopedia.* Cambridge, MA: Blackwell Scientific; 1990:1721–1722.

152. Guttmacher AF, Nichols BL. Teratology of conjoined twins. *Birth Defects.* 1967;3(1):3–9.

153. Ingalls TH, Bazemore MK. Prenatal events antedating the birth of thoracopagus twins. *Arch Environ Health.* 1969;19:358–364.

154. Zimmerman AA. Embryologic and anatomic consideration of conjoined twins. *Birth Defects.* 1967;3:18–27.

155. Herring SW, Rowlatt UF. Anatomy and embryology in cephalothoracopagus twins. *Teratology.* 1981;23:159–173.

156. Machin GA, Sperber GH. Invited editorial comment: lessons from conjoined twins. *Am J Med Genet.* 1987;28:89–97.

157. Spencer R. Conjoined twins: theoretical embryologic basis. *Teratology.* 1992;29:181–184.

158. Singer DB, Rosenberg HS. Pathologic studies of thoracopagus conjoined twins. *Birth Defects.* 1967;3(1):97–105.

159. Marin-Padilla M, Chin AJ, Marin-Padilla TM. Cardiovascular abnormalities in thoracopagus twins. *Teratology.* 1981;23:101–113.

160. Grosse B. Siamese twins born pregnant. *Sun.* 1989;7(47):1,17.

161. Seo JW, Lee YS, Chi JG. Cross-sectional illustration on major types of conjoined twins. *J Korean Med Sci.* 1988;3:19–25.

162. Merwin MC, Wright J. Lateral cephalothoracopagus: a case report. *Teratology.* 1984;29:181–184.

163. Harper RG, Kenigsberg K, Sia CG, Horn D, Stern D, Bongiovi V. Xiphopagus conjoined twins: a 300–year review of the obstetric, morphopathologic, neonatal and surgical parameters. *Am J Obstet Gynecol.* 1980;137:617–629.

164. Ursell PC, Wigger HJ. Asplenia syndrome in conjoined twins: a case report. *Teratology.* 1983;27:301–304.

165. Zake EZN. Case reports of 16 sets of conjoined twins from a Uganda hospital. *Acta Genet Med Gemellol.* 1984;33:75–80.

166. Little J, Bryan EM. Congenital Anomalies. In: MacGillivray I, Campbell DM, Thompson B, eds. *Twinning and Twins.* Chichester: John Wiley; 1988:213–217.

167. Delprado WJ, Baird PJ. Cephalothoracopagus syncephalus: a case report with previously unreported anatomical abnormalities and chromosomal analysis. *Teratology.* 1984;29:1–9.

168. Baron BW, Shermeta DW, Ismail MA, Ben-Ami T, Yousefzadeh D, Carlson N, Amarose AP, Esterley JR. Unique anomalies in cephalothoracopagus janiceps conjoined twins with implications for multiple mechanisms in the abnormal embryogenesis. *Teratology*. 1990;41:9–22.

169. Winston KR, Rockoff MA, Mulliken JB, Strand RD, Murray JE. Surgical division of craniopagi. *Neurosurgery*. 1987;21:782–791.

170. Bucholz RD, Yoon K-W, Shively RE. Temporoparietal craniopagus. Case report and review of the literature. *J Neurosurg*. 1987;66:72–79.

171. Konstantinova BL. Morphological and cytogenetic studies on conjoined twins. *Acta Genet Med Gemellol*. 1976;25:55–58.

172. Siebert JR, Machin GA, Sperber GH. Anatomic findings in dicephalic conjoined twins: implications for morphogenesis. *Teratology*. 1989;40:305–310.

173. Gupta JM. Pyopagus conjoined twins. *Br Med J*. 1966;2:868–871.

174. Albert MC, Drummond DS, O'Neill J, Watts H. The orthopedic management of conjoined twins: a review of 13 cases and report of 4 cases. *J Pediatr Orthop*. 1992;2:300–307.

175. Wiegenstein L, Iozzo RV. Unusual findings in a conjoined ("Siamese") twin placenta. *Am J Obstet Gynecol*. 1980;137:744–745.

176. Bardawil WA, Reddy RL, Bardawil LW. Placental considerations in multiple pregnancy. *Clin Perinatol*. 1988;15(1):28.

177. Leachman RD, Latson JR, Kohler CM, McNamara DG. Cardiovascular evaluation of conjoined twins. *Birth Defects*. 1967;3(1):52–65.

178. Izukawa T, Kidd BSL, Moes CAF, Tyrrell MJ, Ives EJ, Simpson JS, Shandling B. Assessment of the cardiovascular system in conjoined thoracopagus twins. *Am J Dis Child*. 1978;132:19–24.

179. Gerlis LM, Seo J-W, Ho SY, Chi JEG. Morphology of the cardiovascular system in conjoined twins: spatial and sequential segmental arrangements in 36 cases. *Teratology*. 1993;47:91–108.

180. Seo JW, Shin SS, Chi JG. Cardiovascular system in conjoined twins: an analysis of 14 Korean cases. *Teratology*. 1985;32:151–161.

181. Walton JM, Gillis DA, Giacomantonio JM, Hayashi AH, Lau HYC. Emergency separation of conjoined twins. *J Pediatr Surg*. 1991;26:1337–1340.

182. Weston PJ, Ives EJ, Honore RLH, Lees GM, Sinclair DB, Schiff D. Monochorionic diamniotic minimally conjoined twins: a case report. *Am J Med Genet*. 1990;37:558–561.

183. Rajadurai VS, Matthai J, Judhau MA. Omphalopagus twins and twin transfusion syndrome. *Indian J Pediatr*. 1988;55:811–816.

184. Wedberg R, Kaplan C, Leopold G, Porreco R, Renik R, Benirschke K. Cephalothoracopagus (Janiceps) twinning. *Obstet Gynecol*. 1979;54:392–396.

185. Riccardi VM, Bergmann CA. Anencephaly with incomplete twinning (diprosopus). *Teratology*. 1977;16:137–140.

11
Triplets and Higher Multiples

All the aspects of multiple gestation that have been presented in the preceding chapters as applying to twins, apply equally to triplets and higher multiples (multiplets),[1] although the permutations and combinations increase with greater numbers of infants. The caveats to the use of triplets and higher multiples in studies of "nature versus nurture" (Chapter 1) are stronger because zygosity determination is a more complex issue, although the means of zygosity determination are the same as with twins (Chapter 2). The relative roles of monovular and polyovular mechanisms of multiple gestation (Chapter 2) are being modified dramatically by the use of drugs that hyperstimulate the ovary, whether natural or in vitro fertilization occurs, because higher multiples seem to be the rule in these cases. This trend is leading to a reassessment of infertility treatment because of the biologic cost to the mother and fetuses,[1] the cost to society of caring for more tiny babies,[2] and the coping stresses for the families.[3,4] Virtually any combination of single-egg or multiple-egg origins of the fetuses can be represented when there are three or more infants. The actual number and zygosity of infants that are born is further modified by fetal death, both spontaneous and induced (Chapter 5). The patterns of placentation of triplets and greater multiples is potentially as complex as the discussion of twin placentas might suggest (Chapter 3), but a measured stepwise approach with accurately labeled diagrams simplifies the interpretation. Obstetric complications (Chapter 4) are more frequent as the number of fetuses increases. Although greater success is being achieved in supporting gestations with relatively large numbers of infants, prematurity (Chapter 4)

and low birth weight (Chapter 6) are greater problems when there are more than two infants in the uterus. Considerations of anomalies, disorders, and diseases in triplets and higher multiples are basically the same as with twins (Chapters 6 and 7). Also, the lesions of monochorionic monozygosity (Chapters 8, 9, and 10) are just as relevant, and some of the patterns of incomplete or aberrant twinning are actually relatively more common in cases of three fetuses in one gestation.

In the following discussion, triplets are considered in more detail than the higher multiples because of their greater frequency. Information from the literature is augmented with case material from the Survey '91 Review of placentas from surviving multiplets, and autopsies of one or more fetuses or infants from multiplet conceptions. Although the number of cases was not as great as the number of twins that were available for review, the data are presented in some detail as a possible starting point for other reviews in the future, because more information is needed. The emphasis is on features that are or may be particular to the multiplet nature of the conception.

Triplets

There are several problems encountered when one tries to assess the pathology of triplet conceptions specifically. First, triplets occur far less often than twins, and the literature reflects the resultant greater difficulty assessing the same characteristics and relationships that have been reported in such detail for twins in the preceding chapters in this volume.

Second, the advent of assisted reproduction technologies has had a particular impact on the incidence and management of triplet gestations, rendering the statistical rates observed in earlier reports, even when well documented, less appropriate to current practice. Within these constraints, the following discussion reviews triplet gestations in a sequence that parallels the review of twins, focusing on reports and findings related to the "tripletness" of the conception. Relevant details from triplets in the Survey '91 Review are included.

Rates and Origins

The reported rates of occurrence of triplets are difficult to correlate into meaningful generalizations for three reasons. First, depending on the source of data, racial factors are important determinants of triplet zygosity and hence rates,[5] as noted with twins. Reported rates of triplets have ranged from 1 : 612 deliveries in the Yoruba tribe in western Nigeria[6] and 1 : 1,014 deliveries in eastern Nigeria,[7] to 1 : 9,524 in Japan,[8] with rates in the United States ranging from 1 : 1,300 in the southeastern area[9] to 1 : 10,000 in Chicago[9] and in the Collaborative Perinatal Project.[10] Second, almost all reported rates are of triplet deliveries, not triplet conceptions, so the rates of fetal mortality are bypassed. It has been suggested that as many as one-third of spontaneous triplets actually deliver as singletons, but that estimate was made before the routine use of ultrasound.[11] Rates of fetal triplet mortality based on early ultrasound diagnosis of three sacs with fetal heart motions range from 7.7% loss of all three, to 15% loss of two, and 43% loss of one conceptus by 20 weeks' gestation.[12] It is true that these data are from artificially induced multiplets, but they represent the most completely monitored cases and at least are an indication of the possible magnitude of triplet fetal mortality. Third, the increased occurrence of triplets (and higher multiples) after fertility therapies and manipulations is substantial, with reports of up to 83% of triplet deliveries being the result of hormonal ovulation induction.[13] The rate of triplets after in vitro fertilization (IVF) as a contribution to the number of triplets overall cannot be determined from the reported cases, but it does not seem to be as great a proportion. Triplets after IVF occur either from an original triplet conception, or as a result of spontaneous or induced embryofetal loss from a higher multiple.

The possible embryologic origin of triplets is simply an expansion of the possibilities with twins—trizygotic, dizygotic with one zygote providing a monozygotic pair, or monozygotic with twin conceptuses initially, one of which goes through the twinning process again. Systematic zygosity studies of triplets do not appear to have been reported, so that relative rates of the three zygosity patterns are not documented. A statistical estimate, with all the caveats entailed when dealing with small numbers, suggested that dizygotic sets were two to three times as common as either monozygotic or trizygotic sets in the United States and Australia, prior to the use of the new fertility technologies.[5] In a slightly later period in Japan, monozygotic sets were estimated to be about three times as common as dizygotic sets, with trizygotic sets the least common.[5] In contrast, in the same period, the estimate in Nigeria was a combined ratio of monozygotic to dizygotic to trizygotic sets of 1 : 4 : 6.[5] These estimates appear to reflect the racial factors already noted with twins, and the other factors that influence the different twinning processes are discussed in Chapter 2. Spontaneous triplets are sufficiently uncommon that specific epidemiologic associations have not been made beyond a possibly familial neuroendocrine predisposition to multizygotic conceptions.[14]

While it is true that the pathologist has only a partial perspective on rates of triplets, some idea of the load to the laboratory may be of interest. In the Survey '91 Review, one triplet placenta with survival of all infants was seen for every 19 twin placentas where both survived, and there was one triplet set where one or more came to autopsy for every 14 twin sets beyond 20 weeks' gestation where one or more came to autopsy.

Placentation

Examination of triplet placentation is basically no different than of twin placentation, the process simply is extended to include one more set of observations. The procedure has been described in Chapter 3, and there are two key components that warrant particular emphasis when applying the process to triplets—accurate identification of the

FIGURE 11.1. Example of physical setup to examine triplet placentation analogous to the methods described for twin placentas in Chapter 3. Note identification of umbilical cords by 1, 2, and 3 suture ties to indicate birth order.

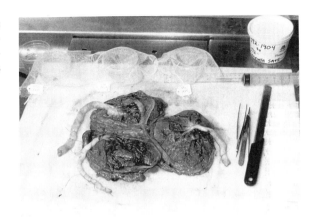

cords, and a systematic stepwise approach to the dissection (Fig. 11.1). The description of the pattern of separating membranes may include up to three relationships, depending on the chorionicity and fusion of the chorionic masses. The patterns of cord insertions and chorionic vascularity, and the proportion of chorionic surface area for each triplet are as important as with twins. In cases with the potential for intertriplet vascular anastomoses, i.e., monoamniotic or diamniotic placentations, the injection and documentation techniques are the same as for twins, with care needed to keep precise track of which vessels belong to which infant. Photographs and line drawings can be invaluable in cases that have a number of important findings.

The *pattern of placentation* in triplets ranges from one disk with a single inner layer of amnion and one outer chorionic shell, monochorionic monoamniotic,[15] to three separate disks and gestational sacs, trichorionic triamniotic.[9] As can be seen from Fig. 11.2, trichorionic membranes are the most frequent, and two separate disks are more common than single or triple masses. When two disks are present, the double disk is twice as likely to be dichorionic as monochorionic. The numbers are too small to make any further comments, except to note the relative prominence of monochorionic disks among the sets where one or more of the triplets comes to autopsy, analogous to the trend observed with twins. The rather different distributions of chorionic patterns noted in Fig. 11.2, based on data in the references cited,[16–19] exemplify the difficulties of collating reported triplet data. The orientations of the three placental masses to each other when fused can vary from side by side, to

wedges of a more circular mass, as displayed by the examples in Fig. 11.3. It can be seen from even these few examples that chorionicity is not predictable from the arrangements of the respective fetal masses, except that monochorionic doubles or triples are fused.

Zygosity assignment related to placentation is not usually assessed specifically in the literature. Monozygosity is usually inferred from monochorionicity, whatever the patterns of amnion, and dizygosity from unlike sex. Same-sex triplets in dichorionic sets, and same-sex pairs and triplets in trichorionic sets require more specific testing as noted in Chapter 2. Based on membrane patterns and recorded fetal sex in the Survey '91 Review cases, at least 68% of the survivor group sets and 56% of the autopsy group sets would have needed additional tests to determine zygosity, a greater proportion than with twins because of the added permutations due to the third conceptus. In one triplet set of three females with dichorionic triamniotic placentation with two disks (Fig. 9.9), the triplet with the separate disk had differently shaped hands and feet and was documented to be blood group O Rh+, and the monochorionic twins were both A Rh+.

Because the numbers were too small, correlation of the pattern of placentation with assisted fertility therapies was not possible from the Survey '91 Review cases. All known hormonally induced polyovulations (all but one with clomiphene), and all known IVF sets were trichorionic, with one-, two-, and three-disk patterns seen, and no predominance of any combinations of fetal sex.

There were additional placental findings reported

Number of disks*	Membrane patterns*											
	TCTA		S	A	DCTA		S	A	MCTA	S	A	DCDA	S	A

Number of disks*	TCTA		DCTA		MCTA		DCDA	
	S	A	S	A	S	A	S	A
1	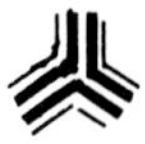 5	3	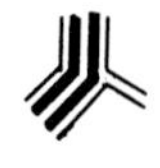 6	1	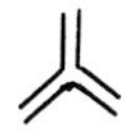 5	4	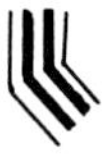 1	1
2	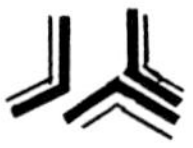 18	0	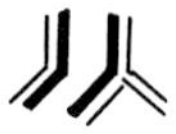 11	3				
3	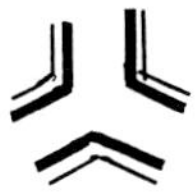 3	3						
Totals†	53.0	33.3	34.7	27.8	10.2	22.2	2.0	5.5

References**

	TCTA	DCTA	MCTA
(16)	75	8	17
(17)	67	33	—
(18)	42	42	16
(19)	12.5	37.5	50

TCTA, trichorionic triamniotic; DCTA, dichorionic triamniotic; MCTA, monochorionic triamniotic; DCDA, dichorionic diamniotic, i.e., one monoamniotic pair; S, Survivor group, Survey '91 Review; A; Autopsy group, Survey '91 Review.

Note: In drawings, the zone represented is the junction of the chorionic sacs from each triplet; immediately adjacent lines suggest the membranes are apposed, where the lines are separated this is meant to represent distinct gestational sacs; heavy line represents chorion, fine line represents amnion.

*Numbers in disk/membrane grid are actual numbers of triplet sets with patterns indicated.

†Percentage of each membrane pattern among all triplet sets in survivor group and autopsy group from Survey '91 Review; is less than 100% in the autopsy group because of incomplete information on a few cases.

**Distribution of membrane patterns reported in references noted in percentages.

FIGURE 11.2. Patterns of placentation in triplets.

in both the survivor group and autopsy group triplets from the Survey '91 Review. *Umbilical cord anomalies* were described more commonly than with twins (Fig. 11.4). Compared to the data in Table 3.3, of 147 surviving triplets, 14.3% had a marginal insertion of the cord, 12.2% had a velamentous insertion (up to 17 cm from the placental margin), and one triplet had a two vessel cord. Compared to Table 3.4, 46.4% of the trichorionic placentas (most commonly the two-disk pattern), 64.7% of the dichorionic triamniotic placentas (both forms), and 60% of the monochorionic triamniotic placentas had cord anomalies when all three triplets survived. Of the affected sets, 55.5% had only one cord anomaly, two sets had all three cord insertions affected (marginal/marginal/velamentous in a dichorionic triamniotic single disk, and all cords with marginal insertions in a dichorionic triamniotic single disk), and the remainder had

combinations of marginal and/or velamentous insertions in equal numbers. The data for the triplets from the autopsy group were incomplete, but at least one-third of the sets had one or more cord anomalies reported, more than half consisting of velamentous insertions. At least 18% of the autopsied triplets had cord anomalies—velamentous insertions, abnormally long cords, and one single-artery cord. It is interesting to note that while velamentous and marginal insertions were more common with triplets than twins, single umbilical artery cords were recorded less often. If this is a real difference, its significance remains to be determined. In 14.2% of the live-born triplet placentations, there were intramembranous vessels looping from the cord insertion site for one of the triplets in each set. These were distinct from those cases with intramembranous vessels associated with velamentous cord insertions. This means that at least 17% of

FIGURE 11.3. Selected examples of triplet placenta patterns. (a) Trichorionic triamniotic single disk—cords had been marked with safety pins, trimmed weight 785 g. Note labeling of umbilical cords with tags on specimen, thick baselines of attachment of dichorionic diamniotic septa between triplets, and accessory lobe triplet A. This was the eighth pregnancy (six living) of a 34-year-old mother, delivered at 35 weeks. A—female 2,220 g; B—male, 2,250 g; C—male 1,700 g; zygosity not assessed. Histologically, portion A was immature for dates, portion B normal, portion C quite ischemic—perhaps accounting for the discordant weight. (b) Trichorionic triamniotic placentation with two disks, cords marked with sutures. Single disk for triplet C, male, 2,320 g, trimmed weight 295 g, microscopically normal; double disk A (female, 2,670 g) and B (female, 2,610 g), trimmed weight 840 g, mildly asymmetric surface areas—40% to A, 60% to B, microscopically normal. Elective section at 35 weeks, 35 year old mother with three prior abortions only. Zygosity of A and B not assessed. (c) Dichorionic triamniotic with two disks, cords identified with sutures. In A/B placenta, the separating (histologically proven) diamniotic layer has been rolled to make it more visible. Trimmed weight 785 g, surface equally vascularized from A and B, solitary arterial anastomosis indicated by arrows—note complete lack of relationship of the vascular equator to the attachment zone of the separating membranes; microscopically normal; A—male, 2,590 g, B—male, 2,680 g. Portion C trimmed weight 360 g, male, 2,560 g, zygosity not assessed, histologically normal.

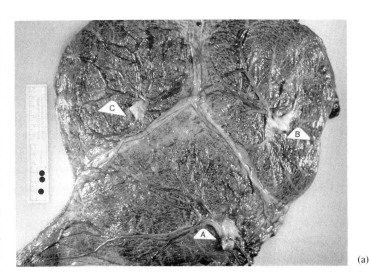

(a)

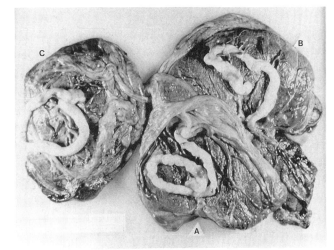

(b)

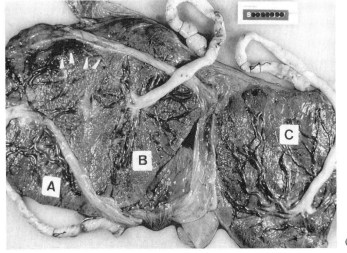

(c)

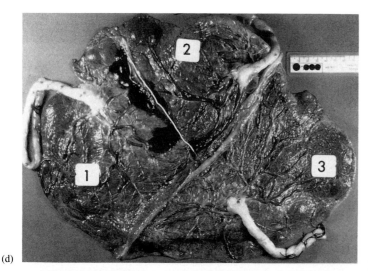

(d)

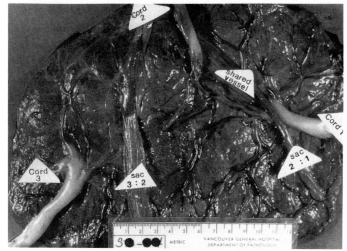

(e)

FIGURE 11.3. *Continued*. (d) Dichorionic triamniotic single disk to compare with (a). Note cords marked. Note prominent baseline for dichorionic diamniotic membranes between triplet 3 (female) and triplets 1 and 2 (males), diamniotic septum line of attachment is indicated with string because it was not prominent enough for the photograph. This was one of the oldest specimens in the series and the dark material is extravasated India ink from injection of anastomoses, one of the problems when using such materials to demonstrate vascular connections. (e) Another example of dichorionic triamniotic single-disk placenta with a different alignment of chorionic masses and membranes. Note alternate way of identifying respective triplet areas and clearly shown vessels. This was the oldest photograph of triplet placentas available from the Survey '91 Review cases, patient data not accessible.

the 147 surviving triplets were theoretically at risk for damage to intramembranous vessels, but in none of these cases was any vascular damage described. It was noted in the discussion of umbilical cord length with twins that the cords are usually shorter than singleton length, but that some of the Survey '91 Review cases had unusually long segments attached to the placenta. With most delivered placentas with surviving infants, the cord length attached to the specimen received is an unknown amount of the total, but there were at least three triplets from different sets with longer than expected cord segments on the placenta—47 to 55 cm at 34 to 35 weeks. Further observations of cord length with triplets may be worthwhile. In the 147 triplets, there was a true knot in only one cord, a hypoplastic umbilical artery in another cord, and moderate to marked cord edema reported in 3.4% of cords.

Vascular anastomoses between the triplets are described below (see Monochorionic Monozygosity), but it can be noted here that they were documented in 94% of monochorionic pairs in dichorionic triamniotic sets, and 80% of monochorionic triamniotic sets in the survivor group, and 60% and 100% of the same respective placental patterns in the autopsy group.

A number of additional gross and microscopic findings were noted that are not necessarily specific to triplet conceptions. Evidence of old premature separation of the placental membranes was recorded in 12.2% of the survivor-group triplet pla-

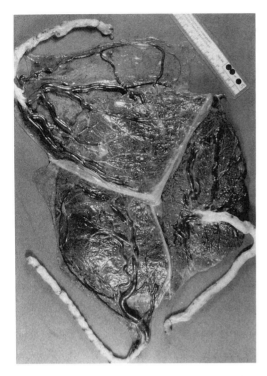

FIGURE 11.4. Example of triplet placenta with cord insertion anomalies. Note the complex velamentous portion of one cord, a less arborized pattern of the other velamentous cord insertion, and normal insertion of the third cord. This was a spontaneous triplet gestation, trichorionic triamniotic, like-sex set at 35 weeks but no other details were available. The cords were not identified at the time of delivery.

oma.[20,21] Both followed gonadotropin stimulation and they terminated spontaneously at 17 weeks and 19 weeks. One was a male/female pair with separate placentas, and the other was a dichorionic diamniotic fused twin placenta with a female/female pair. It is interesting that both these reports come from Japan, where the rate of dizygotic twinning is one of the lowest in the world, and multizygotic triplets are particularly rare.

Obstetric Aspects

As might be expected, all the concerns related to the obstetric aspects of twin pregnancies are equally important or accentuated with triplets. One review noted that triplets are more often in the first completed pregnancy, because up to two thirds of the women had had a history of infertility and required hormonal stimulation to achieve conception.[17] Beyond this difference, there do not appear to be any consistent problems with, or characteristics of, the artificially induced compared to the natural triplet pregnancy.[22] Accurate prenatal diagnosis of triplets using ultrasound requires a thorough examination of the entire uterus to avoid false negatives, and an awareness of scanning artifacts that may create false positives.[23]

Maternal disorders potentially affecting the conceptus have been reviewed in Chapter 4. As with twins, the situation can be complicated by the technical difficulties of assessing and monitoring three fetuses, and the possibility of discordant fetal effects and responses. Reported examples seem to be infrequent, but Rh isoimmunization has been described.[24] No maternal disorders affecting the triplet pregnancy were described in either the survivor or autopsy groups of the Survey '91 Review cases.

Gestational complications of carrying triplets have received the greatest scrutiny in the literature. While some authors have found little or no difference in the rate of antenatal complications with triplet pregnancies compared to twins,[25] that has not been the experience in all reports.[7,12,16,17,26–31] Preeclamptic toxemia has been reported in an average of 23.8% of mothers with triplet pregnancies (range 8-46%), twice the rate with twins,[12] with the HELLP (hemolysis, elevated liver enzymes, low platelets) syndrome three times as often.[12] Placental separation severe enough to lead to delivery

centations, but only once in the autopsy group. This was a bit surprising, considering the frequency of reported vaginal bleeding in early to midpregnancy (see next section). Similarly, evidence of ascending infection—fetal vasculitis and/or chorioamnionitis—was less common than expected, with very mild involvement of triplet A in only 10.2% of survivor-group triplet sets, and mild to moderate involvement of triplet A and occasionally triplet B in less than one third of the autopsy-group sets. Nonspecific villitis, perivillus fibrin, villus edema, chorangioma/chorangiosis, were no more frequent than observed with singletons.

The concept of dizygotic twinning as an explanation for the combination of a fetus and placenta with a distinct *chorioma* is presented in Chapter 3. There are two well-documented reports of dizygotic twins with a separate classical androgenetic chori-

(abruptio placenta) was reported in 7% of two series of triplet gestations, seven times the rate in twins.[12] Gestational diabetes mellitus was mentioned in one report in 38.6% of mothers with triplets, ten times the rate with twins.[12] Maternal anemia was noted on average in one third of the mothers (range 10–70%), twice as often as with twins in one series.[12] A number of other complications are assessed in individual reports and the references cited can be consulted as a detailed presentation of clinical findings is beyond the scope of this review. Serious complications were noted infrequently in the pregnancy histories available in the Survey '91 Review of triplets. One woman had both preeclamptic toxemia and gestational diabetes mellitus, but all three female infants with a dichorionic triamniotic placenta were well grown and did well when delivered by section for preterm labor at 30 weeks. Another woman, with Clomid-induced triplets, had a ruptured appendix and peritonitis at 11 weeks, and a cervical suture was placed at 24 weeks for preterm labor. She delivered a week later and small unlikesex triplets B and C from a trichorionic fused placenta died within hours.

The most important obstetric complication of a triplet gestation appears to be *preterm labor* and delivery. As the numbers of fetuses increase, the incidence of preterm labor increases, it tends to occur earlier, and postponing delivery is less successful.[16] The median reported gestational age of all triplet deliveries (spontaneous or elective) is 31 to 35 weeks, with 6.6% to 29% delivered before 30 weeks, and a remarkably uniform rate of 84.6% to 87% delivered before 37 weeks.[13,17,25,27–29,32,33] Preterm labor has been reported as high as 92.3% in triplets, more than double the 41.5% rate in twins.[12] In most cases, the preterm labor was spontaneous in onset—premature rupture of membranes was reported in 15.4%, not significantly different from the 13.8% with twins.[12] Because of the greater volume of the uterine contents, it might be suspected that a contributing factor to preterm labor would be premature dilatation of the cervix, and therefore that cervical cerclage would be helpful in delaying delivery. The reported experience varies and a consensus seems no more apparent than with twins. It has been suggested that triplet pregnancy per se is not associated with cervical incompetence and that cervical ligation does not prolong gestation.[27,31] In contrast, prophylactic cerclage has been reported to

be associated with significant prolongation of gestation with heavier infants who require less-intensive neonatal care.[34] And finally, a third report suggests that the observations could neither support nor deny the value of cerclage.[28]

Most of the management discussions and variations have been aimed at reducing prematurity because of the concomitant risks to the fetus for neonatal complications. There has been considerable debate about the value of bed rest, enhanced monitoring on an inpatient or outpatient basis, the value of prophylactic tocolysis and corticosteroids, and the best way to deliver the triplets.[6,7,12,13,16,17,22–31,34–37] It appears that despite aggressive prenatal management, the rate of prematurity in pregnancies with three or more fetuses has not changed significantly in recent decades, but perinatal mortality rates have decreased, attributed to improvements in neonatal care.[13,23] Intensive antenatal education and monitoring by nurses on an outpatient basis, with appropriate medical management including tocolysis, and liberal operative delivery, has provided encouraging results with a corrected perinatal survival rate of 95%.[32] Recent experience with the application of Doppler studies of umbilical artery waveforms in triplet pregnancies may assist obstetric management,[38,39] although details of placentation and zygosity would have enhanced the value of the reported studies.

The clinical concerns in triplet pregnancies have been mentioned briefly in order to provide a background for the pathologic findings in the infants and placenta(s). With a history of preterm labor, premature rupture of membranes, or cervical incompetence, the pathologist examining the placenta(s) will be looking for evidence of contributing factors, such as premature separation or ascending infection. Decidual iron containing macrophages in the reflected membranes were noted microscopically in only six placentations from the survivor group of the Survey '91 Review, and only one significant abruption—under triplet B's portion in a case of interval delivery. This was surprising as up to 34.5% of triplet pregnancies have been reported to have episodes of first and second trimester vaginal bleeding.[13] Although 85% of the survivor group delivered before 37 weeks, and there was a history of premature onset of labor and/or premature rupture of membranes in at least 23%, histologic chorioamnionitis was described in only 10.2%, gestational age range 31 to 33 weeks, and was mild in all but one case, where it was focally moderate. Inflammation was limited to triplet A's portion of the placenta. There was localized funisitis in one case of cord prolapse each in the survivor group and the autopsy group. In the autopsy group, early to moderate chorioamnionitis was recorded in 28% of cases, gestational age range 22 to 26 weeks, also mainly in portion A. These data do not seem to reflect an increased risk of ascending infection with triplets in spite of the increased rate of preterm labor.

The significance of the *gestational age* at delivery is the risk of perinatal morbidity and mortality. This is emphasized in all discussions of neonatal outcome of triplets and is exemplified by the Survey '91 data. The median gestational age at delivery of the survivor group was 32 to 33 weeks, and the range was 26 to 37 weeks, with only 10% delivered before 30 weeks. In the autopsy group, the median age was 28 to 29 weeks, the range was 22 to 40 weeks, and 61% had delivered by 30 weeks. The gestational age at delivery did not seem to correlate with placentation in either the survivor or the autopsy group. Trichorionic and dichorionic placentas were seen with equal frequency at all gestational ages, and monochorionic triplets delivered from 28 to 35 weeks' gestation with no clustering. Any differences in this comparison need greater numbers of cases in order to detect significant trends that may have clinical significance.

The *neonatal complications* of prematurity are no different pathologically when they occur in triplets, and the incidence in twins related to birth order, fetal sex, and other factors is discussed in Chapter 4. There are differing reports of the relative frequency of complications in twins and triplets—from no difference,[25] to hyaline membrane disease (HMD) in 19.3% of twins versus 43.6% of triplets,[12] for example. Respiratory distress syndrome (RDS) due to HMD has been reported in 23.7% of triplets (with 50% mortality)[13] to 43% (13.8% mortality),[16] but with no comment on the relation to sex, age, birth order, or weight. One study noted that 73.3% of triplets less than 34 weeks gestational age had RDS, while none greater than 34 weeks were affected; 45.5% of triplets of less than 1,500 g, 36.4% of triplets of 1,501 to 2,000 g, and 11.8% of triplets of more than 2,000 g were affected.[40] In other words, size and gestational age are more

important to morbidity than triplet-ness, although the one may lead to the other. The relative risk for RDS based on birth order seems to be equal.[30] The role of antenatal steroids to induce lung maturation is not clear. In one report, there was no apparent benefit,[16] while another suggested a benefit of reduced severity, although the actual numbers were not considered statistically significant.[13] There were only a few other neonatal complications analyzed in triplets and they followed the same trends as HMD and RDS. One interesting association was absent end diastolic flow in antenatal umbilical artery Doppler studies with subsequent necrotizing enterocolitis in two triplets in one set out of six sets studied.[38] These were male and female triplets but placental details were not provided.

The incidence of complications of prematurity in triplets from the survivor group of the Survey '91 Review is not known, but in the autopsy group they were considered responsible for 48.5% of the mortality beyond 20 weeks' gestation, as defined in Chapter 4. This compares to 30.4% of perinatal and later twin mortality (Table 5.7). The triplet dying of complications of prematurity was more likely male (68.7%), triplet C (43.7%), from a monochorionic placenta (41.6%), at less than 27 weeks' gestation (56.3%), birth weight less than 1,000 g (62.5%), and to have survived fewer than 7 days (68.7%). This pattern is equivalent to what was seen with twins (see Chapter 4), except the triplets affected had been delivered 6 weeks earlier on average and were more often monochorionic. In triplet sets where one died, 62.5% died from complications of prematurity; in sets where two died, both died from complications of prematurity in 80%; in sets where all three triplets died, complications of prematurity affected triplet C in one set and triplets B and C in another, 20% of infants. The pathologic findings were as expected, with early deaths due to hyaline membrane formation with pulmonary barotrauma, and later deaths associated with bronchopulmonary dysplasia and its complications. Just under a third of the triplets lived for 8 days to 3 months before succumbing. Death was hastened in 25% with pulmonary sepsis, all with gram negative organisms; ductus ligation was needed in 12.5%; necrotizing enteropathy was significant in 12.5%; intracranial subependymal cell plate hemorrhage was notable in 18.7%, and pulmonary hemorrhage in 12.5%.

The consensus regarding delivery of triplets seems to favor elective abdominal delivery.[13,16,23,32,35] This preference has arisen from concerns about increased risks for the second and third triplets due possibly to delivery trauma, intrapartum cord prolapse, or hemodynamic changes in uteroplacental blood flow. One factor that might be important to delivery trauma is malpresentation—triplet A is more likely to be vertex, and triplets B and C breech, but all combinations have been seen.[29] Operative delivery was suggested as a way of reducing the perinatal morbidity and mortality of the second and third triplets,[35] although not every review reported equally successful outcomes.[13] Apgar scores and biochemical measures have been used to detect relative differences in triplet outcomes related to mode of delivery, but the reported results are not uniform. Apgar scores have been reported as significantly lower in the third triplet,[40] or independent of birth order.[17,41] Birth order did not appear to influence acid-base status in the absence of any obstetric complication or anesthetic problem.[40,41]

Although delivery trauma is a reasonable concern related to maneuvers that may be needed to deliver malpresenting triplets, the chief risk of problems of labor and delivery is *fetal asphyxia*. The importance of asphyxia as a cause of perinatal triplet death is not clear from the literature, but longer-term disabilities potentially related to problems of labor and delivery have been reported.[13,31] One review of triplets of less than 1,500 g birth weight, followed up for at least 1 year, found 10.5% with severe neuromuscular problems and 21% with mild muscle tone or attention deficit problems. It was not clear what the contributing factors were thought to be—birth order, placentation, and neonatal data were not provided. Another review found that major neurologic handicaps persisted in 4.1%, and all were third-born triplets, but other predisposing factors were not detailed. A more positive review excluded infants with congenital malformations and found only 1.2% of the remaining survivors had a major handicap, nature not specified.[16]

In the Survey '91 Review autopsy series of triplet deaths over 20 weeks' gestation, asphyxia (as defined in Chapter 4) was the cause of death of 15.1%, compared to 8.9% of twins (Table 4.1). There were too few cases to detect meaningful trends. One set of spontaneous monochorionic well-grown males died suddenly in utero at 35 weeks and were delivered the next day. The combined weight was 7,780 g (2,420 g, 2,560 g, 2,800 g); the placenta weighed 660 g. There were fewer chorionic vascular units than normal from all three cords, and intertwin anastomoses on the surface between two of them, but the cords were not identified as to triplet of origin. The main fetal sign of asphyxia was aspirated amniotic debris, but no anatomic cause was found. This case preceded the routine use of fetal monitoring. One 24-week male triplet A (680 g) died 48 minutes after delivery with hypoxic lesions, particularly in the heart. He had a 7-cm-long velamentous cord insertion into the monochorionic triamniotic placenta. His co-triplets died of complications of prematurity—triplet B at 40 days, and triplet C at 12.5 hours. A trichorionic triple-disk female triplet C delivered at 28 weeks suffered from a traumatic breech delivery. She lived 8 weeks, but had intracerebral hemorrhage, leading to hydrocephalus and eventually an infected shunt. There were multiple old cerebral infarcts at the time of autopsy. Other pathologic findings could not be determined as the autopsy was limited to examination of the brain.

Interval delivery, including triplets, has been reviewed in Chapter 4, and the placental features of the interval triplet delivery case from the Survey '91 Review are shown in Fig. 4.4.

Heterotopic pregnancies with twins are discussed in Chapter 4, and heterotopic triplets are also known.[42] In the reported case, male twins were intrauterine and did well when delivered at 34 weeks by emergency section, while the female triplet was intra-abdominal and well grown, but with severe deformations causing lethal respiratory problems. Tubal ectopic pregnancies are not strictly heterotopic, but at least five cases of triplets in tubal gestations have been reported.[43,44] In the two most recent cases, there were monochorionic triamniotic triplets of unstated sex of 7 weeks gestational age size in one, but sex and placentation were not clarified in the other. There were no examples of ectopic or heterotopic triplets in the Survey '91 Review.

Mortality

Triplet mortality statistics are almost always of perinatal/delivered triplets, not of triplet concep-

TABLE 11.1 Triplet mortality.

Reference or source	Timing limits	Intrauterine fetal death*			Neonatal death (Birth–28 days)	Infant death (28–365 days)	Total
		Early (0–13 wks)	Middle (14–26 wks)	Late (27 wks–term)			
17	Live-births				2.3%†		
31	≥20 wks GA		8.1%**		4.7%		
32	>24 wks GA		2.2%		2.8%		
45	NS		5%		12.5%[1]	2.5%[2]	
46	>25 wks GA[3]		6.3%		2.2%		
Survey '91 Review	None						
Totals							
Number of triplets		4 (4)	14 (14)	11 (7)	17 (14)	4 (3)	50 (42)
% of all triplets		(1.9)	(6.7)	(3.4)	(6.7)	(1.9)	(20.3)
% of all triplet pregnancies		(2.8)	(7.2)	(5.8)	(15.9)	(2.9)	(29.0)

Note: Survey '91 Review data comes from 49 triplet pregnancies with all survivors; 18 sets over 20 weeks' gestation with one or more autopsies; 1 set over 20 weeks with autopsy refused; 1 embryonic and 4 fetal sets; one elective reduction set—74 gestations with potentially 222 triplets. The numbers of triplets in parentheses is the number of triplet deaths limited to the same years of acquisition of the survivor placentas, and those numbers are used to derive the percentages of all triplets and percentage of all triplet pregnancies affected by one or more triplet deaths. The total % of all pregnancies affected is less than the sum of the percentages, because of several triplet pregnancies with triplet deaths at different times.

* Intervals of gestational age used in this text.

† Numbers are percentages of triplets dying of all triplets in each age category in each reference.

** Numbers placed between middle and late columns indicate that all fetal deaths were ranked together within the timing limit stated without specifying age, simply defined as "stillbirths."

[1] Neonatal deaths within first week.

[2] Death from 1 weeks to 1 year.

[3] All the mortality reported occurred in 16.9% of the triplet pregnancies in the study.

GA, gestational age; NS, not specified; data from vital statistics register.

tions, so the risk for fetal mortality is not clear, and it is difficult to detect a useful consensus from the available reports for several reasons. Many studies actually limit their mortality data to triplet conceptions that have reached midpregnancy, third trimester, or even live-born delivery. Several studies report no intrauterine fetal death of triplets,[12,13] others report no neonatal mortality,[40] and the term "perinatal mortality" is not clearly defined in many reports. It may be argued that late gestational fetal mortality and neonatal mortality are the only important ones for considerations of obstetric and pediatric/perinatal health care. However, as with twins, there are scientific lessons to be learned from a knowledge of mortality of triplet conceptions as a whole, and grief over loss of a triplet is no less because there are other infants to care for.

Mortality data is presented in Table 11.1, comparing reported rates with the Survey '91 Review triplet data. It should be noted that there are two facts that have influenced the Survey '91 Review data. First, the autopsy data span 20 years, while the survivor placenta data are from 14 years, so two sets of numbers are given, the total deaths for the entire review, and those deaths in the time period for

which data on triplet survivor placentas are available. Rates are calculated using the reduced data set. Second, early and midpregnancy losses represent more recent cases, with an unknown rate of embryonic and early fetal wastage prior to the routine use of ultrasound and the availability of the embryopathology service. Thus, the data suggest that between one-quarter and one-third of triplet conceptions may sustain one or more triplet deaths from conception to delivery and beyond, with up to one-fifth of all conceived triplets succumbing at various times, but this rate of mortality may be an incomplete representation for the reasons stated.

Fetal Mortality

Triplet mortality in the *first trimester* may be considerable. The report of 7.7% loss of all three, 15% loss of two, and 43% loss of one conceptus by 20 weeks' gestation after identification of three sacs with heart motions did not specify the time of loss, but at least some of the triplet wastage would have been in the first trimester.[12] The "vanishing twin" was discussed in Chapter 5, and an "empty sac" has been reported with triplets.[47] Embryofetal triplet

TABLE 11.2. Midpregnancy fetal triplet mortality—Survey '91 Review.

Case	GA	Sex	Weight	Placentation	Comment
1	16	F	149	TCTA-S	Bromocriptene pregnancy; antepartum hemorrhage led to delivery
		F	133		of triplet A; triplets B and C extracted; early ascending
		F	149		infection
2	19	M	150	MCTA	Vaginal bleeding for 1 month prior to delivery; one cord with
		M	149		only two vessels; no comment about anastomoses
		M	160		
3	18	F	232	MCTA	Severe polyhydramnios, cause not determined; no comment
		F	205		about anastomoses
		F	151		
4	21	F	300	MCTA	Premature rupture of membranes with *Escherichia coli* ascending
		F	320		infection; vascular anastomoses mentioned between B and C,
		F	430		but no details
5	22	F	380	TCTA-S	Clomid induced; 42-hour interval delivery of B and C after A,
		M	480		first triplet lived 30 minutes
		M	420		

GA, gestational age in weeks; M, male; F, female; Placentation: TCTA-S, trichorionic triamniotic with three disks; MCTA, monochorionic triamniotic.

death can be spontaneous or induced. The one *spontaneous* loss in the Survey '91 Review was at 7 weeks' gestation, following 4 days of vaginal bleeding. It was a trichorionic conception with fragmented placental tissue, so the arrangement was not determined. One sac was ruptured, but contained an empty amniotic sac, and the other two unruptured sacs had no embryonic tissues at all. *Elective* embryofetal terminations may be associated with triplets in two ways—a higher-order conception is reduced to triplets, or a triplet conception is reduced to twins. Elective reductions of higher-order multiples entail a number of ethical as well as medical concerns and have been reviewed in Chapter 5. The ethical issues and medical rationale for reduction procedures in triplets are even more uncertain.[40,48] Based solely on mortality, there does not seem to be any advantage in reducing triplet conceptions.[40] There was one example of elective first trimester reduction of triplets in the Survey '91 Review, and this has been described in Chapter 5. Selective reduction following identification of one chromosomally abnormal chorionic villus sample in a triplet pregnancy has been reported, but follow-up details were not provided.[49]

Triplet mortality in the *second trimester* is difficult to determine. The latter part of this 14 to 26 weeks gestational age time period becomes part of the reports of perinatal or neonatal mortality, and mortality in the earlier part of the period is rarely recorded. There are two main patterns of *spontane-

ous second trimester fetal death—concordant death with termination of the pregnancy, and death of one or two with creation of a fetus papyraceous. There were five sets with spontaneous concordant triplet fetal death in the Survey '91 Review (Table 11.2, and Fig. 11.5). They were all well preserved, almost all same-sex sets, 60% monochorionic, and 60% female sets. Unfortunately, the possibility of feto-fetal transfusion was not discussed, although the polyhydramnios in case 3, and the weight discordance in case 4 are suggestive. Although well preserved, the placentation in fetal loss cases was often disrupted during the process of removal, and the umbilical cords were not identified as to triplet of origin. As noted in Chapter 5, in the discussion of fetus papyraceous, the incidence of *fetus papyraceous* with triplets has been reported by some authors to be higher than with twins, sometimes with two papyraceous fetuses and a normal survivor (refs. 56–59, Chapter 5). There were no triplet conceptions with a fetus papyraceous in the Survey '91 Review. *Elective* reduction in the second trimester was not identified among the Survey '91 Review cases, but there is one report of selective feticide of a hydrocephalic male triplet at 19 weeks with intracardiac air.[50] He had a separate sac and placental disk from his twin sisters, who did well after abdominal delivery at 35 weeks 5 days.

Fetal death of triplets in the *third trimester* is difficult to ascertain for the reasons noted at the beginning of this section. The different reported rates of stillbirth, as noted from the literature, compared with data from the Survey '91 Review, are presented in Table 11.1, and these are not materially different from the range of rates quoted for twins in Chapter 5. The largest review of late fetal triplet deaths was a series of 89 sets of triplets of more than 25 weeks gestational age, with 16.9% of the pregnancies affected, for a rate of 6.4% of all the triplets.[46] Monochorionicity was important— 26.6% of the 15 sets with fetal deaths were monochorionic triamniotic, and another 40% had a monochorionic pair, although the relationship of fetal outcome to chorionicity in the latter group was not clear in all cases. Half the dichorionic triplet sets were diamniotic, but no specific reference to monoamniotic complications was made. The cause of the 17 fetal deaths in this series could not be determined from the report. There was no relationship to birth order or sex of the triplets, in contrast to other reports. Another review had noted that while 47.5% of all the triplet pregnancies reviewed were same-sex sets, 60.4% of triplet stillbirths were in same-sex sets—possibly a reflection of monochorionicity—and a greater proportion of male triplets succumbed.[45] The same study also noted increasing mortality by birth order, from A to B to C, in a ratio of 1 : 1.2 : 1.3; 21.4% of live-born co-triplets died, almost all from complications of prematurity and low birth weight, compared with 26% in the Survey '91 Review of surviving twins (Table 5.3). This review noted no maternal signs of coagulopathy, and although the majority were delivered within hours of the diagnosis of fetal death, it was for obstetric reasons, and it was suggested that fetal death of one or two triplets should not be the sole indication for delivery.

When one fetus of a multiple pregnancy dies in utero, there is concern for the *potential consequences* to the surviving fetuses, and the durability of the pregnancy, as discussed in Chapter 5. Assessment of the consequences is difficult because of the rarity of discordant triplet fetal death compared to all pregnancies, but the comments made regarding twins are probably applicable to triplets as well. As with twins, one of the key contributors to fetal mortality is monochorionic placentation. In one series of 26 triplet sets, 23% had monochorionic placentas, but 80% of the triplet sets with fetal death had monochorionic placentas.[51] In this same series, 7.7% of all the triplets died in late pregnancy in

utero, affecting 19.2% of the pregnancies. Details of other placental findings, such as chorionic vascular patterns or intertwin anastomoses, were not given, nor was autopsy data provided, and cause of death was not discussed. The intervals from fetal death were not known, but up to 11 weeks passed between diagnosis of death and delivery. The surviving triplets were followed for up to 8 years, and only one had any reported problems, attributed to complications of prematurity. There were no signs of maternal coagulopathy in any case. Discordant fetal death with maternal coagulopathy has been reported in one case.[52] One triplet died at 22 weeks, and maternal coagulopathy was treated successfully with heparin. The second triplet died at 34 weeks with no maternal consequences, and the live-born triplet at 35 weeks had no hematologic problems. No placental data were provided and the cause of death of the two fetuses was not clear from the report.

With the higher proportion of monochorionic placentations, there is the possibility of interfetal transfusion imbalance as a cause of death, in the patterns described in Chapter 9. This would seem to be the case in a set of discordantly grown male twins in a dichorionic triamniotic triplet set, who died at different times and had "clearly common" placental vasculature.[53] The female triplet was normal. Fetofetal transfusion syndrome was assessed as contributing to both stillbirth and neonatal death in a report of two sets of monochorionic twins in dichorionic triplet sets, although the details of placental vasculature were not provided.[50]

In the Survey '91 Review, there were five triplet sets with one or more *spontaneous* late fetal deaths for a total of 10 deaths (Table 11.3). There were too few cases to analyze in the same detail as done for twins in Table 5.3, although a few comparisons can be made. Using the same categories of fresh, macerated less than 1 week, and retained more than 1 week, there were none fresh, 40% macerated, and 60% retained, compared to 35%/40%/25%, respectively, for twins. Unlike the twins, the sex ratio was 1 : 1 overall. All three were affected in two sets, two in one set, and one in two sets. Concordant deaths were all with monochorionic placentations, as was one of the single deaths, a trend of increased fetal mortality with monochorionic placentation noted in twins as well. Asphyxia was listed as the cause of death in 40%, complications of mono-

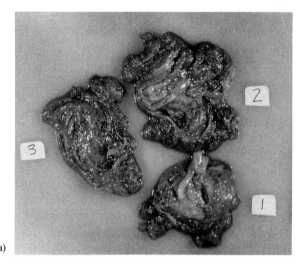

(a)

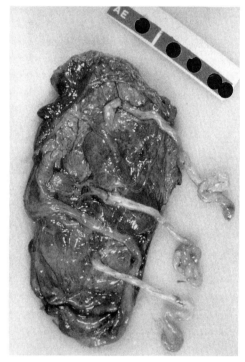

(b)   (c)

FIGURE 11.5. Examples of fetal triplets. (a and b) Case 1,
Table 11.2: Trichorionic triamniotic triple disk (a) with
normal female fetuses (b) delivered at 16 weeks' gestation with evidence of antepartum hemorrhage and early
ascending infection. (c and d) Case 2, Table 11.2:
Monochorionic triamniotic (c) with normal male fetuses
(d) delivered at 19 weeks after 1 month of antepartum
hemorrhage. (e and f) Monochorionic triamniotic placenta (e) with normal female fetuses (f) delivered at 18
weeks, pregnancy marked by polyhydramnios of unidentified cause. Odd pattern of fetal congestion visible in
photograph was not discussed in report. Differential size
of darkest and palest triplets raises question of twin
transfusion, but no comment regarding anastomoses in
placenta was made in report. Case 3, Table 11.2.

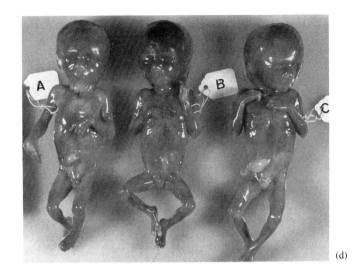

(d)

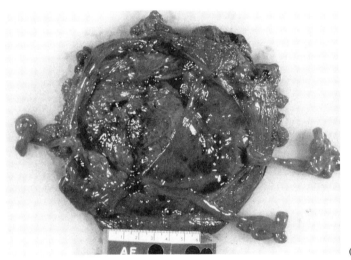

(e)

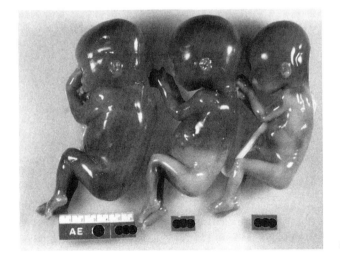

(f)

TABLE 11.3. Late pregnancy fetal triplet mortality (stillbirth)—Survey '91 Review.

Case	GA	Category	Order	Sex	CH	Placentation	Comment
1	40	Retained 4 wks +	B	F	34	DCTA-1	Severely growth retarded twin in monochorionic pair; possibly donor in twin transfusion; also velamentous cord insertion, mural thrombi one umbilical artery
2	35	Macerated 24 hrs	A	M	50	MCTA	All had decreased vascular units on surface of placenta; anastomoses between two—cords not identified; nearly concurrent fetal death with aspirated amniotic debris, cause not determined
			B	M	47		
			C	M	50		
3	31	Retained 10 days	A	F	37	MCTA	Cause fetal death not described; placenta in fragments; A and B anencephalic, C normal
			B	F	33		
			C	F	41		
4	34	Retained macerated	A	M	44	DCDA-1	Monoamniotic twins with entangled cords; both with long umbilical cords—65 cm and 60 cm; B growth retarded
			B	M	29.5		
5	33	Retained 4 weeks	C	F	32	TCTA-3	Growth retarded; very twisted umbilical cord with constriction at abdominal wall; death attributed to cord anomaly

GA, gestational age at delivery; Category: macerated (death less than 1 week prior to delivery); retained (death more than 1 week prior to delivery); interval of retention in utero after fetal death indicated where known. Order: birth order of deceased triplet; Sex: sex of deceased triplet, F, female; M, male. CH, Crown-heel length in centimeters; weight is not used as criterion of growth because of changes due to maceration. Placentation: DC, dichorionic; MC, monochorionic; TC, trichorionic; TA, triamniotic; DA, diamniotic; following number refers to number of disks where more than one possible.

chorionicity in 30%, cause not determined in 30%—compared with approximately 24%, 37%, and 25%, respectively, for stillborn twins. It may be that with greater numbers, the patterns of triplet late fetal mortality would parallel the observations with twins.

There were no *elective* terminations in the third trimester in triplet sets in the Survey '91 Review, nor were any reported cases identified.

Postnatal Mortality

Perinatal (birth to 7 days), neonatal (8 to 28 days), and infant (29 days to 1 year) mortality of triplets has received more literature attention than fetal death. There seems to be a consensus that more postnatal triplets die than twins, but the magnitude and characteristics of this difference were difficult to define. The increased postnatal mortality of triplets compared to twins or singletons has been related most directly to the greater proportion of low birth weight infants from triplet sets. Birth-weight-specific mortality has been reported to compare favorably with that of singletons,[4] and while relative gestational maturity has been suggested as a possible reason,[7] this was not borne out in the analyses.[4] Mortality has been reported to be higher in same-sex sets, of males compared to females, and increasing with birth order from A to C.[13,45] Birth-order–related mortality has been reported to be 3.4% for triplet A, 17.9% for triplet B, and 20.7% for triplet C,[13] although the time interval between deliveries does not appear to be a factor.[7] Other reviews have noted no difference in death rates by birth order.[32,40] Mortality has been related to presentation—9.8% mortality of vertex, 15.8% of breech, and 28.6% of transverse presentations in one report,[13] but 37% mortality in vertex and 25% in breech presentations in another report.[29] Postnatal triplet mortality has been most dramatically related to gestational age and birth weight—no mortality of triplets of 1,500 g or more birth weight, and no mortality of triplets of gestational age 28 weeks or greater in one series, although the relative importance of these two criteria was not clear.[31]

The postnatal mortality of triplets in the Survey '91 Review is detailed in Table 11.4 and category of causes is related to sex, birth order, and placentation in Table 11.5 for comparison with Table 5.7 of twins. Although the number of triplets is far fewer than the number of twins in these two tables, the importance of prematurity and its complications is

TABLE 11.4. Postnatal triplet mortality from Survey '91 Review.

Case	GA	Placentation	Triplet				Diagnosis	Comment
1	31	DCTA	A[1]	F[2]	1100[3]	2d[4]	HMD; sepsis	Anterpartum hemorrhage; "street person"
			C	F	1120	5d	HMD (no sepsis)	
2	29	NS	A	F	980	23d	BPD; sepsis	Clomid conception; PIH and anemia; both babies septic early; no placenta data
			B	M	850	3m	BPD;sepsis	
3	26	NS	B	M	820	33h	HMD,RBT,PH;SEPH	PROM; no placenta data; triplet C very stormy course
			C	M	NS	28d	BPD;PT;DA;++	
4	28	TCTA-3	C	F	1070	8w	Severe cerebral damage	Traumatic breech with fetal asphyxia
5	26	TCTA-1	C	M	680	24h	HMD, RBT	Preterm delivery due to ascending infection
6	27	DCTA-2	A	M	910	32h	HMD	Possible minor element feto-fetal transfusion
7	24	MCTA	A	M	680	48'	Acute hypoxia	Preterm delivery due to ascending infection; all had fewer chorionic vessels than normal; A and C had velamentous cord insertions, C had SUA
			B	M	600	40d	BPD,RBT;CHF;SEPH;NEC	
			C	M	680	12h	HMD,RBT,PH;SEPH	
8	26	DCTA-2	A	F	1100	8h	Recipient	Feto-fetal transfusion syndrome with A and B; case described in Chapter 9
			B	F	580	21h	Donor	
			C	F	840	6h	HMD,RBT	
9	29	MCTA	A	M	1270	3d	Asphyxia;HMD;sepsis	Prolapse of velamentous cord of A after PROM
10	25	TCTA-1	B	M	620	7h	HMD,RBT	Clomid conception; very early ascending infection
			C	F	580	12h	HMD,RBT	
11	22	TCTA-3	A	F	380	30'	Immaturity	Interval delivery; co-triplets stillborn
12	26	TCTA-f	A	M	480	3h	HMD	Clomid conception; ascending infection
13	29	DCTA-2	C	M	1430	67d	BPD;NEC;sepsis	Had own placental mass, cause preterm delivery not defined

GA, gestational age at delivery, in weeks; Placentation: DC, dichorionic; TC, trichorionic; MC, monochorionic; TA, triamniotic; NS, not stated; 1,2,3, number of disks; f, fragmented. Triplets: [1]A,B,C (birth order); [2]F, female, M, male; [3]birth weight in grams; [4]duration of survival (', minutes, h, hours, d, days, w, weeks, m, months). Diagnoses: HMD, hyaline membrane disease; BPD, bronchopulmonary dysplasia; RBT, respiratory barotrauma; PH, pulmonary hemorrhage; SEPH, subependymal cell plate hemorrhage; PT, pneumothorax; DA, patent ductus arteriosus; CHF, congestive heart failure; NEC, necrotizing enterocolitis. Comment: PIH, pregnancy-induced hypertension; PROM, premature rupture of membranes; SUA, single umbilical artery.

TABLE 11.5. Causes of postnatal triplet mortality—Survey '91 autopsy series.

Category	Percentage of total mortality	Ratio of males to females	Ratio of A:B:C birth order	Ratio of monochorionic: dichorionic:trichorionic: unstated placentation
Prematurity sequelae	71.4	2:1	1:1:1.8	1:4:2:2
Asphyxia	9.5	1:1	1:0:1	1:0:1:0
Prematurity/asphyxia	4.8	1:1	1:0:0	1:0:0:0
Immaturity	4.8	0:1	1:0:0	0:0:1:0
Anomalies	–	–	–	–
Monochorionic monozygosity	9.5	0:2	1:1:0	1:1:0:0
Other	–	–	–	–
Undetermined	–	–	–	–

obvious in both groups, with greater risks for males and last-born infants. Monochorionic monozygosity seems less important as a source of potential mortality of triplets than twins, largely because there were no cases of anomalies of monozygotic duplication among the triplet cases reviewed, compared to the number of examples among the sets of twins.

Morbidity

As with twins, there are two categories of triplet morbidity that have attracted attention—fetal growth, and generalized and system-related diseases and disorders. Because triplet mortality seems strongly correlated with fetal growth, as noted in the previous section, triplet growth has been discussed more extensively in the literature.

Growth

There are three aspects to consider when assessing fetal growth in multiple gestation. First, the pattern of growth over time is accessible by competent ultrasound examination,[54] and is a reflection of the intrauterine environment, including the number of conceptuses.[55] Second, birth weights are measurable and are a function not only of the intrauterine environment and number of conceptuses but of gestational age as well.[56,57] Third, interfetal growth discrepancy suggests discordant fetal and/or placental pathology and must be explained, as already noted with twins in Chapter 6. All three aspects can be assessed appropriately only against reliable triplet-specific data, and there has been a recent cluster of reports of studies of large numbers of triplets attempting to provide valid growth data. Even though more recent reviews of triplet growth have had the advantage of much more precise gestational age data, because more than half of the pregnancies are induced with very specific conception times known, the interpretations and conclusions vary somewhat.

The importance of normal values for *fetal growth in utero* is that they would provide a more reliable way of monitoring a triplet pregnancy, so that appropriate care could be provided to maximize fetal survival. No statistically significant difference in second trimester growth of triplets compared to twins or singletons was found using biparietal diam-

eter (BPD), long and short axes of the head, abdominal profile, femur diaphysis length, and thigh circumference, all obtained from ultrasound examination.[58] The conclusion was that triplet growth in utero could be assessed using the same criteria as used for twins and singletons. In contrast, another report suggested that growth patterns of triplets are different from singletons, with slowing of BPD, head circumference and abdominal circumference growth after 28 weeks' gestation, but maintenance of the head circumference/abdominal circumference ratio, and parallel femur growth but on the low side of the singleton range.[54] Tables of ultrasound values for BPD, abdominal circumference, head circumference, head/abdomen circumference ratios, and femur length are available.[54]

The commonest way of assessing fetal growth is by comparison of *birth weights* with age-related normal distributions at the time of delivery. Curves constructed in this fashion for triplets suggest that the average triplet newborn has a weight corresponding to about the 30th percentile of singleton standards from 26 to 35 weeks' gestation, but that it falls progressively thereafter, reaching the 10th percentile at 38 weeks.[56] This would appear to be because triplet growth remains linear from 22 to 38 weeks' gestation, while singleton growth rates become steeper in the last 8 weeks because of greater soft-tissue deposition.[57,59] Birth weight curves for triplets from 21 to 38 weeks are reproduced in Fig. 11.6. The factors that might influence birth weight have been evaluated statistically, and heavier triplets were noted with male infants of older, taller, heavier, multiparous mothers, who gained more weight during pregnancy.[56,60] There were no reported differences between spontaneous or induced triplets.[56,60] The only correlation of birth weight with presentation was that the heaviest infant presented first with greater frequency than would be expected by chance alone.[60] This was interpreted as more likely due to subtle differences in fetal weight affecting fetal presentation, rather than any direct effect of presentation on fetal growth. Correlations with zygosity and placentation patterns are incomplete due to lack of adequate data.

The importance of valid growth standards for triplets is the definition of what is truly small for gestational age (SGA) for triplets. Up to 14% of triplets have been said to be SGA based on singleton standards,[22] up to 16% without an indication of the

FIGURE 11.6. Triplet growth curves (a) Triplet growth from 21 to 38 weeks' gestation.[57] Mean individual triplet birth weights (N = 580) in grams and 95% confidence limits by gestational age at delivery. Number of individual triplets delivered at each gestational week is listed above confidence bands. Regression line of best fit (R = 0.98) is superimposed on data. (b) Triplet growth from 28 to 38 weeks' gestation.[56] (a) Reprinted with permission from Jones JS, Newman RB, Miller MC, Cross-sectional analysis of triplet birth weight, *Am J Obstet Gynecol*, 1991;164(1):137. (b) Reprinted with permission from Elster AD, Bleyl JL, Craven TE, Birth weight standards for triplets, *Obstet Gynecol*, March 1991;77(3):389.

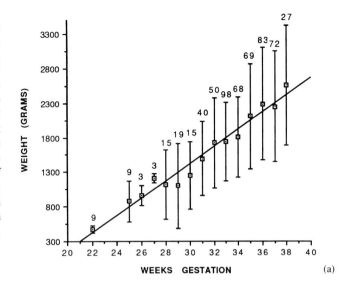

(a)

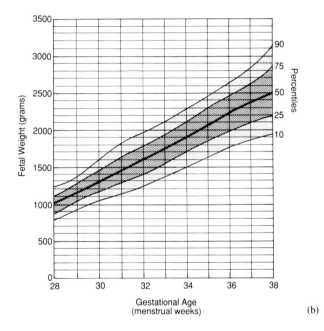

(b)

standards used,[16] and up to 53.3%, again using singleton standards.[25] In other reports, stillborn triplets are not classed as growth retarded, although the reported weights are clearly low.[46,51] In one report, it was noted that 60% of the SGA triplets had monochorionic placentas, but it was not clear how many SGA triplets each monochorionic placenta had.[16] Otherwise, the patterns and causes of SGA triplets are not discussed.

Although the numbers are small, the Survey '91 Review cases of triplets were assessed using the values in Fig. 11.6, and the patterns of growth retardation identified are shown in Table 11.6, calling those triplets SGA who were at or below the 10th percentile. There is always a problem using weight data standards for macerated fetuses, and no linear measurement norms are yet available for triplets. Retained macerated fetuses were assessed as probably growth retarded at death if their crown–heel length was at least 4 weeks behind singleton standards for that gestational age. As might be expected, growth retardation was more prevalent in

TABLE 11.6. Patterns of triplet growth retardation—Survey '91 Review.

	Incidence of sets affected	Placentation T:D:M	Birth order A:B:C*	Sex M:F†	Causes**			
					MM	PDev	PDis	CND
Survivor group	19%	2.5:1:0	0:6:1	1:1.3	28.3%	28.3%	28.3%	28.3%
Autopsy group	50%	4:3:1	1:2.5:2	1:1.8	18%	18%	–	64%

*Relative birth order of affected triplets.

†Ratio of males (M):females(F) affected.

**These add up to more than 100% with the survivor group, because in some cases it was hard to decide which factor was more important.

Incidence: only one triplet affected per survivor set; two sets in autopsy group had two affected.

Placentation: T, trichorionic, D, dichorionic, M, monochorionic. Causes: MM, complications of monochorionic monozygosity—twin transfusion; monoamniotic cords entangled; PDev, developmental lesions of the placental portion of the affected triplet, e.g., single umbilical artery, velamentous cord, abnormally long cord, abnormally spiraled cord, smaller chorionic volume, decreased chorionic vessels; PDis, placental diseases, such as evidence of ischemia, impaired fetal blood flow (hemorrhagic endovasculopathy), perivillus fibrin deposition in placental portion of affected triplet; CND, a cause for smaller size not identified.

the autopsy group. Surprisingly, monochorionic placentation was not as frequent as might be expected for mortality trends, although when present it was usually important. It is not clear why the smaller triplet tended to be the second born, especially in the survivor group, when the lightest of the three was equally A, B, or C in the group as a whole. The heaviest was equally A or B, and half as often C. The importance of placental findings to an interpretation of impaired fetal growth is evident in the survivor group, while the cause of impaired fetal growth was not decided in nearly two-thirds of the autopsy group.

Interfetal size variation in multiple gestations is an important indication of potentially significant fetal and/or placental problems, as noted in Chapter 6. It has been reported that intertriplet growth differences are more pronounced than with twins, and that this may have relevance to antepartum management.[57] In a review of 580 infants from 196 triplet sets, 30.1% of the gestations had an intertriplet discordance of at least 25% as determined by the difference between the largest and smallest members of each triplet set, as a percent of the largest, six times the rate in twins.[57] About 7% of triplet sets had greater than 40% discordance. Unfortunately, no details were provided regarding placental findings in any cases, and potential causes of the discordance were not discussed. A review of ultrasound findings in triplet conceptions in the first trimester suggested that interfetal size variation begins early, but as these were cases for multifetal pregnancy reduction, it is not known if the smaller triplets would have terminated spontaneously, or

carried on as growth retarded fetuses.[61] The Survey '91 Review triplet cases were assessed to evaluate discordant growth analagous to the data for twins in Table 6.3, but this was only possible for the survivor group based on the data available. Compared to the twin data, survivor group triplets that were growth discordant tended to be more discordant—50% were in the marked discordant group (25–39.9% difference), and 31.3% in the moderate group (20–24.9% difference), compared to twin values of 30.3% and 23.9%, respectively. Most of these smaller twins were also SGA, and the characteristics are already outlined in Table 11.6, with no significant changes from that distribution when considering growth discordance.

Disease

The general discussions in Chapters 1 and 6 concerning the interpretation of disease incidence in twins apply to triplets as well. The manifestations of the disorders are no different because they occur in triplets, so perhaps that is why there are few reports of such cases in the literature. The importance of descriptions of diseases in triplets relates to the potential intrinsic natural "experiment" that such occurrence may represent, and what that can tell us about the disease or disorder in question. However, any such evaluation requires precise knowledge of zygosity, and for some conditions, placental findings. There are rare reported cases where it appears that simply the number of infants to be cared for creates overwhelming management problems and malnutrition and neglect occur. An example was one unfortunate woman with two sets of triplets after a set of twins—8 children under the age of 4 years.[30] In other reported cases, one triplet was reported to have died from sudden infant death syndrome at about 10 weeks of age, but sex, birth order, and placentation were not stated[16]; fetal hydrops, unrelated to twin transfusion, in two females in a trichorionic triamniotic triplet set with growth retarded male was not characterized further[46]; and concordant globoid cell leukodystrophy in monozygotic (red cell antigen and HLA types) triplet girls has been reported.[62]

An association of multiple reproduction and teratomas was noted for twins in Chapter 6, and with anomalies of monozygotic duplication in Chapter 10. In this regard, there was an interesting set of female triplets, all blood group A+, but no other assessment of zygosity indicated, who had concurrent bilateral ovarian benign cystic teratomas.[63] There was no comment about other multiple pregnancies or teratomas in relatives, and only one singleton pregnancy was reported from one of the sisters.

In the Survey '91 Review of triplets, there were no instructive examples of disease processes unrelated to complications of prematurity.

Anomalies

The lessons from anomalous development of triplets are simply an extension of those from twins, as noted in Chapter 7, with the possible addition of a "controlled" experiment of nature if the triplets were originally dizygotic with one subsequent monozygotic pair. The frequency of anomalies does not appear to be greater in triplets than twins, although there are few statistics reported, and some studies actually dismiss malformed infants from the discussions.[16] One report noted a rate of 1.1% lethal malformations and 6.9% minor (correctable) malformations in a series of 87 triplets from 29 pregnancies beyond 22 weeks' gestation.[13]

As with twins, knowledge of placentation and zygosity are key components in any analysis. A few examples are provided from the literature by way of illustration. Concordance for the presence of congenital cardiac anomalies, but discordance for some of the details, has been reported in monochorionic female triplets.[64] A set of monochorionic male triplets was discordant for right ventricular endocar-

dial fibroelastosis—present in two of the three—but potential reasons for the asymmetry were not clear.[65] There were reportedly "many anastomoses" between the three fetal circulations on the placenta. Concordant pyloric stenosis in monochorionic male triplets has been reported.[66] Widely varied clinical manifestations of fetal hydantoin syndrome were noted in trichorionic triplets, where the two girls were considered dizygotic on the basis of different hair color, and the boy was the most severely affected.[67] The possibility of differential dosage was suggested, but because the triplets were weight discordant by only 15%, the interpretation was that uterine blood flow, and therefore dosage, would have been similar to all three. The differential manifestations were thus attributed to differing genetic makeup. Examples of discordant Down syndrome in triplets have been attributed to heterozygosity between the normal and affected children.[68,69] Monozygotic heterokaryotic twins are discussed in Chapter 7 and discordant sex in one of three monozygotic triplets has been reported due to the same process.[70] Two normal boys and a girl with features of Turner's syndrome had a monochorionic triamniotic placenta, and 33 identical blood components. Blood lymphocytes were normal homogeneous 46,XY karyotype in all infants. Skin fibroblasts provided the same karyotype in the males, but nonmosaic 45,X in the female.

In the autopsy group of triplets from the Survey '91 Review, there were anomalies noted in half the infants, lethal anomalies in two cases, and minor findings in the remainder. The lethal lesion was concordant anencephaly in two of three female monochorionic triplets. The placenta with these triplets was definitely monochorionic, but the cords had not been identified as to triplet of origin and the parenchyma was sufficiently fragmented that details of cord insertions and interfetal vascular anastomoses could not be determined. Therefore, any potentially contributory placental factors to the discordant anomaly in apparently monozygotic triplets could not be assessed. Other potential causes of monozygotic discordance for anomalies are discussed in Chapter 7. Other than a single umbilical artery in one case, which could be determined at birth, all the minor anomalies identified would not have been detected without autopsy. These consisted of three cases of Meckel's diverticulum, and one each of accessory cervical thymus, abnormal lamination in the right motor cortex of the cerebrum, asymmetric cusps of the aortic valve, a cecum in the right upper quadrant, persistent left superior vena cava to the coronary sinus, and mild unilateral ureterovesical junction stenosis. There was no relation to placentation or fetal sex. One set of monochorionic triamniotic male triplets had different minor anomalies—the abnormal cerebral cortex in A, Meckel's diverticulum in B, and single umbilical artery in C.

Monochorionic Monozygosity

The major area of pathology of multiple pregnancy that is specific to the multifetal nature of the conception consists of those lesions found only with monochorionic monozygosity.

Monoamniotic

Monoamniotic sets of multiples are virtually limited to twins, whether the conception is of two, three, four, or more fetuses at a time. As noted in Chapter 8, it is a challenge to imagine the embryonic events that could lead to three or four fetuses within the same amnion, although normal female triplets from a confirmed monoamniotic monochorionic placenta were delivered spontaneously at 35½ weeks.[71] In contrast, another monochorionic monoamniotic triplet set was aborted spontaneously and all the cords were intertwined.[72] There was a normal fetus, an anencephalic fetus, and a small amorphic chorangiopagus parasiticus fetus, but the sex of the triplets was not stated. In the Survey '91 Review, there were two examples of monoamniotic twins within a dichorionic triplet set. In the survivor group set of spontaneous male triplets, the monoamniotic pair were equally well grown (A—2,580 g, B—2,500 g), at the time of vaginal delivery at 36 weeks. The placenta is shown in Fig. 11.7. The dichorionic co-triplet was normal, 2,360 g, but zygosity was not assessed. The monoamniotic set in the autopsy group is case 9 in Table 8.1 and is shown in Fig. 8.8c.

Vascular Anastomoses

The considerations of anatomy, pathophysiology, consequences, and documentation of interfetal vascular anastomoses are as relevant to monochorionic triplets and monochorionic twins in triplet sets as they are to twins (see Chapter 9), although specific triplet references in the literature are few. Examples of the possible extent of interfetal vascular anastomoses in triplets are presented clearly by Boyd and Hamilton.[19] In one review of triplet mortality in 15 of 89 pregnancies, feto-fetal transfusion was recorded in two sets, one male and one female, both dichorionic diamniotic, suggesting that both affected pairs were monoamniotic.[46] All four fetuses died, three stillborn and one in the day after birth. No further details were given. A third monoamniotic set (sex not stated), in a dichorionic placentation with a separate disc for the co-triplet, was reported with fetal death of the triplets attributed to feto-fetal transfusion.[73] The affected fetuses were said to be deep red/pale at delivery, and of equal length, but 100 g different in weight, 900 g/800 g, at 29½ weeks. Unfortunately, there were no further details regarding the fetal findings at autopsy, and the nature of the interfetal vascular communications were variably described as "superficial" and "villous." This predominance of transfusion syndromes with monoamniotic pairs in triplets is in contrast to the rarity in monoamniotic twin pairs, as noted in Chapters 8 and 9, and remains to be clarified.

In the Survey '91 Review of triplets, 86% of the monochorionic pairs in the survivor group, and 70% of the monochorionic pairs in the autopsy group had demonstrable interfetal vascular anastomoses. In 9% of the survivor group monochorionic sets (all in dichorionic triplet placentas), no anastomoses were found with injection. In the remainder of both groups, the specimens were too fragmented to determine the details or there was no reference to anastomoses. While the numbers are considerably smaller than from the twins reviewed, the patterns of anastomoses recorded in triplets are summarized in Table 11.7. The data are presented in this fashion to serve as a potential guide to others who may wish to review triplet interfetal anastomoses in a comparable manner. In comparison with twins, the triplets are more complex because of the possibility of interfetal anastomoses among all three triplets in monochorionic triamniotic sets, so the different types of placenta are shown separately. In the survivor group with monochorionic triamniotic triplets, all three were involved in vascular connections in three of four sets—A with B and B with C in two sets, and all three connected in one set. The connections in the monochorionic triamniotic sets

FIGURE 11.7. Monoamniotic triplet pairs. This is a placenta from the survivor group. The relationship of the three placental portions can be seen in (a) with triplets A and B the monochorionic pair. Cord A had an estimated 5-cm velamentous insertion (membranes were torn), 20 cm away from the marginal insertion of cord B and the cords were not entangled. The surface area supplied by vessels from cord A was about 40% and from cord B about 60%. Note the absence of any sign of separating membranes between the circulations of A and B (b), and the presence of one 2-mm-diameter venous shunt (v) and one 1-mm-diameter parenchymal shunt from A to B (p). The only microscopic difference was greater villus congestion on side A. The triplets were all male, A—2,580 g, B—2,500 g, C—2,360 g. Trimmed weight of the placenta was 920 g, with about two-thirds of the area to A/B and one-third to C. Mother, 34 years old, first pregnancy, spontaneous triplets, section delivery at 36 weeks. (See Fig. 8.8c for an example of a monoamniotic twin pair in a dichorionic diamniotic triplet placentation from the autopsy group of the Survey '91 Review, where both triplets died at different times as a result of cord entanglement.)

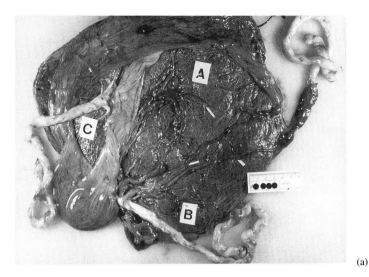

(a)

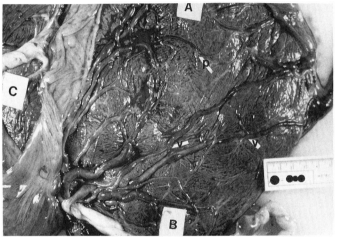

(b)

in the autopsy group involved all three in one set, and only two fetuses in two other sets. A method of representing this complexity is presented in Fig. 11.8. Table 11.7a looks at the number of anastomoses per placenta, as done for twins in Table 9.2, and the data distribution is similar. Table 11.7b compares the distribution of the different types of anastomoses, analogous to Table 9.3, and the relative proportions are roughly parallel between the twins and the dichorionic triamniotic triplet sets. There are too few cases in the autopsy group and dichorionic diamniotic sets to make any comparisons, except for the increased parenchymal anastomoses in the autopsy group, as noted for twins. As with twins in Table 9.5, Table 11.7c indicates that arterial and parenchymal anastomoses, alone and combined, were the most frequent patterns observed. One example of the anastomotic pattern

seen with a monochorionic pair with twin transfusion syndrome in a dichorionic triamniotic placentation is shown in Fig. 9.9b, and an example of extensive intertwin anastomoses without feto-fetal transfusion in Fig. 11.9.

In spite of the frequency of demonstrated interfetal vascular anastomoses in the Survey '91 Review triplet cases, there was no noted clinical evidence of any pattern of twin transfusion syndrome in the survivor group, clear chronic twin transfusion in only one autopsy-group set (described in Chapter 9), and a suggestion in two additional autopsy-group sets that twin transfusion might have been contributory. In one dichorionic triamniotic set, one of the monochorionic pair died at least 4 weeks prior to delivery and was growth retarded for that date. Postmortem autolysis rendered organ weights less helpful than usual, and placental details were not

TABLE 11.7. Interfetal vascular anastomoses in triplet sets—Survey '91 Review.

(a) Number of anastomoses per placenta

Type	Group	1	2	3	4	5	6	7	8
DCTA	S	4	5	2		2	1		
	A		3						
MCTA	S			1	1		2		
	A		2						1
DCDA	S		1						
	A	1							

(b) Types of anastomoses

	Type	Group	Arterial	Venous	Parenchymal	Compound	Total
% (number) of placentas with one or more of each type of anastomosis	DCTA	S	63.2 (12)	15.8 (3)	42.1 (8)	10.5 (2)	* (25)
		A	14.3 (1)		42.8 (3)	14.3 (1)	* (5)
	MCTA	S	15.8 (3)		21.1 (4)	10.5 (2)	* (9)
		A	42.8 (3)		28.6 (2)		* (5)
	DCDA	S		5.3 (1)	5.3 (1)		* (2)
		A		14.3 (1)			* (1)
% (number) of each type of anastomosis in total number of anastomoses	DCTA	S	38.9 (14)	8.3 (3)	44.4 (16)	8.3 (3)	100 (36)
		A	16.7 (1)		66.7 (4)	16.7 (1)	100 (6)
	MCTA	S	15.8 (3)		73.7 (14)	10.5 (2)	100 (19)
		A	27.3 (3)		72.7 (8)		100 (11)
	DCDA	S		50.0 (1)	50.0 (1)		100 (2)
		A		100.0 (1)			100 (1)

*These percentages add up to more than 100% as most placentas had more than one type of anastomosis.

(c) Distribution of combinations of anastomotic types

	DCTA		MCTA		DCDA		Total		Overall
	S	A	S	A	S	A	S	A	number (%)
Arterial + parenchymal	5	1	1	3			6	4	10 (37.0)
Arterial only	5						5		5 (18.5)
Arterial + parenchymal + compound	1		2				3		3 (11.1)
Parenchymal only			1	1			1	1	2 (7.4)
Venous + parenchymal	1						1		2 (7.4)
Venous only						1		1	1 (3.7)
Compound only	1						1		1 (3.7)
Arterial + venous	1						1		1 (3.7)
Parenchymal + compound			1					1	1 (3.7)
Arterial + venous + parenchymal	1						1		1 (3.7)

DCTA, dichorionic triamniotic; MCTA, monochorionic triamniotic; DCDA, dichorionic diamniotic (i.e., one monoamniotic pair); S, survivor group; A, autopsy group.

provided. The stillborn triplet had a velamentous cord insertion with a mural thrombus in one umbilical artery, a potential factor in growth retardation and fetal death, but the dichorionic well-grown normal co-triplet also had a velamentous cord insertion with no apparent consequences. In another dichorionic triamniotic set with one 3-mm arterial and one 3-mm artery to a 2-mm vein parenchymal shunt from triplet B to triplet A in the monochorionic pair, the villus tissue on the arterial side of the parenchymal shunt was more mature than on the venous side, suggesting a chronic imbalance. The triplets were equal size at birth and although triplet A died at 32 hours of age from complications of

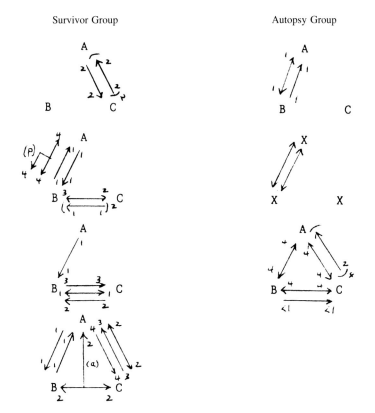

Survivor Group   Autopsy Group

—→ = parenchymal anastomosis with direction artery → vein indicated by arrowhead and size of vessels in millimeters by number.

←—→ = arterial anastomosis with size indicated.

⊢— = compound anastomosis with arterial connection providing a parenchymal shunt in one case (p) and a third arterial connection (a) in another.

( ) = more than one of same type of anastomosis, indicated by superscript.

X = cords not identified, but anastomoses recorded; in this case, one arterial and one venous (hence two double-headed arrows), size not stated.

FIGURE 11.8. Representation of intertriplet vascular anastomoses in monochorionic triamniotic placentas from both the survivor group and the autopsy group of the Survey '91 Review.

prematurity, his heart weight was not increased, suggesting that if there had been any vascular imbalance it must have been acute. Just why feto-fetal transfusion syndromes seem relatively less frequent with triplets than twins is not explained, unless the pressure effects of the third conceptus mass/volume affect the hemodynamics.

There are no definitive reports of triplets with examples of survival with damage following the death of one of a monochorionic pair, where the damage is attributed to complications across inter-fetal anastomoses. There is one interesting case of reportedly dichorionic triamniotic male triplets with a fetus papyraceous and associated well-grown monochorionic triplet with microcephaly and neurologic dysfunction.[74] The findings might suggest that this was a case of feto-fetal transfusion with death of the donor, and then a hypotensive episode, which the co-triplet survived, but with neurologic damage. Unfortunately, this triplet died without autopsy and there were few placental details. The third triplet had no right external auditory meatus and a deformed right external ear, was dizygotic by ABO blood groups, and otherwise normal.

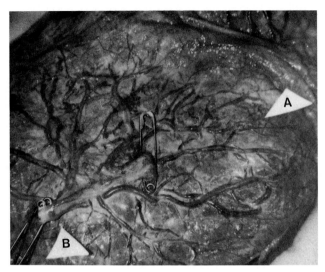

FIGURE 11.9. Vascular anastomoses in monochorionic pair of dichorionic triamniotic triplet set. Cords were identified with sutures. Specimen was a single disk with a surface area of triplets A and B equal to that of C. Trimmed weight, 650 g. Infants delivered at 28 weeks, A—male, 1,210 g, B—male, 1,255 g, C—female, 1,195 g. Cord A has one safety pin, cord B has two pins. The vascular equator was difficult to define due to the great degree of overlap of the respective circulations. As mentioned in the discussion of circulatory patterns with monochorionic twins in Chapter 9, the overlapping pattern of circulations tends to be associated with large numbers of anastomoses and eight were identified in this case, including arterial, parenchymal and compound patterns. (Original photograph was a Polaroid™ snapshot.)

Anomalies of Duplication

It has already been noted in the discussion in Chapter 10 that triplet conceptions seem unusually represented in sets with anomalies of monozygotic duplication. Among the asymmetric duplications, the reported cases with triplets seem to be limited to the *chorangiopagus parasiticus* (CAPP) pattern, with case reports beginning over a century ago.[75] In reported series of CAPP fetuses, 3.5% to 21.5% of the cases occurred in triplet sets,[76–78] and in a review of 340 cases, CAPP fetuses were part of a monozygotic pair occurring within triplets three times as often as among monozygotic pairs alone.[79] Unfortunately, many of the case reports of CAPP fetuses in triplet gestations seem to focus on details other than the pathologic anatomy of the placental membranes and vasculature. There is one intriguing report of apparently monochorionic triamniotic female triplets with a normally grown pair and a third CAPP twin, who was twice their size.[80] The abnormal triplet had a two vessel velamentous cord and one anastomosis was mentioned between the two normal triplets, but additional details of the vascular interconnections were not available. It is not clear which triplet was acting as the pump twin, as neither was described as having any problems neonatally. Two CAPP fetuses as part of a triplet conception have been reported, but the membrane and vascular relationships were not determined and it was said that the normal triplet, who died shortly after birth, had no abnormalities at autopsy.[81] This is somewhat surprising as it (sex not stated) must have been the sole cardiac force for the other two masses and the placenta. Triplets delivered spontaneously at 34 weeks consisted of a normal triplet, pump triplet, and CAPP fetus (sex not stated and no placental details).[82] The pump twin reportedly did well initially but died of heart failure and no abnormality other than "massive cardiac dilatation" was identified at autopsy. Boyd and Hamilton[19] have a very clear photograph of a diamniotic male pair with a CAPP fetus (and a separate disk from a female co-triplet), displaying the direct vascular connections between the pump fetus and the parasitic fetus, and it is a good example of the use of photography to document these anomalies. A case of conjoined CAPP twins in a monochorionic triplet pregnancy has been reported and the surviving male pump twin did well after an episode of neonatal heart failure.[83] The three-vessel cord of the conjoined CAPP fetuses had "prominent vascular anastomoses" to the three-vessel cord of the pump twin. This case seems to be a bridging lesion between asymmetric and symmetric anomalies of monozygotic duplication.

Up to 6% of *conjoined twins* may be part of a triplet set[76] and nine cases of conjoined twins in triplet sets have been reviewed.[84] Two-thirds were thoracopagus twins and the normal triplet was the same sex in all but one case, although zygosity was not stated. Isolated case reports have been presented since that review, but details of placentation, fetal sex, and findings in the conjoined twins are few. A very unusual conjoined twin was dicephalus dibrachius, but also sirenomelic, and probably dichorionic (two disks) with a normal male co-triplet, who died of complications of prematurity (gestational age not stated).[85] The sex of the anomalous twin was not reported. Dicephalus dibrachius dipus twins have been reported with a normal fetus, but sex and placentation were not described.[86] The pregnancy was terminated electively at 15 weeks. Female cephalothoracopagus conjoined twins with well normal male co-triplet have also been identified by ultrasound antenatally.[87] A possible triplet conjunction, thoracopagus twins with perhaps an included fetus-in-fetu or endoparasitic triplet, does not appear to have been confirmed in the scientific literature.[88] There were no examples of abnormalities of monozygotic duplication in the Survey '91 Review of triplets.

Quadruplets and Higher Multiples

The higher multiples of human conception are sufficiently rare that they are often the subject of single case reports. Mayer[89] provides an exhaustive, remarkable, and thoroughly delightful review of probable, possible, and pretentious reports of 6 to 365 "infants" at a single parturition, from the time of Aristoteles to the 20th century. He describes some reasonably well-documented and truly phenomenal examples of fertility, which occurred long before the so-called "fertility drugs." The unfortunate feature of many of the single-case reports is that details of the placental relationships are incomplete, so that zygosity assessment is often uncertain. The zygosity combinations in natural multiples probably represent a random distribution, whereas induced multiples are more likely to be polyovulatory. When zygosity assignment is not pursued at the time of delivery by the methods described in Chapter 2, intricate statistical and probability calculations are sometimes used,[90] but the complexity makes them unattractive to most reviewers, and they do not help with the individual case.

All the considerations discussed to this point with reference to twins and triplets are simply extended by the number of additional fetuses in higher multiples. The psychosocial and societal concerns regarding the biologic cost and economic and emotional burdens of multiplets are considerable.[1,4] The rarity of such sets means that pattern analyses of clinical and pathologic features are limited, particularly beyond quadruplets, and as much as possible needs to be learned from each multiplet set. The following discussion focuses on selected observations of quadruplets and quintuplets, because of their increased occurrence with the assisted reproduction technologies, and refers only briefly to sextuplets and higher multiples.

Quadruplets

The increasing *frequency* of quadruplets is brought out dramatically by noting that only 48 such pregnancies were reported from 1900 to 1952,[55] but two recent reviews were able to assess 10 cases from only one perinatal practice in a 5-year period (May 1986–April 1991),[91] and 71 cases through a support group for mothers of supermultiples from a 10-year period (1980–1989).[92] The role of assisted reproduction technology in this frequency is evidenced by the fact that only 4 of the 81 quadruplet pregnancies in these recent reviews were spontaneous (4.9%), while in a slightly earlier series (1970–1978), one of six (16.7%) was spontaneous.[28] In many smaller reviews, all the quadruplet gestations reported are the result of hormonal therapy, with or without embryo or gamete manipulations.[12,22,93] This frequency has led to two reduction management considerations—reduction of the number of embryos placed in the uterus, and reduction of the number of embryos in the uterus. Part of the problem with preimplantation reduction is that it is difficult to predict the viability of preimplantation embryos,[94] but some centers are electing to replace only two or three embryos and cryopreserve the remainder for future cycles if pregnancy is not established (Zouves C, 1991, personal communication). It was noted in Chapter 5 that there are considerable ethical and medical considerations surrounding elective reductions of established embryos.[23] There are some who consider that with current antenatal and neonatal care, the mortality of quadruplets (and quintuplets) is "too low to justify feticide as life saving for those spared from fetal killing, but only as an elimination of perhaps stressful lives."[95] Others deal with this problem by offering the procedure, using current data to enable more informed decision-making.[93]

The most important information needed to guide decision making in quadruplet (and higher multiple) pregnancies is accurate data on morbidity and mortality. This can be difficult to assess from available reports because data from pregnancies with four, five, or even six fetuses are sometimes combined with triplet data, because of the small numbers, and it is hard to determine if there are increased risks specific to the higher multiples.[16,93] Also, some reports limit their consideration to cases in the latter half of gestation, or record cases with fetal mortality in a manner that is hard to interpret.

Obstetric concerns emphasize gestational complications and premature delivery.[6,12,91–93,96] The concerns about accurate early sonographic diagnosis are pertinent, and one report suggests that even if there are triplets in utero, that does not rule out an ectopic combined heterotopic quadruplet.[97] In this spontaneously conceived case, there was one tubal gestational sac, with viable fetus, which ruptured at 9 weeks and had to be removed, and living triplets in utero, possibly dichorionic triamniotic. Two living infants and one stillborn were delivered at 36 weeks, but no other details were provided. A second similar case is mentioned briefly in one large review.[92] Gestational complications reported with quadruplet pregnancies include gestational diabetes mellitus in 10% to 50%, pregnancy induced hypertension in 17% to 90%, first trimester bleeding in 35%, anemia in 10% to 25%, urinary tract infection in 14% to 17%. Incompetent cervix has been reported leading to cerclage in 14%, but the value of prophylactic elective cerclage seems as debatable as with triplets in the absence of true cervical incompetence. All studies suggest the tendency of preterm labor to occur earlier and be more resistant to tocolysis with increasing numbers of fetuses. In a review of 228 reported quadruplet deliveries in eight series from 1931 to 1991, the mean gestational age at delivery was 31.1 weeks, range 29.7 to 33.2 weeks, median 30.2 weeks.[91] Maternal parity beyond one was associated with longer gestations in several series. An intensive antenatal management protocol in one center was able to prolong gestation to 33 weeks or longer in 60% of the patients.[91] Operative delivery, preferably elective, is the recommended procedure because of the high rate of malpresentations and risk of prolapsed cord. Postpartum hemorrhage has been reported in 21% of mothers with quadruplets.

Reported *fetal/neonatal concerns* have focused on fetal growth, fetal mortality, and perinatal mortality and morbidity.[6,12,91–93,96] As with triplets, fetal growth of quadruplets is in the lower zones reported for singletons, and levels off as the singleton curve begins to accelerate.[90] Mean birth weights have ranged from 1,000 g to 1,700 g, but in some reports the ranges for birth weight given suggest that stillborn fetuses are included in the data. Discordant growth is mentioned, but not detailed or discussed as to cause. Fetal mortality is difficult to ascertain as some studies are limited to later gestations only. Empty gestational sacs have been documented by ultrasound examination, but residues could not be found when the remainder of the conception delivered.[47] In one review, 7% of the quadruplet pregnancies had spontaneous early fetal death of one of the quadruplets, but there were no details of the relevant pathology.[92] The later spontaneous fetal deaths reported have been of one, two, or three of the fetuses, with varying intervals of retention of the dead fetus,[92] or loss of the entire conception.[93] The numbers are small and details scanty, so contributing factors and cause of death are not clear. Neonatal morbidity is related to prematurity with hyaline membrane disease in 88%, pulmonary interstitial emphysema in 25%, bronchopulmonary dysplasia in 66%, patent ductus arteriosus in 75%, intraventricular hemorrhage in 21%, and sepsis in 17%.[96] Another way of looking at neonatal morbidity is to note that 75% of quadruplets in one review required intensive neonatal care, and remained hospitalized up to five times longer than twins.[12] In one report of 268 live-born quadruplets, there was 12.3% neonatal mortality, the majority less than 1,000 g birth weight and less than 28 weeks' gestation,[92] while there was no neonatal mortality in another series.[91] A review of 41 sets of quadruplets from 1975 to 1983 reported that in 17%, all four fetuses/infants died, all survived in 66%, and in 17%, one or more were stillborn or died after birth,[45] but again, contributing factors and cause of death were not discussed. An important question is the nature of long term infant outcome, but the reports are conflicting—no long-term morbidity in 10 cases (interval of follow-up not indicated),[91] compared to neurodevelopmental abnormalities of varying severity in 30% of infants, affecting one or more of the infants in four of seven sets followed for more than 2 years.[93]

FIGURE 11.10. Patterns of quadruplet zygosity with estimated frequencies.

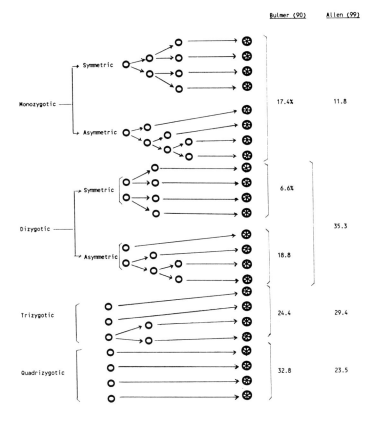

Developmental anomalies and morbidity, other than due to complications of prematurity, have not been reported to any extent even in the large series. Brief reference is made to one case each of Potter's syndrome and neural tube defect–hydrocephalus in stillborn quadruplets,[92] one neonatal death with trisomy 18, coarctation of the aorta and esophageal atresia,[93] double outlet right ventricle with ventricular septal defect and overriding aorta in a stillborn quadruplet,[16] surviving quadruplets with atrial septal defect in one, Down syndrome in another, and unilateral multicystic kidney in a third,[16] and a surviving quadruplet with duplication of one renal pelvis and congenital lung cyst.[12] None of the reports identify sex, birth order, placentation, or zygosity. In one case of trichorionic quadriamniotic 3 + 1 (i.e., three quadruplets shared one disk with a separate disk for the fourth quadruplet) all female quadruplets, one of the monochorionic set had bilateral polycystic kidneys (Potter type 1), and a marginal cord insertion on her portion of the placenta, with fewer chorionic vascular units than normal.[98] Her monochorionic twin had a velamentous cord insertion with fewer chorionic vascular

units, and developed necrotizing enterocolitis requiring bowel resection, but she survived. She had no renal lesions identified, and although twin transfusion was suggested, anastomoses were not described. Sudden infant death syndrome has been reported in one quadruplet from each of two sets, but details, such as birth order, were not given.[92]

Details of *zygosity, placentation,* and complications of *monochorionic monozygosity* in quadruplet pregnancies have not been discussed in most of the reviews, because concern has focused on clinical characteristics and management. Theoretically, there are four patterns of quadruplet zygosity, with the embryos originating from one, two, three, or four ova—monozygotic, dizygotic, trizygotic, and quadrizygotic. Subtypes of conceptions from one or two ova have been termed symmetric or asymmetric, depending on the pattern of subsequent twinning (Fig. 11.10).[89] The relative frequencies of the different patterns of zygosity are based on statistical estimates only; detailed studies using current technology have yet to be correlated and compared with the estimates. All the potential patterns of placentation that such a scheme suggests, based on the

TABLE 11.8. Patterns of quadruplet placentation.

Reference or source	Pattern of placentation*	Fetal sex†	Fetal weights	Comment
19	QCQA-3 + 1	FMF + F	NS	
	QCQA-1	FFFM	NS	
	QCQA-3 + 1	FMM + M	NS	
	TCQA-2 + 2	FM + *MM*[a]	NS	Probably trizygotic
	QCQA-1	FMFF	NS	
	TCQA-1	MF*FF*	NS	
	QCQA-3 + 1	MFM + F	2469/1844/2298 + 1759	All survived
	DCQA-1	*FF*[b]*MM*	[b]199/1861/1986/1589	Probably symmetric dizygotic
	TCQA-1	MF*FF* [a,b]	NS	FP has marginal cord
16	MCQA	NS	NS	Feto-fetal transfusion; no details
	QCQA-NS	NS	NS	Four examples in series, no details
72	TCQA-1	NS	NS	Marginal cord in one of MC pair
98	TCQA-3 + 1	*FFF* + F	1020/1020/1736 + 1475	**
Survey '91 Review	QCQA-1	MFFF	650/620/840/520	See Table 11.9
	QCQA-1	FMMF	860/980/1020/690	See Table 11.9
	QCQA-1 + 2 + 1	FFFF	358/352/370/347	See Table 11.9

*Numbers after letteers refer to disk patterns. e.g., 3 + 1 means 3 chorionic masses in one disk and one separate disk.

†F, female; M, male; + indicated separation of fetuses by sex in relation to pattern of placentation; e.g., FMF + F means one disk had two female and one male quadruplets and a third female had a separate disk; italics represents monochorionic set.

**Separate quadruplet had marginal cord insertion; dichorionic quadruplet from fused disk had normal placenta; one of monochorionic twins had cystic kidneys, marginal core insertion, decreased vascular units, and co-twin had velamentous cord, decreased surface vascular units and hypervascular villi.

[a]Monochorionic twins with demonstrated vascular anastomoses.

[b]One macerated or fetus papyraceous (FP) in monochorionic pair.

NS, not stated; QC, quadrichorionic; QA, quadriamniotic ("quad" is used in preference to "tetra" to avoid confusion with TC, trichorionic, DC, dichorionic, MC, monochorionic).

timing of the twinning process, as outlined in Chapter 3, have been reported,[90] and even monoamniotic triplets in quadruplets have been reported twice (cited in ref. 100). Patterns of placentation are related to zygosity, as discussed in Chapter 3, but zygosity can be predicted from placentation only with monochorionicity or unlike-sex dichorionicity, setting aside the rare twinning mechanisms described in Chapter 2. When placental details are not available, fetal findings have been used. For example, a set of four female infants delivered at 22 weeks who died at the time of birth were said to have had two separate placental masses.[101] Zygosity assessment was based on 52 anthropomorphic measurements, x-ray findings, anatomic findings, and dermatoglyphics, because the placentas were not retained or described. Two sets of monozygotic twins were identified based on these data, but it was not clear what the original zygosity was thought to be, and in fact the implication was that two separate placentas defined them as two distinct sets of twins. Even with current methods, it might be difficult to differentiate the symmetric and asymmetric monozygotic quadruplets. Unfortunately, neither fetal sex nor placentation data are provided in most reviews, and scattered single-case reports are the source of the information available.

Examples of patterns of placentation with quadruplets are presented in Table 11.8. The majority of quadruplet placentations are fused masses, even though quadrichorionic, probably simply reflecting space constraints in the uterus that is trying to accommodate more gestational sacs. Anomalous cord insertions seem to be no more frequent than with twins or triplets, but the numbers of cases with details of cord insertions are few. From the eight cases with photographs or other information[19,98] (Survey '91 Review), there were six marginal and one velamentous cord insertions out of a possible 32, a frequency of about 22%. No two-vessel cords were reported.

Complications of monochorionic monozygosity have been reported infrequently with quadruplets. It is possible that the two cases with a papyraceous monochorionic fetus in Table 11.8 represented twin

TABLE 11.9. Quadruplets from Survey '91 Review—autopsy group.

Case GA Origin	Sex	Age at death	Birth weight (g)	Cause of death	Placentation	Comment
1	M	SB	650	"Immaturity"	TCQA-1; no	Could be asymmetric dizygotic or
26	F	5 hrs	620	"Immaturity"	anastomoses	trizygotic; no studies done;
Spontaneous	F	SB	840	"Immaturity"	described in	findings in monochorionic pair
	F	SB	520	"Immaturity"	MC pair	did not suggest twin transfusion, vessels not described; preterm labor attributed to abruptio placenta
2	F	–	860	Survived	QCQA-1	Old and recent premature separation
27	M	3½ days	980	HMD;SEPH;PIE		of all sacs; accelerated maturity
Pergonal	M	14 hrs	1020	HMD;PH;PIE;SEPH		in C; villus edema, congestion
	F	–	690	Survived		and intravillus hemorrhage in D
3	F	SB	358	Asphyxia	QCQA-1-2-1	Proven trizygosity by ABO, Rh,
22	F	7.5 hrs	352	HMD;SEPH		and DNA studies postmortem; B
Clomid	F	8 hrs	370	HMD;SEPH		and D monozygotic, A and C
	F	13.5 hrs	347	HMD;RPT:SEPH		dizygotic; mother had cone biopsy of cervix 2 years prior to conception; spontaneous onset of labor; multiple foci old premature separation of all sacs

GA, gestational age at delivery in weeks; Origin: whether conception spontaneous or induced, and if so, how. SB, stillborn; M, male; F, female; Cause of death: HMD, hyaline membrane disease; SEPH, subependymal cell plate hemorrhage; PIE, pulmonary interstitial emphysema; PH, pulmonary hemorrhage; RPT, right pneumothorax. Placentation: TC, trichorionic; QA, quadriamniotic; QC, quadrichorionic; MC, monochorionic; numbers after pattern of placentation refer to distribution of chorionic masses as in Table 11.8.

transfusion syndrome—vascular connections were confirmed in one, but could not be assessed in the other.[19] Anastomoses without mention of twin transfusion was noted in the fourth case from ref. 19 on Table 11.8. Feto-fetal transfusion was said to have occurred between two of the four fetuses in a monochorionic quadriamniotic set, but no further details were given.[72] Feto-fetal transfusion was suspected between monochorionic twins in a trichorionic quadriamniotic set, but vascular connections were not described, and modifications of findings on the basis of umbilical cord insertions were considered.[98] Asymmetric duplication does not appear to have been reported with quadruplets, but a conjoined pair in a quadruplet set has been mentioned briefly.[102]

The three sets of quadruplets identified from the Survey '91 Review are detailed in Table 11.9 and portrayed in Fig. 11.11.

Quintuplets

As might be expected, details of quintuplet gestations are even scarcer than of quadruplets. The rarity of surviving quintuplet sets is evidenced by the fact that many are known by name.[6,103] Fortunately, the public interest in quintuplet birth has become more benign and helpful since the commercialization and misguided psychosocial management of the first well-known surviving set, the Dionne quintuplets in Canada in 1934.[104,105] In 1960, it was reported that of the 71 sets of quintuplets in the world literature, two sets were known to have survived (the Dionnes in Canada and the Diligentis in Argentina), three sets were believed to be monozygotic, although 20 sets were same-sex sets, 11 female and 9 male.[106] Since then, there have been more reports of surviving quintuplets in the general press[107,108] than in the scientific literature.[109] Some of the best-documented cases pathologically are the apparently monozygotic sets, perhaps because of the remarkable embryologic ramifications.

Monozygosity of quintuplets has attracted the most attention when it seems that all five were from one egg. Unfortunately, although it was said that the Dionne placenta contained "no separation into sections in any way," and that "blood vessels ramified in all directions from the areas where the cords entered and appeared to intermingle with one

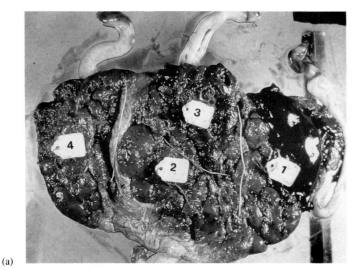

(a)

FIGURE 11.11. Quadruplets from Survey '91 Review. (a) Case 1, Table 11.9. Trichorionic quadriamniotic single-disk placentation with preterm labor associated with premature separation of quadruplet A's portion of the placenta. White cords were used to demarcate the respective fetal zones of the parenchyma. There was no mention of interfetal anastomoses between the two monochorionic quadruplets in the report available and unfortunately no fetal surface photograph was taken in this case, one of the oldest in the Survey Review group. (b and c) Case 2, Table 11.9. Quadrichorionic quadriamniotic with at least partial fusion of all disks.

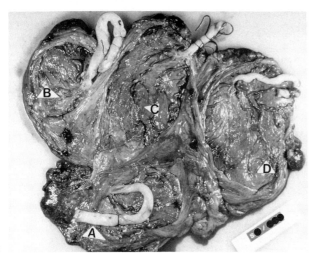

(b)

another," it was never examined pathologically.[103] Blood groups and detailed physical characteristics were the basis for assessing the five female Dionne quintuplets to have been monozygotic. The mechanism was suggested to have been by two sequential symmetric twinning events, followed by a third twinning of one of the four resultant embryos, with specific identification of which quintuplet resulted at which stage, on the basis of the physical observations.[103] Much has been written about the Dionne quintuplets, and their lives have been followed carefully. One important observation relates to the caveats of twin studies noted in Chapter 1, and the discussion in Chapter 7 about influences affecting apparently monozygotic multiples who seem to differ in unexpected ways:

. . . even when individuals have exactly the same hereditary factors, they may begin life with important differences already laid out by environmental discrepancies; and that even if they are reared together in the same way (and with as much calculated uniformity as the Dionnes experienced), their paths are nevertheless destined to diverge to some extent.[104]

In another monochorionic quintuplet set, all died of "immaturity," and interfetal anastomoses were documented, but twin transfusion was not suggested, and no fetal anomalies were identified.[106,110] There is a reference to a monoamniotic quintuplet pregnancy in the mid-1800s (cited in ref. 100), but no other monoamniotic set in quintuplets was identified. A set of monochorionic pentamniotic females had one chorangiopagus parasiticus anomaly, with

FIGURE 11.11. *Continued.* Note how the relationships are more clearly shown after trimming of cords and membranes (c), although both photographs are worth taking. Note the ties marking the umbilical cords. At the time of prosection, the chorionic masses were separated along the lines of attachment of the septal membranes, and fetal/placental weights were: A—860 g/200 g, B—980 g/180 g, C—1,020 g/140 g, D—690 g/225 g. It is interesting that the surviving quadruplets, A and D, were the lightest but had the heaviest placental weights. (d) Case 3, Table 11.9. Quadrichorionic quadriamniotic with equally grown females (d), but severe fragmentation of placental tissues (no photograph taken). Cords were marked so that some portions of parenchyma could be assigned to each infant for purposes of microscopic assessment. Quad A had its own placental mass, about 80 g, quad C had its own mass, about 98 g. Quads B and D shared the dichorionic disk with respective parenchymal masses approximately 75 g and 85 g. Note that zygosity assignment required genetic studies and that although apparently "identical," they were in fact trizygotic. Also, B and D shared a disk and although it had a dichorionic dividing septum, they were proven to be a monozygotic pair.

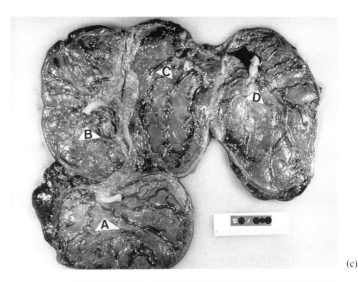

(c)

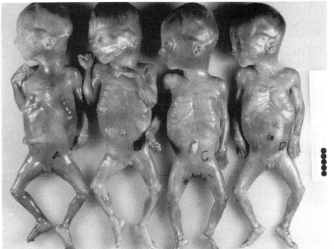

(d)

many vascular connections noted among the fetal circulations.[111]

Reviews of obstetric and neonatal concerns are necessarily limited by the numbers available. Those pregnancies that could be maintained to 32 weeks resulted in five living infants in all six sets in a review of eight cases.[6] In a review of 16 sets of quintuplets from a 12-year period in Japan (1974–1985), all infants were live-born in three sets, all were stillborn in eight sets, and survival in five sets was mixed.[112] There were no same-sex sets in this series, but otherwise no details of placentation or discussion of cause of death was provided.

Elective reduction of quintuplet conceptions has been discussed in Chapter 5, including one case from the Survey '91 Review, the only quintuplet set identified among the cases available.

Six and More

Pregnancies of six or more fetuses are usually mentioned more frequently in the literature on elective reduction procedures, as described in Chapter 5, but there are some detailed case reports of pregnancies with high multiples that continued to delivery.

Hormonally induced sextuplets were delivered by elective section at 34 weeks.[113] These Florentine sextuplets were four boys (birth weights 1,430 g, 1,520 g, 1,540 g, 1,700 g), and two girls (1,150 g,

1,500 g), with a single placental mass that had six chorionic sacs. No neonatal problems were reported and all were doing well at an unstated age thereafter.

The Birmingham septuplets were from a gonadotropin-stimulated conception and were delivered by section at 32 weeks.[114,115] They are the best-documented set located in the literature and can serve as a model of investigation and documentation. The infants were as follows: female, 920 g, died at 20 days, and male, 1,300 g, died at 12 days, both with intestinal obstruction, details not provided; female, 1,410 g, female, 1,250 g, and male, 1,180 g, all survived and did well; female, 1,260 g, died at 1 hour from acute hypovolemia, as her portion of the placenta was cut during delivery; and a fetus papyraceous, probably male, who died at 10 to 11 weeks' gestation based on size, but contributing factors were not suggested. The placenta was a single mass containing seven chorionic sacs, confirmed microscopically. The surface areas were nearly equal, except for the fetus papyraceous, and all viable portions had normal gross and microscopic findings. All circulations were injected and no anastomoses were identified. Zygosity testing consisted of three placental enzymes and nine blood group antigens, and on the basis of the results, the pregnancy was identified to have resulted from six and possibly seven fertilized ova, as the fetus papyraceous could not be assessed.

Another set of septuplets resulting from human menopausal gonadotropin and human chorionic gonadotropin, delivered spontaneously at about mid-pregnancy (dates not clear from report).[116] The first female, 276 g, was stillborn at home. The rest were live-born but died shortly after birth: female, 266 g; male, 410 g; female, 420 g; female, 315 g; male, 240 g; female, 370 g. The placentation was described as one mass with six chorionic sacs and a separate single disk, with most cords having marginal insertions, one with only two vessels. Unfortunately, no zygosity assessment was undertaken and the assumption was that, because they were all in their own chorionic sac, they were septovular in origin. In reality, it is only certain that there were at least two eggs, as there were five females and two males.

In a hormonally induced octuplet pregnancy, section delivery took place at 33 weeks 3 days.[117] The arrangement of placentation, fetal sex, and

birth weights (as used in Table 11.8) was as follows: heptachorionic hepta-amniotic—3 + 1 + 4 (membranes around fetus papyraceous, octuplet 7, were not defined); MMF + F + MM?M (sex of fetus papyraceous not stated); 1,690 g/1,670 g/870 + 570 g (macerated) + 1,980 g/1,510 g/?/510 g (fetus papyraceous 12 cm crown–rump length; last octuplet macerated). Unfortunately, there was no discussion of cause of fetal death or marked weight discordance in the survivors. At 18½ months of age, the relative weight discordance persisted but they were otherwise well. A tracheoesophageal fistula in octuplet 2 was repaired at 54 days of age.

A nonuplet pregnancy resulting from hormonal stimulation was delivered vaginally with forceps or digital assistance after spontaneous onset of labor at 27 weeks' gestation.[118] There were three placental masses—multiplets 1, 2, 3, 4, 7, 8, and 9 shared one, and multiplets 5 and 6 each had one; all sacs had histologically proven amnion and chorion. Assessment of 14 blood group antigens taken with the distribution of fetal sex indicated at least seven ovulations (septazygotic), but the zygosity of the two macerated nonuplets (numbers 2 and 9, both male) was not determined. The seven infants that were live-born were four females and three males, ranged in weight from 420 to 1,000 g, and all died in 21 to 162 hours, with intraventricular hemorrhage in five of them, pulmonary hemorrhage in two of them, and complications of possible meconium ileus in one. The cause of death of the two macerated stillborn infants was not determined.

Concluding Comments

While triplets and higher multiples have been thought to be at greater risk for maternal and fetal morbidity and mortality, the greatest risks, as with twins, are those of prematurity and impaired growth, rather than any risks intrinsic to being a multiplet. While prematurity and low birth weight are more common with greater numbers of fetuses in utero, current trends to enhanced antenatal surveillance, more liberal elective operative delivery, and the availability of advanced neonatal care are providing results with triplets that are approaching the data in twins. Assisted reproduction technologies are providing more opportunity to apply these measures to quadruplets and quintuplets, and some encouraging outcomes are being reported. When six or more embryos are identified, reduction procedures are reported to reduce the numbers to a more viable range, although survival is not universally precluded.

The individual pathologist is unlikely to see many examples of higher multiplets in their experience, although triplets are relatively more common. Because these cases are rare, it is the pathologist's responsibility to provide as much detail as possible concerning findings in the placenta(s) and fetuses/infants who succumb. This can be done in conjunction with clinical evaluation of the survivors. The opportunity to assess the influence of zygosity and placentation on abnormal development and disease in sets with several combinations at one time is one to be cherished and pursued to the furthest possible extent. Consultation with genetics colleagues can be very helpful for zygosity testing, even after fetal death (as in case 3 of quadruplets from the Survey '91 Review). With the new DNA technologies, the patterns of twinning that lead to these high multiples may be clarified, adding to our knowledge of embryology of human multiples.

References.

1. van Duivenboden YA, Merkus JMWM, Verloovevanhurick SP. Infertility treatment: implications for perinatology. *Eur J Obstet Gynecol.* 1991; 42:201–204.

2. AP wireservices. Multiple births costly. *The Globe and Mail.* 1992;July 15:A7.

3. Coping with three, four, or more. (Editorial). *Lancet.* 1990;336:473.

4. Kiely JL, Kleinman JC, Kiely M. Triplets and higher-order multiple births. Time trends and infant mortality. *Am J Dis Child.* 1992;146:862–868.

5. Keith LG, Ameli S, Keith DM. The Northwestern University Triplet Study 1: Overview of the international literature. *Acta Genet Med Gemellol.* 1988;37:55–63.

6. Petrikovsky BM, Vintzileos AM. Management and outcome of multiple pregnancy of high fetal order: literature review. *Obstet Gynecol Surv.* 1989; 44:578–584.

7. Eqwuatu VE. Triplet pregnancy: a review of 27 cases. *Int J Gynecol Obstet.* 1980;18:460–464.

8. Imaizumi Y. Triplets and higher order multiple births in Japan. *Acta Genet Med Gemellol.* 1990;39:295–306.

9. Shanklin DR, Perrin EVDK. Multiple gestation. In: Perrin EVDK, ed. *Pathology of the Placenta.* Vol 5. *Contemporary Issues in Surgical Pathology,* Roth LM, series ed. New York: Churchill Livingstone; 1984:165–182.

10. Myrianthopoulos NC. An epidemiologic survey of twins in a large, prospectively studied population. *Am J Hum Genet.* 1970;22:611–629.

11. Hommel H, Festge B. Drillingsschwangerschaft mit Fetus papyraceus. *Zentralbl Gynakol.* 1979; 101:845–847.

12. Seoud MA-F, Toner JP, Kruithoff C, Muasher SJ. Outcome of twin, triplet, and quadruplet in vitro fertilization pregnancies: the Norfolk experience. *Fertil Steril.* 1992;57:825–834.

13. Weissman A, Yoffe N, Jakobi P, Brandes JM, Paldi E, Blazer S. Management of triplet pregnancies in the 1980's—are we doing better? *Am J Perinatol.* 1991;8:333–337.

14. Gedda L. Twins in History and Science. Springfield: Charles C Thomas; 1961:67–90.

15. Wharton B, Edwards JH, Cameron AH. Monoamniotic twins. *J Obstet Gynecol Br Cwlth.* 1968; 75:158–163.

16. Gonen R, Heyman E, Asztalos EV, Ohlsson A, Pitson LC, Shennan AT, Milligan JE. The outcome of triplet, quadruplet, and quintuplet pregnancies managed in a perinatal unit; obstetric, neonatal and follow-up data. *Am J Obstet Gynecol.* 1990; 162:454–459.

17. Keith LG, Ameli S, Depp OR, Hobart J, Keith DM. The Northwestern University Triplet Study II: fourteen triplet pregnancies delivered between 1981 and 1986. *Acta Genet Med Gemellol.* 1988;37:65–75.

18. Fox H. Pathology of the placenta. In: Bennington JL, ed. *Major Problems in Pathology.* Vol VII. London: WB Saunders; 1978:90.

19. Boyd JD, Hamilton WJ. *The Human Placenta.* Cambridge: W. Heffer; 1970:321–324.

20. Ohmichi M, Tasaka K, Suehara N, Miyake A, Tanizawa O. Hydatidiform mole in a triplet pregnancy following gonadotropin therapy. *Acta Obstet Gynecol Scand.* 1986;65:523–524.

21. Azuma C, Saji F, Takemura M, Ohashi K, Kimura T, Miyake A, Takagi T, Tanizawa O. Triplet pregnancy involving complete hydatidiform mole and two fetuses: genetic analyses by deoxyribonucleic acid fingerprint. *Am J Obstet Gynecol.* 1992;166:664–667.

22. Olofsson P. Triplet and quadruplet pregnancies—a forthcoming challenge also for the "general" obstetrician. *Eur J Obstet Gynecol Reprod Biol.* 1990;35:159–171.

23. Alvarez M, Berkowitz R. Multifetal gestation. *Clin Obstet Gynecol.* 1990;33:79–87.

24. Desjardins PD, Dodds JR, Willoughby HW. Rh-D isoimmunization in a triplet pregnancy. *Can Med Assoc J*. 1972;106:1000–1001.

25. Sassoon DA, Castro LC, Davis JL, Hobel CJ. Perinatal outcome in triplet versus twin gestations. *Obstet Gynecol*. 1990;75:817–820.

26. Daw E. Triplet pregnancy. *Br J Obstet Gynecol*. 1978;85:505–509.

27. Itzkowic D. A survey of 59 triplet pregnancies. *Br J Obstet Gynecol*. 1979;86:23–28.

28. Ron-el R, Caspi E, Schreyer P, Weinraub Z, Arieli S, Goldberg MD. Triplet and quadruplet pregnancies and management. *Obstet Gynecol*. 1981;57:458–463.

29. Holcberg G, Biale Y, Lewenthal H, Insler V. Outcome of pregnancy in 31 triplet gestations. *Obstet Gynecol*. 1982;59:472–476.

30. Syrop CH, Varner MW. Triplet gestation: maternal and neonatal implications. *Acta Genet Med Gemellol*. 1985;34:81–88.

31. Lipitz S, Reichman B, Paret G, Modan M, Shalev J, Serr DM, Mashiach S, Frenkel Y. The improving outcome of triplet pregnancies. *Am J Obstet Gynecol*. 1989;161:1279–1284.

32. Newman RB, Hamar C, Miller MC. Outpatient triplet management: a contemporary review. *Am J Obstet Gynecol*. 1989;161:547–555.

33. Michlewitz H, Kennedy J, Kawada C, Kennison R. Triplet pregnancies. *J Reprod Med*. 1981;26:243–246.

34. Hutson JM, Creatura C, Edersheim TG. Prophylactic circlage in triplet pregnancy (Abstract). *Am J Obstet Gynecol*. 1992;166:408.

35. Feingold M, Cetrulo C, Peters M, Chaudhary A, Shmoys S, Geifman O. Mode of delivery in multiple birth of higher order. *Acta Genet Med Gemellol*. 1988;37:105–109.

36. Loucopoulos A, Jewelewicz R. Management of multifetal pregnancies: sixteen years' experience at the Sloane Hospital for Women. *Am J Obstet Gynecol*. 1982;143:902–905.

37. Wiggins DA, Elliott JP. Oligohydramnios in each sac of a triplet gestation caused by Motrin—fulfilling Koch's postulates. *Am J Obstet Gynecol*. 1990;162:460–461.

38. Rafla NM. Surveillance of triplets with umbilical artery velocimetry waveforms. *Acta Genet Med Gemellol*. 1989;38:301–304.

39. Giles W, Trudinger BJ, Cook CM, Connelly AJ. Umbilical artery waveforms in triplet pregnancy. *Obstet Gynecol*. 1990;75:813–816.

40. Creinin M, Katz M, Laros R. Triplet pregnancy: changes in mortality and morbidity. *J Perinatol*. 1991;11:207–212.

41. Antoine C, Kirshenbaum NW, Young BK. Bio-

chemical differences related to birth order in triplets. *J Reprod Med*. 1986;31:330–332.

42. Cario GM, Carlton MA. An unusual set of triplets: twin intrauterine pregnancy with singleton extrauterine pregnancy. *Aust NZ J Obstet Gynecol*. 1984;24:51–54.

43. Forbes DA, Natale A. Unilateral tubal triplet pregnancy. Report of a case. *Obstet Gynecol*. 1968;31:360–362.

44. Singhal AM, Chin VP. Unilateral triplet ectopic pregnancy. A case report. *J Reprod Med*. 1992;37:187–188.

45. Botting BJ, Davies IM, MacFarlane AJ. Recent trends in the incidence of multiple births and associated mortality. *Arch Dis Child*. 1987;62:941–950.

46. Børlum K-G. Third-trimester fetal death in triplet pregnancies. *Obstet Gynecol*. 1991;77:6–9.

47. Gindoff PR, Yeh M-N, Jewelewicz R. The vanishing sac syndrome. Ultrasound evidence of pregnancy failure in multiple gestations, induced and spontaneous. *J Reprod Med*. 1986;31:322–325.

48. Holder AR, Henifin MS. Selective termination of pregnancy. *Hastings Cent Rep*. 1988;Feb/Mar:21–22.

49. Appelman Z, Cuspi B. Chorionic villi sampling and selective termination of a chromosomally abnormal fetus in a triplet pregnancy (Abstract). *Fetal Diag Ther*. 1991;6:165.

50. Shalev E, Issakov D, Feldman E, Zuckerman H. Selective feticide of hydrocephalic fetus in triplets pregnancy. In: Schenker JG, Weinstein D, eds. *The Intrauterine Life—Management and Therapy*. Amsterdam: Elsevier Science; 1986:53–54.

51. Gonen R, Heyman E, Asztalos E, Milligan JE. The outcome of triplet gestations complicated by fetal death. *Obstet Gynecol*. 1990;75:175–178.

52. Skelly H, Marivate M, Norman R, Kenoyer G, Martin R. Consumptive coagulopathy following fetal death in triplet pregnancy. *Am J Obstet Gynecol*. 1982;142:595–596.

53. Sakala EP. Intrauterine demise of two fetuses in an unsuspected triplet pregnancy. A case report. *J Reprod Med*. 1986;31:1055–1060.

54. Weissman A, Jakobi P, Yoffe N, Zimmer EZ, Paldi E, Brandes JM. Sonographic growth measurements in triplet pregnancies. *Obstet Gynecol*. 1990;75:324–328.

55. McKeown T, Record RG. Observations on fetal growth in multiple pregnancy in man. *J Endocrinol*. 1952;8:386–389.

56. Elster AD, Bleyl JL, Craven TE. Birth weight standards for triplets under modern obstetric care in the United States, 1984–1989. *Obstet Gynecol*. 1991;77:387–393.

57. Jones JS, Newman RB, Miller MC. Cross-sectional analyses of triplet birth weight. *Am J Obstet Gynecol*. 1991;164:135–140.

58. Hata T, Deter RL, Hill RM. Individual growth curve standards in triplets: prediction of third-trimester growth and birth characteristics. *Obstet Gynecol*. 1991;78:379–384.

59. Hata T, Deter RL, Hill RM. Reduction of soft tissue deposition in normal triplets. *J Clin Ultrasound*. 1991;19:541–545.

60. Newman RB, Jones JS, Miller MC. Influence of clinical variables on triplet birth weight. *Acta Genet Med Gemellol*. 1991;40:173–179.

61. Isada NB, Sorokin Y, Drugan A, Johnson MP, Zador IE, Evans MI. First trimester interfetal size variation in multifetal pregnancies (MFP) (Abstract). *Am J Obstet Gynecol*. 1991;164:346.

62. Arroyo HA, Grippo J, Taratuto A, Duffau J, Chamoles N. Krabbe disease in monozygotic triplets. *Dev Med Child Neurol*. 1991;33:1101–1103.

63. Feld D, Labes J, Nathanson M. Bilateral ovarian dermoid cysts in triplets. *Obstet Gynecol*. 1966;27:525–528.

64. Akimoto N, Satow Y, Lee JY, Sumida H, Okamoto N, Akagi T. Autopsy case of the monozygotic triplets with conotruncal anomalies (Abstract). *Teratology*. 1986;34:480.

65. Siebold H, Mohr W, Lehmann WD, Lang D, Spanel R, Schwarz J. Fibroelastosis of the right ventricle in two brothers of triplets. *Pathol Res Pract*. 1980;170:402–409.

66. Janik JS, Nagaraj HS, Lehocky R. Pyloric stenosis in identical triplets. *Pediatrics*. 1982;70:282–283.

67. Bustamante SA, Stumpff LC. Fetal hydantoin syndrome in triplets. A unique experiment of nature. *Am J Dis Child*. 1978;132:978–979.

68. Shiono H. Down's syndrome with twinning in one triplet. *Am J Dis Child*. 1977;131:522–524.

69. Liberfarb RM, Atkins L, Holmes LB. Down syndrome in two of three triplets. *Clin Genet*. 1978;14:261–264.

70. Dallapiccola B, Stomeo C, Ferranti G, Di Lecce A, Purpura M. Discordant sex in one of three monozygotic triplets. *J Med Genet*. 1985;22:6–11.

71. Sinykin MB. Monoamniotic triplet pregnancy with triple survival. *Obstet Gynecol*. 1958;12:78–82.

72. Benirschke K, Kaufmann P. Pathology of the Human Placenta. 2nd ed. New York: Springer Verlag; 1990:720–728.

73. Pons JC, Olivennes F, Fernandez H, Ramdin I, Mayenga JM, Bessis R, Papiernik E. Transfusion syndrome in a triplet pregnancy. *Acta Genet Med Gemellol*. 1990;39:389–393.

74. Roos FJ, Roter AM, Molina FA. A case of triplets including anomalous twins and a fetus compressus. *Am J Obstet Gynecol*. 1957;73:1342–1345.

75. Simons JP, Gowen GA. Fetus amorphus. Report of a case. *Surg Gynecol Obstet*. 1925;41:171–179.

76. Schinzel AAGL, Smith DW, Miller JR. Monozygotic twinning and structural defects. *J Pediatr*. 1979;95:921–930.

77. Sato T, Kaneko K, Konuma S, Sato I, Tamada T. Acardiac anomalies: review of 88 cases in Japan. *Asia-Oceana J Obstet Gynecol*. 1984;10:45–52.

78. van Allen MI, Smith DW, Shepard JW. Twin reversed arterial perfusion. (TRAP) sequence: a study of 14 pregnancies with acardius. *Semin Perinatol*. 1983;7:285–293.

79. James WH. A note on the epidemiology of acardiac monsters. *Teratology*. 1978;16:211–216.

80. Landy HJ, Larsen JW, Schoen M, Larsen ME, Kent SG, Weingold AB. Acardiac fetus in a triplet pregnancy. *Teratology*. 1988;37:1–6.

81. San Filippo J, Bianchine JQ, Walsh A, Badawy S. Acardius myelocephalus. Two monsters in a triplet pregnancy. *NY State J Med*. 1979;79:245–247.

82. Ginsberg NA, Appelbaum M, Rabin SA, Caffarelli MA, Kuuspalu M, Daskal JL, Verlinsky Y, Strom CM, Barton JJ. Term birth after midtrimester hysterotomy and selective delivery of an acardiac twin. *Am J Obstet Gynecol*. 1992;167:33–37.

83. Amatuzio JC, Gorlin RJ. Conjoined acardiac monster. *Arch Pathol Lab Med*. 1981;105:253–255.

84. Tan K-L, Tock EPC, Dawood MY, Ratnam SS. Conjoined twins in a triplet pregnancy. *Am J Dis Child*. 1971;122:455–458.

85. Vestergaard P. Triplets pregnancy with a normal foetus and a dicephalus dibrachius sirenomelius. *Acta Obstet Gynecol Scand*. 1972;51:93–94.

86. Apuzzio JJ, Ganesh VV, Chervenak J, Sama JC. Perinatal diagnosis of dicephalus conjoined twins in a triplet pregnancy. *Am J Obstet Gynecol*. 1988;159:1214–1215.

87. Koontz WL, Layman L, Adams A, Lavery JP. Antenatal sonographic diagnosis of conjoined twins in a triplet pregnancy. *Am J Obstet Gynecol*. 1985;153:230–231.

88. Grosse B. Siamese twins born pregnant. *Sun*. 1989;47(7):1,17.

89. Mayer CF. Sextuplets and higher multiparous births. A critical review of history and legend from Aristoteles to the 20th century. *Acta Genet Med Gemellol*. 1952;1:118–135,242–275.

90. Bulmer MG. *The Biology of Twinning in Man*. Oxford: Clarendon Press; 1970:95–109.

91. Elliott JP, Radin TG. Quadruplet pregnancy: contemporary management and outcome. *Obstet Gynecol*. 1992;80:421–424.

92. Collins MS, Bleyl JA. Seventy-one quadruplet

pregnancies: management and outcome. *Am J Obstet Gynecol*. 1990;162:1384–1392.

93. Lipitz S, Frenkel Y, Watts C, Ben-Rafael Z, Barkai G, Reichman B. High order multifetal gestation—management and outcome. *Obstet Gynecol*. 1990;76:215–218.

94. Goldman JA, Feldberg D, Ashkenazi J, Shelef M, Dicker D, Hart J. Multiple pregnancy after in-vitro fertilization and embryo transfer: report of a quadruplet pregnancy and delivery. *Hum Reprod*. 1987;2:511–515.

95. Versmold HT. Outcome of grand multiplets: is there a case for selective feticide? (Abstract). *Fetal Diagn Ther*. 1991;6:165.

96. Campbell WA, Cusick W, Vintzileos AM, Rodis JF, Turner GW, Egan JFX, McLean D. Outcome of quadruplet pregnancies using early hospitalization (Abstract). *Am J Obstet Gynecol*. 1991;164:319.

97. Rowland DM, Geagan MB, Paul DA. Sonographic demonstration of combined quadruplet gestation, with viable ectopic and concomitant intrauterine triplet pregnancies. *J Ultrasound Med*. 1987;6:89–91.

98. Shanklin DR. Placentation and perils of multiple pregnancy. UT Memphis Perinatal Mortality Conference, No. 57, Feb 15, 1989.

99. Allen G. A differential method for estimation of type frequencies in triplets and quadruplets. *Am J Hum Genet*. 1960;12:210–244.

100. Quigley JK. Monoamniotic twin pregnancy. A case record with review of the literature. *Am J Obstet Gynecol*. 1935;29:354–362.

101. Diddle AW, Burford TH. Study of set of quadruplets. *Anat Rec*. 1935;61:281–293.

102. Adair FL. Fetal malformations in multiple pregnancy. *Am J Obstet Gynecol*. 1930;20:539–552.

103. Newman HH. *Multiple Human Births. Twins, Triplets, Quadruplets and Quintuplets*. New York: Doubleday, Doran; 1940:98–103.

104. Scheinfeld A. *Twins and Supertwins*. Philadelphia: JB Lippincott; 1967:208–211.

105. Jones N. Quints shocked the world in 1934. *The Province*. 1991;November 1:A57.

106. Gibbs CE, Boldt JW, Daly JW, Morgan HC. A quintuplet gestation. *Obstet Gynecol*. 1960;16:464–468.

107. Greenwalt J. Thankful for five tiny blessings. *People Weekly*, 1988;Feb 15:92–100.

108. Sarick L. Nation's first test-tube quintuplets arrive 11 weeks ahead of schedule. *The Globe and Mail*, 1988;Feb 8:A2.

109. Berbos JN, King BF, Janusz A. Quintuple pregnancy. Report of a case. *JAMA*. 1964;188:813–816.

110. Neubecker RD, Blumberg JM, Townsend FM. A human monozygotic quintuplet placenta. Report of a specimen. *J Obstet Gynecol Br Cwlth*. 1962;69:137–139.

111. Hamblen EC, Baker RD, Derieux GD. Roentgenographic diagnosis and anatomic studies of quintuplet pregnancy. *JAMA*. 1937;109:10–12.

112. Imaizumi Y. Stillbirth rate and weight at birth of quintuplets in Japan. *Acta Genet Med Gemellol*. 1989;38:65–69.

113. Giovannucci-Uzielli ML, Vecchi G, Donzelli GP, D'Ancona VL, Lapi E. The history of the Florentine sextuplets: obstetric and genetic considerations. In: Gedda L, Parisi P, Nance WE, eds. Twin Research 3: Twin Biology and Multiple Pregnancy. *Prog Clin Biol Res*. 1981;69A:217–220.

114. Aiken RA. An account of the Birmingham "sextuplets." *J Obstet Gynecol Br Cwlth*. 1969;76:684–691.

115. Cameron AH, Robson EB, Wade-Evans T, Wingham J. Septuplet conception: placental and zygosity studies. *J Obstet Gynecol Br Cwlth*. 1969;76:692–698.

116. Turksoy RN, Toy BL, Rogers J, Papageorge W. Birth of septuplets following human chorionic gonadotropin administration in Chiari-Frommell syndrome. *Obstet Gynecol*. 1967;30:692–698.

117. Serreyn R, Thiery M, Vandekerckhove D. Outcome of an octuplet pregnancy. *Arch Gynecol*. 1984;234:283–293.

118. Garrett WJ, Carey HM, Stevens LH, Climie CR, Osborn RA. A case of nonuplet pregnancy. *Aust NZ J Obstet Gynecol*. 1976;16:193–199.

Author Index

Subject Index